Handbook of Orthopedic Surgery

Handbook of Orthopedic Surgery

Editor: Lucius Graves

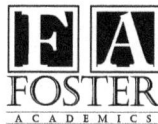

FA FOSTER
ACADEMICS

www.fosteracademics.com

www.fosteracademics.com

FA
FOSTER
ACADEMICS

Cataloging-in-Publication Data

Handbook of orthopedic surgery / edited by Lucius Graves.
    p. cm.
Includes bibliographical references and index.
ISBN 978-1-63242-766-3
1. Orthopedic surgery. 2. Orthopedics. 3. Surgery, Operative. I. Graves, Lucius.
RD732.5 .H36 2019
617.3--dc23

Foster Academics,
118-35 Queens Blvd., Suite 400,
Forest Hills, NY 11375, USA

ISBN 978-1-63242-766-3 (Hardback)

Contents

Preface

This book aims to highlight the current researches and provides a platform to further the scope of innovations in this area. This book is a product of the combined efforts of many researchers and scientists, after going through thorough studies and analysis from different parts of the world. The objective of this book is to provide the readers with the latest information of the field.

Orthopedic surgery is a branch of surgery. It studies the disorders and diseases related to the musculoskeletal system. The treatment methods used by orthopedic surgeons to treat the disorders related to the musculoskeletal system are both surgical and nonsurgical. Some of the common sub-branches associated with orthopedic surgery include spine surgery, hand and upper extremity, total joint reconstruction, foot and ankle surgery, pediatric orthopedics, surgical sports medicine and musculoskeletal oncology. Spinal fusion is a very common orthopedic surgical technique. It is used to join two or more vertebrae, at the time, when the disc wears out. The various sub-fields of orthopedic surgery along with technological progress that have future implications are glanced at in this book. It studies, analyzes and upholds the pillars of orthopedic surgery and its utmost significance in modern times. This book, with its detailed analyses and data, will prove immensely beneficial to professionals and students involved in this area at various levels.

I would like to express my sincere thanks to the authors for their dedicated efforts in the completion of this book. I acknowledge the efforts of the publisher for providing constant support. Lastly, I would like to thank my family for their support in all academic endeavors.

Editor

Accuracy of MRI diagnosis of early osteonecrosis of the femoral head: a meta-analysis and systematic review

Ya-Zhou Zhang[†], Xu-Yang Cao[†], Xi-Cheng Li[*][iD], Jia Chen, Yue-Yuan Zhao, Zhi Tian and Wang Zheng

Abstract

Objective: To evaluate the overall diagnostic value related to magnetic resonance imaging (MRI) in patients with early osteonecrosis of the femoral head.

Methods: By searching multiple databases and sources, including PubMed, Cochrane, and Embase database, by the index words updated in December 2017, qualified studies were identified and relevant literature sources were also searched. The qualified studies included prospective cohort studies and cross-sectional studies. Heterogeneity of the included studies were reviewed to select proper effect model for pooled weighted sensitivity, specificity, and diagnostic odds ratio (DOR). Summary receiver operating characteristic (SROC) analyses were performed for meniscal tears.

Results: Forty-three studies related to diagnostic accuracy of MRI to detect early osteonecrosis of the femoral head were involved in the meta-analysis. The global sensitivity and specificity of MRI in early osteonecrosis of the femoral head were 93.0% (95% CI 92.0–94.0%) and 91.0% (95% CI 89.0%–93.0%), respectively. The global positive likelihood ratio and global negative likelihood ratio of MRI in early osteonecrosis of the femoral head were 2.74 (95% CI 1.98–3.79) and 0.18 (95% CI 0.14–0.23), respectively. The global DOR was 27.27 (95% CI 17.02–43.67), and the area under the SROC was 93.38% (95% CI 90.87%–95.89%).

Conclusions: This review provides a systematic review and meta-analysis to evaluate the diagnostic accuracy of MRI in early osteonecrosis of the femoral head. Moderate to strong evidence indicated that MRI appears to be significantly associated with higher diagnostic accuracy for early osteonecrosis of the femoral head.

Keywords: Meta-analysis, Early osteonecrosis of the femoral head, Magnetic resonance imaging, Diagnostic accuracy

Background

Avascular Necrosis of Femur Head (ANFH), or osteonecrosis of the femoral head, is a pathologic process, which was first seen in the weight-bearing area of the femur. The stress can lead to bone trabecular structure injury (microfracture) and influence the repair process of the femur, and if not managed timely, it leads to the collapse and deformation of the femur. With many etiological factors, ANFH results from interruption of blood supply to the bone and then leads to ischemic necrosis. ANFH can be divided in traumatic ANFH and non-traumatic ANFH with the non-traumatic ANFH further dividing into steroid-induced and alcoholic non-traumatic ANFH and so on. The timely treatment of early ANFH could promote the recovery the disease. However, in the late stage, it results in femur collapse, loss of hip function, and a very poor outcome that affects the quality of life. Therefore, the early diagnosis of ANFH is of great significance [1–3].

Several methods for early diagnosis of ANFH have been proposed, including MRI, SPECT, CT, X-ray, DSA, and laser Doppler with different characteristics. MRI has been characterized as being non-invasive, rapid and high sensitive, and commonly used by many clinicians [4–6]. Furthermore, MRI has been used in many studies in the

* Correspondence: zccsfh@163.com

[†]Ya-Zhou Zhang and Xu-Yang Cao contributed equally to this work.

Department of Orthopedics, Heibei General Hospital, No. 348 Heping East Road, Shijiazhuang 050051, Hebei, China

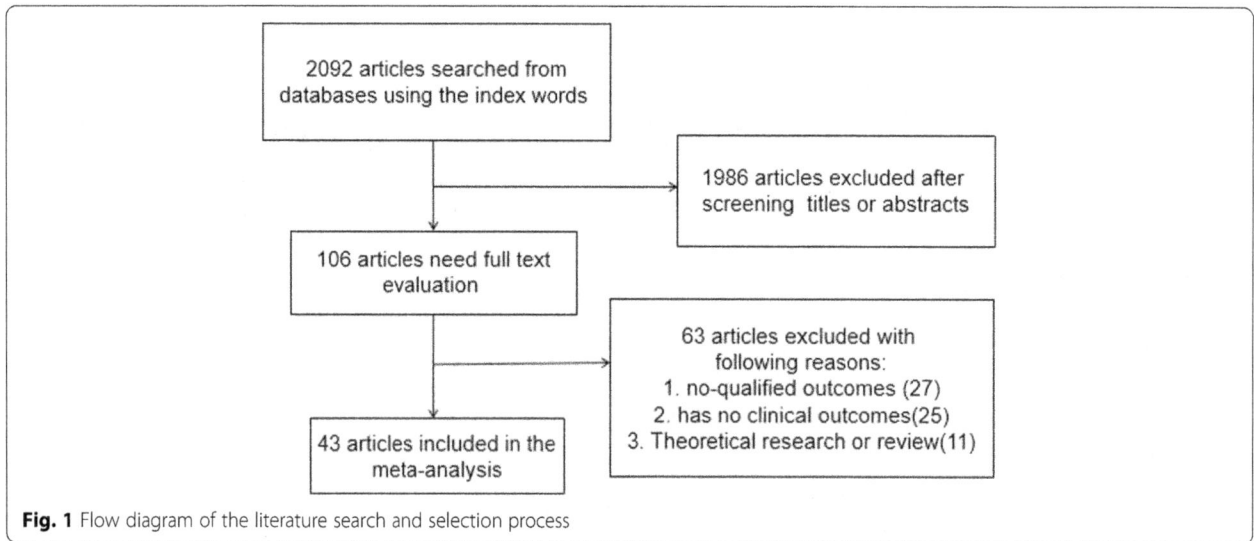

Fig. 1 Flow diagram of the literature search and selection process

diagnosis of early ANFH. Therefore, in this paper, a systematic review and meta-analysis of all qualified studies were performed to explore the diagnosis accuracy of MRI in early ANFH.

Methods
Search strategy
The following electronic databases were searched from their inception to December 2017: The Cochrane, PubMed, Embase database, for all the qualified trails that analyze the diagnostic accuracy of MRI of early osteonecrosis of the femoral head. Other related articles and reference materials were also identified for additional available studies. The literatures were searched independently by two investigators, and a third investigator was involved to reach an agreement.

Study selection
The studies that met the following criteria were included in our review: (1) prospective cohort study or cross-sectional study; (2) the research objects are patients suspected with early osteonecrosis of the femoral head without other serious diseases; (3) the studies provided the data of true positive (TP), false positive (FP), false negative (FN), and true negative (TN); and (4) the publications were only available in English and Chinese.

The studies that met the following criteria were excluded in our review: (1) repeat publications, or shared content and results; (2) case report, theoretical research, conference report, systematic review, meta-analysis, expert comment, and economic analysis; (3) the outcomes were not relevant; and (4) two or more results of the TP, FP, FN, and TN were zero.

Data extraction and quality assessment
Two independent investigators extracted the following data based on predefined criteria. Differences were settled by discussion with a third reviewer. The analyses data were extracted from all the included studies and consisted of two parts: basic information and main outcomes. The first part was about the basic information: the author name, the sample size, the percentage of male, and the age. The second part was the clinical outcomes. A 2×2 contingency table was constructed for each selected study; the results corresponding to the gold standard and MRI were selected as positive or negative. The data included true positive (TP), false positive (FP), false negative (FN), and true negative (TN). In studies in which one single cell in the 2×2 contingency table had a value of 0, 0.5 were added to all of the cells for calculation. Sensitivity, specificity, and likelihood ratio were calculated respectively, and the diagnostic odds ratio (DOR) was used as the measure of diagnostic accuracy. A DOR value of 1 indicates a test without discriminatory power, and the higher the DOR value is, the greater the degree of relevance of the assessed diagnostic test. The studies were performed by two reviewers independently. Any arising difference was resolved by discussion.

Statistical analysis
All statistical analyses were performed in the STATA 10.0 (TX, USA). Chi-squared and I^2 tests were used to assess the heterogeneity of clinical trial results and determine the analysis model (fixed-effects model or random-effects model). When the chi-squared test P value was ≤ 0.05 and I^2 test value was $> 50\%$, it was defined as high heterogeneity and assessed by random-effects model. When the

chi-squared test P value was > 0.05 and I^2 tests value was $\leq 50\%$, it was defined as acceptable heterogeneity data and assessed by fixed-effects model. For further assessment of heterogeneity, diagnostic threshold analysis was performed based on the correlation (Spearman's) between the logit of sensitivity and the logit of [1-specificity]. When a threshold effect occurs, the sensitivity and specificity of the investigated study exhibits negative correlation (or a positive correlation between sensitivity and [1-specificity]). Therefore, a strong positive correlation between sensitivity and [1-specificity] suggests the presence of a threshold effect. When heterogeneity caused by threshold effect was observed, a summary receiver operating characteristic (SROC) curve was plotted. This method was appropriate given that the global sensitivity and specificity values were overestimated. In such cases, analysis of the ROC panel points, as well as analysis of the SROC curve, was recommended. Deeks' Funnel Asymmetry Plot was used to identify the publication bias.

Results

Characteristics of included studies

A total of 2092 articles were searched by the indexes. After screening the titles and abstracts, 1986 articles were excluded, leaving 106 articles for further selection. During full-text screening, 63 articles were excluded due to the following criteria: unqualified outcomes [7], theoretical research or review [8], and has non clinical outcome [9]. At last, 43 studies [7–50] with 3133 hips were involved in the final meta-analysis. The selection process was presented in Fig. 1. The main characteristics of the included studies were summarized in Table 1. The basic information included number of hips, age, and gender.

Diagnostic accuracy

All the included studies reported the results of the accuracy of MRI of early osteonecrosis of the femoral head. Based on the correlation (Spearman's $R = -0.209$, $P = 0.589$) between the logit of sensitivity and the logit of [1-specificity], there was no threshold effect.

Based on the chi-squared test ($Q = 166.45$, $P = 0.000$) and I^2 tests ($I^2 = 74.6\%$), heterogeneity was high, so we chose the random-effects model to analyze the sensitivity. The global sensitivity was 93.0% (95% CI 92.0–94.0%, Fig. 2). Based on the chi-squared test ($Q = 144.43$, $P = 0.000$) and I^2 tests ($I^2 = 70.9\%$), heterogeneity was high. Therefore, we chose the random-effects model to analyze the specificity, and the global specificity was 91.0% (95%CI 89.0–93.0%, Fig. 3).

Based on the chi-squared test ($Q = 125.33$, $P = 0.000$) and I^2 tests ($I^2 = 66.5\%$), heterogeneity was high, so we

Table 1 The basic characteristics description of included studies

Study	No. of hip	Gender	Age
Genez BM 1998	11	4 M, 3F	11–35
Robinson HJ 1989	96	–	–
Hauzeur JP 1989	49	–	–
Zhang X 1994	30	26 M	24–58
Ryu JS 2002	32	14 M, 10 F	39.5
Liu Jihua 2004	72	40 M, 8 F	43.6
Chen Lei 2005	62	3 M, 21 F	31.8
Zhou Hongmei 2006	91	23 M, 18 F	30–60
Xie Zhongwei 2010	68	34 M, 16 F	34
Sun Lili 2015	50	36 M, 14 F	50.1
Fang Wu 2017	35	20 M, 15 F	57.1
Feng Zhanyou 2017	71	33 M, 38 F	61.5
Cheng Houpei 2016	65	40 M, 25 F	41.14
Qiu Pengdong 2012	59	31 M, 23 F	38.5
Zheng Liwen 2013	98	35 F, 21 M	38.2
Cui Baoli 2014	114	–	32.3
Xie Yan 2014	81	37 M, 32 F	31–62
Jia Hong 2017	40	25 M, 15 F	56.6
Zhang Kaixiang 2016	100	62 M, 38 F	42.3
Lin Chen 2017	42	–	52.87
Lu Chun 2016	52	28 M, 24 F	51.2
Ding Qinmei 2011	62	31 M, 15 F	41.2
Chen Longhua 2015	196	75 M, 45 F	58.4
Luo Zian 2017	93	39 M, 21 F	32.3
Tan Zhihong 2016	131	54 M, 32 F	58.68
Wang Yuli 2017	50	38 M, 12 F	53.8
Wang Wenbin 2012	72	29 M, 11 F	52.5
Liu Xianzhi 2017	29	16 M, 13 F	52.26
Liu Feng 2017	43	25 M, 18 F	58.14
Guo Hongbin 2017	70	39 M, 31 F	44.86
Lin Yi 2015	90	30 M, 20 F	45.6
Wang Linhong 2014	183	60 M, 40 F	47
Fang Chaohui 2014	122	56 M, 38 F	64.8
Li Yan 2014	98	69 M, 29 F	51.52
Liu Dailiang 2015	86	23 M, 20 F	55.36
Xiang Zhenghua 2014	61	35 M, 26 F	52.8
Wu Shiping 2017	75	51 M, 24 F	40.7
Wang Kun 2017	56	34 M, 22 F	38.74
Cai Huaiwei 2017	69	45 M, 24 F	54.6
Li Yanming 2015	37	–	52.6
Ji Xuewen 2017	50	28 M, 22 F	48.3
Wang Sihe 2013	86	32 M, 27 F	32.4
Shen Wen 2014	56	21 M, 15 F	45.3

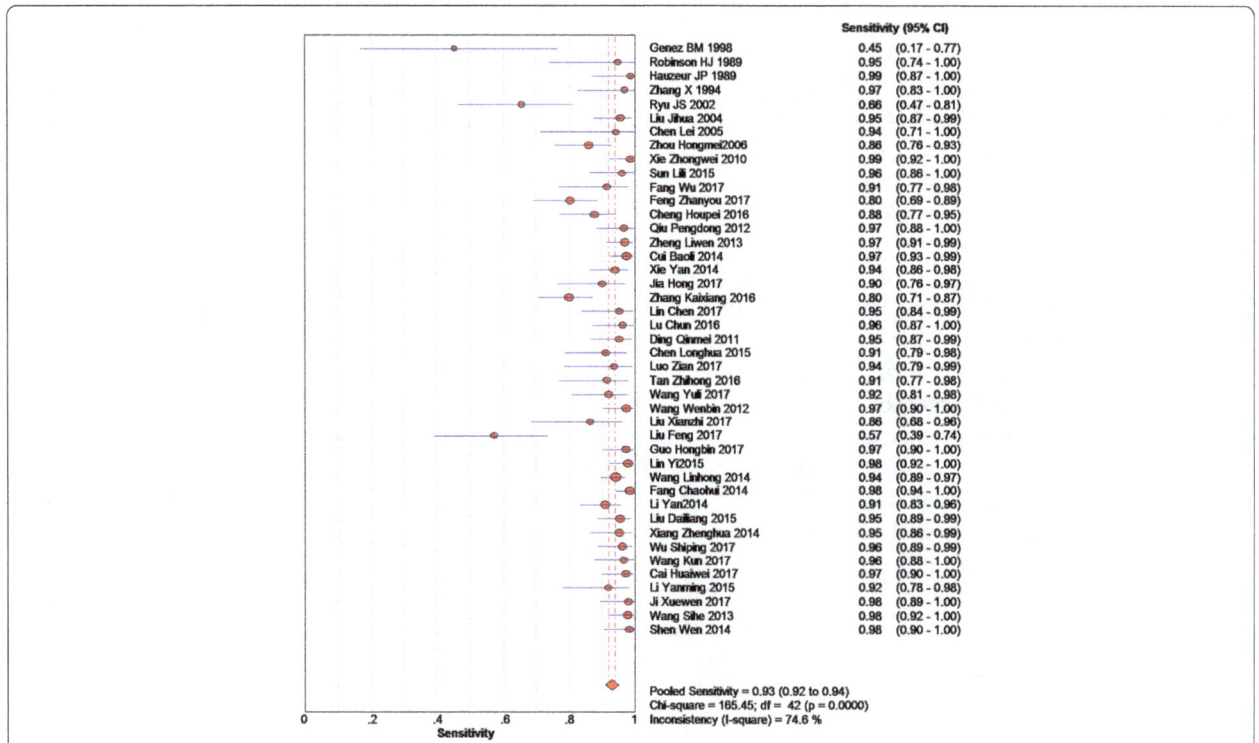

	Sensitivity (95% CI)
Genez BM 1998	0.45 (0.17 - 0.77)
Robinson HJ 1989	0.95 (0.74 - 1.00)
Hauzeur JP 1989	0.99 (0.87 - 1.00)
Zhang X 1994	0.97 (0.83 - 1.00)
Ryu JS 2002	0.66 (0.47 - 0.81)
Liu Jihua 2004	0.95 (0.87 - 0.99)
Chen Lei 2005	0.94 (0.71 - 1.00)
Zhou Hongmei 2006	0.86 (0.76 - 0.93)
Xie Zhongwei 2010	0.99 (0.92 - 1.00)
Sun Lili 2015	0.96 (0.86 - 1.00)
Fang Wu 2017	0.91 (0.77 - 0.98)
Feng Zhanyou 2017	0.80 (0.69 - 0.89)
Cheng Houpei 2016	0.88 (0.77 - 0.95)
Qiu Pengdong 2012	0.97 (0.88 - 1.00)
Zheng Liwen 2013	0.97 (0.91 - 0.99)
Cui Baoli 2014	0.97 (0.93 - 0.99)
Xie Yan 2014	0.94 (0.86 - 0.98)
Jia Hong 2017	0.90 (0.76 - 0.97)
Zhang Kaixiang 2016	0.80 (0.71 - 0.87)
Lin Chen 2017	0.95 (0.84 - 0.99)
Lu Chun 2016	0.96 (0.87 - 1.00)
Ding Qinmei 2011	0.95 (0.87 - 1.00)
Chen Longhua 2015	0.91 (0.79 - 0.98)
Luo Zian 2017	0.94 (0.79 - 0.99)
Tan Zhihong 2016	0.91 (0.77 - 0.98)
Wang Yuli 2017	0.92 (0.81 - 0.98)
Wang Wenbin 2012	0.97 (0.90 - 1.00)
Liu Xianzhi 2017	0.86 (0.68 - 0.96)
Liu Feng 2017	0.57 (0.39 - 0.74)
Guo Hongbin 2017	0.97 (0.90 - 1.00)
Lin Yi 2015	0.98 (0.92 - 1.00)
Wang Linhong 2014	0.94 (0.89 - 0.97)
Fang Chaohui 2014	0.98 (0.94 - 1.00)
Li Yan 2014	0.91 (0.83 - 0.96)
Liu Dailiang 2015	0.95 (0.89 - 0.99)
Xiang Zhenghua 2014	0.95 (0.86 - 0.99)
Wu Shiping 2017	0.96 (0.89 - 0.99)
Wang Kun 2017	0.96 (0.88 - 1.00)
Cai Huaiwei 2017	0.97 (0.90 - 1.00)
Li Yanming 2015	0.92 (0.78 - 0.98)
Ji Xuewen 2017	0.98 (0.89 - 1.00)
Wang Sihe 2013	0.98 (0.92 - 1.00)
Shen Wen 2014	0.98 (0.90 - 1.00)

Pooled Sensitivity = 0.93 (0.92 to 0.94)
Chi-square = 165.45; df = 42 (p = 0.0000)
Inconsistency (I-square) = 74.6 %

Fig. 2 Forest plot showing the sensitivity values of MRI of early osteonecrosis of the femoral head

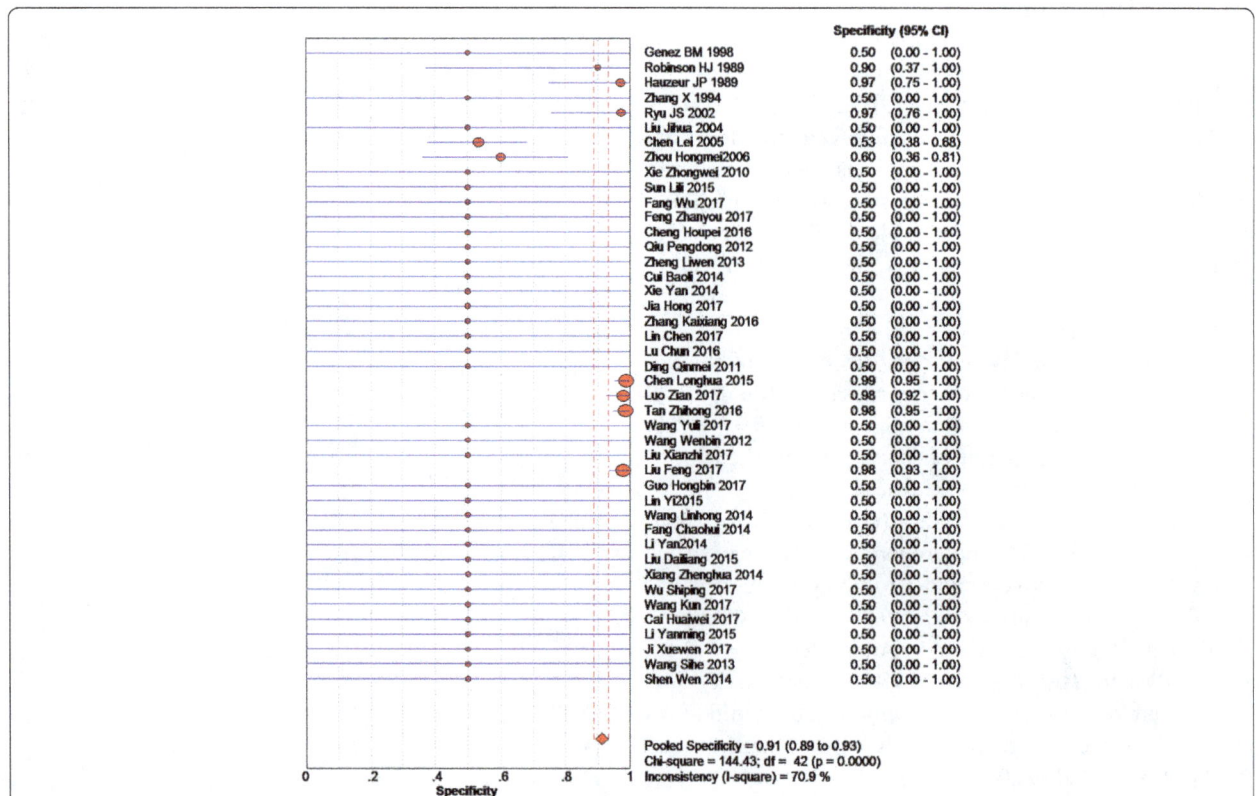

	Specificity (95% CI)
Genez BM 1998	0.50 (0.00 - 1.00)
Robinson HJ 1989	0.90 (0.37 - 1.00)
Hauzeur JP 1989	0.97 (0.75 - 1.00)
Zhang X 1994	0.50 (0.00 - 1.00)
Ryu JS 2002	0.97 (0.76 - 1.00)
Liu Jihua 2004	0.50 (0.00 - 1.00)
Chen Lei 2005	0.53 (0.38 - 0.68)
Zhou Hongmei 2006	0.60 (0.36 - 0.81)
Xie Zhongwei 2010	0.50 (0.00 - 1.00)
Sun Lili 2015	0.50 (0.00 - 1.00)
Fang Wu 2017	0.50 (0.00 - 1.00)
Feng Zhanyou 2017	0.50 (0.00 - 1.00)
Cheng Houpei 2016	0.50 (0.00 - 1.00)
Qiu Pengdong 2012	0.50 (0.00 - 1.00)
Zheng Liwen 2013	0.50 (0.00 - 1.00)
Cui Baoli 2014	0.50 (0.00 - 1.00)
Xie Yan 2014	0.50 (0.00 - 1.00)
Jia Hong 2017	0.50 (0.00 - 1.00)
Zhang Kaixiang 2016	0.50 (0.00 - 1.00)
Lin Chen 2017	0.50 (0.00 - 1.00)
Lu Chun 2016	0.50 (0.00 - 1.00)
Ding Qinmei 2011	0.50 (0.00 - 1.00)
Chen Longhua 2015	0.99 (0.95 - 1.00)
Luo Zian 2017	0.98 (0.92 - 1.00)
Tan Zhihong 2016	0.98 (0.95 - 1.00)
Wang Yuli 2017	0.50 (0.00 - 1.00)
Wang Wenbin 2012	0.50 (0.00 - 1.00)
Liu Xianzhi 2017	0.50 (0.00 - 1.00)
Liu Feng 2017	0.98 (0.93 - 1.00)
Guo Hongbin 2017	0.50 (0.00 - 1.00)
Lin Yi 2015	0.50 (0.00 - 1.00)
Wang Linhong 2014	0.50 (0.00 - 1.00)
Fang Chaohui 2014	0.50 (0.00 - 1.00)
Li Yan 2014	0.50 (0.00 - 1.00)
Liu Dailiang 2015	0.50 (0.00 - 1.00)
Xiang Zhenghua 2014	0.50 (0.00 - 1.00)
Wu Shiping 2017	0.50 (0.00 - 1.00)
Wang Kun 2017	0.50 (0.00 - 1.00)
Cai Huaiwei 2017	0.50 (0.00 - 1.00)
Li Yanming 2015	0.50 (0.00 - 1.00)
Ji Xuewen 2017	0.50 (0.00 - 1.00)
Wang Sihe 2013	0.50 (0.00 - 1.00)
Shen Wen 2014	0.50 (0.00 - 1.00)

Pooled Specificity = 0.91 (0.89 to 0.93)
Chi-square = 144.43; df = 42 (p = 0.0000)
Inconsistency (I-square) = 70.9 %

Fig. 3 Forest plot showing the specificity values of MRI of early osteonecrosis of the femoral head

	Positive LR (95% CI)
Genez BM 1998	0.92 (0.20 - 4.18)
Robinson HJ 1989	5.55 (0.92 - 33.36)
Hauzeur JP 1989	16.99 (2.53 - 114.07)
Zhang X 1994	1.90 (0.47 - 7.63)
Ryu JS 2002	11.73 (1.72 - 80.07)
Liu Jihua 2004	1.90 (0.47 - 7.59)
Chen Lei 2005	1.96 (1.40 - 2.75)
Zhou Hongmei2006	2.11 (1.25 - 3.58)
Xie Zhongwei 2010	1.96 (0.49 - 7.83)
Sun Lili 2015	1.90 (0.48 - 7.62)
Fang Wu 2017	1.81 (0.45 - 7.25)
Feng Zhanyou 2017	1.60 (0.40 - 6.42)
Cheng Houpei 2016	1.74 (0.43 - 6.99)
Qiu Pengdong 2012	1.92 (0.48 - 7.67)
Zheng Liwen 2013	1.93 (0.48 - 7.72)
Cui Baoli 2014	1.94 (0.48 - 7.76)
Xie Yan 2014	1.87 (0.47 - 7.47)
Jia Hong 2017	1.78 (0.44 - 7.15)
Zhang Kaixiang 2016	1.59 (0.40 - 6.40)
Lin Chen 2017	1.88 (0.47 - 7.55)
Lu Chun 2016	1.91 (0.48 - 7.63)
Ding Qinmei 2011	1.89 (0.47 - 7.56)
Chen Longhua 2015	54.85 (15.98 - 188.23)
Luo Zian 2017	34.66 (10.16 - 118.25)
Tan Zhihong 2016	47.67 (13.90 - 163.48)
Wang Yuli 2017	1.82 (0.45 - 7.31)
Wang Wenbin 2012	1.93 (0.48 - 7.73)
Liu Xianzhi 2017	1.70 (0.42 - 6.85)
Liu Feng 2017	21.48 (7.35 - 62.74)
Guo Hongbin 2017	1.93 (0.48 - 7.72)
Lin Yi2015	1.95 (0.49 - 7.78)
Wang Linhong 2014	1.88 (0.47 - 7.50)
Fang Chaohui 2014	1.96 (0.49 - 7.84)
Li Yan2014	1.81 (0.45 - 7.24)
Liu Dailiang 2015	1.90 (0.47 - 7.59)
Xiang Zhenghua 2014	1.89 (0.47 - 7.56)
Wu Shiping 2017	1.91 (0.48 - 7.64)
Wang Kun 2017	1.91 (0.48 - 7.65)
Cai Huaiwei 2017	1.93 (0.48 - 7.72)
Li Yanming 2015	1.82 (0.45 - 7.29)
Ji Xuewen 2017	1.94 (0.49 - 7.77)
Wang Sihe 2013	1.94 (0.49 - 7.77)
Shen Wen 2014	1.95 (0.49 - 7.79)

Random Effects Model
Pooled Positive LR = 2.74 (1.98 to 3.79)
Cochran-Q = 125.33; df = 42 (p = 0.0000)
Inconsistency (I-square) = 66.5 %
Tau-squared = 0.7085

Positive LR   0.01   1   100.0

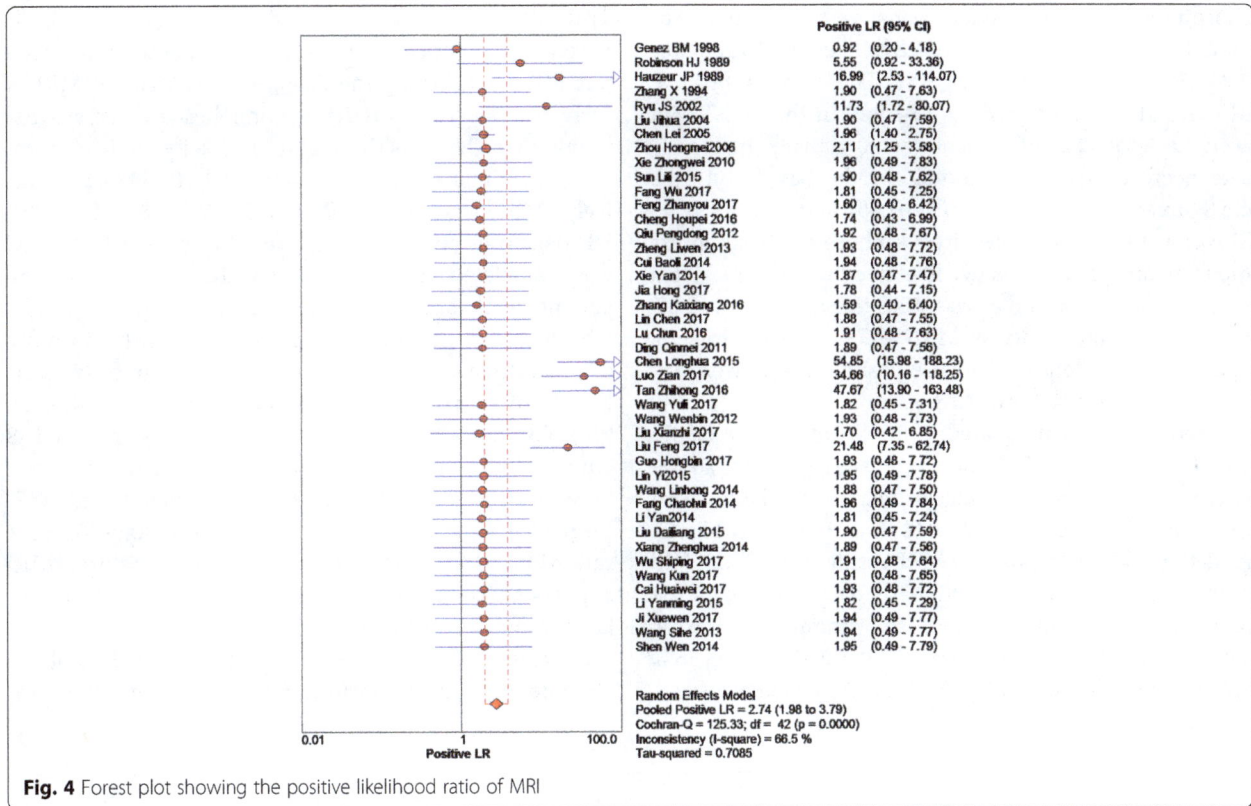

Fig. 4 Forest plot showing the positive likelihood ratio of MRI

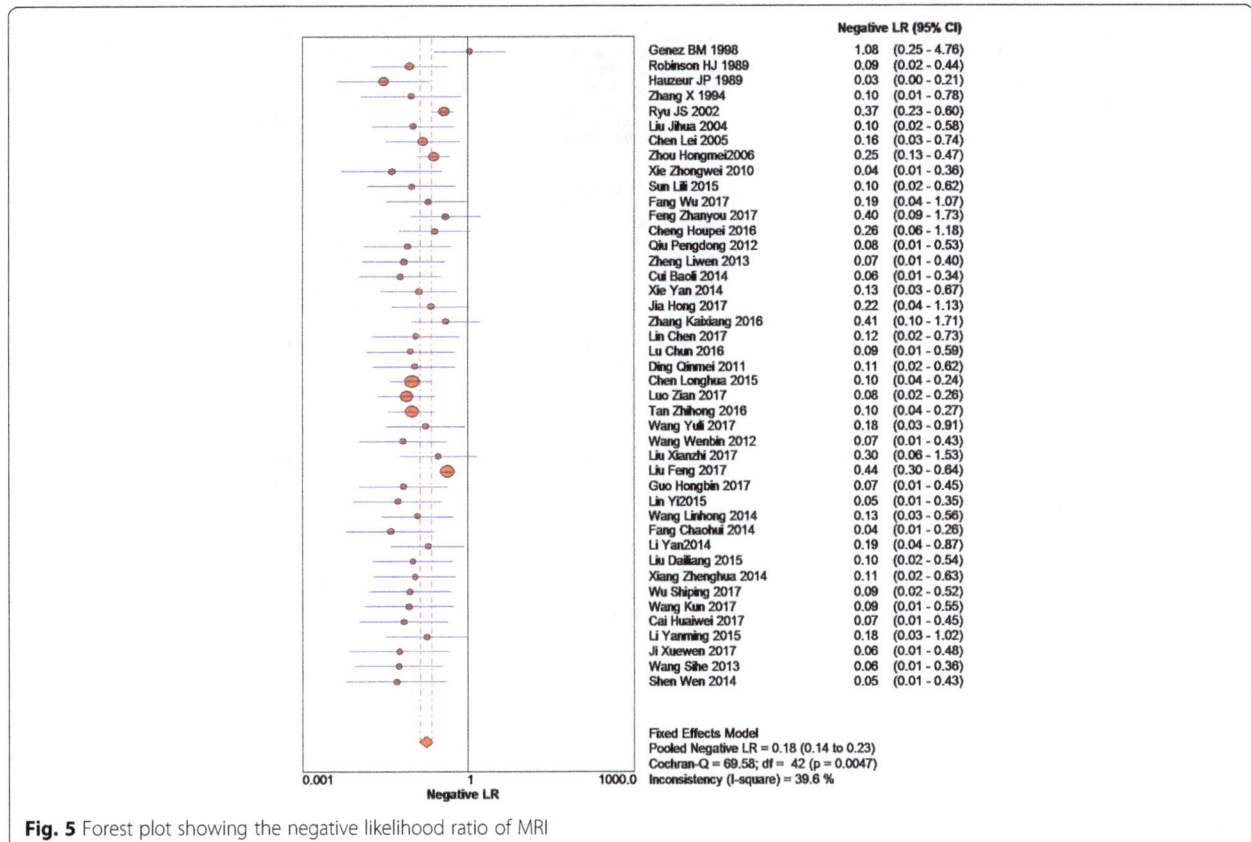

	Negative LR (95% CI)
Genez BM 1998	1.08 (0.25 - 4.76)
Robinson HJ 1989	0.09 (0.02 - 0.44)
Hauzeur JP 1989	0.03 (0.00 - 0.21)
Zhang X 1994	0.10 (0.01 - 0.78)
Ryu JS 2002	0.37 (0.23 - 0.60)
Liu Jihua 2004	0.10 (0.02 - 0.58)
Chen Lei 2005	0.16 (0.03 - 0.74)
Zhou Hongmei2006	0.25 (0.13 - 0.47)
Xie Zhongwei 2010	0.04 (0.01 - 0.36)
Sun Lili 2015	0.10 (0.02 - 0.62)
Fang Wu 2017	0.19 (0.04 - 1.07)
Feng Zhanyou 2017	0.40 (0.09 - 1.73)
Cheng Houpei 2016	0.26 (0.06 - 1.18)
Qiu Pengdong 2012	0.08 (0.01 - 0.53)
Zheng Liwen 2013	0.07 (0.01 - 0.40)
Cui Baoli 2014	0.06 (0.01 - 0.34)
Xie Yan 2014	0.13 (0.03 - 0.67)
Jia Hong 2017	0.22 (0.04 - 1.13)
Zhang Kaixiang 2016	0.41 (0.10 - 1.71)
Lin Chen 2017	0.12 (0.02 - 0.73)
Lu Chun 2016	0.09 (0.01 - 0.59)
Ding Qinmei 2011	0.11 (0.02 - 0.62)
Chen Longhua 2015	0.10 (0.04 - 0.24)
Luo Zian 2017	0.08 (0.02 - 0.26)
Tan Zhihong 2016	0.10 (0.04 - 0.27)
Wang Yuli 2017	0.18 (0.03 - 0.91)
Wang Wenbin 2012	0.07 (0.01 - 0.43)
Liu Xianzhi 2017	0.30 (0.06 - 1.53)
Liu Feng 2017	0.44 (0.30 - 0.64)
Guo Hongbin 2017	0.07 (0.01 - 0.45)
Lin Yi2015	0.05 (0.01 - 0.35)
Wang Linhong 2014	0.13 (0.03 - 0.56)
Fang Chaohui 2014	0.04 (0.01 - 0.26)
Li Yan2014	0.19 (0.04 - 0.87)
Liu Dailiang 2015	0.10 (0.02 - 0.54)
Xiang Zhenghua 2014	0.11 (0.02 - 0.63)
Wu Shiping 2017	0.09 (0.02 - 0.52)
Wang Kun 2017	0.09 (0.01 - 0.55)
Cai Huaiwei 2017	0.07 (0.01 - 0.45)
Li Yanming 2015	0.18 (0.03 - 1.02)
Ji Xuewen 2017	0.06 (0.01 - 0.48)
Wang Sihe 2013	0.06 (0.01 - 0.36)
Shen Wen 2014	0.05 (0.01 - 0.43)

Fixed Effects Model
Pooled Negative LR = 0.18 (0.14 to 0.23)
Cochran-Q = 69.58; df = 42 (p = 0.0047)
Inconsistency (I-square) = 39.6 %

Negative LR   0.001   1   1000.0

Fig. 5 Forest plot showing the negative likelihood ratio of MRI

chose random-effects model to analyze the positive likelihood ratio, and the global positive likelihood ratio was 2.74 (95% CI 1.98–3.79, Fig. 4). Therefore, a positive MRI result was increased by 2.74-fold in the odds of an accurate diagnosis of patients who actually had early osteonecrosis of the femoral head. Based on the chi-squared test ($Q = 69.58$, $P = 0.005$) and I^2 tests ($I^2 = 39.6\%$), with low heterogeneity, we chose the fixed-effects model to analyze the negative likelihood ration. The global negative likelihood ratio was 0.18 (95% CI 0.14–0.23, Fig. 5), indicating the use of MRI, which was close to zero. Specifically, the odds of a false-positive result were increased by only a factor of 0.18.

Based on the chi-squared test ($Q = 59.71$, $P = 0.037$) and I^2 tests ($I^2 = 29.7\%$), heterogeneity was low, so we chose the fixed-effects model to analyze the DOR, with the global DOR being 27.27 (95% CI 17.02–43.67, Fig. 6). And the odds of a positive MRI result were 27.27-fold higher among individuals with early osteonecrosis of the femoral head compared to those without the disease. The area under the SROC was 93.38% (AUC = 93.38%; 95% CI 90.87%–95.89%, Fig. 7), indicating high accuracy.

Conclusions

Several systematic reviews and meta-analysis have been published concerning the diagnostic accuracy of MRI of early osteonecrosis of the femoral head. Li et al. [51] found that the sensitivity and specificity of MRI were 95%(95% CI 94–96%) and 77%(95% CI 70–83%), respectively. Moreover, the DOR was 31.89%(95% CI 17.32–58.70%), and the AUC under the SROC was 0.9166. MRI was associated with high diagnostic accuracy in the patients with suspected early ANFH. Song et al. [52], who included 21 articles, reported that MRI was more effective than CT in diagnosing ANFH. Significant statistical difference was identified between them (OR, 0.13; 95% CI 0.03–0.51). Su et al. [53], who included 8 studies of 515 patients, found the ANFH positive rate between CT and MRI was statistically significant (OR, 0.12; 95% CI 0.04–0.33), so as the early stage positive rate (OR, 0.45; 95% CI 0.26–0.78). Therefore, MRI appears to be a promising diagnostic tool for avascular necrosis of the femoral head.

However, there were several limitations in this analysis: (1) differences in the inclusion and exclusion criteria for

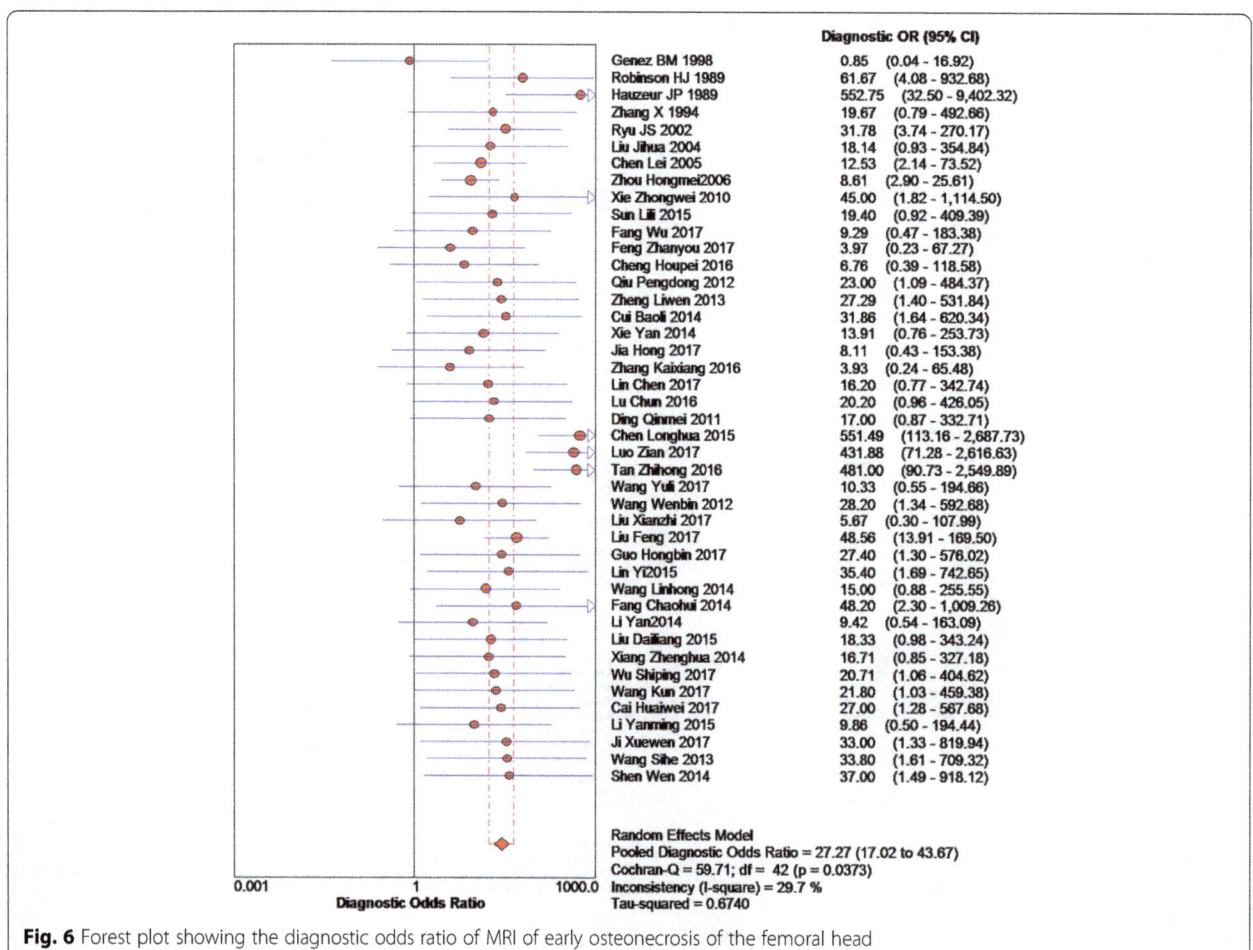

	Diagnostic OR (95% CI)
Genez BM 1998	0.85 (0.04 - 16.92)
Robinson HJ 1989	61.67 (4.08 - 932.68)
Hauzeur JP 1989	552.75 (32.50 - 9,402.32)
Zhang X 1994	19.67 (0.79 - 492.66)
Ryu JS 2002	31.78 (3.74 - 270.17)
Liu Jihua 2004	18.14 (0.93 - 354.84)
Chen Lei 2005	12.53 (2.14 - 73.52)
Zhou Hongmei 2006	8.61 (2.90 - 25.61)
Xie Zhongwei 2010	45.00 (1.82 - 1,114.50)
Sun Lili 2015	19.40 (0.92 - 409.39)
Fang Wu 2017	9.29 (0.47 - 183.38)
Feng Zhanyou 2017	3.97 (0.23 - 67.27)
Cheng Houpei 2016	6.76 (0.39 - 118.58)
Qiu Pengdong 2012	23.00 (1.09 - 484.37)
Zheng Liwen 2013	27.29 (1.40 - 531.84)
Cui Baoli 2014	31.86 (1.64 - 620.34)
Xie Yan 2014	13.91 (0.76 - 253.73)
Jia Hong 2017	8.11 (0.43 - 153.38)
Zhang Kaixiang 2016	3.93 (0.24 - 65.48)
Lin Chen 2017	16.20 (0.77 - 342.74)
Lu Chun 2016	20.20 (0.96 - 426.05)
Ding Qinmei 2011	17.00 (0.87 - 332.71)
Chen Longhua 2015	551.49 (113.16 - 2,687.73)
Luo Zian 2017	431.88 (71.28 - 2,616.63)
Tan Zhihong 2016	481.00 (90.73 - 2,549.89)
Wang Yuli 2017	10.33 (0.55 - 194.66)
Wang Wenbin 2012	28.20 (1.34 - 592.68)
Liu Xianzhi 2017	5.67 (0.30 - 107.99)
Liu Feng 2017	48.56 (13.91 - 169.50)
Guo Hongbin 2017	27.40 (1.30 - 576.02)
Lin Yi 2015	35.40 (1.69 - 742.65)
Wang Linhong 2014	15.00 (0.88 - 255.55)
Fang Chaohui 2014	48.20 (2.30 - 1,009.26)
Li Yan 2014	9.42 (0.54 - 163.09)
Liu Dailiang 2015	18.33 (0.98 - 343.24)
Xiang Zhenghua 2014	16.71 (0.85 - 327.18)
Wu Shiping 2017	20.71 (1.06 - 404.62)
Wang Kun 2017	21.80 (1.03 - 459.38)
Cai Huaiwei 2017	27.00 (1.28 - 567.68)
Li Yanming 2015	9.86 (0.50 - 194.44)
Ji Xuewen 2017	33.00 (1.33 - 819.94)
Wang Sihe 2013	33.80 (1.61 - 709.32)
Shen Wen 2014	37.00 (1.49 - 918.12)

Random Effects Model
Pooled Diagnostic Odds Ratio = 27.27 (17.02 to 43.67)
Cochran-Q = 59.71; df = 42 (p = 0.0373)
Inconsistency (I-square) = 29.7 %
Tau-squared = 0.6740

0.001   1   1000.0
Diagnostic Odds Ratio

Fig. 6 Forest plot showing the diagnostic odds ratio of MRI of early osteonecrosis of the femoral head

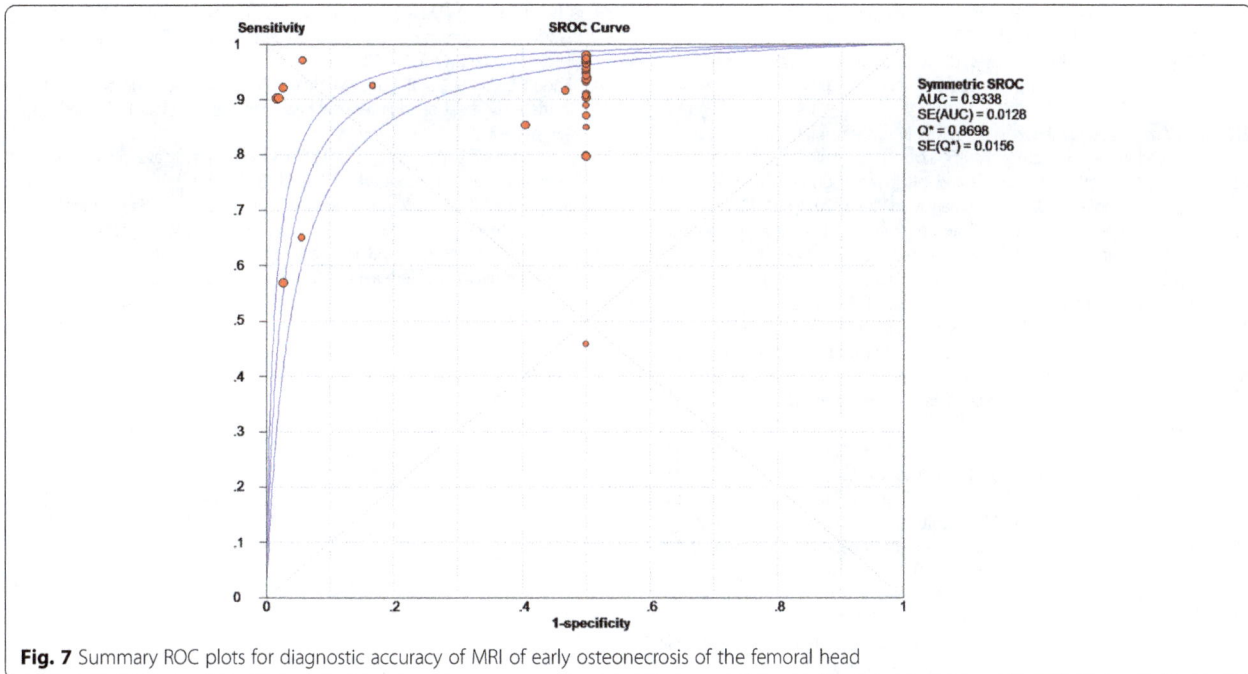

Fig. 7 Summary ROC plots for diagnostic accuracy of MRI of early osteonecrosis of the femoral head

patients, (2) different patients with previous disease and treatments were unavailable, (3) all the included studies were from English and Chinese articles, which may be the source of bias, (4) the fluency of technicians between different studies varied, and (5) pooled data were used for analysis, and individual patients' data were unavailable, which limited a more comprehensive analysis.

In summary, in this systematic review and meta-analysis, MRI as a diagnostic method is associated with higher accuracy for detecting ANFH. More studies and randomized controlled trails with high-quality and large samples are warranted for further evaluation.

Abbreviations
ANFH: Avascular Necrosis of Femur Head; FN: False negative; FP: False positive; MRI: Magnetic resonance imaging; SROC: Summary receiver operating characteristic; TN: True negative; TP: True positive

Authors' contributions
YZZ have made substantial contributions to the conception and design of the study. XYC and XCL searched the literature, extracted data from the collected literature, and analyzed the data. JC and WZ wrote the manuscript. YYZ and ZT revised the manuscript. All authors approved the final version of the manuscript.

Competing interests
The authors declare that they have no competing interests.

References
1. Mankin HJ. Nontraumatic necrosis of bone (osteonecrosis). N Engl J Med. 1992;326(22):1473–9.
2. Castro FP Jr, Barrack RL. Core decompression and conservative treatment for avascular necrosis of the femoral head: a meta-analysis. Am J Orthop. 2000; 29(3):187–94.
3. Hong YC, Zhong HM, Lin T, Shi JB. Comparison of core decompression and conservative treatment for avascular necrosis of femoral head at early stage: a meta-analysis. Int J Clin Exp Med. 2015;8(4):5207–16.
4. Nakamura T, Matsumoto T, Nishino M, Tomita K, Kadoya M. Early magnetic resonance imaging and histologic findings in a model of femoral head necrosis. Clin Orthop Relat Res. 1997;334:68–72.
5. Ficat RP. Idiopathic bone necrosis of the femoral head. Early diagnosis and treatment. J Bone Joint Surg Br Vol. 1985;67(1):3–9.
6. Jawad MU, Haleem AA, Scully SP. In brief: Ficat classification: avascular necrosis of the femoral head. Clin Orthop Relat Res. 2012;470(9):2636–9.
7. Li YM. Comparative analysis of CT and MRI in diagnosis of femoral head necrosis. World Latest Med Inform. 2015;40:140.
8. Sun LL. Comparative study of CT and MRI in diagnosis of 100 cases of femoral head necrosis. China Health Stand Manag. 2015;10:29–30.
9. Wang YL. The value of contrast MRI and CT in the early diagnosis of femoral head necrosis. Chin J Trauma Disabil Med. 2017;25(21):47–8.
10. Zheng LW, Chen RH, Chen YH. The application value of CT and MRI in early diagnosis of osteonecrosis of the femoral head. China Mod Doct. 2013; 51(11):90–1.
11. Cui BG. The application value of CT and MRI in early diagnosis of osteonecrosis of the femoral head. Mod Med Imageol. 2014;23(4):366–9.
12. Xie Y. The value of CT and MRI in the diagnosis of early femoral head necrosis. Chin J Mod Drug Appl. 2014;8(2):70–1.
13. Jia H, Xiao YX, Zhang J, An L. The value of CT and MRI in the diagnosis of femoral head necrosis. Gansu Med J. 2017;36(5):377–8.
14. Fang W, Yang WJ, Liang TH, Huang RS. Application value of CT and MRI in the diagnosis of early femoral head necrosis. J Baotou Med Coll. 2017;33(1):55–6.
15. Feng ZY, Ma Z, Qu JX, Chen W. CT and magnetic resonance imaging (MRI) in the diagnosis of femoral head necrosis in comparison. Mod Diagn Treat. 2017;28(12):2293–5.
16. Zhang KX. MRI and CT diagnosis of avascular necrosis of the femoral head. World Clin Med. 2016;10(8):238.
17. Zi LL. Comparative analysis of CT and MRI in the diagnosis of early necrosis of femoral head. Mod Diagn Treat. 2015;(9):2093–4.
18. Qiu PD. Comparative analysis of CT and MRI in the diagnosis of early necrosis of femoral head. Modern Medical Imageology. 2012;21(5):315–6.

19. Lin C, Ren CP. Clinical value of MRI in the diagnosis of early necrosis of femoral head. J Med Imag. 2017;27(6):1203–5.

20. Sheng W. Comparative analysis of diagnostic value of X - ray, CT and MRI in early diagnosis of avascular necrosis of femoral head. Mod Diagn Treat. 2014;2:352–3.

21. Lu C. Analysis on diagnosis value of MRI in early femoral head necrosis. Chin Foreign Med Res. 2016;14(19):56–7.

22. Ding QM. Comparison of X-ray, CT and MRI in the diagnosis of early avascular necrosis of femoral head. Chin J Primary Med Pharm. 2011;18(6):784–5.

23. Wang SH. Application of spiral CT and high field MRI in the early diagnosis of adult femoral head necrosis. Jiangxi Med J. 2013;12:1288–9.

24. Chen LH. Clinical value of CT and MRI in diagnosis of early osteonecrosis of femoral head in adults. Mod Inst Med Treat. 2015;(2):8–10.

25. Luo ZA. Clinical value of CT and MRI in diagnosis of early osteonecrosis of femoral head in adults. China Med Device Inform. 2017;23(16):93–4.

26. Tan ZH, Wu Y, Zhang PM, Li XL. Clinical value of CT and MRI in diagnosis of early osteonecrosis of femoral head in adults. Mod Med Imageol. 2016;25(2):342–3.

27. Ji XW. Patients with avascular necrosis of the femoral head using MRI, spiral CT examination contrast. China Reflexology. 2017;26(7):154–6.

28. Cai HW. Comparison of multislice spiral CT and MRI in the clinical diagnosis of femoral head necrosis. Int Med Health Guid News. 2017;23(5):731–3.

29. Wang WB. Comparative study of CT and MRI in patients with femoral head necrosis. Chin J CT MRI. 2012;10(6):102–3.

30. Liu XZ, Mu CL. Femoral head necrosis in patients with a comparative study of CT and mri diagnosis. J Imag Res Med Appl. 2017;1(7):7–8.

31. Liu F. Comparative analysis of CT and MRI radiological diagnosis of femoral head necrosis. Mod Diagn Treat. 2017;28(13):2476–7.

32. Guo HB. Comparative analysis of CT and MRI in diagnosis of avascular necrosis of femoral head. Pract Clin J Integ Tradit Chin West Med. 2017;17(8):98–9.

33. Lin Y. Comparison of CT and magnetic resonance imaging in diagnosis and treatment of femoral head necrosis. Guide China Med. 2015;9:149–50.

34. Wang LH. Effect of CT and MRI in diagnosing femoral head necrosis. Contemp Med. 2014;32:150–1.

35. Fang CH. Diagnostic value of two methods of MRI and CT in avascular necrosis of femoral head. China Med Pharm. 2014;13:109–11.

36. Li Y. MRI combined with CT in the diagnosis of avascular necrosis of the femoral head. J Med Imaging. 2014;24(9):1596–8.

37. Zhang J, Peng WX, Y. YF. Observation on the MRI diagnosis on ischemic bone necrosis and surgical treatment. Chin Commun Doct. 2016;32(29):129–30.

38. Liu DL. The value of CT and MRI examination in the early diagnosis of adult femoral head necrosis. Med Inf. 2015;43:347.

39. Xiang ZH. Low field strength MRI diagnosis of avascular necrosis of femoral head. China Foreign Med Treat. 2014;22:188–9.

40. Wu SP. Diagnostic value of multislice spiral CT and mill on femoral head necrosis. Henan Med Res. 2017;26(17):3164–5.

41. Wang K. Evaluation of the value of multislice spiral CT and MRI in the diagnosis of femoral head necrosis. Diet Health. 2017;4(19):323.

42. Xie ZW, Yuan YH. Early diagnosis of avascular necrosis of femoral head in adults. Chin J Lab Diagn. 2010;14(8):1317–9.

43. Genez BM, Wilson MR, Houk RW, Weiland FL, Unger HR Jr, Shields NN, et al. Early osteonecrosis of the femoral head: detection in high-risk patients with MR imaging. Radiology. 1988;168(2):521–4.

44. Robinson HJ Jr, Hartleben PD, Lund G, Schreiman J. Evaluation of magnetic resonance imaging in the diagnosis of osteonecrosis of the femoral head. Accuracy compared with radiographs, core biopsy, and intraosseous pressure measurements. J Bone Joint Surg Am. 1989;71(5):650–63.

45. Hauzeur JP, Pasteels JL, Schoutens A, Hinsenkamp M, Appelboom T, Chochrad I, et al. The diagnostic value of magnetic resonance imaging in non-traumatic osteonecrosis of the femoral head. J Bone Joint Surg Am. 1989;71(5):641–9.

46. Zhang X, Hu CM, Zhao GK, Sun L, Qin DM. The value of magnetic resonance imaging in the early diagnosis of noninvasive avascular necrosis of femoral head. Chin J Surg. 1994;32(9):523–5.

47. Ryu JS, Kim JS, Moon DH, Kim SM, Shin MJ, Chang JS, et al. Bone SPECT is more sensitive than MRI in the detection of early osteonecrosis of the femoral head after renal transplantation. J Nuclear Med. 2002;43(8):1006–11.

48. Liu JH, Zhang SP, Wang SH, Zuo SY. Comparative study of radionuclide scanning and MRI in diagnosis of avascular necrosis of femoral head in early adults. Acta Acad Med Qingdao Univ. 2006;42(4):285–8.

49. Chen L, Hong N, Du XK. Avascular necrosis in severe acute respiratory syndrome: MR imaging with radionuclide correlation. Chin J Med Imag Technol. 2005;21(2):298–300.

50. Zhou HM, Li RG, Cui B, Tang FM, Huang BL. Diagnostic value of CT and MRI in the early stage of adult femoral head necrosis. J Qiqihar Univ Med. 2006; 12(7):529–31.

51. Li YX, Jiang PQ. Meta-analysis of MRI diagnosis of early avascular necrosis of femoral head. Chin Foreign Med Res. 2013;30:143–6.

52. Song WT, Li Z, Li XM, Yang XF. Meta-analysis of CT and MRI diagnosis of avascular necrosis of femoral head. J Pract Radiol. 2010;26(2):221–6.

53. Su JJ, Wu GY, Zhu L, Liu GB. Meta-analysis of CT and MRI diagnosis of avascular necrosis of femoral head. J New Med. 2011;21(3):178–84.

2

WALANT for distal radius fracture: open reduction with plating fixation via wide-awake local anesthesia with no tourniquet

Ying-Cheng Huang[1,2], Chien-Jen Hsu[1], Jenn-Huei Renn[1], Kai-Cheng Lin[1], Shan-Wei Yang[1], Yih-Wen Tarng[1], Wei-Ning Chang[1] and Chun-Yu Chen[1,2,3*]

Abstract

Background: The wide-awake local anesthesia no tourniquet (WALANT) technique is applied during various hand surgeries. We investigated the perioperative variables and clinical outcomes of open reduction and internal fixation (ORIF) for distal radius fractures under WALANT.

Methods: From January 2015 to January 2017, 60 patients with distal radius fractures were treated, and 24 patients (40% of all) were treated with either a volar or a dorsal plate via WALANT procedure. Of these 24 patients, 21 radius fractures were fixed with a volar plate, and the other 3 were fixed with a dorsal plate. Radiographs; range of motions; visual analog scale (VAS); quick disabilities of the arm, shoulder, and hand (Quick DASH) questionnaire; and time to union were evaluated.

Results: One of the 24 patients could not tolerate the WALANT procedure and was reported as a failed attempt at WALANT. In the cohort, 23 patients successfully received distal radius ORIF under WALANT procedure. The average age is 60.9 (range, 20–88) years. The average operation time was 64.3 (range, 45–85) minutes, the average blood loss was 18.9 (range, 5–30) ml, and the average of duration of hospitalization is 1.8 (range, 1–6) days. The average postoperative day one VAS was 1.6 (range, 1–3). The average time of union was 20.7 (range, 15–32) weeks. The mean follow-up period was 15.1 (range, 12–24) months. Functional 1-year postoperative outcomes revealed an average Quick DASH score of 7.60 (range, 4.5–13.6) and an average wrist flexion and extension of 69.6° (range, 55–80°) and 57.4° (range, 45–70°). There was no wound infection, neurovascular injury, or other major complication noted.

Conclusions: WALANT for distal radius fracture ORIF is a method to control blood loss by the effects of local anesthesia mixed with hemostatic agents. Without a tourniquet, the procedure prevents discomfort caused by tourniquet pain. Without sedation, patients could perform the active range of motion of the injured wrist to check if there is impingement of implants. It eliminates the need of numerous preoperative examinations, postoperative anesthesia recovery room care, and side effects of the sedation. However, patients who are not amenable to the awake procedure are contraindications.

Keywords: Distal radius fracture, WALANT, Wide awake, No tourniquet

* Correspondence: iergy2000@gmail.com
[1]Department of Orthopedics, Kaohsiung Veterans General Hospital, No. 386, Dazhong 1st Rd., Zuoying Dist., Kaohsiung City 81362, Taiwan, Republic of China
[2]Department of Orthopedic Surgery, National Defense Medical Center, Taipei, Taiwan, Republic of China
Full list of author information is available at the end of the article

Background

Many minor procedures of the hand and wrist, such as carpal tunnel release and trigger finger release, could be performed with local anesthesia without sedation and could even be performed safely on an outpatient basis, but the common need of a tourniquet can cause pain and discomfort without general anesthesia or brachial plexus block. More recently, a newer technique called wide-awake local anesthesia no tourniquet (WALANT) in which lidocaine and epinephrine are injected for local anesthesia and vasoconstriction, respectively, has been increasingly used by hand surgeons [1, 2]. This technique enables the surgery to be performed with the patient fully awake and without a tourniquet, which allows intraoperative assessment of function during surgery.

Distal radius fracture is a common fracture associated with high-energy trauma in young adults or osteoporotic injury in the elderly [3, 4]. The use of a locking plate to treat such fractures has gained favor recently and helps maintain anatomical structure and facilitate earlier return to normal daily activities [5, 6]. However, plating for distal radius fractures usually requires more surgical time than that for minor hand surgeries as well as a bloodless surgical field to achieve the anatomical reduction. Typically, a tourniquet is used to minimize blood loss, and because of the long duration of surgery and tourniquet-related patient discomfort, open reduction and internal fixation (ORIF) has classically been performed under general anesthesia or brachial plexus block.

We have been using the WALANT technique since January 2015 to perform plating for distal radius fracture, but at present, there is no relevant literature on WALANT for this purpose. The purpose of this retrospective study was to investigate the perioperative variables and clinical outcomes of open reduction and internal fixation (ORIF) for distal radius fractures under WALANT technique, including the operation time, the blood loss, the duration of hospitalization, the time of union, the range of motion of the diseased wrist, the pain, and the functional outcome score 1 year postoperatively.

Methods

From January 2015 to January 2017, 60 patients with distal radius fractures were treated. We excluded patients with concomitant injuries that needed further operative procedure under general anesthesia or spinal anesthesia, such as long bone fracture and traumatic cerebral hemorrhage, and those with peripheral vascular disease or allergy to lidocaine. However, cerebral hemorrhage not requiring surgical intervention was not considered a contraindication to WALANT, and these patients were still therefore included. The other reasons for not participating in the study group included the patient is willing for general anesthesia and the patients who felt lots of anxiety.

The patients were counseled clearly before consenting WALANT surgery. Before the decision of WALANT surgery, the patients were told honestly that the WALANT procedure required at least five needle punctures during the administration of anesthesia. The whole procedure and information about the composite of local injection solution including hemostatic agent were clearly explained.

Regarding other classical anesthesia options, the pros and cons were also informed. The use of sedation of general anesthesia might give rise to the postoperative vomiting and nausea (PONV), and the tourniquet pain and PONV during the recovery time might need extra consumption of medication for symptomatic control. Regional anesthesia like ultrasound-guided axillary brachial plexus block performed by the anesthesiologist for distal radius fracture ORIF is technically demanding, and the risk of unintentional intravascular injection or nerve injury was also told. The WALANT procedure was purely performed by an orthopedist, which saved the use of sedation and tourniquet, as well as lowered the risk of nerve injury.

There were 17 patients with concomitant injuries needing further operative procedures. Nineteen patients were offered WALANT procedure but refused, and the reason for not participating in the study group included the patient is willing for general anesthesia ($n = 15$) and the patients who felt lots of anxiety ($n = 4$). Finally, 24 patients (40%) with distal radial fractures consented to WALANT surgery via fixation with volar plating or dorsal plating, and the other 36 patients were treated under general anesthesia (Fig. 1). The institutional review board of Kaohsiung General Veterans Hospital approved this retrospective study (IRB number: VGHKS17-CT8-13), and informed consent was obtained from all patients.

Anteroposterior and lateral wrist radiographs were obtained on the first admission following trauma. All fracture patterns were recorded according to the Arbeitsgemeinschaft für Osteosynthesefragen/Orthopedic Trauma Association (AO/OTA) fracture classification system.

The indication for using volar plate fixation and dorsal plate depended on the fracture pattern and the surgeon's preference. According to the AO/OTA fracture classification system, of all the patients, 10 cases were classified as extra-articular fracture (6 cases of A2 type, 4 cases of A3 type), and the other 14 cases were intra-articular fractures (3 cases of B2 type, 5 cases of B3 type, 2 cases of C1 type, 3 cases C2 type, and 1 case of C3 type) (Table 1).

In our study, 24 patients were treated with either one or the other. Twenty-one patients were treated with volar plate fixation. Only three patients were treated with dorsal plate fixation, whose distal radius fractures

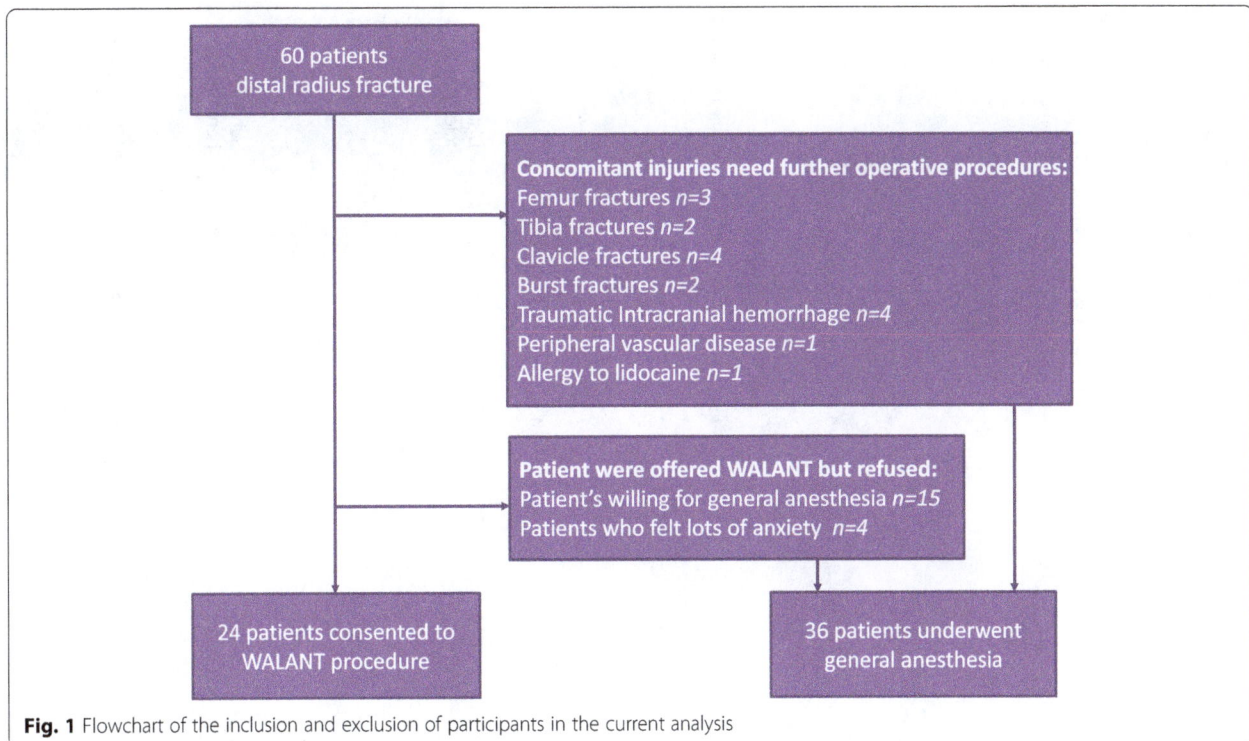

Fig. 1 Flowchart of the inclusion and exclusion of participants in the current analysis

contained the small fragment of the dorsal rim and needed definite dorsal buttress so as to avoid radiocarpal subluxation. Regarding the volar column plate implants, 18 cases used the Synthes 2.4-mm LCP Distal Radius System (DePuy Synthes; Johnson & Johnson Family of Companies, MA, USA), 2 cases used the Civic Locking Plate and Screw System (Microwave Precision, Taiwan), and 1 case used the Aplus Distal Radius Locking Plate System (APlus Biotechnology Corporation, Taiwan). On the other hand, dorsal plating using the 2.4-mm LCP Distal Radius System with a right angle L-shaped plate (DePuy Synthes; Johnson & Johnson Family of Companies, MA, USA) was performed in three cases.

Surgical procedure: preparation

In our institution, the solution used in the WALANT technique consisted of 1 ml of epinephrine (1:1000) and 20 ml of 2% lidocaine, which were mixed with normal saline to give a total of 40 ml, that is, the solution of 1% lidocaine mixed with 1:40000 epinephrine for later injection (Fig. 2). A set of baseline parameters, including heart rate, blood pressure, respiratory rate, and oxygen saturation, was obtained during the entire surgery. At the same time, preoperative intravenous antibiotics with 1 g cefazolin were given for each patient as prophylaxis. The amount of blood loss was based upon the amount in a suction container in the operation room.

Surgical procedure: hematoma block and local anesthetic injection

The protocol using the WALANT technique in our case series started with a hematoma block via a 3–5 ml 1% lidocaine injection from the dorsal site into the fracture site to minimize the discomfort due to sterilization and manipulation procedures for the fractured wrist [7–10]. Subcutaneous injection with 1% lidocaine mixed with 1:40000 epinephrine approximately 5–10 ml was administered directly onto the operative volar or dorsal region of the distal radius. A needle smaller than 25 G was used to perform subcutaneous injection to minimize the injection discomfort (Fig. 3). Then, the injured forearm was sterilized and prepared for surgery while the surgeons waited approximately 18 min to perform the incision for a good hemostatic effect.

Volar plating

The procedure started with a longitudinal skin incision approximately 4 to 5 cm along the flexor carpi radialis (FCR) tendon. The sheath was opened, and the FCR was retracted toward the ulna to deepen the incision between the flexor pollicis longus and radial artery to achieve exposure of the pronator quadratus (PQ) [11]. An additional 5 ml of 1% lidocaine mixed with 1:40000 epinephrine was injected beneath the PQ, and the surgery halted about 30 s while the local anesthetic took effect within the PQ, which was later split and elevated for fracture reduction,

Table 1 Demographic data of the patients and their radiological and clinical outcomes

No.	Age	Sex	Side	AO/OTA classification	Type of approach	OP time (min)	Blood loss (ml)	Duration of hospitalization (days)	Time to union (weeks)	Flexion (degrees)	Extension (degrees)	Postop d1 VAS	Quick DASH score	Follow-up period (months)	Remarks
1	69	F	L	C2	Volar plating	75	5	2	16	60	50	3	4.5	14	
2	57	F	R	A2	Volar plating	60	10	5	16	75	65	1	4.5	20	Subdural hemorrhage
3	71	F	R	B3	Volar plating	45	5	1	24	80	65	2	6.8	12	
4	64	F	L	B2	Dorsal plating	65	20	1	22	75	65	1	9.1	17	
5	20	M	L	B3	Volar plating	75	10	2	20	70	60	1	4.5	18	
6	70	F	R	C2	Volar plating	60	20	1	16	60	45	3	4.5	13	
7	88	F	R	A2	Volar plating	55	10	1	24	75	60	1	6.8	14	
8	63	F	R	A2	Volar plating	90	50	2	24	70	65	3	11.4	13	Shift to general anesthesia
9	80	M	L	A2	Volar plating	70	20	2	28	75	60	1	9.1	24	
10	40	M	R	B3	Volar plating	70	30	1	32	55	55	1	6.8	12	
11	46	F	R	B3	Volar plating	60	20	1	20	75	70	1	4.5	14	
12	65	M	L	C1	Volar plating	60	30	2	16	70	50	3	6.8	16	Distal ulna fracture
13	70	F	R	B2	Dorsal plating	85	20	1	22	70	60	1	6.8	15	
14	76	F	R	B2	Dorsal plating	65	25	2	20	75	45	1	9.1	12	
15	73	F	L	A3	Volar plating	70	30	1	16	70	60	3	9.1	12	
16	46	M	L	B3	Volar plating	60	20	6	18	60	65	1	11.4	24	Subdural hemorrhage
17	65	F	L	C1	Volar plating	60	30	2	24	65	45	2	11.4	12	
18	70	M	R	A3	Volar plating	85	20	1	22	70	50	2	9.1	15	
19	76	F	R	C2	Volar plating	65	25	2	15	60	55	1	9.1	15	

Table 1 Demographic data of the patients and their radiological and clinical outcomes *(Continued)*

No.	Age	Sex	Side	AO/OTA classification	Type of approach	OP time (min)	Blood loss (ml)	Duration of hospitalization (days)	Time to union (weeks)	Flexion (degrees)	Extension (degrees)	Postop d1 VAS	Quick DASH score	Follow-up period (months)	Remarks
20	73	F	L	A3	Volar plating	70	30	1	20	80	60	2	4.5	15	
21	23	M	R	A2	Volar plating	55	10	3	24	80	70	1	4.5	18	Multiple rib fractures
22	26	M	R	A2	Volar plating	50	5	2	22	65	50	2	6.8	12	
23	57	M	L	C3	Volar plating	70	10	1	20	60	45	2	13.6	12	
24	75	F	R	A3	Volar plating	50	30	1	20	75	70	1	11.4	12	

VAS visual analog scale, *Quick DASH* quick disabilities of the arm, shoulder, and hand, *ORIF* open reduction internal fixation, *CRIF* close reduction internal fixation

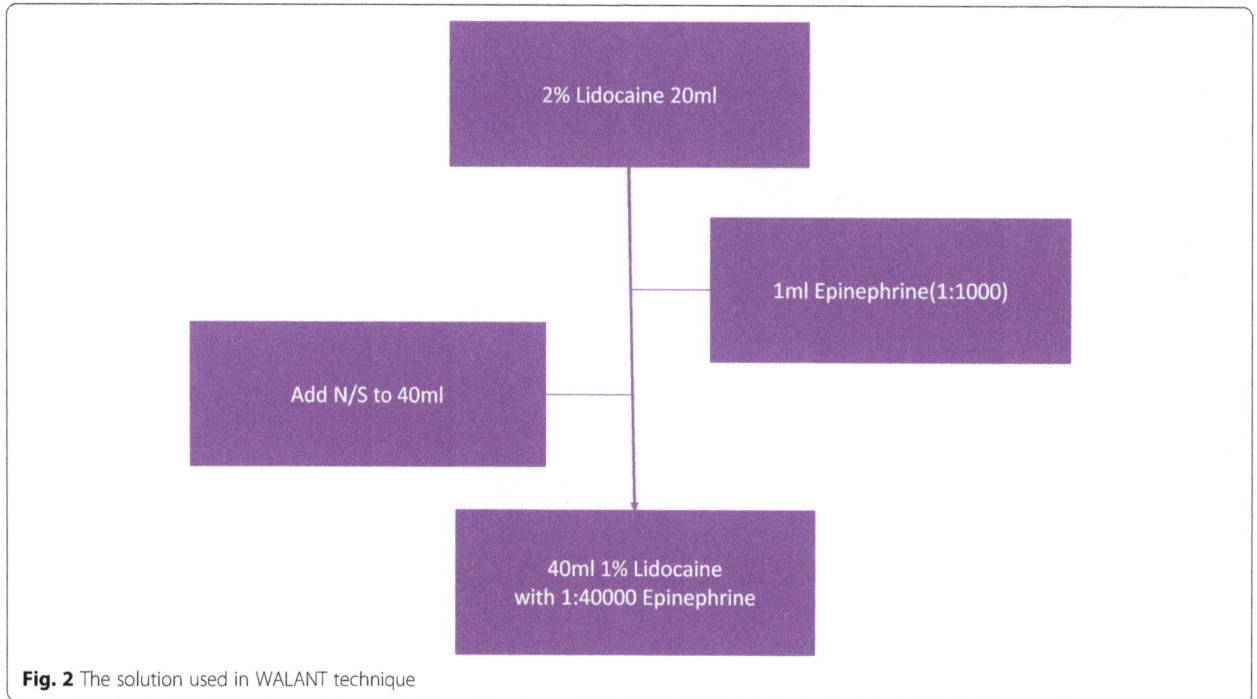

Fig. 2 The solution used in WALANT technique

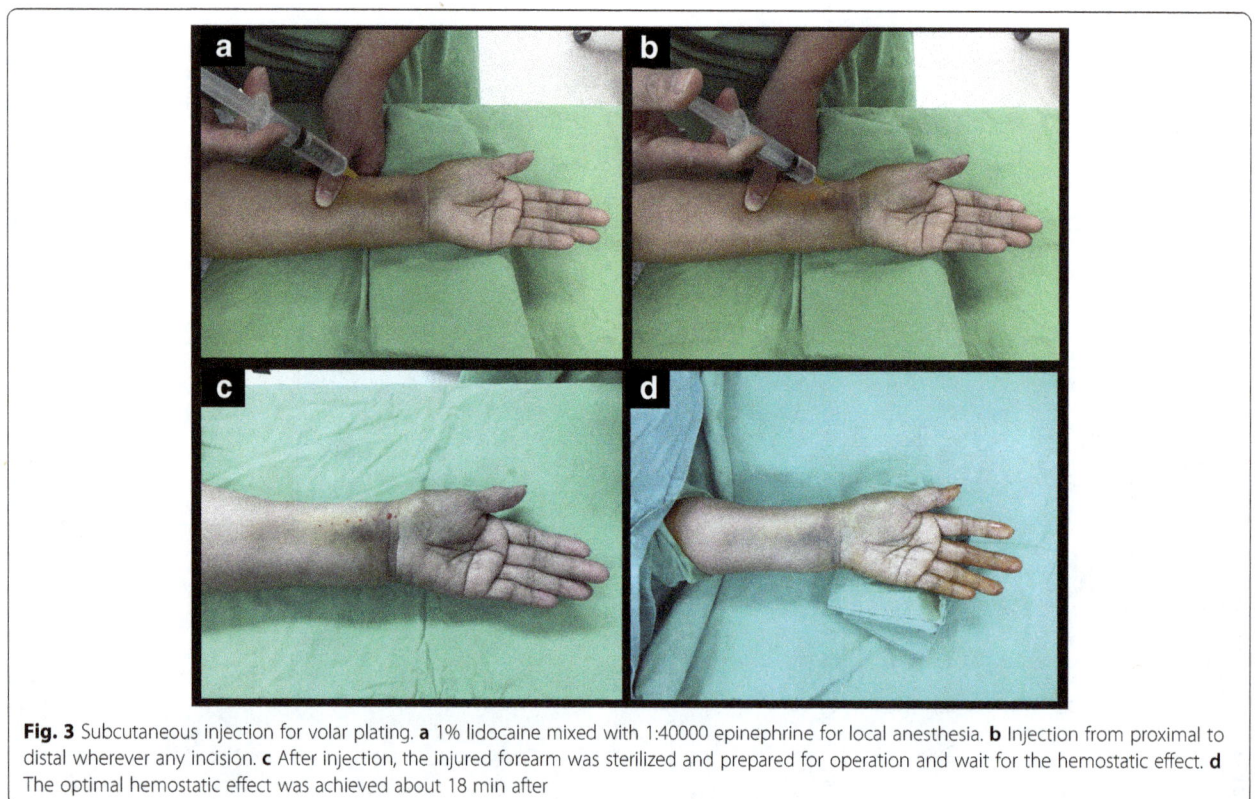

Fig. 3 Subcutaneous injection for volar plating. **a** 1% lidocaine mixed with 1:40000 epinephrine for local anesthesia. **b** Injection from proximal to distal wherever any incision. **c** After injection, the injured forearm was sterilized and prepared for operation and wait for the hemostatic effect. **d** The optimal hemostatic effect was achieved about 18 min after

plate placement, drilling procedures, and screw fixations (Fig. 4).

Dorsal plating

Using a single dorsal skin incision along the line between the third and fourth compartments, the extensor retinaculum was carefully dissected. An additional 5 ml of 1% lidocaine mixed with 1:40000 epinephrine was injected beneath the retinaculum to infiltrate the tendon sheath and the periosteum of the intermediate column. Then, the extensor retinaculum was opened as far as needed for later fracture reduction, plate placement, drilling procedures, and screw fixations.

Postoperative care and follow-up

Postoperative treatment following the surgical procedure for the patients was standardized. Regular oral tramadol 37.5 mg/acetaminophen 325 mg combination tablets (Ultracet®) two times a day was the protocol for postoperative pain control medication for each patient (usually about 10 days after operation). Immobilization with a short arm splint for 1 week was performed for each patient. The patients were taught to use a consecutive passive wrist motion with flexion and extension from the removal of the splint to postoperative 1 month, under weekly outpatient department close follow-up. Then, active training of a range of motion (ROM) using objects weighing up to 5 kg was started since the second month

postoperatively. There was no implant removal after surgery during follow-up of these patients. All patients performed exercise on their own and were followed up for ≥ 12 months postoperatively.

According to the clinician, the patients achieved clinical union without pain or any clinical symptom postoperatively. Anteroposterior (AP) and lateral wrist radiographs were obtained for the radiographic evaluation of the bone union, in which the fracture gap disappeared on the AP and lateral views, which was also confirmed by the radiologist's report of the plain film at the same time. The functional outcomes by using the quick disabilities of the arm, shoulder, and hand (Quick DASH) questionnaire [12] were evaluated 1 year postoperatively, and the maximum ROM at the wrist was also recorded at our outpatient department monthly.

Results

The demographic information, perioperative variables, and clinical outcomes are presented in Table 1. One of the 24 patients could not tolerate the WALANT procedure and was reported as a failed attempt at WALANT. Regarding the other 23 patients under WALANT procedure, the average age is 60.9 (range, 20–88) years. Concerning the time from injury to surgery, 7 patients were arranged for the operation on the same day, and the other 16 patients received the procedure on the next day. The average surgical time was 64.3 min (range, 45–

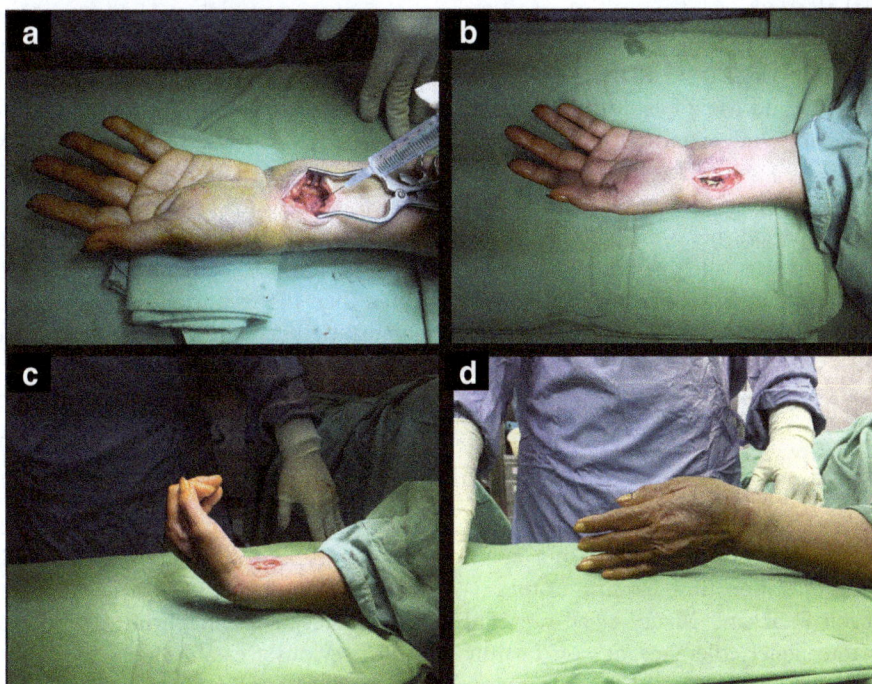

Fig. 4 Henry approach via WALANT technique. **a** Before splitting the pronator quadrates, we injected an additional 5 ml of 1% lidocaine mixed with 1:40000 epinephrine beneath it for later procedures. **b** Volar ORIF with plating. **c** The patient was required to perform active range of motion with wrist extension and flexion. **d** Perform radial and ulna deviation

85 min). The average amount of blood loss during surgery was 18.9 ml (range, 5–30 ml). The average duration of hospitalization was 1.8 days (range, 1–6 days). The average time to union for each radius was 20.7 weeks (range, 15–32 weeks). The average follow-up period was 15.1 months (range, 12–24 months).

The patient who could not endure the subcutaneous injection and felt very nervous under an awake status agreed to receive general anesthesia to complete the surgery, which was still performed without a tourniquet. The operation time of the patient was more than the average of the other 23 patients under WALANT procedure (90 vs. 64.3 min).

In our study, there was a victim of multiple rib fractures, two minimal subdural hemorrhages not requiring surgical intervention, one patient with a distal radius and ulna fracture receiving percutaneous pinning for distal ulnar fracture in addition to volar plating of the radius. Despite the associated injuries, they still underwent the WALANT procedure for distal radius fracture fixation successfully.

The average postoperative day 1 visual analog scale score was 1.6 (range, 1–3). Postoperative pain control medication is mainly Ultracet 500 mg two times a day during hospitalization, as well as the medication sent home with. During outpatient department follow-up, almost all the patients undergoing WALANT procedure claimed that no extra medication for pain was needed.

The average Quick DASH score of the 23 injured radii was 7.60 (range, 4.5–13.6). The patient with the highest Quick DASH score of 13.6 was a 57-year-old male with a C3-type distal radius fracture. It was particularly difficult for him to turn a key and use a fork with his injured wrist. The average flexion and extension of each wrist were 69.6° (range, 55–80°) and 57.4° (range, 45–70°), respectively.

During the follow-up period, none of the patients received secondary interventions, such as bone grafting or shockwave treatment, and all patients achieved union. No wound infection, finger necrosis, palpitation, or other complication was found in our study.

Discussion

The use of a tourniquet for hemostatic effect has been popular in simple hand surgeries, such as tendon repair or transfer, transverse carpal ligament release, and full-thickness skin grafts. However, the patients could not tolerate very long operation time because of tourniquet pain. Hutchinson et al. and Maury et al. reported studies about the tourniquet tolerance among healthy volunteers, in which the average tolerance to forearm tourniquet was 13 and 25 min, respectively, with temporary pain and paresthesia [13, 14]. Prolonged tourniquet usage may give rise to nerve injury or severe neurological deficit [15]. Thus, a wide-awake local anesthesia with no tourniquet procedure was developed. The WALANT technique has been used in different hand surgeries, particularly in soft tissue repair or reconstruction [1, 16–20]. In addition, finger fractures could be also treated by closed reduction and percutaneous pinning under WALANT technique [21]. The WALANT technique has several advantages, including simplifying the preparations for surgeries, lowering the risk of general anesthesia, and saving time in the postoperative recovery room. Furthermore, it may reduce medical costs of preoperative evaluation of general anesthesia, shorten hospitalization days, decrease opioid agent consumption, and save medical resources [16]. To our knowledge, no study has been reported regarding the management of distal radius fractures by using ORIF with the WALANT technique.

In previous studies, Lalonde reported that the effective concentration of the hemostatic agent is from 1:400000 epinephrine in treating tendon repair on wrist surgery to 1:100000 epinephrine in surgical dissection and manipulation for fractured bones [16]. The optimal time delay between local injection and incision to minimize bleeding depends on the maximal vasoconstriction [22], occurring approximately 25.9 min after injection of 1:100000 epinephrine beneath the skin [23]. In the present study, we performed the surgeries over the wrist not only for soft tissue dissection but also for bony procedures, such as reduction with forceps and manipulation with limb traction. Unlike treating finger fractures which may only need fixation with percutaneous pinning or open reduction at a small area, orthopedic surgeons had to manage blood loss due to the transection through the subcutaneous vessel from a relatively larger operation field as well as bleeding from the bone marrow in the fracture sites. Therefore, the regimen of the WALANT technique in our study for distal radius fractures is 1:40000 epinephrine, which is more concentrated than that reported in previous studies to meet the hemostatic effects during the whole operation [16]. The time delay between the local injection and incision in our study was 18 min, which provided sufficient time for the medical staff to sterilize the diseased limb before the surgeons' incision and achieve a hemostatic effect during the whole operation. Otherwise, after the initial hematoma block combined with preventive injection underneath the PQ muscle, bony procedures, such as drilling and screwing into bones, could be performed without any discomfort.

The safety of epinephrine use in hand surgeries has been previously established [24]. Cyanosis of the distal fingers due to epinephrine use has been previously reported, but procaine acidity was found to be the culprit for finger loss [25, 26]. Even when procaine has been confirmed as the real cause of necrosis, there still have been concerns about the possible vasoconstriction caused by epinephrine in the human finger, and phentolamine has been used to reverse the vasoconstriction in rare cases of necrosis onset. Nodwell and Lalonde reported that the white finger can be reversed by subcutaneous injection of 1 mg of phentolamine in 220 cc of saline wherever the epinephrine is injected [27]. Certainly, this situation seldom occurs. However, if there is a suspicion of cyanosis of the distal finger related to the epinephrine use, the vasoconstriction can be reversed. In our study, we injected the more concentrated epinephrine cocktail into the distal radius area instead of the distal fingers, and there was no remarkable ischemia sign or finger necrosis. Epinephrine-induced cardiac ischemia has been rarely reported, even with a high dose of 1:1000 epinephrine [28]. In our study, no complication such as finger necrosis, palpitation, or allergy was found.

Without tourniquet use, hemostatic control could still be achieved, and no patient received a blood transfusion in our study. The average blood loss was only 18.9 ml. In fact, such a small amount of blood loss does not interfere with the whole procedure. In Ruxasagulwong's prospective trial [29] regarding common minor orthopedic hand soft tissue surgery (including carpal tunnel syndrome, de Quervain's disease, and trigger finger), even though there was a more surgical field bleeding in the wide-awake group without tourniquet application, the amount of blood loss in the conventional group with tourniquet use was significantly higher because of vasodilatation with a moderate amount of bleeding after the release of tourniquet pressure prior to skin suture to check for bleeding. It is worth mentioning that the amount of blood loss under the WALANT technique may be relatively less than the uncalculated blood loss after tourniquet release.

Lalonde et al. reported that carpal tunnel release and trigger finger release were minor surgeries, which could be performed in procedure rooms under field sterility with very low infection rates [2, 30]. In our hospital, the fracture fixation under WALANT technique was still performed in the main operation room with well-equipped tools and image intensifier. Preoperative intravenous antibiotics with 1 g cefazolin were still given to each patient as prophylaxis for the purpose of infection prevention. In addition, all patients stayed in the hospital at least one night, and we could teach the patients how to care for the surgical wound. Therefore, no wound infection was encountered in our study.

When we performed minor orthopedic hand soft tissue surgery such as trigger finger release, the patient is asked to performed metacarpal-phalangeal joint flexion to confirm the adequate release of A1 pulley. Similarly, when distal radius ORIF under WALANT technique was performed, the patient was asked to performed wrist and finger motions to confirm the stability of fracture

fixation and to see if there was an impingement of implant (Additional files 1 and 2: Videos S1 and S2).

Health costs have continued to increase over time [31]. Assessments of cost savings and patient satisfaction also have been reported and need to be discussed [32]. Furthermore, the National Health Insurance Administration-Ministry of Health and Welfare has already started bundling payments of selected orthopedic diagnosis-related groups (DRG) in Taiwan for a period of time. The hospitals receive a single index code with the same payment for a particular DRG, in order to reduce the cost as possible. One of the main costs for the payment is the stays of patient's hospitalization. In the present study, the average operation time was 64.3 min (range, 45–85 min), and the average of duration of hospitalization was 1.8 days (range, 1–6 days). Two patients with subdural hemorrhage had relatively longer hospital stays than the average (5 and 6 days, respectively), because they needed more days for the complete observation of head injuries. For cost efficiency, WALANT eliminates the need for sedation, which means that there is no need for numerous preoperative examinations, specialists monitoring intraoperative sedation, postoperative anesthesia recovery room care, and that there will be less incidence of nausea, vomiting, or unwanted side effects of opiates or sedation. Dr. Lalonde claimed that patients could spend less time at the hospital for the procedure because there is no anesthesia recovery time, and the patients could talk to their surgeon during the WALANT procedure for advice on how to avoid complications, when to return to work, and how to take pain medication. Additionally, the patients do not need preoperative anesthetic assessment visits, chest X-rays, and needle pricking for blood tests, and the patients do not need to fast prior to general anesthesia, change medication schedules (such as required for patients with diabetes under regular oral hyperglycemic drug control), discontinue anticoagulation medication, or a caregiver during the evening shift [33].

Some patients, such as uremia patients with ipsilateral wrist fractures and arteriovenous shunts who should not be subjected to tourniquet applications, those with chronic occlusive pulmonary disease or severe congestive heart failure and other cardiovascular problems with difficulties in extubation after general anesthesia, may benefit from surgeries under the WALANT technique. In addition to the benefits mentioned above, doctors can perform surgery with the patient awake and directly examine them for active ROM and tendon function of the injured limbs and reduce the rate of impingement or of usual complications, such as tendon irritation (even that caused by compression of the plate), which cannot be achieved under general anesthesia.

Discussions with the patients were made regarding the rehabilitation plans, to provide education concerning wound care, and about the return to work after surgery, which increases patient's sense of safety and builds their confidence for achieving a good recovery [34]. Adequate explanations about the whole procedure are necessary for patients who are about to receive distal radius ORIF under the WALANT technique. In our case series, even after we fully discussed the discomfort caused by local injection before surgery, one patient still felt very unwell and requested shifting to general anesthesia. Therefore, surgeons should evaluate the patient's personality prior to the WALANT technique for ORIF of distal radius because patients with psychological problems or lots of anxiety are contraindications for the WALANT procedure. For those who are not amenable to the awake procedure, ORIF of distal radius under general anesthesia is still recommended.

This study had several limitations, including its retrospective nature and small sample size. In addition, there was no control group of patients treated with general anesthesia without a tourniquet. Further comparative analyses of distal radius ORIF under the WALANT technique and under general anesthesia without a tourniquet with a large group of consecutive patients are warranted.

Conclusions
Patients receiving the WALANT surgery for distal radius ORIF do not require sedation, which allows the patients to communicate with the doctors during the procedure and perform active movement of the operated limb to examine if there is an impingement of implants, as well as save the need of numerous preoperative examinations, specialists monitoring intraoperative sedation, postoperative anesthesia recovery room care, and the side effects of opiates or sedation. Without tourniquet use, tourniquet pain can be avoided and blood loss can be controlled by epinephrine injection. No complications such as infection or implant failure were observed in our case series. Most importantly, a sufficient explanation of the whole procedure is necessary for patients who are about to receive distal radius ORIF under the WALANT technique. Patients who are not amenable to the awake procedure are contraindications.

Abbreviations
DRG: Diagnosis-related groups; GA: General anesthesia; WALANT: Wide-awake local anesthesia no tourniquet

Authors' contributions
All authors made substantive intellectual contributions to this study to qualify as authors. Y-CH, C-YC, and J-HR designed the study. An initial draft of the manuscript was written by Y-CH. K-CL, S-WY, and Y-WT re-drafted the parts of the manuscript, C-JH and W-NC provided helpful advice on the final revision. All authors were involved in writing the manuscript. All authors read and approved the final manuscript.

Competing interests
The authors declare that they have no competing interests.

Author details
[1]Department of Orthopedics, Kaohsiung Veterans General Hospital, No. 386, Dazhong 1st Rd., Zuoying Dist., Kaohsiung City 81362, Taiwan, Republic of China. [2]Department of Orthopedic Surgery, National Defense Medical Center, Taipei, Taiwan, Republic of China. [3]Department of Occupational Therapy, Shu-Zen Junior College of Medicine and Management, Kaohsiung, Taiwan, Republic of China.

References
1.   Lalonde D, Martin A. Epinephrine in local anesthesia in finger and hand surgery: the case for wide-awake anesthesia. J Am Acad Orthop Surg. 2013; 21(8):443–7.
2.   Lalonde D, Eaton C, Amadio PC, et al. Wide-awake hand and wrist surgery: a new horizon in outpatient surgery. Instr Course Lect. 2015;64:249–59.
3.   Liporace FA, Adams MR, Capo JT, et al. Distal radius fractures. J Orthop Trauma. 2009;23(10):739–48.
4.   Diaz-Garcia RJ, Oda T, Shauver MJ, et al. A systematic review of outcomes and complications of treating unstable distal radius fractures in the elderly. J Hand Surg [Am]. 2011;36(5):824–35.e2.
5.   Chung KC, Watt AJ, Kotsis SV, et al. Treatment of unstable distal radial fractures with the volar locking plating system. J Bone Joint Surg Am. 2006; 88(12):2687–94.
6.   Jupiter JP, Marent-Huber M, LCP Study Group, et al. Operative management of distal radial fractures with 2.4-millimeter locking plates. A multicenter prospective case series. J Bone Joint Surg Am. 2009;91(1):55–65.
7.   Gottlieb M, Cosby K. Ultrasound-guided hematoma block for distal radial and ulnar fractures. J Emerg Med. 2015;48(3):310–2.
8.   Tageldin M, Alrashid M, Khoriati A, et al. Periosteal nerve blocks for distal radius and ulna fracture manipulation—the technique and early results. J Orthop Surg Res. 2015;10:134.
9.   Ketonis C, Ilyas A, Liss F. Pain management strategies in hand surgery. Orthop Clin North Am. 2015;46(3):399–408.
10. Ceran C, Aksam B, Aksam E, et al. Selective nerve block combined with tumescent anesthesia. J Hand Surg [Am]. 2015;40(12):2339–44.
11. Protopsaltis T, Ruch D. Volar approach to distal radius fractures. J Hand Surg [Am]. 2008;33(6):958–5.
12. Hudak PL, Amadio PC, Bombardier C, et al. Development of an upper extremity outcome measure: the DASH (disabilities of the arm, shoulder, and head). Am J Ind Med. 1996;29(6):602–8.
13. Hutchinson DT, McClinton MA. Upper extremity tourniquet tolerance. J Hand Surg [Am]. 1993;18(2):206–10.
14. Maury A, Roy W. A prospective, randomized, controlledtrial of forearm versus upper arm tourniquet tolerance. J Hand Surg (Br). 2002;27(4):359–60.
15. Flatt AE. Tourniquet time in hand surgery. Arch Surg. 1972;104(2):190–2.
16. Lalonde D. Minimally invasive anesthesia in wide awake hand surgery. Hand Clin. 2014;30(1):1–6.
17. Hagert E, Lalonde D. Wide-awake wrist arthroscopy and open TFCC repair. J Wrist Surg. 2012;1(1):55–60.
18. Nakanishi Y, Omokawa S, Kobata Y, et al. Ultrasound-guided selective sensory nerve block for wide-awake forearm tendon reconstruction. Plast Reconstr Surg Glob Open. 2015;3(5):e392.
19. Lalonde D. Wide-awake extensor indicis proprius to extensor pollicis longus tendon transfer. J Hand Surg [Am]. 2014;39(11):2297–9.
20. Gunasagaran J, Sean ES, Shivdas S, et al. Perceived comfort during minor hand surgeries with wide awake local anaethesia no tourniquet (WALANT) versus local anaethesia (LA)/tourniquet. J Orthop Surg (Hong Kong). 2017;25(3):1–4.
21. Xing S, Tang J. Surgical treatment, hardware removal, and the wide-awake approach for metacarpal fractures. Clin Plast Surg. 2014;41(3):463–80.
22. Mckee D, Lalonde D, Thoma A, et al. Achieving the optimal epinephrine effect in wide awake hand surgery using local anesthesia without a tourniquet. Hand (N Y). 2015;10(4):613–5.
23. McKee D, Lalonde D, Thoma A, et al. Optimal time delay between epinephrine injection and incision to minimize bleeding. Plast Reconstr Surg. 2013;131(4):811–4.

24. Mann T, Hammert W. Epinephrine and hand surgery. J Hand Surg [Am]. 2012;37(6):1254–6.

25. Lalonde D, Bell M, Benoit P, et al. A multicenter prospective study of 3,110 consecutive cases of elective epinephrine use in the fingers and hand: the Dalhousie Project clinical phase. J Hand Surg [Am]. 2005;30(5):1061–7.

26. Thomson C, Lalonde D, Denkler K, et al. A critical look at the evidence for and against elective epinephrine use in the finger. Plast Reconstr Surg. 2007;119(1):260–6.

27. Nodwell T, Lalonde DH. How long does it take phentolamine to reverse adrenaline-induced vasoconstriction in the finger and hand? A prospective randomized blinded study: the Dalhousie Project experimental phase. Can J Plast Surg. 2003;11(4):187.

28. Cunnington C, McDonald J, Singh R. Epinephrine-induced myocardial infarction in severe anaphylaxis: is nonselective β-blockade a contributory factor? Am J Emerg Med. 2013;31(4):759.e1–2.

29. Ruxasagulwong S, Kraisarin J, Sananpanich K. Wide awake technique versus local anesthesia with tourniquet application for minor orthopedic hand surgery: a prospective clinical trial. J Med Assoc Thail. 2015;98(1):106–10.

30. LeBlanc MR, Lalonde DH, Thoma A, et al. Is main operating room sterility really necessary in carpal tunnel surgery? A multicenter prospective study of minor procedure room field sterility surgery. Hand. 2011;6(1):60–3.

31. Whiting P, Rice C, Avilucea F, et al. Patients at increased risk of major adverse events following operative treatment of distal radius fractures: inpatient versus outpatient. J Wrist Surg. 2017;6(3):220–6.

32. Rhee P, Fischer M, Rhee L, McMillan H, Johnson A. Cost savings and patient experiences of a clinic-based, wide-awake hand surgery program at a military medical center: a critical analysis of the first 100 procedures. J Hand Surg [Am]. 2017;42(3):e139–47.

33. Lalonde D. Conceptual origins, current practice, and views of wide awake hand surgery. J Hand Surg Eur Vol. 2017;42(9):886–95.

34. Lalonde D. Wide awake local anaesthesia no tourniquet technique (WALANT). BMC Proc. 2015;9(Suppl 3):A81.

3

Effectiveness and safety of glucosamine and chondroitin for the treatment of osteoarthritis: a meta-analysis of randomized controlled trials

Xiaoyue Zhu[1], Lingli Sang[2], Dandong Wu[2], Jiesheng Rong[3] and Liying Jiang[4*]

Abstract

Objective: To assess the symptomatic effectiveness and safety of oral symptomatic slow-acting drugs (SYSADOAs) on the treatment of knee and/or hip osteoarthritis, such as chondroitin, glucosamine, and combination treatment with chondroitin plus glucosamine.

Methods: We searched electronic database including PubMed, Embase, Cochrane Library, and the reference lists of relevant articles. An updated meta-analysis was performed to assess the effectiveness of these slow-acting drugs for osteoarthritis.

Results: Twenty-six articles describing 30 trials met our inclusion criteria and were included in the meta-analysis. The estimates between chondroitin and placebo showed that chondroitin could alleviate pain symptoms and improve function. Compared with placebo, glucosamine proved significant effect only on stiffness improvement. However, the combination therapy did not have enough evidence to be superior to placebo. Additionally, there was no significant difference in the incidence of AEs and discontinuations of AEs when compared with placebo.

Conclusions: Given the effectiveness of these symptomatic slow-acting drugs, oral chondroitin is more effective than placebo on relieving pain and improving physical function. Glucosamine showed effect on stiffness outcome. Regarding on the limited number of combination therapy, further studies need to investigate the accurate effectiveness. This information accompanied with the tolerability and economic costs of included treatments would be conducive to making decisions for clinicians.

Keywords: Osteoarthritis, Glucosamine, Chondroitin, Treatment

Background

Osteoarthritis (OA), characterized by progressive cartilage matrix degradation, subchondral bone sclerosis, and osteophyte formation, is the most common form of arthritis [1, 2]. Globally, the prevalence of OA, particularly of the large weight-bearing joints such as the knee and hip, is also predicted to grow [3]. Presently, OA has emerged as one of the major public health concerns and continues to affect about 10% of men and 18% of women over 60 years of age [1].

Previous studies suggest that aging, genetic predisposition, obesity, inflammation, and excessive mechanical loading predispose to OA occurrence and development [4]. The structural changes result in joint pain and stiffness, swelling, and tenderness, which can eventually lead to disability and affect the quality of life of patients [5]. Treatment strategies of OA include both non-pharmacological and pharmacological therapies. Among pharmacological therapies, analgesics and non-steroidal anti-inflammatory drugs (NSAIDs) are current treatment options for OA because of their well-established effectiveness. However, they act as symptomatic treatments without offering disease modification of OA, and they are accused for increased risk adverse events, including the gastrointestinal and/or cardiovascular system

* Correspondence: J_meili@126.com
[4]Shanghai Key Laboratory for Molecular Imaging, Shanghai University of Medicine & Health Sciences, Shanghai, People's Republic of China
Full list of author information is available at the end of the article

[6]. For this reason, attention has recently been focused on an ideal treatment, which can improve the clinical symptoms of OA with better tolerability and safety profiles, such as symptomatic slow-acting drugs (SYSADOAs) [7].

Glucosamine and chondroitin, as important medicine in those SYSADOA, are naturally occurring compounds in the body functioning as the principal substrates in the biosynthesis of proteoglycan [8, 9]. It is suggested that glucosamine and chondroitin are both partially absorbed and then reaches the joints, exerting on relieving joint pain and slowing the rate of joint destruction and cartilage loss. They are two main categories of agents potentially or theoretically acting as chondroprotective agents and disease-modifying OA drugs (DMOADs) [8, 10]. The effectiveness based on the result of RCT published in 2013 suggested that consumption of chondroitin for certain dosage has a positive effect on pain relief and function improvement [7]. Recently, a trial conducted in 2017 demonstrated a lack of superiority of chondroitin and glucosamine combination therapy over placebo [11]. Although many studies have shown a significant treatment effect, accompanied with remarkable safety, there is still controversy regarding the effectiveness of these putative DMOADs compared with placebo [7, 11]. International guidelines for the management of OA had given an equivocal recommendation of glucosamine and chondroitin, and they are not recommended according to Osteoarthritis Research Society International (OARSI) guidelines published in 2014 [12].

Therefore, based on existing evidence, a study needs to be updated and critically evaluates the current evidence-based information about the administration of glucosamine and chondroitin for the treatment of knee or hip OA. In our study, a relatively comprehensive meta-analysis was performed to assess the effectiveness and safety of putative DMOADs.

Methods

Search strategy

We conducted this meta-analysis following the PRISMA extension statement [13]. We systematically searched electronic database including PubMed, Embase, and Cochrane Library based on logic combination of keywords and text words associated with OA to extract concerned RCTs from inception to May 22, 2018. The Internet-based search used the following terms: "arthritis," "osteoarthritis," "OA," "joint disease," "glucosamine," "GH," "GS," "chondroitin," "CH," "CS," and the corresponding free terms. The search was restricted to English language and studies of human participants. We then screened reference lists of all obtained articles, including relevant reviews, to avoid missing relevant articles. And, we also searched ClinicalTrials.gov for progressive trials.

Inclusion and exclusion criteria

Studies were included if they met the following criteria: (1) RCTs; (2) studies about primary hip and/or knee OA patients with clinical and/or radiologic diagnosis; (3) studies covering at least two of the following oral treatments: glucosamine, chondroitin, or the two in combination against placebo; and (4) extractable data reporting the pain, function, stiffness, and the adverse events (AEs) of patients.

The exclusion criteria were as follows: (1) studies of non-randomized and/or uncontrolled trials, (2) treatment methods described unclearly, (3) interventions combined with non-steroidal anti-inflammatory drugs, (4) studies or data reported repeatedly, and (5) trial arms with sub-therapeutic doses (< 1500 mg/day of glucosamine and < 800 mg/day of chondroitin (according to dosage licensed in Europe)) [14].

Data extraction

Two investigators (X.Y.Z and L.L.S) independently assessed all studies for eligibility and extracted data in accordance with a preconfigured form from each study. Any disagreements were resolved through discussion with a third reviewer (L.Y.J). For each study, patients' characteristics including mean age, sex, mean duration of symptom, BMI, duration of follow-up, type of outcome (pain, function, stiffness, and AEs), trial design, trial size, details of intervention, treatment duration, and results were individually extracted. Data of intention-to-treat analysis was employed whenever possible.

Quality assessment

The Cochrane Risk of Bias Tool was used to evaluate the methodological quality of the included studies (version 5.3) [15]. The tool evaluated seven potential risks of bias: random sequence generation, allocation concealment, blinding of participants, blinding of outcome assessment, incomplete outcome data, selective reporting, and other bias. Each item was judged by the following criteria: low risk of bias, uncertain risk of bias, and high risk of bias. Whenever studies included three or more high risk of bias, it was considered as poor methodological quality. Two reviewers (X.Y.Z and L.L.S) checked the profile of each included study independently.

Outcome measures

The primary outcomes of this meta-analysis were pain intensity, function improvement, and stiffness score from baseline to the end of treatment. The secondary outcome was safety of studies. We preferred to the scale that was recognized to be the highest on the hierarchy of those suggested outcomes when more than one pain scales were given for a trial. Among these scales, global pain has precedence over pain on walking and the Western Ontario and McMaster Universities Osteoarthritis Index (WOMAC) pain subscale [16, 17].

Similarly, the data of function and stiffness was extracted with the same method. If global function score was not reported, the walking disability, function subscale of WOMAC, or Lequesne Index would be applied instead.

The standard mean difference (SMD) was used to calculate the difference between two interventions because different studies assessed the same outcome by employing different scales. SMD expresses the size of the intervention effect in each study relative to the variability observed in that study by dividing the pooled SD of the differences between two interventions [18, 19]. The effect size was transformed back to the different units of the WOMAC Visual Analogue Scale (VAS), the most commonly used scale based on a media pooled SD of 2.5 cm to assess pain on the scale of 0 to 10 cm. A standardized WOMAC function score (0–10) was transformed by SMD, which based on a median pooled SD of 2.1 units. A change of 2 points on the 0–10 scale was interpreted clinically significant improvement [20]. The negative effect size indicated a better treatment effect on pain relief and function improvement.

Statistical analysis

All results summarized using STATA software (version 13.1, StataCorp, College Station, TX). For continuous outcomes, SMD with 95% credible interval (CI) was used to present the effect size. For counting data, we calculated relative risk (RR) with 95% CI. The heterogeneity between studies was tested using the Q statistics. $P < 0.1$ was considered statistically significant. And, I^2 was used to quantify the inconsistency among the potentially disparate sources of studies. A random-effects model was used if $I^2 > 50\%$. A subgroup analysis was conducted because there were different types of SYSADOA. Publication bias was examined through visual inspection of funnel plot asymmetry. A sensitivity analysis was performed to evaluate the effect of each study on the combined effect size by omitting each study.

Results

Study selection and characteristics

A flowchart of study search and selection was presented in Additional file 1: Figure S1. We identified 1407 references in our literature search and out of 97 potentially eligible studies, 26 articles describing 30 trials met our inclusion criteria and were included in the meta-analysis [7, 11, 21–44]. All trials were published as full journal articles and all trials used a placebo control. Only two articles compared the effectiveness among glucosamine, chondroitin, and the two in combination with placebo at one time [29, 33]. Therefore, 14 RCTs were employed to assess the effectiveness of oral glucosamine, 12 studies were included in the analysis of oral chondroitin, and 4 trials were used to estimate the effectiveness in the subgroup of the combination of glucosamine and chondroitin. Characteristics of included studies were shown in Table 1. All of these included studies were published in English language. A total of 7172 participants were enrolled in this meta-analysis for the pain outcome. Most trials included patients with only knee OA, 1 trial [42] included patients with knee or the hip OA, and 1 trial [31] included patients with the only hip OA. The average age of the patients ranged between 42.65 and 67.09 years (median, 62.28 years), and the percentage of women ranged from 28 to 93% (median, 65%). The average duration of symptoms was reported in 14 trials [11, 21–25, 27–32, 41, 42] and ranged from 1.60 years to 12.98 years (median, 8.05 years).

Risk of bias

Risk of bias in those included studies was summarized in Additional file 1: Figure S2. All studies were judged as low risk of bias for blinding to patients. Randomization was mentioned in all trails. Nevertheless, 6% did not report details of adequate sequence generation. All studies were judged as low risk of bias for blinding for patients, while 65% for blinding to outcome assessment. In addition, 15% trails did not describe the method of allocation concealment and 92% reported complete outcome data. None of the studies was thought to have poor methodological quality.

Pain

All studies (7127 patients) contributed to the meta-analysis of pain-related outcomes for the putative DMOADs compared with placebo (Table 1). Fourteen trials (2845 randomized patients) compared glucosamine with placebo [21–34]. Twelve trials (3082 randomized patients) compared chondroitin with placebo [7, 29, 33, 35–43]. Four trials (1200 randomized patients) compared the two in combination with placebo [11, 29, 33, 44].

The meta-analysis identified an overall effect size of − 0.071 (95% CI, − 0.228 to 0.085). When the SMD was transformed, glucosamine showed no significant effect compared with placebo (effect size, − 0.263 cm [95% CI, − 0.635 to 0.113 cm]). However, chondroitin showed better effect compared with placebo (effect size, − 0.540 cm [95% CI, − 0.900 to − 0.178 cm]). Glucosamine plus chondroitin presented no significant effect when compared with placebo (effect size, 1.980 cm [95% CI, − 0.740 to 4.700 cm]) (Table 2). A funnel plot based on studies on the effect size was generated to detect the potential publication bias, and it manifested a significant asymmetry in Additional file 1: Figure S3.

Function

Twenty-five trials (6667 patients) contributed to the meta-analysis of physical function. Table 2 showed estimates across different treatments compared with placebo.

Table 1 Characteristics of the included studies for osteoarthritis of knee and/or hip

Study, year	Treatment (daily dose)	Participants randomized (n)	Treatment duration (weeks)	Symptom duration (year)	Mean age (year)	Female (%)	OA grade	Joint	Pain outcome extracted	Timepoint extracted (weeks)
Glucosamine vs placebo										
Noack 1994 [21]	G(1500 mg)/ placebo	126/126	1–4	2.00–10.00	55.00	60	I–III	Knee	Lequesne global scale	4
Houpt 1999 [22]	G(1500 mg)/ placebo	58/60	1–8	8.30	64.46	62	NA	Knee	WOMAC	12
Reginster 2001 [23]	G(1500 mg)/ placebo	106/106	1–144	7.80	65.75	76	II–III	Knee	WOMAC	144
Pavelka 2002 [24]	G(1500 mg)/ placebo	101/101	1–144	10.55	62.35	79	II–III	Knee	WOMAC	144
Braham 2003 [25]	G(1500 mg)/ placebo	24/22	1–12	12.98	42.65	28	I–III	Knee	KPS	12
McAlinton 2004 [26]	G(1500 mg)/ placebo	101/104	1–12	NA	> 65.00	64	NA	Knee	WOMAC	12
Cibere 2004 [27]	G(1500 mg)/ placebo	71/66	1–24	1.60	64.48	56	≥ 2	Knee	WOMAC	24
Usha 2004 [28]	G(1500 mg)/ placebo	30/28	1–12	3.05	51.03	NA	I–III	Knee	VAS	12
Clegg 2006 [29]	G(1500 mg)/ placebo	317/313	1–24	9.95	58.40	63	II–III	Knee	WOMAC	24
Herrero-Beaumont 2007 [30]	G(1500 mg)/ placebo	106/104	1–12	7.30	63.94	93	II–III	Knee	WOMAC	24
Rozendaal 2008 [31]	G(1500 mg)/ placebo	111/111	1–12	11.70	63.40	69	> 2	Hip	WOMAC	96
Giordano 2009 [32]	G(1500 mg)/ placebo	30/30	1–12	6.30	57.65	70	I–III	Knee	WOMAC	24
Fransen 2014 [33]	G(1500 mg)/ placebo	152/151	1–48	> 2.00	60.90	83	NA	Knee	WOMAC	96
Kwoh 2014 [34]	G(1501 mg)/ placebo	98/103	1–12	NA	52.23	49	0–4	Knee	WOMAC	24
Chondroitin vs Placebo										
Bucsi 1998 [35]	C(1200 mg)/ placebo	39/46	1–12	> 0.50	59.95	60	I–III	Knee	VAS	24
Bourgeois 1998 [36]	C(1200 mg)/ placebo	83/44	1–13	NA	63.35	76	I–III	Knee	VAS	13
Uebelhart 1998 [37]	C(1200 mg)/ placebo	23/23	1–48	NA	58.50	52	I–III	Knee	VAS	48
Mazieres 2001 [38]	C(1200 mg)/ placebo	63/67	1–12	NA	67.09	75	II–III	Knee	Pain at rest	12
Uebelhart 2004 [39]	C(1200 mg)/ placebo	54/56	1–12	NA	63.45	81	I–III	Knee	Husskisson visual analogue score for pain	12
Michel 2005 [40]	C(1200 mg)/ placebo	150/150	1–96	NA	62.80	51	I–III	Knee	WOMAC	96
Clegg 2006 [29]	C(1200 mg)/ placebo	318/313	1–24	9.60	58.20	64	II–III	Knee	WOMAC	24
Mazieres 2006 [41]	C(1200 mg)/ placebo	153/154	1–24	6.40	66.00	70	II–III	Knee	Pain at rest	24
Kahan 2009 [42]	C(1200 mg)/ placebo	309/313	1–12	6.30	62.30	68	I–III	Knee/ hip	WOMAC	12
Wildi 2011 [43]	C(800 mg)/ placebo	35/34	1–48	> 0.50	62.26	59	I–III	Knee	WOMAC	48

Table 1 Characteristics of the included studies for osteoarthritis of knee and/or hip *(Continued)*

Study, year	Treatment (daily dose)	Participants randomized (n)	Treatment duration (weeks)	Symptom duration (year)	Mean age (year)	Female (%)	OA grade	Joint	Pain outcome extracted	Timepoint extracted (weeks)
Zegels 2013 [7]	C(1200 mg)/ placebo	236/117	1–12	NA	65.17	65	NA	Knee	Global pain	12
Fransen 2014 [33]	C(800 mg)/ placebo	151/151	1–48	> 2.00	60.05	83	NA	Knee	WOMAC	96
Glucosamine + Chondroitin vs Placebo										
Clegg 2006 [29]	G + C(1500 + 1200 mg)/ placebo	317/313	1–24	9.80	58.40	63	II–III	Knee	WOMAC	24
Fransen 2014 [33]	G + C(1500 + 800 mg)/ placebo	151/151	1–48	> 2.00	60.65	85	NA	Knee	WOMAC	96
Lugo 2016 [44]	G + C(1500 + 1200 mg)/ placebo	65/58	1–12	NA	52.84	54	II–III	Knee	WOMAC	24
Roman-Blas 2017 [11]	G + C(1500 + 1200 mg)/ placebo	80/78	1–24	6.20	65.99	84	II–III	Knee	Global pain	24

G glucosamine, *C* chondroitin, *G + C* glucosamine + chondroitin, *NA* not available, *WOMAC* Western Ontario and McMaster Universities, *KPS* Knee Pain Scale, *VAS* Visual Analogue Scale

In general, the summary of DMOADs had a better effect compared with placebo. The overall effect size was −0.090 (95% CI, −0.242 to 0.061). After being transformed, the effect size for the subgroup of chondroitin versus placebo was −0.462 units (95% CI, −0.752 to −0.170 units). Meanwhile, other comparisons presented no significant effect.

Stiffness

Thirteen trials (4079 patients) contributed to the outcome of stiffness. The overall difference in stiffness improvement versus placebo was −0.142 (95% CI, −0.301 to 0.017) for the summary of these treatments, −0.305

(95% CI, −0.609 to 0.002) for glucosamine, 0.026 (95% CI, −0.073 to 0.126) for chondroitin and −0.070 (95% CI, −0.214 to 0.074) for the combination of glucosamine and chondroitin (Table 2). In terms of stiffness, only glucosamine showed statistical significance when compared with placebo.

Safety

Twenty studies reported the withdrawals of patients due to AEs. Eight studies reported the number of patients with AEs such as diarrhea, abdominal pain, nausea, headache, and others. Figure 1 showed the results of safety and tolerability including the number of withdrawals due to AEs.

Table 2 Effect sizes of symptomatic outcomes

Outcomes	Interventions	No. of studies	Test of association			Test of heterogeneity		
			SMD	95% CI	P value	Model	I^2 (%)	P value
Pain	G vs. PBO	14	−0.105	(−0.254, 0.045)	0.170	Random	72.50	0.000
	C vs. PBO	12	−0.216	(−0.360, −0.071)	0.003	Random	70.80	0.000
	G + C vs. PBO	4	0.792	(−0.296, 1.880)	0.153	Random	98.50	0.000
	Overall	30	−0.071	(−0.228, 0.085)	0.369	Random	90.10	0.000
Function	G vs. PBO	11	−0.126	(−0.264, 0.012)	0.073	Random	64.10	0.002
	C vs. PBO	10	−0.220	(−0.358, −0.081)	0.002	Random	68.30	0.001
	G + C vs. PBO	4	0.556	(−0.368, 1.480)	0.238	Random	98.00	0.000
	Overall	25	−0.090	(−0.242, 0.061)	0.242	Random	89.00	0.000
Stiffness	G vs. PBO	8	−0.305	(−0.609, −0.002)	0.048	Random	89.00	0.000
	C vs. PBO	3	0.026	(−0.073, 0.126)	0.604	Fixed	31.70	0.232
	G + C vs. PBO	2	−0.070	(−0.214, 0.074)	0.340	Fixed	0.00	0.582
	Overall	13	−0.142	(−0.301, 0.017)	0.081	Random	82.90	0.000

G glucosamine, *C* chondroitin, *G + C* glucosamine + chondroitin, *PBO* placebo

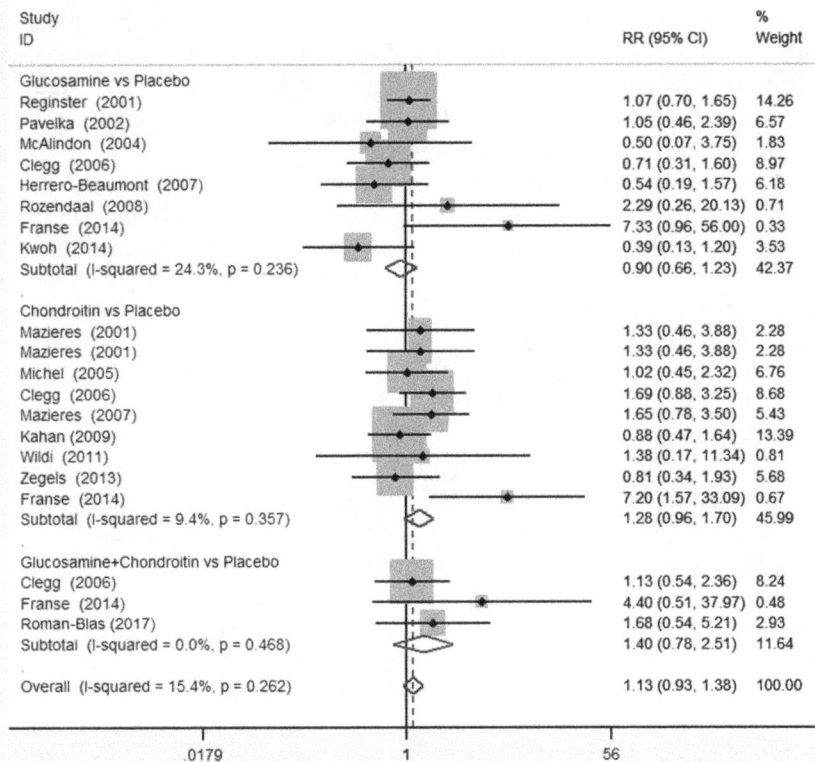

Fig. 1 Forest plot of RR and 95% CIs of studies of adverse events. RR relative risk, 95% CI confidence interval, G + C glucosamine + chondroitin

There was no significant difference in the comparison between any options versus placebo. In addition, six specific kinds of AEs were also analyzed by meta-analysis, and the results were presented in Table 3. The meta-analysis of those studies showed that there was no statistically significant difference between the group of SYSADOAs and placebo group.

Sensitivity analysis
We also conducted sensitivity analyses for those outcomes to confirm the robustness of the results. Sensitivity analysis of sample size and methodological quality of included studies did not show any major change in view of pain, function, and stiffness (Additional file 1: Table S1).

Discussion
In this study, we performed four individual outcome-oriented meta-analyses of randomized control trials selected on the basis of their high methodologic quality, assessing the effectiveness and safety of glucosamine, chondroitin, and the combination for the treatment of knee and/or hip OA. In our meta-analysis, the pooled effect sizes suggested that these SYSADOAs showed no significant effect on the outcome of pain, function, and stiffness compared with placebo. However, the estimates between chondroitin and placebo showed that chondroitin could alleviate pain symptoms and improve function. Compared with placebo, glucosamine proved significant effect only on the sapect of stiffness improvement. Whereas, in this

Table 3 Risk ratio (95% CI) of specific adverse effects between different treatment groups

Comparison	GI AE	CV AE	CNS AE	MU AE	Infection	Skin AE	Others
G vs PBO	0.99(0.79, 1.23)	NA	0.72(0.46, 1.10)	1.52(0.88, 2.63)	1.07(0.50, 2.32)	0.80(0.38, 1.68)	1.21(0.98, 1.48)
C vs PBO	0.35(0.14, 0.87)	1.13(0.45, 2.84)	0.79(0.37, 1.67)	NA	0.98(0.72, 1.34)	1.00(0.41, 2.45)	NA
G + C vs PBO	2.79(0.30, 26.00)	NA	1.86(0.36, 9.74)	2.79(0.30, 26.00)	2.79(0.12, 67.10)	NA	4.66(0.23, 94.79)
Overall	0.92(0.74, 1.13)	1.13(0.45, 2.84)	0.77(0.54, 1.11)	1.58(0.93, 2.70)	1.01(0.76, 1.35)	0.88(0.50, 1.55)	1.22(1.00, 1.50)

G glucosamine, C chondroitin, G + C glucosamine + chondroitin, PBO placebo, NA not available, GI gastrointestinal, CV cardiovascular, CNS central nervous system, MU musculoskeletal

head-to-head meta-analysis, the combination of glucosamine and chondroitin did not have enough evidence to be superior to placebo. There was no significant difference in the incidence of AEs and discontinuations of AEs for these SYSADOAs when compared with placebo.

Glucosamine and chondroitin are dietary supplements commonly used by those OA patents and are recommended by physician for purported analgesic and chondroprotective effects [45]. Glucosamine was considered as a water-soluble amino monosaccharide, which was one of the most abundant monosaccharides in the human body and is in high quantities in articular cartilage. Chondroitin was a major component of the extracellular matrix of articular cartilage, which played an important role in creating considerable osmotic pressure. In this way, it could provide cartilage with resistance and elasticity to resist tensile stresses during loading condition [46]. Chondroitin and glucosamine were tested in several clinical trials of osteoarthritis. In spite of the controversy surrounding the SYSADOAs, they were commonly used to control symptoms of OA in western countries. Therefore, an understanding of chondroitin and glucosamine consumption is of significance for public health.

In the previous meta-analysis, Richy and colleagues combined 7 trials of glucosamine and 8 trials of chondroitin for osteoarthritis treatment demonstrated comparable efficacies of chondroitin and glucosamine and a highly significant effectiveness of glucosamine on all involved outcomes when compared with placebo, which was contrary with our results of glucosamine and the combination therapy [47]. Collectively, their study showed that chondroitin was considered effective on pain relief, which was consistent with our finding. Additionally, a pair-wise meta-analysis of chondroitin by Monfort and colleagues suggested that chondroitin present a slight to moderate efficacy in the symptomatic treatment of OA, with an excellent safety profile [48]. The subgroup of our study covering 12 RCTs of chondroitin present that chondroitin showed significant effect in both outcome of pain and function improvement. In our study, only 4 RCTs met the criteria of combination therapy and were included in the subgroup of this meta-analysis. And glucosamine and chondroitin combination therapy failed to reduce joint pain and function improvement; this may due to original data restraints. However, this finding was similar to a least RCT publish in 2017. Roman-Blas and his colleagues indicated that chondroitin and glucosamine combination therapy failed to reduce joint pain [11]. But in the subgroup of patients with moderate-to-severe knee pain of their RCT, significant relief of joint pain with this combination therapy was observed.

Considering the reasons above, we do not oppose the use of chondroitin, although chondroitin were not recommended according to Osteoarthritis Research Society International (OARSI) guidelines published in 2014. In fact, we recommend that the future guidelines would reconsider the oral treatment option of chondroitin for the treatment of OA in the clinical feature. In terms of the aspect of safety, the current study provides valuable information to help physicians make treatment decisions for OA patients.

It was worth mentioning that a comprehensive and rigorous literature search strategy was performed in our meta-analysis, which insured that it was unlikely to miss other relevant trials. All the methods were strict inclusion and exclusion criteria to demonstrate the effectiveness and significance of our conclusions. In our meta-analysis, dosage was strictly restricted and the RCTs included should met these criteria, so the results could be comparable and reasonable. To minimize bias, studies selection, quality assessment, and data extraction were completed by two reviewers independently. What is more, several sensitivity analyses of low quality were conducted to make the results more sensible and comprehensive.

There are several limitations in this meta-analysis that need to be considered. Firstly, the quality of original data resulted in some limitation of the quality of our analysis. Secondly, in this study, there is potential publication bias. Some unpublished papers and abstracts were not taken into consideration because of unavailable data. The language might also introduce a bias. Actually, we selected only the English language. Thirdly, several specific adverse effects of interventions cannot be proven due to the inadequate reporting of adverse event data. Moreover, the numbers of RCTs between combination therapy of glucosamine and chondroitin were limited. Researches on SYSADOAs are still required due to the limitations on the quality and quantity of the available evidence.

Conclusion

In conclusion, in accordance with our results, it can be definitively stated that oral chondroitin in recommended dosage is more effective than placebo on relieving pain and improving physical function. Compared with placebo, glucosamine showed significant effect on the outcome of stiffness. In the aspect of safety, both compounds are well tolerated. Actually, combination therapy is definitely common in clinical practice, and treatment intervention on OA patients like the combination of SYSADOAs was also usual in clinical experience. Our study would help highlight the potential role of SYSADOAs. Further studies of the glucosamine and chondroitin combination therapy need to explore the effectiveness for an accurate characterization of osteoarthritis treatment and their possible mechanism. Therefore, the above information, along with the safety profile should be conducive to clinicians in decision making.

Abbreviations

AEs: Adverse effects; DMOADs: Disease-modifying OA drugs; NSAIDs: Non-steroidal anti-inflammatory drugs; OA: Osteoarthritis; OARSI: Osteoarthritis Research Society International; RR: Relative risk; SYSADOAs: Symptomatic slow-acting drugs

Funding

This study was supported by the Research Innovation Program for College Graduates of Jiangsu Province (YKC16019) and Jiangsu Students' Platform for Innovation and Entrepreneurship Training Program (201710304058).

Authors' contributions

All authors certified that they have participated in the conceptual design of this work, the analysis of the data, and the writing of the manuscript to take public responsibility for it. XZ drafted the protocol and wrote the final paper. LJ contributed to the research design and made critical revisions. LS and DW participated in data collection. JR participated in the data analysis. All authors reviewed the final version of the manuscript and approve it for publication.

Competing interests

The authors declare that they have no competing interests.

Author details

[1]Baoshan Center for Disease Control and Prevention, Shanghai, People's Republic of China. [2]Department of Epidemiology, School of Public Health, Nantong University, Nantong, Jiangsu Province, People's Republic of China. [3]Department of Orthopedics Surgery, The Second Affiliated Hospital of Harbin Medical University, Harbin, Heilongjiang Province, People's Republic of China. [4]Shanghai Key Laboratory for Molecular Imaging, Shanghai University of Medicine & Health Sciences, Shanghai, People's Republic of China.

References

1. Glyn-Jones S, Palmer AJ, Agricola R, et al. Osteoarthritis. Lancet. 2015; 386(9991):376–87.
2. Lotz M, Martel-Pelletier J, Christiansen C, et al. Value of biomarkers in osteoarthritis: current status and perspectives. Ann Rheum Dis. 2013;72(11): 1756–63.
3. Felson DT, Zhang Y. An update on the epidemiology of knee and hip osteoarthritis with a view to prevention. Arthritis Rheum. 1998;41(8):1343–55.
4. arc OC, arc OC, Zeggini E, et al. Identification of new susceptibility loci for osteoarthritis (arcOGEN): a genome-wide association study. Lancet. 2012; 380(9844):815–23.
5. Nuesch E, Dieppe P, Reichenbach S, Williams S, Iff S, Juni P. All cause and disease specific mortality in patients with knee or hip osteoarthritis: population based cohort study. Bmj. 2011;342:d1165.
6. Essex MN, O'Connell MA, Behar R, Bao W. Efficacy and safety of nonsteroidal anti-inflammatory drugs in Asian patients with knee osteoarthritis: summary of a randomized, placebo-controlled study. Int J Rheum Dis. 2016;19(3):262–70.
7. Zegels B, Crozes P, Uebelhart D, Bruyere O, Reginster JY. Equivalence of a single dose (1200 mg) compared to a three-time a day dose (400 mg) of chondroitin 4&6 sulfate in patients with knee osteoarthritis. Results of a randomized double blind placebo controlled study. Osteoarthr Cartil. 2013;21(1):22–7.
8. Persiani S, Rotini R, Trisolino G, et al. Synovial and plasma glucosamine concentrations in osteoarthritic patients following oral crystalline glucosamine sulphate at therapeutic dose. Osteoarthr Cartil. 2007;15(7):764–72.
9. Conte A, Volpi N, Palmieri L, Bahous I, Ronca G. Biochemical and pharmacokinetic aspects of oral treatment with chondroitin sulfate. Arzneimittelforschung. 1995;45(8):918–25.
10. Verbruggen G, Goemaere S, Veys EM. Chondroitin sulfate: S/DMOAD (structure/disease modifying anti-osteoarthritis drug) in the treatment of finger joint OA. Osteoarthr Cartil. 1998;6 Suppl A:37–8.
11. Roman-Blas JA, Castañeda S, Sánchez-Pernaute O, Largo R, Herrero-Beaumont G. Combined treatment with chondroitin sulfate and glucosamine sulfate shows no superiority over placebo for reduction of joint pain and functional impairment in patients with knee osteoarthritis: a six-month multicenter, randomized, double-blind, Placebo-Controlled Clinical Trial. Arthritis Rheumatol. 2017;69(1):77–85.
12. McAlindon TE, Bannuru RR, Sullivan MC, et al. OARSI guidelines for the non-surgical management of knee osteoarthritis. Osteoarthr Cartil. 2014;22(3):363–88.
13. Panic N, Leoncini E, Belvis G D, et al. Evaluation of the endorsement of the Preferred Reporting Items for Systematic reviews and Meta-Analysis (PRISMA) statement on the quality of published systematic review and meta-analyses[J]. Plos One. 2013;8(12):e83138.
14. European Medicines Agency. EMEA public statement on the suspension of the marketing authorisation for Bextra (valdecoxib) in the European Union [online]. (2005) Available at: http://www.ema.europa.eu/docs/en_GB/ document_library/Public_statement/2009/12/WC500018391.pdf.
15. Green JPTHaS. Corchrane Reviewers' Handbook 5.1.0. Review Manage 2011.
16. Juni P, Reichenbach S, Dieppe P. Osteoarthritis: rational approach to treating the individual. Best Pract Res Clin Rheumatol. 2006;20(4):721–40.
17. Juhl C, Lund H, Roos EM, Zhang W, Christensen R. A hierarchy of patient-reported outcomes for meta-analysis of knee osteoarthritis trials: empirical evidence from a survey of high impact journals. Arthritis. 2012;2012:136245.
18. Cooper HM, Hedges LV. The handbook of research synthesis. New York: Russell Sage Foundation; 1994.
19. Cooper HM, Hedges LV, Valentine JC. The handbook of research synthesis and meta-analysis. 2nd ed. New York: Russell Sage Foundation; 2009.
20. Bannuru RR, Schmid CH, Kent DM, Vaysbrot EE, Wong JB, McAlindon TE. Comparative effectiveness of pharmacologic interventions for knee osteoarthritis: a systematic review and network meta-analysis. Ann Intern Med. 2015;162(1):46–54.
21. Noack W, Fischer M, Forster KK, Rovati LC, Setnikar I. Glucosamine sulfate in osteoarthritis of the knee. Osteoarthr Cartil. 1994;2(1):51–9.
22. Houpt JB, McMillan R, Wein C, Paget-Dellio SD. Effect of glucosamine hydrochloride in the treatment of pain of osteoarthritis of the knee. J Rheumatol. 1999;26(11):2423–30.
23. Reginster JY, Deroisy R, Rovati LC, et al. Long-term effects of glucosamine sulphate on osteoarthritis progression: a randomised, placebo-controlled clinical trial. Lancet. 2001;357(9252):251–6.
24. Pavelká K, Gatterová J, Olejarová M, Machacek S, Giacovelli G, Rovati LC. Glucosamine sulfate use and delay of progression of knee osteoarthritis: a 3-year, randomized, placebo-controlled, double-blind study. Arch Intern Med. 2002;162(18):2113–23.
25. Braham R, Dawson B, Goodman C. The effect of glucosamine supplementation on people experiencing regular knee pain. Br J Sports Med. 2003;37(1):45.
26. McAlindon T, Formica M, LaValley M, Lehmer M, Kabbara K. Effectiveness of glucosamine for symptoms of knee osteoarthritis: results from an internet-based randomized double-blind controlled trial. Am J Med. 2004;117(9):643–9.
27. Cibere J, Kopec JA, Thorne A, et al. Randomized, double-blind, placebo-controlled glucosamine discontinuation trial in knee osteoarthritis. Arthritis Rheum. 2004;51(5):738–45.
28. Usha PR, Naidu MU. Randomised, double-blind, parallel, placebo-controlled study of oral glucosamine, methylsulfonylmethane and their combination in osteoarthritis. Clin Drug Investig. 2004;24(6):353–63.
29. Clegg DO, Reda DJ, Harris CL, et al. Glucosamine, chondroitin sulfate, and the two in combination for painful knee osteoarthritis. N Engl J Med. 2006; 354(8):795–808.
30. Herrero-Beaumont G, Ivorra JA, Del Carmen Trabado M, et al. Glucosamine sulfate in the treatment of knee osteoarthritis symptoms: a randomized, double-blind, placebo-controlled study using acetaminophen as a side comparator. Arthritis Rheum. 2007;56(2):555–67.
31. Rozendaal RM, Koes BW, van Osch GJ, et al. Effect of glucosamine sulfate on hip osteoarthritis: a randomized trial. Ann Intern Med. 2008;148(4):268–77.
32. Giordano N, Fioravanti A, Papakostas P, Montella A, Giorgi G, Nuti R. The efficacy and tolerability of glucosamine sulfate in the treatment of knee osteoarthritis: a randomized, double-blind, placebo-controlled trial. Curr Ther Res. 2009;70(3):185–96.

33. Fransen M, Agaliotis M, Nairn L, et al. Glucosamine and chondroitin for knee osteoarthritis: a double-blind randomised placebo-controlled clinical trial evaluating single and combination regimens. Ann Rheum Dis. 2015;74(5):851–8.

34. Kwoh CK, Roemer FW, Hannon MJ, et al. Effect of oral glucosamine on joint structure in individuals with chronic knee pain: a randomized, placebo-controlled clinical trial. Arthritis Rheum. 2014;66(4):930–9.

35. Bucsi L, Poór G. Efficacy and tolerability of oral chondroitin sulfate as a symptomatic slow-acting drug for osteoarthritis (SYSADOA) in the treatment of knee osteoarthritis. Osteoarthr Cartil. 1998;6 Suppl A(5):31–6.

36. Bourgeois P, Chales G, Dehais J, Delcambre B, Kuntz JL, Rozenberg S. Efficacy and tolerability of chondroitin sulfate 1200 mg/day vs chondroitin sulfate 3 x 400 mg/day vs placebo. Osteoarthr Cartil. 1998;6(Suppl A):25–30.

37. Uebelhart D, Thonar EJ, Delmas PD, Chantraine A, Vignon E. Effects of oral chondroitin sulfate on the progression of knee osteoarthritis: a pilot study. Osteoarthr Cartil. 1998;6 Suppl A(21):39–46.

38. Mazieres B, Combe B, Van AP, Tondut J, Grynfeltt M. Chondroitin sulfate in osteoarthritis of the knee: a prospective, double blind, placebo controlled multicenter clinical study. J Rheumatol. 2001;28(1):173–81.

39. Uebelhart D, Malaise M, Marcolongo R, et al. Intermittent treatment of knee osteoarthritis with oral chondroitin sulfate: a one-year, randomized, double-blind, multicenter study versus placebo. Osteoarthr Cartil. 2004;12(4):269–76.

40. Michel BA, Stucki G, Frey D, et al. Chondroitins 4 and 6 sulfate in osteoarthritis of the knee: a randomized, controlled trial. Arthritis Rheum. 2005;52(3):779–86.

41. Mazieres B, Hucher M, Zaim M, Garnero P. Effect of chondroitin sulphate in symptomatic knee osteoarthritis: a multicentre, randomised, double-blind, placebo-controlled study. Ann Rheum Dis. 2007;66(5):639–45.

42. Kahan A, Uebelhart D, De VF, Delmas PD, Reginster JY. Long-term effects of chondroitins 4 and 6 sulfate on knee osteoarthritis: the study on osteoarthritis progression prevention, a two-year, randomized, double-blind, placebo-controlled trial. Arthritis Rheum. 2009;60(2):524–33.

43. Wildi LM, Raynauld JP, Martelpelletier J, et al. Chondroitin sulphate reduces both cartilage volume loss and bone marrow lesions in knee osteoarthritis patients starting as early as 6 months after initiation of therapy: a randomised, double-blind, placebo-controlled pilot study using MRI. Ann Rheum Dis. 2011;70(6):982–9.

44. Lugo JP, Saiyed ZM, Lane NE. Efficacy and tolerability of an undenatured type II collagen supplement in modulating knee osteoarthritis symptoms: a multicenter randomized, double-blind, placebo-controlled study. Nutr J. 2016;15:14.

45. DiNubile NA. Glucosamine and chondroitin sulfate in the management of osteoarthritis. Commentary Postgrad Med 2009;121(4):48–50.

46. Jomphe C, Gabriac M, Hale TM, et al. Chondroitin sulfate inhibits the nuclear translocation of nuclear factor-kappaB in interleukin-1beta-stimulated chondrocytes. Basic Clin Pharmacol Toxicol. 2008;102(1):59–65.

47. Richy F, Bruyere O, Ethgen O, Cucherat M, Henrotin Y, Reginster JY. Structural and symptomatic efficacy of glucosamine and chondroitin in knee osteoarthritis: a comprehensive meta-analysis. Arch Intern Med. 2003; 163(13):1514–22.

48. Monfort J, Martel-Pelletier J, Pelletier J-P. Chondroitin sulphate for symptomatic osteoarthritis: critical appraisal of meta-analyses. Curr Med Res Opin. 2008;24(5):1303–8.

4

Cross-cultural adaptation and validation of the VISA-A questionnaire for Chilean Spanish-speaking patients

Andres Keller[1], Pablo Wagner[1,2], Guillermo Izquierdo[1], Jorge Cabrolier[1], Nathaly Caicedo[1], Emilio Wagner[1*] and Nicola Maffulli[3]

Abstract

Background: The purpose of this study is to translate, culturally adapt, and validate the VISA-A questionnaire for Chilean Spanish speakers with Achilles tendinopathy (AT), which has been originally developed for English-speaking population.

Methods: According to the guidelines published by Beaton et al., the questionnaire was translated and culturally adapted to Chilean patients in six steps: initial translation, synthesis of the translation, back translation, expert committee review, test of the pre-final version (cohort $n = 35$), and development of VISA-A-CH. The resulting Chilean version was tested for validity on 60 patients: 20 healthy individuals (group 1), 20 patients with a recently diagnosed AT (group 2), and 20 with a severe AT that already initiated conservative treatment with no clinical improvement (group 3). The questionnaire was completed three times by each participant: at the time of study enrollment, after an hour, and after a week of the initial test.

Results: All six steps were successfully completed for the translation and cultural adaptation of the VISA-A-CH. VISA-A-CH final mean scores in the healthy group was significantly higher than those in the other groups. Group 3 had the lowest scores. Validity showed excellent test-retest reliability (rho $c = 0.999$; Pearson's $r = 1.000$) within an hour and within a week (rho $c = 0.837$; Pearson's $r = 0.840$).

Conclusions: VISA-A was translated and validated to Chilean Spanish speakers successfully, being comparable to the original version. We believe that VISA-A-CH can be recommended as an important tool for clinical and research settings in Chilean and probably Latin-American Spanish speakers.

Keywords: VISA-A, Achilles tendinopathy, Score validation, Spanish validation

Background

Achilles tendinopathy (AT) is the most common cause of posterior heel pain [1–3] in athletes and non-athletes [4]. The activities most related to this pathology are those involving jumping and running [4, 5]. The incidence of AT has been increasing in the last decades, with a prevalence of 10% in runners [4, 6]. In terms of its clinical presentation, pain in the middle portion of the Achilles tendon during and after physical activity, increased volume in the involved region of the tendon, and morning stiffness are frequent. The above symptoms usually decrease when the patient reduces the load or the level of activity but tend to recur when the activity is resumed [7, 8]. For these reasons, AT is a frequent cause of limitation in the physical activity of patients, with the consequent negative impact on their general health.

Despite the high incidence and its multi-factorial etiology [9], the decision to undertake conservative or operative treatment in patients with AT is still under debate [10], though surgical treatment is generally recommended only following failure of conservative measures [11, 12]. Regardless of the management path chosen, the aim of treatment is to return the patient to clinical and functional wellbeing. The achievement of these objectives can be difficult to compare

* Correspondence: ewagner@alemana.cl; emiliowagner@gmail.com
[1]Department of Orthopedics, Universidad del desarrollo - Clinica Alemana de Santiago, Vitacura 5951, 7650568 Santiago, Chile
Full list of author information is available at the end of the article

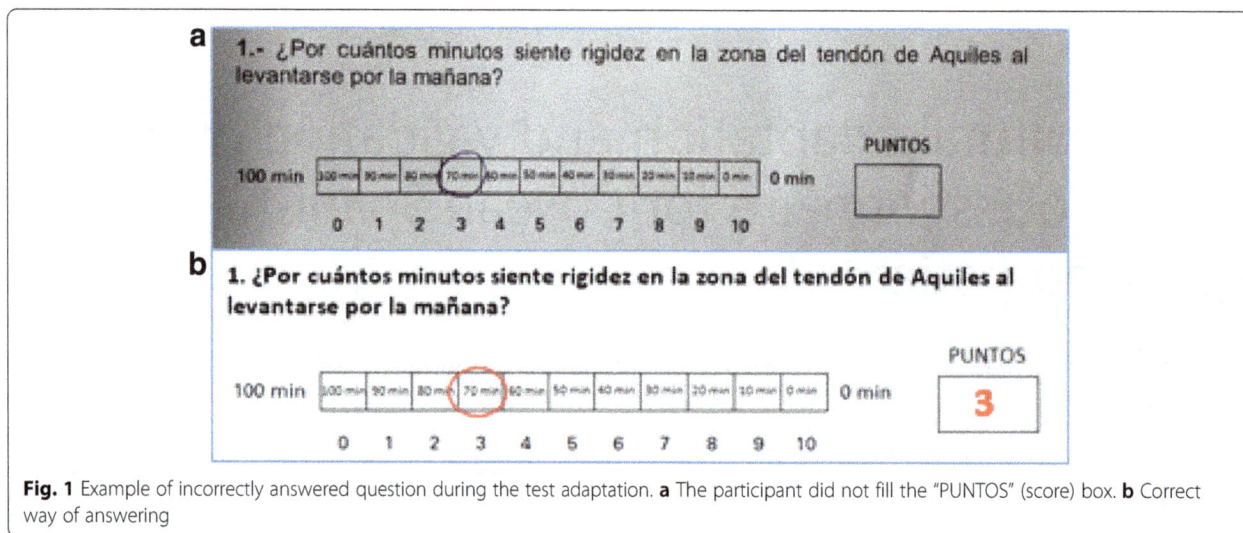

Fig. 1 Example of incorrectly answered question during the test adaptation. **a** The participant did not fill the "PUNTOS" (score) box. **b** Correct way of answering

objectively between different studies, mainly because of the ways in which they are measured, and possible difference in severity and clinical presentation of the condition.

A simple, self-administered questionnaire was developed by the Victorian Institute of Sports Assessment to be completed by patients with AT, called VISA-A (Victorian Institute of Sport Assessment-Achilles Questionnaire), which assesses several aspects such as: pain (questions 1–3), function (questions 4–6), and activity (questions 7 and 8). For this reason, it can be used to determine the clinical severity of the condition and provide a guide for treatment, as well as to monitor the effects of treatment, constituting a validated, reliable, and accurate tool to specifically evaluate patients with AT [13]. Moreover, it is useful to compare results between different studies [14–17]. The questionnaire was developed for English-speaking populations: this is the reason why it is necessary to translate, culturally adapt, and validate [18] the VISA-A in other languages. This has already been the case for the Swedish- [14], Italian- [16], and German-speaking populations [19].

The purpose of this study was to translate, culturally adapt, and validate the VISA-A questionnaire for the Spanish-speaking Chilean population with AT.

Methods

According to the guidelines published by Beaton et al. [18], the questionnaire was translated and culturally adapted to Spanish-speaking Chilean patients in six steps.

Step 1. Initial translation: two bilingual translators whose mother tongue was Spanish developed two independent translations. One of the translators had medical knowledge of the concepts and terms (an orthopedic surgeon with specialization in foot and ankle); the other translator had no medical knowledge or relation with health care system (native translator).

Step 2. Synthesis of translation: both translators agreed on their translations and developed a common translation (preliminary translation V1.0).

Step 3. Retrograde translation: with the preliminary version V1.0 in hand and blind to the original version (VISA-A), two non-medically expert translators whose mother tongue was English translated the questionnaire back into English.

Step 4. Expert committee: a committee was organized with the participation of the original translators, other expert translators, orthopedic surgeons with experience in foot and ankle surgery, and other health care professionals, to review all translations and to develop the pre-final version of the questionnaire (V2.0).

Step 5. Test of the V2.0 questionnaire: this stage ensured that the adapted version was equivalent to the original version. The questionnaire was completed by a cohort of 35 people. Later, they were interviewed to discuss errors, what they understood of each question, and the difficulty to answer them.

Table 1 VISA-A-CH scores of patients with AT (group 2) at different time points

Answer time (hours)	N	Min	p50	Max	Mean
0	20	28	71	100	67.16
1	20	29	70.5	100	67.33
168	20	28	69.5	100	65.27

Table 2 VISA-A-CH scores of patients with AT and failure to conservative treatment (group 3)

Answer time (hours)	N	Min	p50	Max	Mean
0	20	14	22.5	40	24.7
1	20	14	22.5	40	24.7
168	20	14	23.5	35	26

Step 6. Development of the final version (VISA-A-CH): after analyzing the opinions, doubts, and suggestions of the interviewees, corrections were made to V2.0 in each one of its items, with the final version being developed V3.0 (VISA-A-CH) (Additional file 1).

After the translation and cultural adaptation, the VISA-A-CH questionnaire was subjected to validation.

After approval by the local ethics committee, the VISA-A-CH was prospectively delivered to 60 patients divided into three groups: group 1, 20 healthy patients with no AT symptoms and signs (control group); group 2, 20 patients with a recently diagnosed AT; and group 3, 20 patients with severe AT who already initiated conservative management with no clinical improvement. These patients were all older than 18, and all had been selected and evaluated by a trained foot and ankle orthopedic surgeon in a single center in Santiago, Chile. Informed consent was obtained from all individual participants included in the study.

The questionnaire was completed anonymously three times by each participant: at the time of study enrollment (time 0), after 1 h (time + 1), and after 1 week of the initial test (time + 7).

Descriptive statistics were calculated, using percentile, mean, and standard deviation. The questionnaires (three each participant, 180 in total) were evaluated using mixed models to control intra- and inter-patient variability. We used significance level of 95%, and the data were processed with software STATA version 14.0.

Results

To develop the translation and cultural adaptation of the questionnaire (step 5 from the "Methods" section), initially, a cohort of 23 men and 12 women with age of 18 to 50 years were interviewed to check for score structure and reading comprehension. Half of them were fourth year medical students from a Chilean University. The other half were firefighters from the regional fire station. Each participant was given a copy of VISA-A-CH V2.0 to read and respond as directed. At the end of the survey, feedback on the questionnaire was requested.

Twenty-seven participants (77%) did not answer the questionnaire in a structural correct form (i.e., ticking the relevant box) as shown in Fig. 1.

Regarding the comprehension of the questions, all the participants reported having no problem understanding what was being asked.

On the other hand, 16 participants (45%) reported that in some of the questions there was no precise alternative for someone healthy and asymptomatic (for example, the maximum score for question no. 7 was: "Yes, I do sport or physical activity to the same or even to a higher level since the discomfort began"). Healthy participants have never experienced any discomfort. However, as expected, they responded correctly with the maximum score for those questions.

For the validation stage of VISA-A-CH, three groups were selected to complete the questionnaire as explained

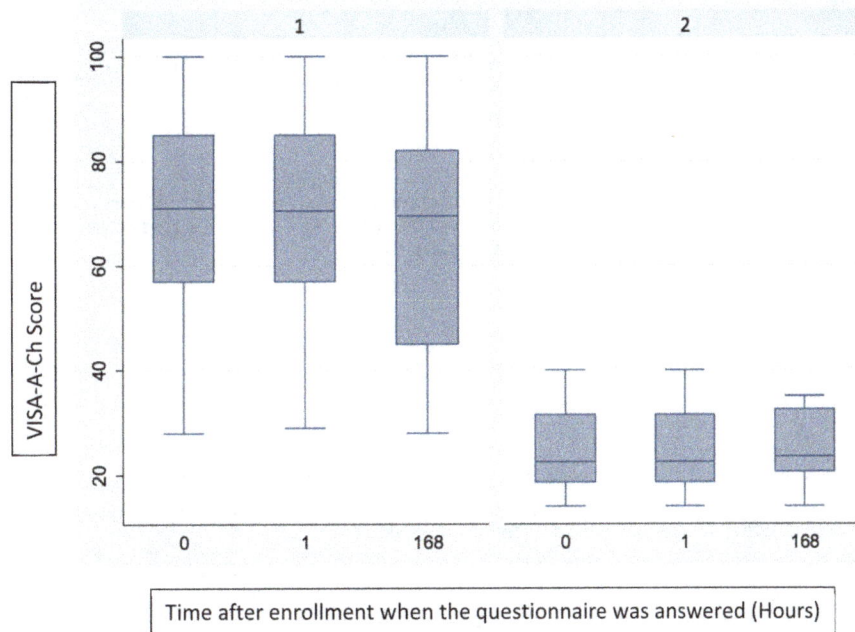

Fig. 2 Figure showing scores (*y* axis) in groups 2 and 3 throughout time (*x* axis, in hours). 0, 1, and 168 h (7 days). Column 1, group 2; column 2, group 3

in the "Methods" section: group 1: 20 healthy subjects, 10 men and 10 women, with a mean age of 38 years (range 20–55); group 2: 20 patients with a recently diagnosed AT, 13 men and 7 women, with a mean age of 41 years (25–49); and group 3: 20 patients with a severe AT that already initiated conservative treatment with no clinical improvement, 14 men and 6 women, with a mean age of 43 years (29–51).

The control group obtained 100 points in all measurements at all time points (at the time of enrollment, after 1 h, and after a week). Group 3 had the lowest scores of all the groups at all time points (time 0, + 1, + 7). Tables 1 and 2 show the scores of groups 2 and 3 (Tables 1 and 2). When comparing questionnaire results in groups 2 and 3, the p value of 0.335 indicates that there was no significant change in re-test scores at an hour (rho $c = 0.999$; Pearson's $r = 1000$) or at a week from diagnosis (rho $c = 0.837$; Pearson's $r = 0.840$). Figure 2 depicts the scores obtained by the patients in groups 2 and 3 at different time points, showing no change. The final version of the VISA-A-CH questionnaire is shown in Figs. 3, 4, and 5.

Discussion

With the multinational advance of research, it is necessary when comparing studies to have equivalent scoring systems, questionnaires, and results [20, 21]. In the case of self-administered questionnaires, comparing results between studies with different language and culture populations may lead to systematic errors if these assessment tools are not equivalent to the original [22]. Since most questionnaires are developed in English, they have to be validated in other languages. This is not just a translation issue: when the questionnaire is used in another country or with immigrants, it must necessarily be culturally adapted. Beaton et al. developed a clinical guideline for cultural translation and adaptation of self-report scores [18]. It has progressive stages of translation, synthesis,

Visa-A-Ch: Cuestionario de puntaje para tendón de Aquiles del Instituto de Victoria.

En este cuestionario, el término dolor se refiere específicamente al dolor de la región del tendón de Aquiles.

Conteste en los casilleros de respuesta y luego coloque el puntaje de cada pregunta en la casilla PUNTOS.

1.- ¿Por cuántos minutos siente rigidez en la zona del tendón de Aquiles al levantarse por la mañana?

PUNTOS

100 min | 100 min | 90 min | 80 min | 70 min | 60 min | 50 min | 40 min | 30 min | 20 min | 10 min | 0 min | 0 min

0 1 2 3 4 5 6 7 8 9 10

2.- ¿Una vez que ha entrado en calor durante el dia, siente dolor al estirar completamente el tendón de Aquiles cuando apoya la punta de los pies en el borde de un escalón? (manteniendo la rodilla estirada)

PUNTOS

dolor severo [ ] sin dolor

0 1 2 3 4 5 6 7 8 9 10

3.- ¿Después de caminar en terreno plano por 30 minutos, presenta dolor durante las siguientes dos horas? (si no es capaz de caminar en terreno plano por 30 minutos debido al dolor, conteste 0 en esta pregunta).

PUNTOS

dolor severo [ ] sin dolor

0 1 2 3 4 5 6 7 8 9 10

Fig. 3 Image of the final version of the VISA-A-CH questionnaire

4.- ¿Siente dolor al bajar escaleras a paso normal?

PUNTOS

dolor severo [ ] [ ] [ ] [ ] [ ] [ ] [ ] [ ] [ ] [ ] [ ] sin dolor

0 1 2 3 4 5 6 7 8 9 10

5.- ¿Siente dolor al colocarse en punta de pies en una superficie plana 10 veces seguidas, o inmediatamente después?

PUNTOS

dolor severo [ ] [ ] [ ] [ ] [ ] [ ] [ ] [ ] [ ] [ ] [ ] sin dolor

0 1 2 3 4 5 6 7 8 9 10

6.- ¿Cuántos saltos en un solo pie puede realizar sin dolor?

PUNTOS

0 saltos [ ] [ ] [ ] [ ] [ ] [ ] [ ] [ ] [ ] [ ] [ ] 10 saltos

0 1 2 3 4 5 6 7 8 9 10

7.- ¿Se encuentra actualmente practicando algún deporte o algún tipo de actividad física? Si no tiene molestias en la zona del tendón de Aquiles marque 10 puntos.

0 [ ] No, ninguno.

4 [ ] Si, pero el deporte o actividad física ha sufrido modificaciones o adaptaciones debido al dolor.

7 [ ] Si, realizo deporte o actividad física sin restricciones, pero no en el mismo nivel desde que comenzaron las molestias.

10 [ ] Si, realizo deporte o actividad física al mismo o incluso a un nivel superior desde que comenzaron las molestias.

PUNTOS

Fig. 4 Image of the final version of the VISA-A-CH questionnaire

reverse translation, expert committee, test of the questionnaire, and development of the final version.

The VISA-A, originally developed in English, is a reliable and reproducible questionnaire to compare results among patients with different degrees of AT severity. We have to remember it is not a diagnostic tool, but a valid way to measure the condition of the Achilles tendon. Its continuous numerical score has the potential to be used in clinical and research settings, but it was not designed to be a diagnostic tool [13]. Although the translation of the VISA-A was not difficult, cultural adaptation in relation to how to complete the questionnaire was the first inconvenience we encountered. Although the score of these evaluations was not affected, it showed how unclear it was in its filling instructions (77% of respondents did not respond in the boxes requested). For this reason, the VISA-A-CH developers added an instruction phrase on how to fill it: "Answer in the answer boxes and then fill the box labeled PUNTOS (translation for score) with the score for each question." When analyzing test-retest reliability, no significant changes were found between the scores obtained in all patient groups. They all had scores not statistically different at time 0, + 1 and + 7. A week after diagnosis, groups 2 and 3 patients, despite the medical indications and the schedule of eccentric exercises given to the patients, showed no change in score, perhaps highlighting that, despite the correct exercises having been prescribed and implemented, in the short term, the symptoms of AT do not change.

We point out that the use of the VISA-A-CH is likely to transcend the country where it was developed, namely Chile, and be used in all the Spanish-speaking countries in Latin America. We are aware of the linguistic differences which have developed during centuries between the Spanish language spoken in Spain and that of Latin America. In this respect, we suspect that a separate cross-cultural adaptation will be needed for Spain.

8.- Por favor, responda sólo una pregunta ya sea 8A, 8B o 8C, según corresponda:

Si usted **no tiene dolor** al realizar deportes que exigen al tendón de Aquiles, por favor responda sólo la pregunta **8A**.

Si usted **tiene dolor** al realizar deportes que exigen al tendón de Aquiles, pero éste **no le impide terminar esas actividades**, por favor responda sólo la pregunta **8B**.

Si usted **tiene dolor** al realizar deportes que exigen al tendón de Aquiles, y éste **le impide terminar esas actividades**, por favor responda sólo la pregunta **8C**.

8A. Si usted no tiene dolor al realizar deportes que exigen al tendón de Aquiles, ¿Por cuánto tiempo puede entrenar o practicar?

0 min	1–10 min	11–20 min	21–30 min	>30 min	PUNTOS
0	7	14	21	30	

O

8B. Si usted tiene algo de dolor al realizar deportes que exigen al tendón de Aquiles, pero éste no le impide terminar esas actividades, ¿Por cuánto tiempo puede entrenar o practicar?

0 min	1–10 min	11–20 min	21–30 min	>30 min	PUNTOS
0	4	10	14	20	

O

8C. ¿Si usted tiene dolor al realizar deportes que exigen al tendón de Aquiles, y éste le impide terminar esas actividades, por cuánto tiempo puede entrenar o practicar?

0 min	1–10 min	11–20 min	21–30 min	>30 min	PUNTOS
0	2	5	7	10	

Fig. 5 Image of the final version of the VISA-A-CH questionnaire

Regarding the limitations of the study, the number of participants in the different stages was established according to previous studies of cultural adaptation to other languages, without calculation of sample size. On the other hand, it should be noted that the patients and controls included in both the translation and validation stages are of the same socioeconomic level, not including patients with other education/cultural levels.

activity highlight the utility of VISA-A-CH for patients with AT. This type of studies is fundamental for subsequent clinical work without methodological errors that occur when patients are evaluated with questionnaires that have not been properly translated and culturally adapted.

Conclusions

In conclusion, the VISA-A questionnaire was successfully translated and culturally adapted to a Chilean Spanish-speaking populace, carefully following the published guidelines for this process. The ability to measure aspects such as pain and functionality in physical

Funding

The authors received no financial support for the research, authorship, and/or publication of this article.

Authors' contributions

AK helped with the study design, organization, translation and adaptation, data analysis, and review. PW helped with the manuscript redaction, data analysis, edition, review, and submission. GI performed the translation organization, validation, and patient interaction. JC performed the translation organization, validation, and patient interaction. NC and GI performed the translation organization, validation, and patient interactions. EW, senior author responsible for team planning, performed the analysis and manuscript edition and final approval. NF, senior author, cooperated with the idea, research planning, manuscript edition, and approval. All authors read and approved the final manuscript.

Competing interests

The authors declare that they have no competing interests.

Author details

[1]Department of Orthopedics, Universidad del desarrollo - Clinica Alemana de Santiago, Vitacura 5951, 7650568 Santiago, Chile. [2]Universidad de los Andes - Hospital Militar de Santiago, Santiago, Chile. [3]Centre for Sports and Exercise Medicine, Barts and The London School of Medicine and Dentistry, Mile End Hospital, London, UK.

References

1. Schepsis AA, Jones H, Haas AL. Achilles tendon disorders in athletes. Am J Sports Med. 2002;30:287–305.
2. Maffulli N, Khan KM, Puddu G. Overuse tendon conditions: time to change a confusing terminology. Arthroscopy. 1998;14:840–3.
3. Lohrer H. Rare causes and differential diagnoses of Achilles tendinitis. Sportverletz Sportschaden. 1991;5:182–5.
4. Kvist M. Achilles tendon injuries in athletes. Sports Med. 1994;18(3):173–201.
5. Stanish WD, Curwin S, Mandell S. Tendinitis: its etiology and treatment. New York: Oxford University Press; 2000.
6. Myerson MS, McGarvey W. Disorders of the insertion of the Achilles tendon and Achilles tendinitis. J Bone Joint Surg Am. 1998;80-A:1814–24.
7. Maffulli N, Sharma P, Luscombe KL. Achilles tendinopathy: aetiology and management. J R Soc Med. 2004;97(10):472–6.
8. Paavola M, Kannus P, Jarvinen TA, Khan K, Jozsa L, Jarvinen M. Achilles tendinopathy. J Bone Joint Surg Am. 2002;84-A(11):2062–76.
9. Sorosky B, Press J, Plastaras C, Rittenberg J. The practical management of Achilles tendinopathy. Clin J Sport Med. 2004;14(1):40–4.
10. Andres BM, Murrell GA. Treatment of tendinopathy: what works, what does not, and what is on the horizon. Clin Orthop Relat Res. 2008;466:1539–54.
11. Jonsson P, Alfredson H, Sunding K, Fahlstrom M, Cook J. New regimen for eccentric calf-muscle training in patients with chronic insertional Achilles tendinopathy: results of a pilot study. Br J Sports Med. 2008;42(9):746–9.
12. Roos EM, Engstrom M, Lagerquist A, Soderberg B. Clinical improvement after 6 weeks of eccentric exercise in patients with mid-portion Achilles tendinopathy—a randomized trial with 1-year follow-up. Scand J Med Sci Sports. 2004;14(5):286–95.
13. Robinson JM, Cook JL, Purdam C, Visentini PJ, Ross J, Maffulli N, Taunton JE, Khan KM. The VISA-A questionnaire: a valid and reliable index of the clinical severity of Achilles tendinopathy. Br J Sports Med. 2001;35:335–41.
14. Silbernagel KG, Thomee R, Karlsson J. Cross-cultural adaptation of the VISA-A questionnaire, an index of clinical severity for patients with Achilles tendinopathy, with reliability, validity and structure evaluations. BMC Musculoskelet Disord. 2005;6:12.
15. Jonge S, de Vos RJ, van Schie HT, Verhaar JA, Weir A, Tol JL. One year follow-up of a randomised controlled trial on added splinting to eccentric exercises in chronic midportion Achilles tendinopathy. Br J Sports Med Jul. 2010;44(9):673–7.
16. Maffulli N, Longo UG, Testa V, Oliva F, Capasso G, Denaro V. Italiant translation of the VISA-A score for tendinopathy of the main body of the Achilles tendon. Disabil Rehabil. 2008;30:1635–9.
17. Silbernagel KG, Thomee R, Eriksson BI, Karlsson J. Continued sports activity, using a pain-monitoring model, during rehabilitation in patients with Achilles tendinopathy: a randomized controlled study. Am J Sports Med. 2007;35:897–906.
18. Beaton DE, Bombardier C, Guillemin F, Ferraz MB. Guidelines for the process of cross-cultural adaptation of self-report measures. Spine. 2000;25(24):3186–91.
19. Lohrer H, Nauck T. Cross-cultural adaptation and validation of the VISA-A questionnaire for German-speaking Achilles tendinopathy patients. BMC Musculoskelet Disord. 2009;10:134. Erratum in: BMC Musculoskelet Disord 2010;11:37
20. Guillemin F, Bombardier C, Beaton D. Cross-cultural adaptation of health related quality of life measures: literature review and proposed guidelines. J Clin Epidemiol. 1993;46:1417–32.
21. Herdman M, Fox-Rushby J, Badia X. A model of equivalence in the cultural adaptation of HRQoL instruments: the universalist approach. Qual Life Res. 1998;7:323–35.
22. Gonzalez-Calvo J, Gonzalez VM, Lorig K. Cultural diversity issues in the development of valid and reliable measures of health status. Arthritis Care Res. 1997;10:448–56.

5

Biomechanical analysis between Orthofix® external fixator and different K-wire configurations for pediatric supracondylar humerus fractures

Wen-Chao Li[1]*, Qing-Xu Meng[2], Rui-Jiang Xu[1], Gang Cai[1], Hui Chen[1] and Hong-Juan Li[3]

Abstract

Background: Closed reduction and percutaneous fixation are considered as the optional treatments for displaced supracondylar humerus fractures. However, there was no published report about the biomechanical analysis in Orthofix® external fixator. In this study, we developed a model of supracondylar humerus fractures and compared the biomechanical analysis of external fixator and different K-wires configurations in order to evaluate the stability of external fixator in supracondylar humerus fractures.

Methods: We developed an anatomic humerus model by third-generation synthetic composite, and 60 synthetic humeris were osteotomized to simulate the humeral transverse supracondylar fracture. Those fractures were reduced and fixed by external fixator or K-wires, and then biomechanical analysis was performed in extension, varus, valgus, and internal and external rotation loading. A paired-sample t test was used to evaluate the distance at the fracture site between the external fixator and K-wire configurations.

Results: During all direction loading, there was a significant statistical difference between external fixator and K-wires ($P < 0.001$ for all pairwise comparisons). In extension and internal rotation loading, the external fixator and three crossed K-wires had no comparable stiffness values ($P = 0.572$; $P = 0.795$), and both were significantly greater than two crossed and lateral K-wires ($P < 0.05$). In external rotation loading, there was no significance between the external fixator and K-wire configurations except two lateral K-wires ($P > 0.05$). In valgus loading, the stability of the external fixator was less than that of three crossed K-wires ($P = 0.001$) but was not significantly different with those of two crossed or three lateral K-wires ($P = 0.126$; $P = 0.564$). In varus loading, the stability of the external fixator was larger than those of two and three lateral K-wires ($P = 0.000$; $P = 007$).

Conclusions: External fixator could provide enough stability for pediatric supracondylar humerus fractures without the injury of the ulnar nerve. Besides, it could enhance the rotational stiffness of the construct in rotation loading to avoid the complication of cubitus varus.

Keywords: Supracondylar humerus fracture, Pediatric, Biomechanical stability, External fixation

* Correspondence: liwenchao301@163.com
[1]Department of Pediatric Surgery, Chinese People's Liberation Army General Hospital, Beijing 100853, China
Full list of author information is available at the end of the article

Background

Supracondylar fracture of the distal humerus is a common fracture in the pediatric population, accounting for approximately 60% of all fractures of the elbow [1]. Since1948, Swenson firstly described two K-wires of different sizes for closed reduction of supracondylar humerus fractures [2]. The classical treatment of displaced supracondylar humeral fractures is closed reduction and percutaneous fixation of Kirschner wires (K-wires). Previous studies have shown that medial and lateral crossed-pin fixation provided more stability in biomechanical analysis than two lateral pin fixation [3]. However, crossed K-wire placement is associated with the risk of iatrogenic ulnar nerve injury up to 3 to 4%. Lee et al. [4] reported that three lateral divergent or parallel pin fixations were effective and safe in avoiding iatrogenic ulnar nerve injury in supracondylar humeral fractures. In Bogdan et al.'s [5] study, the humero-ulnar external fixation is a good alternative to lateral or crossed pinning in supracondylar humeral fractures. The optional K-wire configuration could provide the adequate stability of fracture without the risk of neurovascular injury.

The biomechanical analysis in different configurations, including two cross, two divergent lateral, three divergent lateral, a medial and two lateral, and external fixator with radially K-wire, were performed in supracondylar humerus fractures [6–9]. In our department, we performed the closed reduction and percutaneous fixation of the Orthofix® external fixator in the treatment for supracondylar humerus fractures with successful clinical outcomes. However, there have been no published reports of biomechanical analysis in Orthofix® external fixator in supracondylar humerus fractures. In this study, we developed the model of supracondylar humerus fractures and compared the biomechanical analysis between the external fixator and K-wire configurations in order to evaluate the stability of the external fixator in supracondylar humerus fractures.

Methods

Specimen preparation

The anatomic humerus model was developed using a third-generation synthetic composite for this study (Sawbones #3404; Pacific Research Laboratories, Vashon Island, WA) (Model #1028; Pacific Research Laboratories Inc., Vashon, WA, USA). Sixty synthetic humeri were osteotomized at the level of the coronoid and olecranon fossae to simulate a humeral transverse supracondylar fracture. A 10° oblique osteotomy was created with a standardized jig starting at the proximal edge of the olecranon fossa descending to the coronoid fossa.

After the reduction of fracture fragment, the fracture was then fixed by stainless steel K-wires. We used 1.5-mm K-wires for children with weight less than 15 kg and 2-mm K-wires for other children. Prof Wen-Chao Li had performed the surgery of fracture reduction by radiography-guided fluoroscopy. The external fixator and four different K-wire configurations were used for stabilizing the supracondylar humerus fracture (Fig. 1).

I.   Two crossed K-wires [2]: a medial and a lateral K-wire.
II. Two lateral divergent K-wires [10]: a lateral pin was placed parallel to the lateral metaphyseal flare of the humerus. The second pin crossed the osteotomy site at the medial edge of the coronoid fossa.
III. Three lateral divergent K-wires [9]: two lateral divergent K-wires combined with a K-wire placed between the two divergent pins.
IV. A medial and two lateral divergent K-wires (three crossed K-wires) [7]: two lateral divergent pins combined with a medial K-wire.
V.   External fixator: the first screw was inserted into the osteoepiphysis of capitulum humeri parallel to the articular surface of the distal humeral. The second screw in the distal fracture was parallel to the first

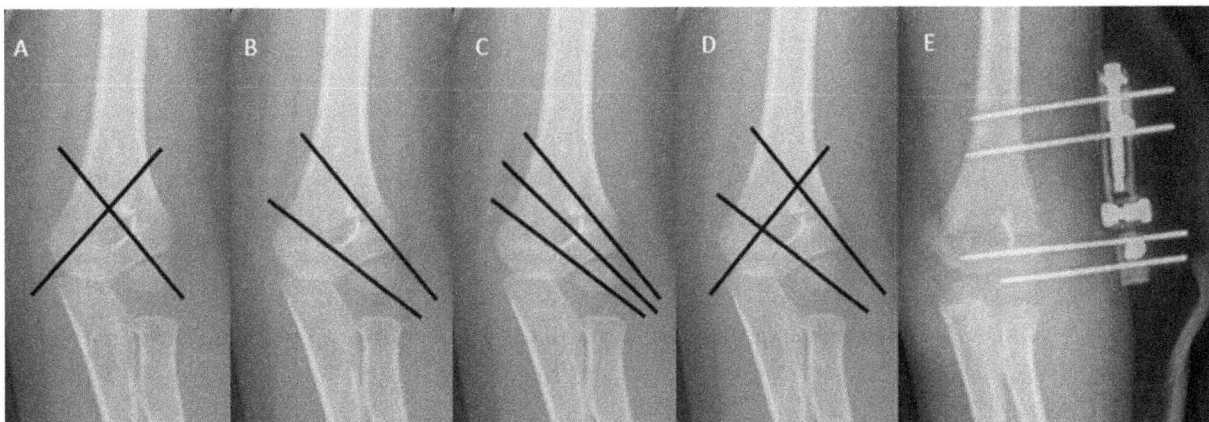

Fig. 1 Schematic of the four K-wire configurations and the external fixator. **a** Two crossed K-wires. **b** Two lateral divergent K-wires. **c** Three lateral divergent K-wires. **d** A medial and two lateral divergent K-wires (three crossed K-wires). **e** External fixator

screw. Both screws pass through the middle metaphysis of the distal end of the humerus and were fixed to the external fixing frame. The others screws were inserted in the proximal fracture. Those screws was fixed in the predesigned position of external fixator. The size of screw in the external fixator is 2 mm.

The specimens with reduction fracture by different fixations were fluoroscopically imaged to ensure consistent orientation between K-wires. Each group including 12 specimens of different fixations were tested in biomechanical analysis by MTS 858 MiniBionix materials testing machine (MTS, Eden Prairie, MN, USA). The testing sequence of five fixations in each group was varied to minimize sequencing effects. We performed the mechanical tests in each fixation to evaluate the different directions of loading: flexion, extension, varus, valgus, internal, and external rotation.

The proximal end of each humerus was embedded with a commercially available two-part epoxy resin and placed into a custom testing machine to provide secure fixation of the specimen during testing. The distal fragment was placed in a custom mold to allow free motion through the fracture site during testing without influencing the position of the K-wires. In the test of extension, varus, and valgus, the load was applied to and measured from the distal fragment at a quasi-static displacement rate of 0.5 mm/s to a maximum of 5 mm. Load (N) and displacement (mm) were measured at the distal fragment and recorded at 10 Hz using an MTS Sintech 1/G material testing machine (MTS Corporation). In the test of internal and external rotations, the custom molds at the distal fragment of the fracture were clamped with two flat plates. Torsion was applied at a quasi-static angular displacement rate of 0.5°/s to an end point of ± 10° using an MTS 858 Minibionix (MTS Corporation, Eden Prairie, MN). Torque (Nm) and angular rotation (mm) were recorded at 10 Hz.

Statistical analysis
Analysis of variance with repeated measurements was used to evaluate differences in the stiffness values of the external fixator and different K-wire configurations. A P value of 0.05 or less was considered statistically significant. Multiple t test comparisons were performed to determine differences among the separate fixation when significance was found. A paired-sample t test was used to evaluate differences in the distance between the different fixations at the fracture site for the external fixator and K-wire configurations.

Results
During the test of all the loading conditions, there were no instances of permanent displacement of the fracture

resulting in loss of fixation or pin deformation. During the extension loading, there was a significant statistical difference between K-wires and the external fixator ($P = 0.000$ for all pairwise comparison). The external fixator and three crossed K-wires had no comparable stiffness values (average ± standard deviation, 7.5 ± 1.4 and 7.9 ± 1.7 N/mm, respectively), and both were significantly greater than two crossed and lateral K-wires. Two lateral K-wires were significantly smaller than other groups ($P < 0.05$). Two crossed with stiffness value of 6.2 ± 1.0 N/mm was larger than two lateral crossed, but smaller than three crossed K-wires and external fixator (Table 1).

The maximal loads and torques required to produce the prescribed displacement and rotation exhibited similar trends to the stiffness results. During the varus and valgus loading, there was significant statistical difference between all K-wires of configurations and external fixator ($P < 0.001$). The stiffness of three crossed K-wires (21.2 ± 3.1 Nm/mm; 17.9 ± 2.3 Nm/mm) was larger than that of two lateral K-wires (14.1 ± 2.0 Nm/mm, $P < 0.001$; 13.5 ± 1.7 Nm/mm, $P < 0.001$) and three lateral K-wires (15.4 ± 2.3 Nm/mm, $P < 0.001$; 15.8 ± 2.0 Nm/mm, $P = 0.042$), and there was no significant difference between three and two crossed K-wires (20.4 ± 2.4 Nm/mm, $P = 0.526$; 16.7 ± 2.1 Nm/mm, $P = 0.238$). In varus loading, there was no significant difference between the stiffness of the external fixator (18.9 ± 2.9 Nm/mm) and three crossed K-wires (21.2 ± 3.1 Nm/mm, $P = 0.015$) or two crossed K-wires (20.4 ± 2.4 Nm/mm, $P = 0.042$). But the stiffness of the external fixator was larger than that of two lateral K-wires (14.1 ± 2.0 Nm/mm, $P = 0.000$) and three lateral K-wires (15.4 ± 2.3 Nm/mm, $P = 0.007$). In valgus loading, the stiffness of the external fixator (15.3 ± 1.8 Nm/mm) was less than that of three crossed K-wires (17.9 ± 2.3 Nm/mm, $P = 0.001$) (Table 2).

During the internal and external rotation loading, there were significant statistical differences between all K-wires of configurations and the external fixator ($P < 0.001$). There was no significant difference between three crossed K-wires and the external fixator ($P > 0.05$). In internal rotation loading, the stiffness in both fixations (117 ± 18 Nmm/degree; 119 ± 16 Nmm/degree) was larger than those of two and three crossed K-wires and three lateral K-wires ($P < 0.05$). In external rotation loading, the stiffness in both fixations (121 ± 16 Nmm/degree; 120 ± 19 Nmm/degree) was not significantly different with two crossed and three lateral K-wires ($P > 0.05$), but larger than that of two lateral K-wires ($P < 0.001$). During all the five loading conditions, there was a trend for two crossed K-wires to have a greater stiffness value than two lateral K-wires ($P < 0.05$), and three lateral K-wires had a

Table 1 Construct stiffness data in extension loading direction for different K-wire configurations or external fixator

Extension loading	Magnitudes (N/mm)	ANOVA (P)	Comparison (P)				
	Mean ± SD†		(I)	(II)	(III)	(IV)	(V)
Two crossed K-wires (I)	6.2 ± 1.0	0.000	–	0.048	0.605	0.028	0.013
Two lateral K-wires (II)	5.1 ± 1.3		–	–	0.038	0.000	0.000
Three lateral K-wires (III)	6.5 ± 1.5		–	–	–	0.140	0.066
Three crossed K-wires (IV)	7.5 ± 1.4		–	–	–	–	0.572
External fixator (V)	7.9 ± 1.7		–	–	–	–	–

Italicized values are significantly different between two groups ($P < 0.05$)
†The values are given as mean ± standard deviation

similar statistically significant difference except for varus loading ($P = 0.194$) (Table 3).

Discussion

Supracondylar humeral fractures are common in children and account for 13~16% of all pediatric fractures. The goals of the treatment for displaced supracondylar humerus fracture are closed or open anatomical reduction and maintaining the reduction of fracture without iatrogenic nerve injury [11]. Those previous studies have reported biomechanical analysis with different K-wire configurations in supracondylar humeral fractures. However, there have been no published reports of biomechanical analysis in the external fixator in supracondylar humerus fractures. In our study, we developed a model of supracondylar humerus fractures and compared biomechanical analysis in the external fixator with different K-wire configurations to evaluate the stability of the external fixator in the humerus fracture. In this study, there was no significant difference between the external fixator and three crossed K-wires in extension, rotation, and varus loading ($P > 0.05$), and the stability of the

external fixator was less than that of three crossed K-wires in valgus loading ($P = 0.001$). Besides, the external fixator provided more stability than two crossed K-wires in extension ($P = 0.013$) and internal rotation ($P = 0.021$) loading and was not significantly different than two crossed K-wires in other direction loading ($P > 0.05$).

It is well known that two crossed K-wires could provide anatomical reduction and the stability of fixation to lower the incidence of Volkmann ischemia with the elbow less than 90°. However, ulnar nerve injury is a common complication when the K-wire is inserted in the medial direction. Those previous studies reported that the frequency of iatrogenic ulnar nerve injuries by the medial placement of K-wires ranges from 1.4 to 15.6% [12]. Babal et al. [13] concluded that the medial pin carried the greater overall risk of nerve injury as compared with the lateral pin-only construct and that the ulnar nerve was at risk of injury in patients who had medial pins. Brauer et al. [14] reported the probability of iatrogenic nerve injury was 1.84 times higher with medial and lateral pins than that with lateral entry pin. In extension loading, Feng et al. reported that the two

Table 2 Construct stiffness data in varus and valgus loading directions for different K-wire configurations or external fixator

Varus loading	Magnitudes (Nm/mm)	ANOVA (P)	Comparison (P)				
	Mean ± SD†		(I)	(II)	(III)	(IV)	(V)
Two crossed K-wires (I)	20.4 ± 2.4	0.000	–	0.000	0.000	0.526	0.224
Two lateral K-wires (II)	14.1 ± 2.0		–	–	0.194	0.000	0.000
Three lateral K-wires (III)	15.4 ± 2.3		–	–	–	0.000	0.007
Three crossed K-wires (IV)	21.2 ± 3.1		–	–	–	–	0.104
External fixator (V)	18.9 ± 2.9		–	–	–	–	–
Valgus loading	Magnitudes (Nm/mm)	ANOVA (P)	Comparison (P)				
	Mean ± SD†		(I)	(II)	(III)	(IV)	(V)
Two crossed K-wires (I)	16.7 ± 2.1	0.000	–	0.000	0.339	0.238	0.126
Two lateral K-wires (II)	13.5 ± 1.7		–	–	0.012	0.000	0.033
Three lateral K-wires (III)	15.8 ± 2.0		–	–	–	0.042	0.564
Three crossed K-wires (IV)	17.9 ± 2.3		–	–	–	–	0.001
External fixator (V)	15.3 ± 1.8		–	–	–	–	–

Italicized values are significantly different between two groups ($P < 0.05$)
†The values are given as mean ± standard deviation

Table 3 Construct stiffness data in internal rotation and external rotation loading direction for different K-wire configurations or external fixator

Internal rotation loading	Magnitudes (Nmm/degree) Mean ± SD[†]	ANOVA (P)	Comparison (P)				
			(I)	(II)	(III)	(IV)	(V)
Two crossed K-wires (I)	101 ± 16	*0.000*	–	*0.024*	0.769	*0.039*	*0.021*
Two lateral K-wires (II)	84 ± 15			–	*0.032*	*0.000*	*0.000*
Three lateral K-wires(III)	99 ± 14				–	*0.022*	*0.008*
Three crossed K-wires (IV)	117 ± 18					–	0.795
External fixator (V)	119 ± 16						–
External rotation loading	Magnitudes (Nmm/degree) Mean ± SD[†]	ANOVA (P)	Comparison (P)				
			(I)	(II)	(III)	(IV)	(V)
Two crossed K-wires (I)	108 ± 15	*0.000*	–	*0.032*	0.451	0.077	0.134
Two lateral K-wires (II)	93 ± 14			–	*0.005*	*0.000*	*0.000*
Three lateral K-wires (III)	102 ± 14				–	0.249	0.432
Three crossed K-wires (IV)	121 ± 16					–	0.900
External fixator (V)	120 ± 19						–

Italicized values are significantly different between two groups (P < 0.05)
[†]The values are given as mean ± standard deviation

lateral divergent pins were less stable than the two crossed pins [9], which was similar with the result of our study (P < 0.05). The external fixator and three crossed K-wires had no comparable stiffness values (7.5 ± 1.4 N/mm; 7.9 ± 1.7 N/mm, respectively), and both were significantly greater than two crossed and lateral K-wires. The external fixator could be regulated in extension direction by a spanner. Besides, the external fixator could provide the stability of the distal and proximal fracture by those screws.

Configurations using lateral-only entry K-wires have been recommended to decrease the risk of iatrogenic injury to the ulnar nerve. Zionts et al. [15] compared the stability provided by different pin configurations and demonstrated that crossed-pin configuration provides the most stable torsional fixation, followed by the fixation achieved with two and three lateral pins. In our study, two crossed K-wire configuration was significantly stiffer than two lateral divergent K-wires, especially in varus and valgus direction loading. Adding a third lateral K-wire to the crossed or two lateral K-wire configuration could provide more stability in the fracture than previous K-wires, but the difference was not significant in the same directions. This finding suggests that the surgeon faced with a biomechanically unstable fracture pattern or a less-than-anatomic reduction may use additional lateral K-wires to supplement biomechanical stability. In Larson et al.'s study [16], the three crossed-pin construct was most stable in the fracture followed by three lateral pins, and two lateral divergent pins demonstrated the least torsional stability. However, Srikumaran et al. [8] reported that gross observation suggests that the addition of a third lateral pin to the crossed configuration increased

cortical destruction, making the construct less stable in extension. In valgus loading, the stiffness of the external fixator (15.3 ± 1.8 Nm/mm) was less than that of the three crossed K-wires (17.9 ± 2.3 Nm/mm, P = 0.001). The screws in the external fixator with good elasticity were likely to bend as a result of interval of fracture fragment during the external loading. Therefore, the stability of the external fixator was less than that of the three crossed K-wires. However, during varus loading, the internal of fracture fragments was compressed without displacement, and the screws were kept to maintain the stability of the fracture fragment. Therefore, there was no significant difference between the stiffness of the external fixator (18.9 ± 2.9 Nm/mm) and the three crossed K-wires (21.2 ± 3.1 Nm/mm, P = 0.015).

Mechanical rotation stability of the different fixations in supracondylar humeral fracture is a major factor to avoid the development of cubitus varus. Cubitus varus has been considered as being just a cosmetic problem by many authors. The ulnar insertion of an anti-rotation wire into the distal fragment reinforces the stability if internal rotation loading is applied and stabilizes the ulnar column of the distal humerus [17]. Wang et al. [18] reported that there was no statistical difference between the two medial pins and the two crossed-pin configurations (P = 0.06 and 0.75, respectively) in internal and external rotation testing, but they were significantly greater than two lateral pins (P = 0.003 and 0.004; P = 0.001 and 0.02, respectively). In our study, the crossed K-wires provided more stability than two lateral K-wires (P = 0.024; P = 0.032), which was similar with the previous study. Besides, the stiffness of two lateral K-wires (84 ± 15 Nmm/degree; 93 ± 14 Nmm/degree) was less than those of the external fixator and other three K-wire configurations ($P < 0.05$). The external fixator could provide more stability and resistance to internal rotation than two and three crossed K-wires ($P = 0.021$; $P = 0.008$), while in external rotation loading, the external fixator was not statistically significantly different with two and three crossed K-wires ($P = 0.134$; $P = 0.432$).

In Feng et al.'s study [9], two medial divergent pins and two crossed pins had comparable stiffness values and both were significantly greater than two lateral pins during the rotation loading, which was similar with our study ($P = 0.024$; $P = 0.032$). Previous biomechanical studies have shown that crossed pins provide greater rotational stability than both parallel lateral and divergent lateral pin constructs for transverse fractures [10, 19]. Bloom et al. [20] reported that the addition of the third K-wire compared with an anatomically reduced two crossed K-wire configuration resulted in increased stiffness of the model for all loading directions. Besides, the external fixator could provide similar resistance to internal and external rotation loading with three crossed K-wires. The above biomechanical analysis showed that the external fixator could provide enough rotation loads and torques in supracondylar humeral fractures.

In this article, we evaluated the biomechanical analysis in the external fixator and K-wire configuration for the displaced supracondylar humerus fractures. However, this study has significant limitations. In our study, we performed the synthesis models to evaluate the biomechanical analysis of fracture reduction techniques, but the transverse osteotomy of the humeral model could not account for the variability of fracture line in clinical fracture. The next study should be performed in a coronal medial obliquity and lateral obliquity model. The surrounding of the fracture including the muscle, periosteum, vessel, and nerve could contribute to the choice of fracture and fragment stability. The model in our study without structural variation or inconsistency was desirable as it mainly involves relative comparisons of stiffness. In experiment study, we could evaluate the biomechanical analysis in the single direction loading in the synthesis model. However, the physiological loading in clinical usually contain two or three directions loading. The complex direction loading in the fracture model can be performed by computer-assisted analysis. The external fixator and different K-wire configurations is performed to evaluate the biomechanical analysis to select the proper fixation.

Conclusions

The external fixator could provide enough stability without the injury of the ulnar nerve in treatment of a supracondylar humeral fracture to reduce the displacement of the fragments. Besides, it enhances the rotational stiffness of the construct in rotation loading to avoid the complication of cubitus varus. The stability of the external fixator was less than that of three crossed K-wires in valgus loading, but there was no significant difference between the external fixator and two crossed K-wires. Long-term results of this new variation of the external fixator will be evaluated in a clinical setting.

Abbreviation
K-wire: Kirschner wire

Funding
This work was supported by the National Natural Science Foundation of China (81702169), Nursery Foundation of People's Liberation Army General Hospital (17KMM12), and Clinical Support Foundation of People's Liberation Army General Hospital (2017FC-TSYS-2043 and 2017FC-TSYS-3015).

Authors' contributions
WCL made contributions to the experiment designs, collected the clinical data, performed the statistical analysis, and drafted the manuscript. RJX and QXM helped in collecting the clinical data and participated in the design of the study. GC, HC, and HJL participated in the statistical analysis. All authors read and approved the final manuscript.

Competing interests
The authors declare that they have no competing interests.

Author details
[1]Department of Pediatric Surgery, Chinese People's Liberation Army General Hospital, Beijing 100853, China. [2]Department of Basic Surgery, Affiliated Hospital of Hebei University, Baoding 071002, China. [3]Department of Orthopaedic, Yu Huang Ding Hospital of Yantai, Yantai 370600, China.

References
1. Basaran SH, Ercin E, Bayrak A, Bilgili MG, Kizilkaya C, Dasar U, et al. The outcome and parents-based cosmetic satisfaction following fixation of paediatric supracondylar humerus fractures treated by closed method with or without small medial incision. Springerplus. 2016;5:174.
2. Swenson AL. The treatment of supracondylar fractures of the humerus by Kirschner-wire transfixion. J Bone Joint Surg Am. 1948;30A(4):993–7.
3. Reising K, Schmal H, Kohr M, Kuminack K, Sudkamp NP, Strohm PC. Surgical treatment of supracondylar humerus fractures in children. Acta Chir Orthop Traumatol Cechoslov. 2011;78(6):519–23.
4. Lee YH, Lee SK, Kim BS, Chung MS, Baek GH, Gong HS, et al. Three lateral divergent or parallel pin fixations for the treatment of displaced supracondylar humerus fractures in children. J Pediatr Orthop. 2008; 28(4):417–22.
5. Bogdan A, Quintin J, Schuind F. Treatment of displaced supracondylar humeral fractures in children by humero-ulnar external fixation. Int Orthop. 2016;40(11): 2409–415.

6. Hohloch L, Konstantinidis L, Wagner FC, Strohm PC, Sudkamp NP, Reising K. Biomechanical comparison of different external fixator configurations for stabilization of supracondylar humerus fractures in children. Clin Biomech. 2016;32:118–23.

7. Silva M, Knutsen AR, Kalma JJ, Borkowski SL, Bernthal NM, Spencer HT, et al. Biomechanical testing of pin configurations in supracondylar humeral fractures: the effect of medial column comminution. J Orthop Trauma. 2013; 27(5):275–80.

8. Srikumaran U, Tan EW, Belkoff SM, Marsland D, Ain MC, Leet AI, et al. Enhanced biomechanical stiffness with large pins in the operative treatment of pediatric supracondylar humerus fractures. J Pediatr Orthop. 2012;32(2):201–5.

9. Feng C, Guo Y, Zhu Z, Zhang J, Wang Y. Biomechanical analysis of supracondylar humerus fracture pinning for fractures with coronal lateral obliquity. J Pediatr Orthop. 2012;32(2):196–200.

10. Hamdi A, Poitras P, Louati H, Dagenais S, Masquijo JJ, Kontio K. Biomechanical analysis of lateral pin placements for pediatric supracondylar humerus fractures. J Pediatr Orthop. 2010;30(2):135–9.

11. Ducic S, Bumbasirevic M, Radlovic V, Nikic P, Bukumiric Z, Brdar R, et al. Displaced supracondylar humeral fractures in children: comparison of three treatment approaches. Srp Arh Celok Lek. 2016;144(1–2):46–51.

12. Kalenderer O, Reisoglu A, Surer L, Agus H. How should one treat iatrogenic ulnar injury after closed reduction and percutaneous pinning of paediatric supracondylar humeral fractures? Injury. 2008;39(4):463–6.

13. Babal JC, Mehlman CT, Klein G. Nerve injuries associated with pediatric supracondylar humeral fractures: a meta-analysis. J Pediatr Orthop. 2010; 30(3):253–63.

14. Brauer CA, Lee BM, Bae DS, Waters PM, Kocher MS. A systematic review of medial and lateral entry pinning versus lateral entry pinning for supracondylar fractures of the humerus. J Pediatr Orthop. 2007;27(2):181–6.

15. Zionts LE, McKellop HA, Hathaway R. Torsional strength of pin configurations used to fix supracondylar fractures of the humerus in children. J Bone Joint Surg Am. 1994;76(2):253–6.

16. Larson L, Firoozbakhsh K, Passarelli R, Bosch P. Biomechanical analysis of pinning techniques for pediatric supracondylar humerus fractures. J Pediatr Orthop. 2006;26(5):573–8.

17. Jain AK, Dhammi IK, Arora A, Singh MP, Luthra JS. Cubitus varus: problem and solution. Arch Orthop Trauma Surg. 2000;120(7–8):420–5.

18. Wang X, Feng C, Wan S, Bian Z, Zhang J, Song M, et al. Biomechanical analysis of pinning configurations for a supracondylar humerus fracture with coronal medial obliquity. J Pediatr Orthop B. 2012;21(6):495–8.

19. Gaston RG, Cates TB, Devito D, Schmitz M, Schrader T, Busch M, et al. Medial and lateral pin versus lateral-entry pin fixation for type 3 supracondylar fractures in children: a prospective, surgeon-randomized study. J Pediatr Orthop. 2010;30(8):799–806.

20. Bloom T, Robertson C, Mahar AT, Newton P. Biomechanical analysis of supracondylar humerus fracture pinning for slightly malreduced fractures. J Pediatr Orthop. 2008;28(7):766–72.

6

Tranexamic acid is associated with selective increase in inflammatory markers following total knee arthroplasty (TKA)

Andrea L. Grant[1,2], Hayley L. Letson[2], Jodie L. Morris[1,2], Peter McEwen[1,2], Kaushik Hazratwala[1,2], Matthew Wilkinson[1,2] and Geoffrey P. Dobson[2]* ⓘ

Abstract

Background: Tranexamic acid (TXA) is commonly used in orthopedic surgery to reduce excessive bleeding and transfusion requirements. Our aim was to examine if TXA was required in all osteoarthritis patients undergoing TKA surgery, and its possible effects on systemic inflammation and coagulation properties.

Methods: Twenty-three patients (Oxford Score 22–29) were recruited consecutively; 12 patients received TXA before (IV, 1.2 g/90 kg) and immediately after surgery (intra-articular, 1.4 g/90 kg). Inflammatory mediators and ROTEM parameters were measured in blood at baseline, after the first bone-cut, immediately after surgery, and postoperative days 1 and 2.

Results: After the bone cut and surgery, TXA significantly increased MCP-1, TNF-α, IL-1β and IL-6 levels compared to non-TXA patients, which was further amplified postoperatively. During surgery, TXA significantly prolonged EXTEM clot times, indicating a thrombin-slowing effect, despite little or no change in clot amplitude or fibrinogen. TXA was associated with three- to fivefold increases in FIBTEM maximum lysis (ML), a finding counter to TXA's antifibrinolytic effect. Maximum lysis for extrinsic and intrinsic pathways was < 8%, indicating little or no hyperfibrinolysis. No significant differences were found in postoperative hemoglobin between the two groups.

Conclusions: TXA was associated with increased systemic inflammation during surgery compared to non-TXA patients, with further amplification on postoperative days 1 and 2. On the basis of little or no change in viscoelastic clot strength, fibrinogen or clot lysis, there appeared to be no clinical justification for TXA in our group of patients. Larger prospective, randomized trials are required to investigate a possible proinflammatory effect in TKA patients.

Keywords: Tranexamic acid, Total knee arthroplasty, Coagulation, Inflammation, Orthopaedic surgery, Trauma

Background

A common perioperative complication during knee and hip surgery is excessive bleeding and the need for blood products [1, 2]. Serine protease inhibitor aprotonin was removed from world markets in 2007 and led to renewed interest in tranexamic acid (TXA) for reducing blood loss during major surgery [3, 4]. TXA is a synthetic lysine analog that reduces active bleeding by blocking the 5 lysine-binding sites on plasminogen, which prevents plasmin formation and decreases fibrinolysis [3, 5]. TXA has a plasma half-life of ~ 2 h, and its antifibrinolytic effects may last up to 7–8 h in the circulation, and ~ 17 h in most tissues [6].

In orthopaedic surgery, two injections of TXA are commonly used; one is given intravenously before the operation, and another in the knee joint on deflation of the tourniquet [7–9]. In a recent large retrospective cohort study, involving 872,416 patients, Poeran and colleagues concluded that TXA was effective in reducing the need for blood transfusions during total hip or knee arthroplasty [10]. However, despite the overwhelming evidence, the same authors cautioned that "we cannot provide support for the ubiquitous use of TXA in all

* Correspondence: geoffrey.dobson@jcu.edu.au
[2]Heart, Trauma and Sepsis Research Laboratory, College of Medicine and Dentistry, James Cook University, 1 James Cook Drive, Townsville, Queensland 4811, Australia
Full list of author information is available at the end of the article

patients requiring joint arthroplasty, as the differential impact on complications among patient subpopulations remains to be studied" [10]. A number of ongoing concerns include timing, dose, route of delivery (IV, oral, topical), and whether all patients should receive the drug [2, 8, 11]. Furthermore, there remains the risk of thromboembolic events [3, 12], and there is an increased awareness in the literature that TXA-specific lysine residues are not specific to reducing blood loss [13], but are involved in other metabolic and signalling events, protein-protein interactions and post-translational modifications [14]. In some cases, TXA can increase bleeding in brain independent of the tPA effect by binding to plasminogen in the presence of increased levels of urokinase plasminogen activator (uPA), which facilitates plasmin formation and the propensity to bleed [4, 15]. In 2017, we also showed that TXA administration in medium-risk cardiac surgery patients led to anomalous clot behaviour after a sternotomy, lower platelet numbers after surgery, and little or no difference in fibrinolysis compared to non-TXA patients [16].

A number of studies and many reviews have suggested that TXA may have anti-inflammatory properties via inhibition of plasmin-mediated activation of complement, monocytes, and neutrophils and may also improve platelet function [17, 18]. However, the evidence is weak, and since mediators of inflammation are associated with increased risk of thrombosis, and vice versa [13, 19], further studies are warranted. We hypothesized based on our previous cardiac surgery study [16] that TXA may have anomalous effects on coagulation properties during surgery, alter the patient's inflammatory status and may not be required for all TKA patients. Thus, the aim of the present study was to examine the effects of TXA on coagulation and inflammation prior to, during, and following surgery, and assess if TXA was required in all patients undergoing elective TKA surgery.

Methods

Approvals

Informed consent was obtained prospectively from all participants, and the study was approved by the Institutional Human Research Ethics Committee (MHS20140812-03). The research undertaken strictly adhered to the Code of Ethics (Declaration of Helsinki) of the World Medical Association for trials involving humans. This study was an analytic, prospective, observational cohort (level II) investigation in which patient groups were separated non-randomly by treatment, with exposure occurring after the initiation of anesthesia.

Subjects and procedures

Twenty-three patients (6 male, 17 female) undergoing TKA across three private practices were recruited to participate in the study (Table 1). The inclusion

Table 1 Demographics, comorbidities and pre-operative, perioperative and post-operative values (6 weeks) in non-TXA and TXA groups

	Non-TXA	TXA	p value
Age (years)	69 ± 1	65 ± 1	0.092
Weight (kg)	91 ± 5	90 ± 6	0.930
No. of patients	11	12	
Gender	M = 4	M = 2	
	F = 7	F = 10	
Osteoarthritis	11	12	
TXA administration:			
IV Infusion (mg/kg)	NA	13.5 ± 0.6	
IA Injection (mg/kg)	NA	15.5 ± 0.7	
Preoperative:			
Hemoglobin (HgB) g/L	136 ± 4	137 ± 4	0.980
Anesthetic:			
General only	0	1	
General + Spinal	11	11	
Perioperative:			
Tourniquet time (Min)	62 ± 11	27 ± 6	0.023*
Surgical time (Min)	107 ± 6	104 ± 4	0.566
Postoperative:			
HgB g/L day 1	121 ± 3§	122 ± 3§	0.787
HgB g/L day 2	111 ± 2§	121 ± 5§	0.093

Data represent mean ± SEM *$p < 0.05$ between non-TXA and TXA group; §$p < 0.05$ compared to preoperative value

criteria were patients who were diagnosed with primary knee osteoarthritis (OA). The exclusion criteria were patients with (1) rheumatoid OA, (2) autoimmune disorders, (3) recent or recurrent infections with antibiotic treatment, or (4) contraindication for TXA use (thrombotic disorder and hematuria). Two of the three surgeons routinely use TXA perioperatively, and the remaining surgeon performed all surgeries for the non-TXA group.

All patients with exception of one TXA patient received both spinal and general anesthesia (Table 1). The anesthetic procedure included intravenous administration midazolam (0.02 mg/kg) and propofol target-controlled infusion (2–5 mg/kg/h) with fentanyl (75–85 μg) as required. A tourniquet was inflated prior to the first midline skin incision and a medial parapatellar access was used to expose the joint capsule. After the bone cut, an intra-articular cocktail comprising Ropivacaine (400 mg), Ketorolac (30 mg), Adrenaline (1 mg), and Methylprednisolone (40 mg) in a total volume of 200 ml of saline was injected into the sub-synovial space, ligaments and muscles around the knee. All unilateral TKA surgery was assisted with Precision Computer Navigation (Stryker®). Implanted prosthesis (cruciate retaining) were cemented (PALACOS® R+G), Heraeus Medical, Germany). After implantation and tourniquet deflation, the capsule was closed.

TXA administration

Following induction of anesthesia and prior to skin incision, an intravenous bolus injection of TXA (1.2 g per 90-kg patient) was administered (Fig. 1, Table 1). After the operation and before skin closure, a second TXA bolus (15.5 g/kg body wt.) was injected in the intra-articular space in saline (i.e., 1.0 g TXA/10 ml saline).

Clinical assessments

Patients were assessed preoperatively and followed up at 6 weeks postoperative for clinical assessments (goniometry for range of movement (ROM) as well as pain scores), and patient reported outcome measures, which included the Knee injury and Osteoarthritis Outcomes Score (KOOS), Oxford Knee Score (OKS), EuroQol (EQ-5D 3L) and Forgotten Joint Score (FJS) (Table 1). Practice nurses used the Angulus ROM iPhone app, which provides flexion and extension values by recording and measuring movement in both a horizontal and vertical plane.

Blood sampling

Peripheral venous blood was collected from patients at three time points: (1) baseline, prior to anesthesia, (2) ~ 10 min after the first bone cut, and (3) ~ 30 min following skin closure. Blood was also collected from patients on days 1 and 2 postoperative. Whole blood (1.8 ml) was collected in 3.2% sodium-citrate vacutainers (BD Australia) for coagulation assessment, and 4 ml was collected into K_2EDTA vacutainers (BD Australia) and centrifuged (1500 rpm, 15 min, 4 °C). Plasma was removed and snap-frozen in liquid nitrogen and stored at − 80 °C for cytokine measurements.

Rotational thromboelastometry

Rotational thromboelastometry (ROTEM®, Tem International, Munich, Germany) was performed on ROTEM® delta according to the manufacturer's instructions and described in Letson and Dobson [20] and Solomon and colleagues [21] (Fig. 2). Assays were run for 60 min. Hyperfibrinolysis was defined as a maximum lysis index greater than or equal to 15% [20, 22].

Cytokine analysis

Milliplex® Human Cytokine/Chemokine Magnetic Bead Panel (Lot #: 2875005, Abacus ALS, Meadowbrook, Queensland) in combination with the Magpix® analyser (Luminex Corporation, Austin, Texas, USA) were used to measure plasma levels of monocyte chemotactic protein (MCP)-1, tumor necrosis factor alpha (TNF-α), interleukin (IL)-6, IL-8, IL-1β, IL-1 receptor antagonist (IL-1RA), IL-4 and IL-10 at baseline, 10 min after bone cut, in recovery, and on days 1 and 2 after surgery. Assays were carried out according to the manufacturer's instructions with samples measured in duplicate. Detection ranges for all analytes were 3.2–10,000 pg/ml. Assay sensitivities (minimum detectable concentration, pg/ml), intra-assay precision (%CV) and inter-assay precision (n = 6 assays; %CV) for each analyte were MCP-1: 1.9, 1.5, 7.9; TNFα: 0.7, 2.6, 13.0; IL-6: 0.9, 2.0, 18.3; IL-8: 0.4, 1.9, 3.5; IL-1β: 0.8, 2.3, 6.7; IL-1RA: 8.3, 2.1, 10.7; IL-4: 4.5; 2.9, 14.7; IL-10: 1.1, 1.6, 16.8.

Statistics

A priori power analysis to determine sample sizes was conducted using G-power3 program to minimize type 1 errors and was based on differences between coagulation parameters prior to and at surgery end [16]. A sample size of 10 patients in each group was sufficient for statistically valid comparisons to be made with respect to TXA vs non-TXA treatments with the power set at 0.8

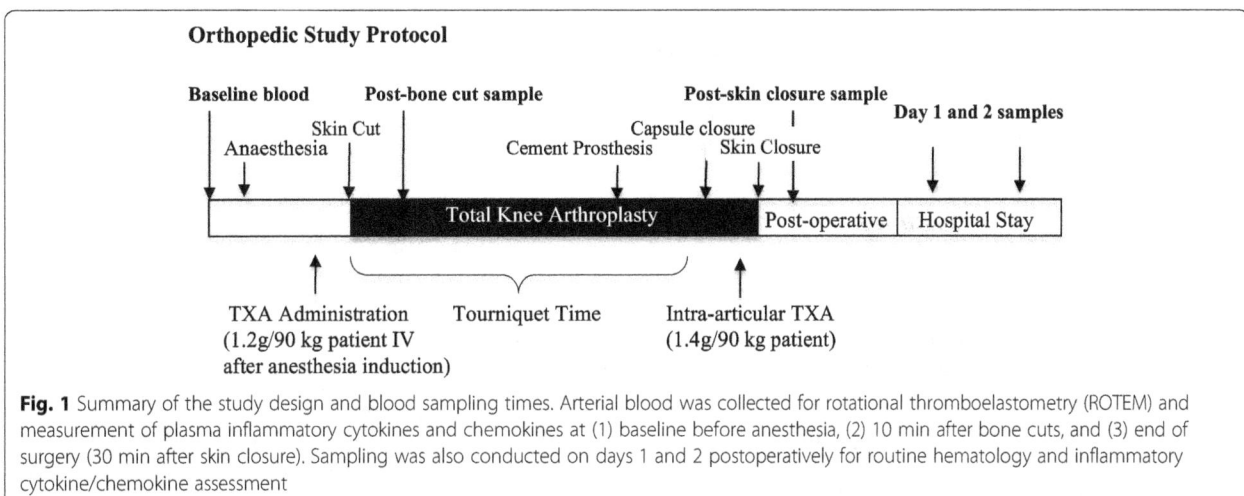

Fig. 1 Summary of the study design and blood sampling times. Arterial blood was collected for rotational thromboelastometry (ROTEM) and measurement of plasma inflammatory cytokines and chemokines at (1) baseline before anesthesia, (2) 10 min after bone cuts, and (3) end of surgery (30 min after skin closure). Sampling was also conducted on days 1 and 2 postoperatively for routine hematology and inflammatory cytokine/chemokine assessment

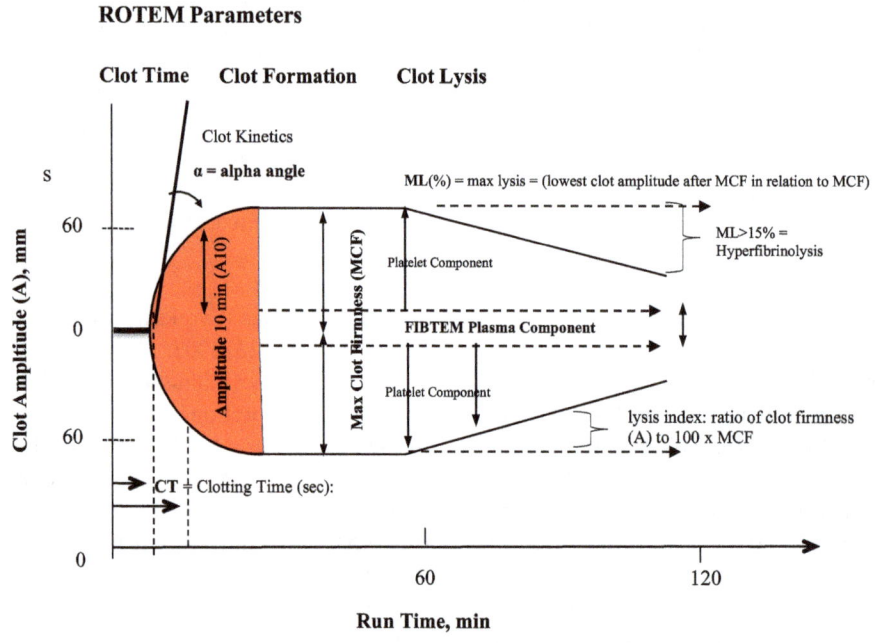

ROTEM Parameters

ROTEM Parameter	Units	Description
EXTEM		Extrinsically-activated test with tissue factor (TF). This pathway is similar to the extrinsic or TF-activated clotting pathway.
FIBTEM		Fibrin-based EXTEM but with the platelet inhibitor cytochalasin D.
INTEM		Intrinsically-activated test using ellagic acid. This pathway is similar to the intrinsic or contact activation pathway.
Clotting Time (CT)	Sec	Time to clot amplitude of 2 mm = initiation of clot formation from beginning of test. Provides information on speed of thrombin, platelet, fibrin formation; also, influenced by clotting factors, anti-coagulants.
Clot Formation Time (CFT)	Sec	Run time from CT until 20 mm clot amplitude. Provides information on kinetics and propagation of clot formation. CFT is influenced by platelet level/function and fibrinogen level and ability to polymerize.
alpha-angle	°	Angle of tangent between 0 mm and the curve when the clot firmness is 20 mm. A lower angle may indicate poor platelet function, low platelet count, fibrin polymerization disorders or low fibrinogen.
Clot Amplitude (e.g. A10)	mm	Clot amplitude 10 min after CT = clot firmness and predictor of MCF
Maximum Clot Firmness (MCF)	mm	Maximum clot amplitude which provided information on clot strength or firmness or clot quality. MCF influenced by platelet function, properties of fibrinogen and fibrin, and presence of Factor XIII
Lysis Index (e.g. LI-30)	%	Percentage of remaining clot stability in relation to the MCF value at 30 min after CT.
Maximum Lysis, (ML)	% of MCF	Percent of clot firmness lost during 2-hour measurement. Abnormal ML at 30 minutes possibly indicates fibrinolysis. ML >15% is indicator of hyperfibrinolysis

Fig. 2 Schematic of a ROTEM Trace showing the key coagulation parameters measuring clot initiation, propagation and clot breakdown or lysis, and definitions of the major ROTEM parameters used in the study

and alpha level at 0.05. SPSS Statistics 24.0 was used for all data analysis (IBM, Armonk, NY). Data normality was assessed using Shapiro-Wilks test, with Levene's test used to determine equality of variances. Independent samples t tests were used for between-groups comparison for normally distributed data. Within group differences were analysed with paired samples t tests. Non-normally distributed data was compared using a Mann-Whitney U test. MILLIPLEX Analyst 5.1 software (Luminex Corporation, Austin, Texas, USA), which analyses data with a 5 parametric logistic weighted curve fit, was used to determine cytokine concentrations. Area under the curve (AUC) was determined for changes in plasma cytokine levels across each of the five time points assessed. The mean AUC for each cytokine was compared for non-TXA and TXA patients using an independent-t test with Welch's correction. All values are expressed as mean ± standard error of the mean (SEM) with significance set at $p < 0.05$.

Results

Perioperative characteristics

There were no significant preoperative differences in patient demographic or clinical parameters (Table 1). Tourniquet time was significantly less in TXA patients compared to non-TXA patients, with no significant differences in surgical times (Table 1). Lower tourniquet times may be due to differences in surgical procedures among surgeons; however, it is important to note that possible longer ischemic times in non-TXA patients may exacerbate postoperative inflammation; however, it was less than TXA-treated patients in our cohort (see below). No differences in preoperative knee biomechanic measures were observed, with the exception of significantly higher extension (5° vs. 2°) in the non-TXA group (Table 2). At 6 weeks postoperative, patients within each group demonstrated significant improvements in KOOS measures compared to baseline, with no significant differences between scores for non-TXA and TXA patients (Table 2).

Table 2 Preoperative and postoperative (6 weeks) range of motion (ROM) and patientreported outcome measures (PROM) in non-TXA and TXA groups

	Non-TXA	TXA	p value
Preoperative:			
ROM			
Flexion (°)	115 ± 5	121 ± 5	0.411
Extension (°)	5 ± 1	2 ± 1	0.046*
KOOS Total	46 ± 6	41 ± 4	0.470
KOOS Pain	10 ± 2	8 ± 1	0.417
KOOS Function	32 ± 4	29 ± 3	0.457
KOOS Movement	4 ± 0.7	4 ± 0.4	1.000
OKS	22 ± 3	29 ± 3	0.457
EQ5D 3L VAS	64 ± 7	67 ± 4	0.760
Postoperative 6 weeks:			
ROM			
Flexion (°)	104 ± 5	110 ± 4§	0.297
Extension (°)	7 ± 1	4 ± 1	0.134
KOOS Total	26 ± 4§	17 ± 3§	0.096
KOOS Pain	5 ± 1§	4 ± 1§	0.304
KOOS Function	18 ± 3§	11 ± 2§	0.098
KOOS Movement	3 ± 0.5	2 ± 0.3§	0.063
OKS	27 ± 2	32 ± 2	0.097
EQ5D 3L VAS	67 ± 7	75 ± 4	0.339
FJS	62 ± 4	52 ± 6	0.170

Data represents mean ± SEM
KOOS The Knee Injury and Osteoarthritis Outcomes Score, OKS Oxford Knee Score, EQ5D (3L) EuroQol 5-Dimension 3-Level Assessment, FJS Forgotten Joint Score. p < 0.05 between non-TXA and TXA group; §p < 0.05 compared with preoperative value

Inflammatory status before, during and following surgery

There were no significant differences in baseline plasma inflammatory mediators between non-TXA and TXA patients (Fig. 3). At surgery end and postoperative days 1 and 2, patients that received TXA had significantly higher plasma levels of MCP-1 compared to non-TXA patients (Fig. 3). Area-under-the-curve (AUC) analysis over 3 days supported this finding ($p = 0.013$) (Fig. 4). TNF-α was also significantly higher in TXA patients at each of the time points assessed (Fig. 3), and supported by AUC analysis ($p = 0.010$). IL-6 was significantly higher immediately after surgery and 1.8-times higher than non-TXA group on day 2 postoperative, but did not reach significance. Similarly, IL-8, a chemokine attractant for neutrophils and lymphocytes, and inducible by TNF-α and IL-1β [23], was 1.8 times higher on day 2 ($p = 0.085$) in TXA versus non-TXA patients. Levels of IL-1β, an inflammation amplifier, were also elevated in plasma of TXA patients after the first bone cut and at surgery end (Fig. 3). However, despite a ninefold increase in IL-1β in TXA patients compared to the non-TXA group at day 2 postoperative (Fig. 3) and a threefold higher AUC value (Fig. 4; $p = 0.064$), these differences were not significant. Plasma levels of IL-1RA remained unchanged throughout surgery through to postoperative day 2 (Fig. 3). Plasma IL-4 levels were higher in TXA patients compared to non-TXA patients after the first bone cut and at surgery end, with levels continuing to increase on day 2. The AUC for IL-4 was significantly higher (8 times) for TXA than non-TXA patients ($p = 0.042$, Fig. 4). After surgery, the anti-inflammatory cytokine IL-10 peaked in both patient groups, and then decreased on days 1 and 2, with a trend toward higher values of IL-10 in plasma from non-TXA compared to TXA patients (1.45 to 2.2 times higher) (Fig. 3).

Coagulation parameters
EXTEM

In non-TXA patients after the first bone cut and at surgery end, CT and α-angles were similar to baseline (Table 3), although CFTs fell by ~20% (96 to 76 s) suggesting a slowing of clot elongation (Fig. 2). Clot amplitudes underwent little or no change in non-TXA patients (Fig. 5), as did clot lysis (LI30, LI45 or ML) (Table 3). In direct contrast, TXA led to significant increases in CT after the bone cut and surgery compared to non-TXA patients, with no additional coagulation changes observed (Table 3, Fig. 5).

FIBTEM

Following surgery, TXA led to a significant increase (1.4 times) in FIBTEM CT compared to non-TXA patients ($p = 0.004$) (Table 3). There were no differences in FIBTEM amplitudes at baseline, after bone cut and at surgery end

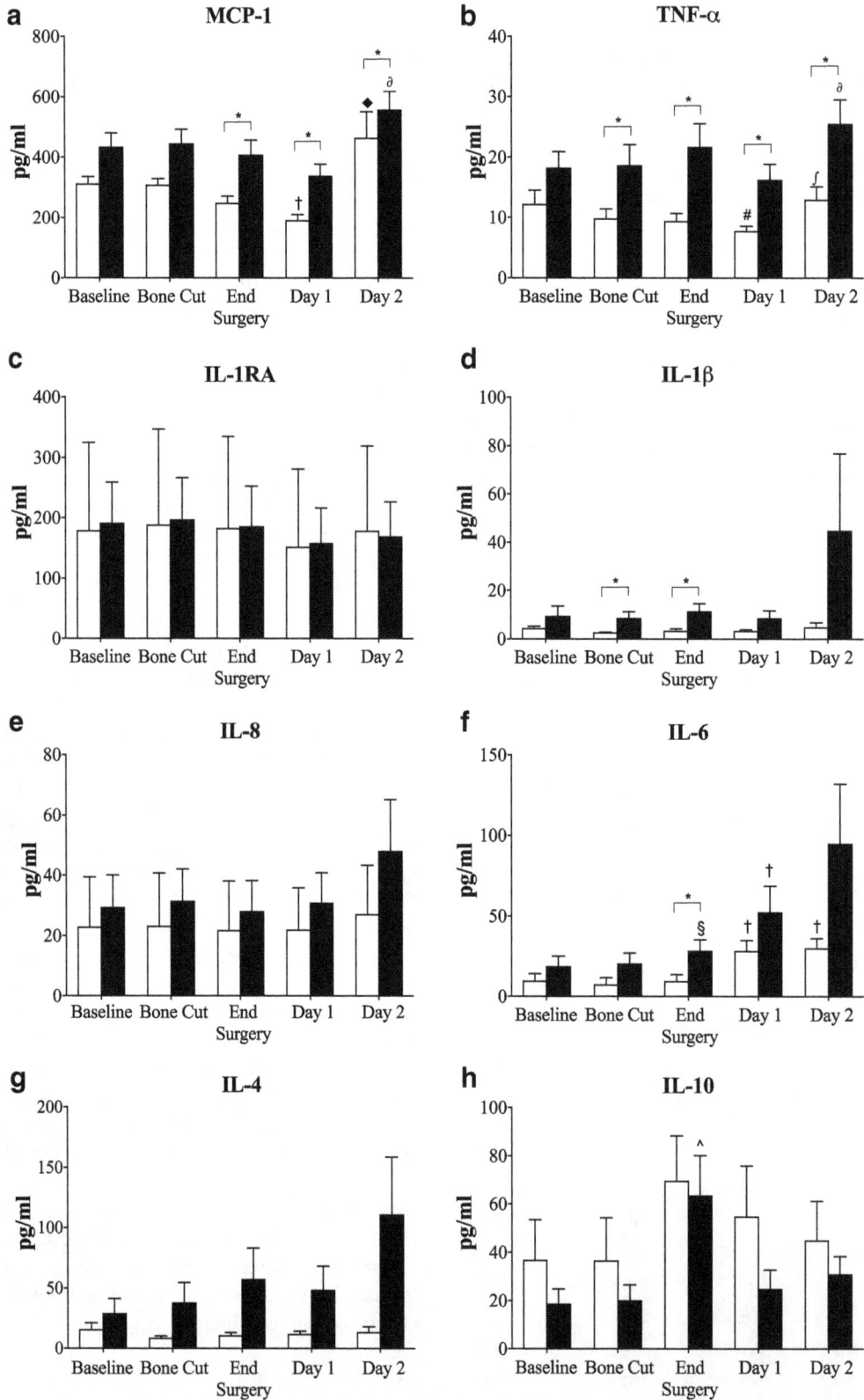

Fig. 3 (See legend on next page.)

(See figure on previous page.)
Fig. 3 Plasma levels of inflammatory cytokine/chemokines **a** MCP-1, **b** TNF-α, **c** IL-1RA, **d** IL-1β, **e** IL-8, **f** IL-6, **g** IL-4, and **h** IL-10 at baseline, after bone cuts, surgery end, day 1 and day 2. White square: non-TXA group; black square: TXA group. Data is expressed as mean ± S.E.M. *$p < 0.05$ compared with corresponding non-TXA patients, $^+p < 0.05$ compared to baseline, bone cut, end surgery and day 1, $^†p < 0.05$ compared to baseline, bone cut and end surgery; $^#p < 0.05$ compared to baseline; $^∫p < 0.05$ compared to end surgery and day 1; $^§p < 0.05$ compared to bone cut; $^∧p < 0.05$ compared to baseline and bone cut

(Fig. 5), indicating that fibrinogen concentration remained unchanged during TKA surgery. TXA also increased maximum lysis following the first bone cut (0.5% to 2.8%, $p = 0.389$) and at surgery end (0.4 to 1.1%. $p = 0.140$); however, these differences were not significant (Table 3).

INTEM

In both TXA and non-TXA patients, CT values were lower than their respective baseline values after the first bone cut or at surgery end, with no statistical difference between groups (Table 3). There were also no differences in clot amplitude at any time point (Fig. 5). Clot lysis was also comparable between the groups and ranged from 4.1 to 6.8%, indicating little or no hyperfibrinolysis.

Discussion

Antifibrinolytics are widely used in orthopaedic surgery to reduce excessive bleeding and minimize transfusion

requirements and re-exploration [5]. In our pilot study in OA patients undergoing TKA, we report:

- Elevated baseline plasma levels of MCP-1 and TNF-α relative to healthy, aged-matched human values, indicating the presence of low-grade systemic inflammation prior to surgery.
- After the first bone cut and surgery end, MCP-1, TNF-α, IL-1β and IL-6 (after surgery) were significantly increased in TXA compared to non-TXA patients, with differences further amplified at postoperative days 1 and 2. TXA appeared to exacerbate the surgical stress inflammatory response.
- EXTEM CT was prolonged in TXA patients after the first bone cut and at surgery end, indicating a thrombin-slowing effect on clot initiation, despite little or no change in clot amplitude or fibrinogen levels.

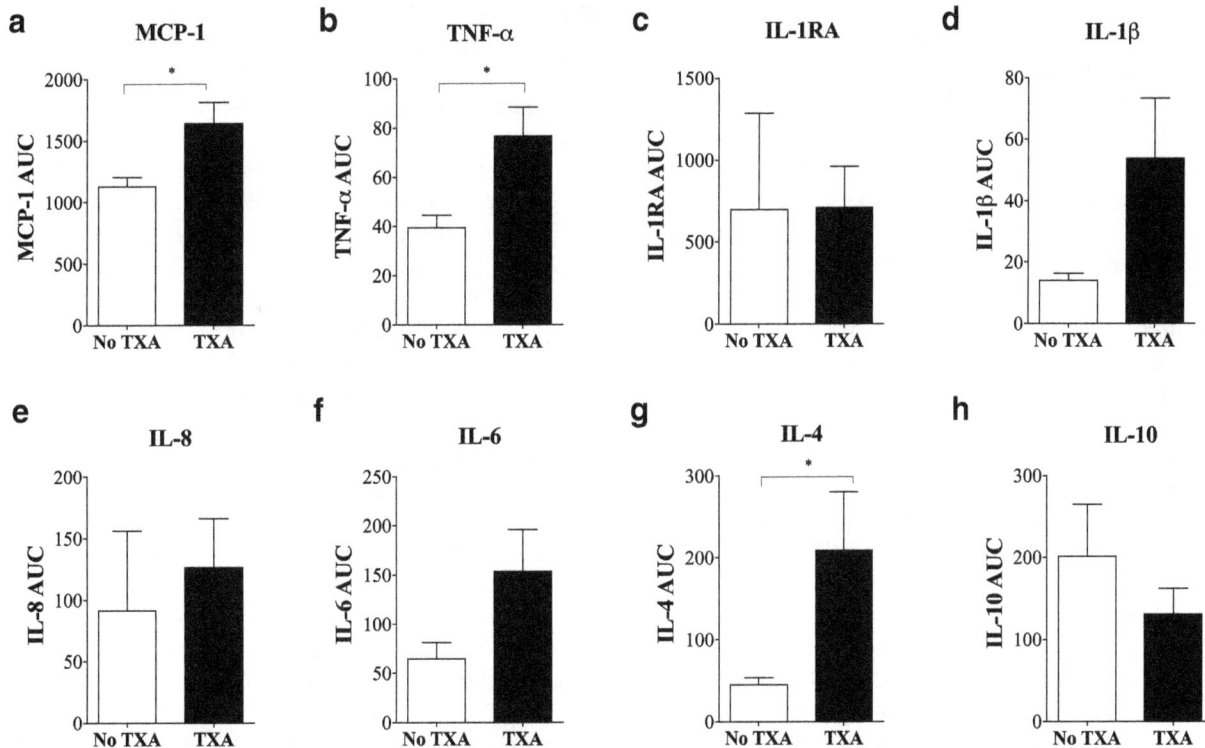

Fig. 4 Area under the curve (AUC) for **a** MCP-1, **b** TNF-α, **c** IL-1RA, **d** IL-1β, **e** IL-8, **f** IL-6, **g** IL-4, and **h** IL-10 based on plasma cytokine levels kinetics from baseline to day 2 postoperative. White square: non-TXA group; black square: TXA group. Data is expressed as mean ± S.E.M. *$p < 0.05$ compared with corresponding non-TXA patients

Table 3 Clot kinetics and lysis parameters for TXA and non-TXA patients at baseline, after bone cut, and end of surgery as measured on EXTEM, FIBTEM and INTEM tests

Test	Group	Time	CT (s)	CFT (s)	Alpha Angle (°)	LI30 (%)	LI45 (%)	ML (%)
EXTEM	Non-TXA	Baseline	59 ± 3	96 ± 2	72 ± 3	100 ± 0	98.1 ± 0.4	3.1 ± 1.0
		Bone Cut	53 ± 1	76 ± 7	76 ± 2*	100 ± 0	97.4 ± 0.5	6.3 ± 0.8*
		Surgery End	51 ± 3	75 ± 7	73 ± 3	100 ± 0	98.7 ± 0.3¥	3.9 ± 0.6¥
	TXA	Baseline	64 ± 4	70 ± 7	76 ± 1	98.8 ± 1.2	95.6 ± 1.9	7.9 ± 1.9
		Bone Cut	59 ± 5	67 ± 6	78 ± 1	99.8 ± 0.3	97.3 ± 0.6	6.5 ± 1.0
		Surgery End	65 ± 3¶	89 ± 14	73 ± 2	100 ± 0	98.3 ± .4	4.4 ± 0.8
FIBTEM	Non-TXA	Baseline	59 ± 6	884 ± 476	76 ± 1	99.1 ± 0.9	99.3 ± 0.7	1.4 ± 1.3
		Bone Cut	53 ± 3	797 ± 604	73 ± 2	100 ± 0	99.9 ± .10	0.5 ± 0.3
		Surgery End	49 ± 2	1483 ± 576	67 ± 7	99.9 ± 0.1	100 ± 0	0.4 ± 0.2
	TXA	Baseline	66 ± 5	1020 ± 480	74 ± 2	100 ± 0	99.5 ± 0.23	1.1 ± 0.4
		Bone Cut	54 ± 4*	403 ± 300	76 ± 1*	98.8 ± 0.7	98.3 ± 1.1	2.8 ± 1.3
		Surgery End	68 ± 5¶	480 ± 301	70 ± 2	99.9 ± 0.1	99.8 ± 0.2	1.1 ± 0.4
INTEM	Non-TXA	Baseline	204 ± 15	104 ± 16	71 ± 2	99.7 ± 0.3	97.7 ± 0.7	4.6 ± 1.0
		Bone Cut	164 ± 10*	71 ± 8*	76 ± 2*	99.7 ± 0.2	96.6 ± 0.5	6.3 ± 0.6
		Surgery End	162 ± 13*	69 ± 10*	73 ± 2	100 ± 0	98.3 ± 0.4	4.1 ± 0.8
	TXA	Baseline	170 ± 11	69 ± 8¶	76 ± 2¶	99.7 ± 0.1	95.9 ± 0.5	6.8 ± 0.8
		Bone Cut	149 ± 8*	65 ± 4	77 ± 1	99.8 ± 0.1	97 ± 0.6*	5.8 ± 0.7
		Surgery End	154 ± 12	101 ± 31	73 ± 4	100 ± 0*	97.9 ± 0.4§	4.8 ± 0.7§

Data represent mean ± SEM. *CT* clot time, *CFT* clot formation time, *LI* lysis index, *ML* maximum lysis. $n = 12$ for TXA group; $n = 11$ for non-TXA group. *$p < 0.05$ compared with baseline; ¥$p < 0.05$ compared with Bone Cut; §$p < 0.05$ compared with baseline and bone cut; ¶$p < 0.05$ compared non-TXA group

- In TXA patients there was a tendency for increased FIBTEM maximum lysis during surgery, a finding that is counter to TXA's antifibrinolytic effect.
- Maximum lysis in EXTEM and INTEM was < 5% and < 7%, respectively during surgery, indicating little or no hyperfibrinolysis, and supported by similar falls in hemoglobin levels (11–19%) on days 1 and 2 postoperative relative to baseline. These data question the need for TXA in this surgical setting.

Low-grade inflammation in OA patients

In chronic OA patients, joint inflammation appears to be expressed systemically as a low-grade inflammatory state [24–29]. We found that baseline levels of plasma MCP-1 (CCL2) were up to four times higher than in aged-matched healthy individuals (95–168 pg/ml) [30, 31], and TNF-α levels almost three times higher than in normal humans (~ 5 pg/ml) [31, 32] (Fig. 3). MCP-1 is a chemokine that regulates recruitment of immune cell traffic from the circulation to sites of inflammation in OA patients [33, 34], and has been implicated in articular cartilage degradation and pain [27, 35]. TNF-α is another potent inflammatory mediator involved in OA progression [36, 37], contributing to cartilage loss through its suppression of collagen and proteoglycan synthesis [24, 36, 38]. Notwithstanding the difficulty of finding aged-matched healthy human data, our data

suggest the OA patients in the current study presented with a low-grade systemic inflammation.

TXA exacerbates inflammation in response to surgical stress

We report significant increases in plasma IL-1β and TNF-α in TXA patients after the first bone cut and at surgery end compared to patients that did not receive TXA (Fig. 3). At the end of surgery, TNF-α and IL-1β continued to increase in TXA patients and were accompanied by significantly higher IL-6 and MCP-1 compared to non-TXA patients (Fig. 3). Although the cytokine increases were small, they indicate a heightened inflammatory state in the TXA patients, and heightened surgical stress response [39–41]. During this early period in knee or hip surgery, Hall and colleagues have confirmed activation of the surgical stress response involving the hypothalamic–pituitary–adrenal (HPA) axis, with concomitant increases in plasma cortisol and catecholamines [42]. In TKA, the stress response is most likely activated from multiple neural, hormonal and metabolic inputs including danger signals (e.g. alarmins) from, soft tissue and bone resection, and firing of afferent nerves, that are detected by resident and circulating immune cells, and the brain respectively [40].

In addition to TXA exacerbating the inflammatory response *during* surgery, another key finding was the

Tranexamic acid is associated with selective increase in inflammatory markers following total knee...

51

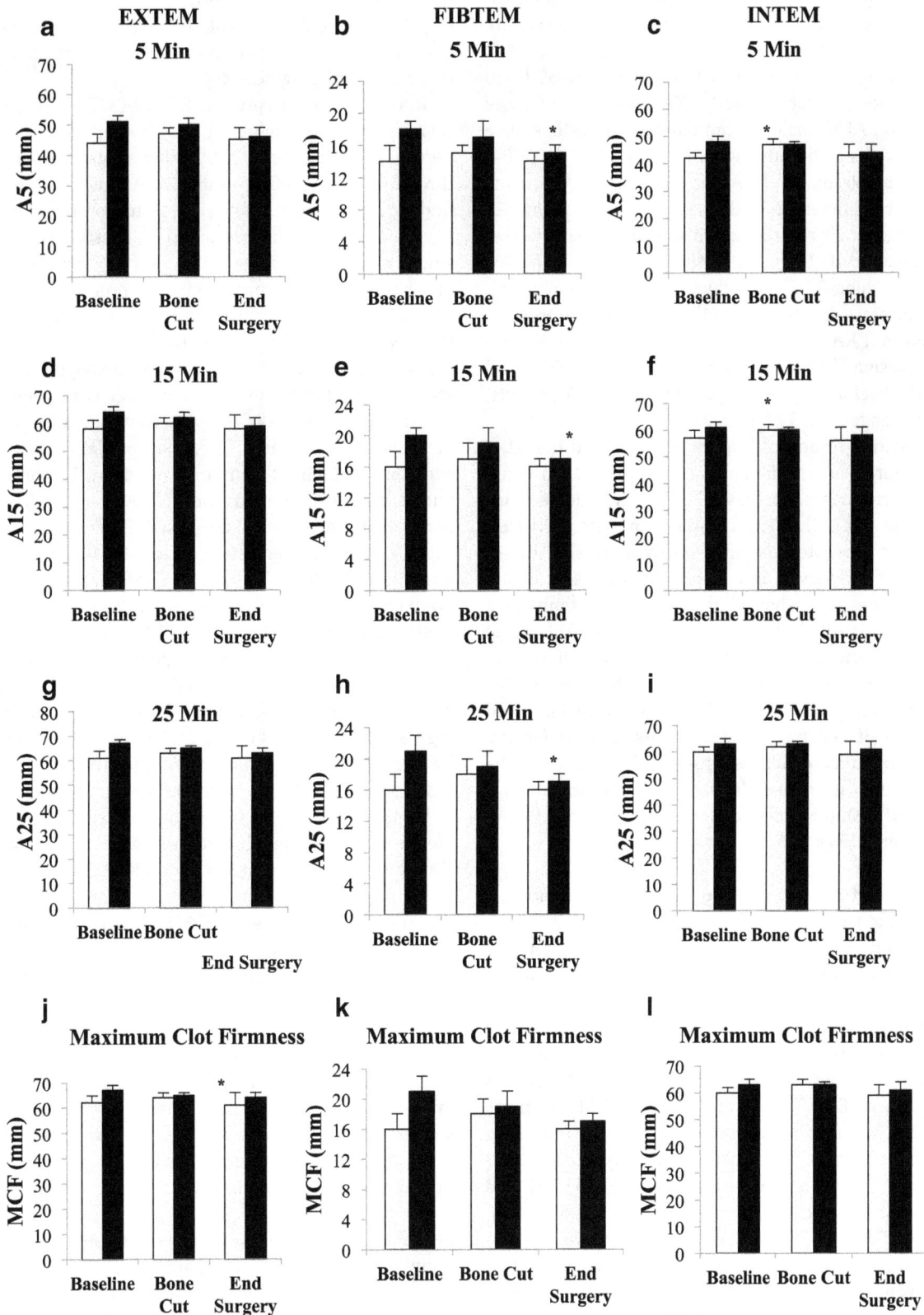

Fig. 5 EXTEM, FIBTEM and INTEM clot amplitudes at 5 (A5, mm), 15 (A15, mm), 25 min (A25, mm) and Maximum Clot Firmness (MCF, mm) at baseline, after bone cuts, surgery end, day 1 and day 2. White square: non-TXA group; black square TXA group. Data expressed as mean ± S.E.M. *p < 0.05 compared to baseline

apparent amplifying effect of TXA on inflammatory cytokine levels over the first two postoperative days (Fig. 3). We found increased concentrations of plasma MCP-1, TNF-α, IL-1β, IL-6, IL-8, and IL-4 and decreased IL-10 levels in patients that received TXA compared to those that did not. AUC analysis from baseline to postoperative day 2 showed significantly higher levels of MCP-1, TNF-α and IL-4 in plasma of TXA than in non-TXA patients (Fig. 4). The differences in IL-4 are of particular interest since it is generally regarded as an anti-inflammatory cytokine, similar to IL-10 and IL-13 [43]. In this role, IL-4 is known to inhibit TNF-α production and IL-1β synthesis and to increase IL-1RA [43, 44]. However, the opposite occurred in TXA patients in our study. At postoperative day 2, plasma TNF-α levels were twofold higher, and IL-1β was fivefold higher compared to non-TXA patients, with no change in IL-1RA (Fig. 2).

Recently, Major and colleagues also reported that IL-4 was not purely an anti-inflammatory cytokine, but could prime macrophages, increase TNF-α and increase inflammation [44]. IL-4, in combination with GM-CSF, can further promote inflammation by increasing differentiation of monocytes into dendritic cells [44]. Bellini and colleagues also showed that IL-4 can stimulate a unique circulating leukocyte subpopulation (0.1–0.5%) of bone marrow-derived stem cells known as fibrocytes that leave the blood and enter the site of healing and differentiate into fibroblasts/myofibroblasts with increased production of cell matrix components, growth factors, and inflammatory cytokines [45–47]. Therefore, in the current study, it is possible that IL-4 contributes to a heightened systemic inflammatory response observed in TXA patients (Figs 3, 4).

TXA prolonged clot times during surgery and had no effect on clot lysis

In our study, baseline ROTEM clotting parameters for OA patients were similar to normal healthy individuals [22, 31, 32, 48]. In contrast to a low-grade inflammatory state at baseline in our OA groups, it appears that there were no apparent coagulation defects. However, after the first bone cut and surgery end, the non-TXA patients had decreased EXTEM, FIBTEM and INTEM clot times (9 to 21% falls relative to baseline) (Table 3), indicating increased thrombin availability. This was further supported by 22 and 34% decreases in EXTEM CFT and INTEM CFT, respectively, with little or no change in α-angles (Table 3). The shift in CT and CFT was associated with no effect on clot amplitude or strength (Fig. 3) but a twofold increase (3.1 to 6.3%) in maximum lysis in EXTEM ($p = 0.021$) and 1.4 times (4.6 to 6.3%) in INTEM after the bone cut (Table 3). Notably, the increases in fibrinolysis in non-TXA patients were within the range of normal values, with 15% often used as a

guide to indicate hyperfibrinolysis [20, 22]. Thus, in non-TXA patients, surgical stress appeared to decrease clot times and thrombin availability without changes in other ROTEM parameters.

However, in TXA patients, EXTEM CT at surgery end was significantly higher (1.3-fold) than non-TXA patients, indicating that TXA during surgical stress has a thrombin-slowing effect (Table 3). We reported a similar finding in cardiac surgery after a sternotomy with TXA having a twofold increase in CT (all tests) [16]. In that study, we speculated that TXA may (1) reduce the rate of prothrombin-thrombin conversion, or (2) inhibit one or more of the polypeptide cleavage reactions, and thereby slow the fibrinogen to fibrin conversion [16]. Interestingly, since TXA is a lysine analogue, reducing the prothrombin-thrombin conversion is possible since the kringle-2 domain of the prothrombin complex is rich in lysine residues, and TXA may partially block these sites thus reducing thrombin production. In contrast to our cardiac surgery study, both TXA and non-TXA patients had significantly decreased INTEM CT during surgery in the current study (Table 3), highlighting differences in TXA with clotting factors or pathway selection. Importantly, and in agreement with our previous study, we found no difference in EXTEM or INTEM clot lysis in TXA and non-TXA patients. This finding suggests that perhaps the beneficial effect of TXA published in a large number of randomized controlled trials involving nearly 1 million patients [10] might not be reflected by the absence of evidence of hyperfibrinolysis with ROTEM (and TEG). In addition, we found no difference in hemoglobin levels between the groups postoperatively (Table 1), suggesting blood loss was similar for both TXA and non-TXA patients after TKA surgery.

TXA paradoxically increases FIBTEM maximum lysis after bone cut and surgery

Another interesting trend observed in the present study was that TXA increased maximum lysis in FIBTEM after the bone cut (5-fold higher) and the end of surgery (~ 3-fold higher) compared to non-TXA patients (Table 3). The FIBTEM test is EXTEM with platelet inhibition (see Fig. 2), and these paradoxical results suggest that TXA weakens, not strengthens, the fibrin network in the absence of platelet contribution. This pro-fibrinolytic effect of TXA was not due to falling levels of fibrinogen because there was no change in FIBTEM amplitudes (Fig. 5). Currently, we do not know the underlying mechanisms for this effect of TXA on maximum lysis. Platelets normally support the formation of a dense, stable fibrin network from αIIbβ3 integrin interactions and the fibrin network [49]. In the absence of platelets, it appears that lysine residues play a role in securing fibrin density and stability in the FIBTEM clot, which is decreased in the presence of TXA. While this observation may be clinically silent under normal hematological conditions, it has the potential to become a significant problem in major surgery or various trauma states, where platelet numbers may decrease or platelet activation is impaired numbers or function.

Potential clinical significance: a call for precision-based medicine

An important finding in the present study was that there appeared to be no clinical advantage of using TXA in our patient group undergoing elective TKA. Without evidence of hyperfibrinolysis (Table 3), there is no clinical justification for TXA use because there is no excessive bleeding [4]. In addition, TXA administration appeared to have a potentially untoward pro-inflammatory effect during and after surgery, which may be linked to a more pronounced TXA-induced stress response to the trauma of surgery. This may be clinically significant since Galvez and colleagues recently demonstrated that patients with OA already have a diminished ability to tolerate surgical stress [29], which the authors associated with a pre-existing low-grade chronic systemic inflammation [40, 42]. Our study further underscores a number of outstanding questions on TXA use in major surgery: (1) Would a single dose administration of TXA have less effect to increase inflammation and stress response to surgery? (2) What laboratory tests should be used to drive TXA use in elective or emergency surgery? and (3) What is the scientific basis for using TXA in orthopaedic surgery? In our view, *TXA should not be viewed as a one-size-fits-all approach to elective surgery*; rather it should be incorporated into a more precision-based set of guidelines [4, 50, 51]. The potential harmful effects of TXA on promoting inflammation warrant further investigation.

Limitations of the study

A major limitation of our pilot study was its lack of randomization, blinding and small patient numbers. Our postoperative period was also limited and requires extension beyond day 2 when joint swelling is at a maximum, and 10–14 days when adhesions begin to form. Given surgically induced inflammation is also linked to postoperative pain and fragmented sleep patterns following TKA [42, 52, 53], these additional metrics should be included in future studies. Another limitation was that we did not measure plasma stress hormones, which may be higher in patients with higher inflammatory status during and following surgical stress [39–42]. We also do not know the effect of the cocktail components that were injected around the knee after the bone cut on TXA's effect to change some ROTEM parameters and/or inflammatory markers. In vitro studies are also required

to examine TXA's effect on fibrinogen with and without platelets, and role of lysine residues using rapid-kinetic monitoring, X-ray crystallography, nuclear magnetic resonance and electron microscopy techniques. Notwithstanding these limitations, our study provides a springboard for a larger prospective, randomized trial to further elucidate the effects of TXA on inflammation and the surgical stress response to TKA, the outcomes of which may have implications for other pediatric and adult elective and emergency surgeries.

Conclusions

In moderate-to-severe OA patients, TXA led to prolongation of EXTEM CT after the first bone cut and end of surgery compared to non-TXA patients, despite little or no change in clot strength or fibrinogen levels. Maximum lysis in EXTEM and INTEM was < 10% in both TXA and non-TXA patients, indicating little or no hyperfibrinolysis and thus questioning the need for TXA in our patient group. TXA was also associated with increased systemic inflammation, with rising plasma levels of proinflammatory cytokines in the first 2 days after TKA surgery.

Abbreviations

IL-4: Interleukin 4; A10: Clot amplitude after 10 min; IL-1RA: Interleukin-1 receptor antagonist; CFT: Clot formation time; CT: Clot time; EXTEM: Extrinsically activated test with tissue factor; FIBTEM: Fibrin-based EXTEM with platelet inhibition; IL-1: Interleukin 1 beta; IL-10: Interleukin 10; IL-6: Interleukin 6; IL-8: Interleukin 8; INTEM: Intrinsically activated test using ellagic acid; LI: Lysis index; MCF: Maximum Clot Firmness; MCP-1: Monocyte chemoattractant protein-1; ML: Maximum lysis; ROTEM: Rotational Thromboelastometry; TKA: Total knee arthroplasty; TNF-α: Tumor necrosis factor alpha; tPA: Tissue plasminogen activator; TXA: Tranexamic acid; uPA: Urokinase plasminogen activator

Acknowledgements

We would like to thank Dr. De Wet Potgieter for assistance with ROTEM and thank College of Medicine and Dentistry, James Cook University (JCU), and the Mater Hospital, Townsville, for internal funding that supported the study. We also thank Ms. Regina Hanson, Mrs. Alicia Harris and Ms. Anna Grimley for their coordination of patient recruitment for the study. We are grateful to Ms. Shannon McEwen, Dr. Varaguna Manoharan, Dr. Ryan Bishal-Faruque and Dr. Genevieve Graw for their assistance with sample collection.

Funding

The study received no specific funding from external agencies in the public, commercial or not-for-profit sectors. The study was supported by internal funds from the Orthopaedic Research Institute of Queensland to ALG and the College of Medicine and Dentistry. The support or funding bodies had no involvement in study design; in the collection, analysis, and interpretation of data; in the writing of the report; or in the decision to submit the paper for publication.

Authors' contributions

AG, HL and JM carried out the ROTEM measurements and data collection. GD and HL conceived the study, and participated in its design and coordination. GD drafted the manuscript. JM and HL carried out the cytokine analysis. PM, KH and MW carried out the surgery and participated in the study design. AG and HL performed the statistical analysis. All authors read and approved the final manuscript.

Competing interests

The authors declare that they have no competing interests.

Author details

[1]The Orthopaedic Research Institute of Queensland (ORIQL), 7 Turner St, Pimlico, Townsville, Queensland 4812, Australia. [2]Heart, Trauma and Sepsis Research Laboratory, College of Medicine and Dentistry, James Cook University, 1 James Cook Drive, Townsville, Queensland 4811, Australia.

References

1. Carling MS, Jeppsson A, Eriksson BI, Brisby I. Transfusions and blood loss in total hip and knee arthroplasty: a prospective observational study. J Orthop Surg and Res. 2015;10:48.
2. Leitner L, Musser E, Kastner N, Friesenbichler J, Hirzberger D, et al. Impact of preoperative antithrombotic therapy on blood management after implantation of primary total knee arthroplasty. Sci Rep. 2016;6:1–5.
3. Walsh M, Shreve J, Thomas S, Moore E, Moore H, et al. Fibrinolysis in trauma: "myth," "reality," or "something in between". Semin Thromb Hemost. 2017;43:200–12.
4. Dobson GP, Doma K, Letson H. Clinical relevance of a p-value: Does TXA save lives after trauma or post-partum hemorrhage? J Trauma Acute Care Surg. 2018;84(3):532–6.
5. Walterscheid Z, O'Neill C, Carmouche J. Tranexamic acid in adult elective orthopaedic and complex spinal surgery: a review. Surg Rehabil. 2017;1:1–4.
6. Dunn CJ, Goa KL. Tranexamic acid: a review of its use in surgery and other indications. Drugs. 1999;57:1005–32.
7. Tanaka N, Sakahashi H, Sato E, Hirose K, Ishima T, et al. Timing of the administration of tranexamic acid for maximum reduction in blood loss in arthroplasty of the knee. J Bone Joint Surg Br. 2001;83:702–5.
8. Lin ZX, Woolf SK. Safety, efficacy, and cost-effectiveness of tranexamic acid in orthopedic surgery. Orthopedics. 2016;39:119–30.
9. Pabinger I, Fries D, Schöchl H, Streif W, Toller W. Tranexamic acid for treatment and prophylaxis of bleeding and hyperfibrinolysis. Wien Klin Wochenschr. 2017;129:303–16.
10. Poeran J, Rasul R, Suzuki S, Danninger T, Mazumdar M, et al. Tranexamic acid use and postoperative outcomes in patients undergoing total hip or knee arthroplasty in the United States: retrospective analysis of effectiveness and safety. BMJ. 2014;349:g4829.
11. Danninger T. Memtsoudis SG Tranexamic acid and orthopedic surgery—the search for the holy grail of blood conservation. Ann Transl Med. 2015;3:77.
12. Binz S, McCollester J, Thomas S, Miller J, Pohlman T, et al. CRASH-2 study of tranexamic acid to treat bleeding in trauma patients: a controversy fueled by science and social media. J Blood Transfus. 2015;2015:874920.
13. Draxler DF, Sashindranath M, Metcalf RL. Plasmin: a modulator of immune function. Semin Thromb Hemost. 2017;43:143–53.
14. Lanouette S, Mongeon V, Figeys D, Couture J-F. The functional diversity of protein lysine methylation. Mol Syst Biol. 2014;10:724.
15. Medcalf RL. The traumatic side of fibrinolysis. Blood. 2015;125:2457–8.
16. Sharma R, Letson HL, Smith S, Dobson GP. Tranexamic acid leads to paradoxical coagulation changes during cardiac surgery: a pilot rotational thromboelastometry study. J Surg Res. 2017;217:100–12.
17. Jimenez JJ, Iribarren JL, Lorente L, Rodriguez JM, Hernandez D, et al. Tranexamic acid attenuates inflammatory response in cardiopulmonary bypass surgery through blockade of fibrinolysis: a case control study followed by a randomized double-blind controlled trial. Crit Care. 2008;11:R117.
18. Robertshaw HJ. An anti-inflammatory role for tranexamic acid in cardiac surgery? Crit Care. 2008;12:105.
19. Fay WF. Linking inflammation and thrombosis: role of C-reactive protein. World J Cardiol. 2010;26:365–9.
20. Letson HL, Dobson GP. Correction of acute traumatic coagulopathy with small-volume 7.5% NaCl adenosine, lidocaine and Mg2+ (ALM) occurs within 5 min: a ROTEM analysis. J Trauma Acute Care Surg. 2015;78:773–83.
21. Solomon C, Ranucci M, Hochleitner G, Schöchl H, Schlimp CJ. Assessing the methodology for calculating platelet contribution to clot strength (platelet component) in thromboelastometry and thrombelastography. Anesth Analg. 2015;121:868–78.
22. Lang T, Bauters A, Braun S, Pötzsch B, von Pape K, et al. Multi-Centre investigation on reference ranges for ROTEM thromboelastometry. Blood Coagul Fibrinolysis. 2005;16:301–10.
23. Pierzchala AW, Kusz DJ, Hajduk G. CXCL8 and CCL5 expression in synovial fluid and blood serum in patients with osteoarthritis of the knee. Arch Immunol Ther Exp. 2011;59:151–5.
24. Kapoor M, Martel-Pelletier J, Lajeunesse D, Pelletier JP, Fahmi H. Role of proinflammatory cytokines in the pathophysiology of osteoarthritis. Nat Rev Rheumatol. 2011;7:33–42.
25. Denoble AE, Huffman KM, Stabler TV, Kelly SJ, Hershfield MS, et al. Uric acid is a danger signal of increasing risk for osteoarthritis through inflammasome activation. Proc Natl Acad Sci U S A. 2011;108:2088–93.
26. Rainbow R, Ren W, Zeng L. Inflammation and joint tissue interactions in OA: implications for potential therapeutic approaches. Arthritis. 2012;2012:741582.
27. Scanzello CR, Goldring SR. The role of synovitis in osteoarthritis pathogenesis. Bone. 2012;51:249–57.
28. Attur M, Statnikov A, Samuels J, Li Z, Alekseyenko AV, et al. Plasma levels of interleukin-1 receptor antagonist (IL1Ra) predict radiographic progression of symptomatic knee osteoarthritis. Osteoarthr Cartil. 2015;23:1915–24.
29. Galvez I, Torres-Piles S, Hinchado MD, Alvarez-Barrientos A, Torralbo-Jimenez P, et al. Immune-neuroendocrine dysregulation in patients with osteoarthritis: a revision and a pilot study. Endocr Metab Immune Disord Drug Targets. 2017;17:78–85.
30. Mariani E, Cattini L, Neri S, Malavolta M, Mocchegiani E, et al. Simultaneous evaluation of circulating chemokine and cytokine profiles in elderly subjects by multiplex technology: relationship with zinc status. Biogerontology. 2006;7:449–59.
31. Kim HO, Kim HS, Youn JC, Shin EC, Park S. Serum cytokine profiles in healthy young and elderly population assessed using multiplexed bead-based immunoassays. J Transl Med. 2011;9:113.
32. Stowe RP, Peek MK, Cutchin MP, Goodwin JS. Plasma cytokine levels in a population-based study: relation to age and ethnicity. J Gerontol A Biol Sci Med Sci. 2010;65:429–33.
33. Deshmane SL, Kremlev S, Amini S, Sawaya BE. Monocyte chemoattractant protein-1 (MCP-1): an overview. J Interf Cytokine Res. 2009;29:313–26.
34. Xu Y-K, Ke Y, Lin J-H. The role of MCP-1-CCR2 ligand-receptor axis in chondrocyte degradation and disease progress in knee osteoarthritis. Biol Res. 2015;48:64.
35. Harris Q, Seto J, O'Brien K, Lee PS, Kondo C, et al. Monocyte chemotactic protein-1 inhibits chondrogenesis of synovial mesenchymal progenitor cells: an in vitro study. Stem Cells. 2013;31:2253–65.
36. Lee AS, Ellman MB, Yan D, Kroin JS, Cole BJ, et al. A current review of molecular mechanisms regarding osteoarthritis and pain. Gene. 2013;527:440–7.
37. Larsson S, Englund M, Struglics A, Lohmander LS. Interleukin-6 and tumor necrosis factor alpha in synovial fluid are associated with progression of radiographic knee osteoarthritis in subjects with previous meniscectomy. Osteoarthr Cartil. 2015;23:1906–14.
38. Silvestri T, Pulsatelli L, Dolzani P, Frizziero L, Facchini A, et al. In vivo expression of inflammatory cytokine receptors in the joint compartments of patients with arthritis. Rheumatol Int. 2006;26:360–8.
39. Weledji EP. Cytokines and postoperative hyperglycaemia: from Claude Bernard to enhanced recovery after surgery. Int J Surg Res. 2014;3:1–6.
40. Dobson GP. Addressing the global burden of trauma in major surgery. Front Surg. 2015;2:43.
41. Aasvang EK, Luna IE, Kehlet H. Challenges in postdischarge function and recovery: the case of fast-track hip and knee arthroplasty. Brit J Anaesth. 2015;115:861–6.
42. Hall GM, Peerbhoy D, Shenkin A, Parker CJ, ., Salmon P Hip and knee arthroplasty: a comparison and the endocrine, metabolic and inflammatory responses. Clin Sci (Lond) 2000:98:71–79.

43. Fernandes JC, Martel-Pelletier J, Pelletier JP. The role of cytokines in osteoarthritis pathophysiology. Biorheology. 2002;39:237–46.

44. Major J, Fletcher JE, Hamilton TA. IL-4 pretreatment selectively enhances cytokine and chemokine production in lipopolysaccharide-stimulated mouse peritoneal macrophages. J Immunol. 2002;168:2456–63.

45. Bellini A, Marini MA, Bianchetti L, Barczyk M, Schmidt M, et al. Interleukin (IL)-4, IL-13, and IL-17A differentially affect the profibrotic and proinflammatory functions of fibrocytes from asthmatic patients. Mucosal Immunol. 2012;5:140–9.

46. Abe R, Donnelly SC, Peng T, Bucala R, Metz CN. Peripheral blood fibrocytes: differentiation pathway and migration to wound sites. J Immunol. 2001;15: 7556–62.

47. Chen D, Zhao Y, Li Z, Shou K, Zheng X, et al. Circulating fibrocyte mobilization in negative pressure wound therapy. J Cell Mol Med. 2017;21: 1513–22.

48. Spiezia L, Bertini D, Boldrin M, Radu C, Bulato C, et al. Reference values for thromboelastometry (ROTEM®) in cynomolgus monkeys (Macaca fascicularis). Thromb Res. 2010;126:e294–7.

49. Wolberg AS. Plasma and cellular contributions to fibrin network formation, structure and stability. Haemophilia. 2010;16:7–12.

50. Letson HL, Dobson GP. Tranexamic acid for post-partum haemorrhage in the WOMAN trial. Lancet. 2017;390:1581–2.

51. Maslove DM, Lamontagne F, Marshall JC, Heyland DK. A path to precision in the ICU. Crit Care. 2017;21:79.

52. Miller RE, Miller RJ, Malfait A-M. Osteoarthritis joint pain: the cytokine connection. Cytokine. 2014;70:185–93.

53. Grosu I, Lavand'homme P, Thienpont E. Pain after knee arthroplasty: an unresolved issue. Knee Surg Sports Traumatol Arthrosc. 2014;22:1744–58.

7

Delayed total hip arthroplasty after failed treatment of acetabular fractures: an 8- to 17-year follow-up study

Tao Wang[1], Jun-Ying Sun[2*], Jun-Jun Zha[2], Chao Wang[2] and Xi-Jiang Zhao[1*]

Abstract

Background: Delayed total hip arthroplasty (THA) is a reliable procedure following failed treatment of acetabular fractures. The aim of the present study was to evaluate the influence of the type of fracture treatment and modern ceramic bearing on the clinical outcomes of delayed THA.

Methods: Between January 1997 and January 2008, 33 patients (33 hips) underwent cementless THA after failed acetabular fractures. Twenty-one were initially treated by open reduction internal fixation (ORIF) and 12 had non-ORIF. Joint articulation was either conventional metal-on-polyethylene (MOP) or ceramic-on-ceramic (COC). Intraoperative measures and preoperative and follow-up clinical, radiological, and functional outcomes were compared between the ORIF and non-ORIF groups.

Results: Surgery duration, blood loss, and transfusion requirement were greater in the ORIF group than in the non-ORIF group ($p < 0.05$). Significant improvement in Harris Hip Scores was seen post-surgery in both groups. However, a significant difference in the mean Harris Hip Score was not observed between the two groups ($p = 0.57$). Six patients in the ORIF group required acetabular reconstructive procedures to address bony defects compared to seven patients in the non-ORIF group ($p = 0.09$). The rate of anatomical restoration was 58.3% (7/12) in the non-ORIF group and 42.9% (9/21) in the ORIF group ($p = 0.12$). Radiolucent lines were observed in the MOP group and none in the COC group. Overall survival rate was similar in both groups ($p = 0.85$): 89.3% in the ORIF group and 87.5% in the non-ORIF group.

Conclusion: Delayed THA with previous acetabular fractures is a challenging procedure. Initial fracture treatment does not influence the outcome of delayed THA, and modern ceramic bearing has promising results in the long-term follow-up.

Keywords: Acetabular fracture, Total hip arthroplasty, Cementless cup, Ceramic-on-ceramic

Background

Acetabular fractures are serious injuries which can lead to progressive impairment of hip function [1]. Anatomic reduction with rigid internal fixation of the acetabulum has been shown to restore hip function and prevent long-term complications. Unfortunately, many patients with fractures of the acetabulum still suffer posttraumatic arthritis or femoral head necrosis regardless of whether operative or non-operative intervention was chosen as the initial treatment. These irreparable complications may occur as a result of residual articular incongruity, early articular cartilage

* Correspondence: sunjunyingsuda@163.com; ouyang520@jiangnan.edu.cn
[1]Department of Orthopedic Surgery, Affiliated Hospital of Jiangnan University, 200 Huihe Rd, Wuxi 214062, Jiangsu, China
[2]Department of Orthopedic Surgery, The First Affiliated Hospital of Soochow University, 188 Shizi Street, Suzhou 215006, Jiangsu, China

damage, inaccurate placement of implant fixation, and disruption of femoral head blood provision. Even when near-anatomic reductions are achieved, the reported incidence of posttraumatic arthritis has been varied between 27 and 37% [2], with the incidence of subsequent total hip arthroplasty (THA) ranging from 8 to 23% [2–4].

When posttraumatic arthritis and femoral head necrosis occur, THA is a rational salvage procedure. Retained internal fixation implants, scar tissue, and residual acetabulum bone defects cause subsequent THAs to be more complex than routine THA [5, 6]. Moreover, the results of these THAs presented to be inferior to THA performed after primary osteoarthritis [7–9], attributable to the extent of loss of bone stock and abnormal anatomy after trauma [9–11]. Therefore, some authors recommended that initial open reduction internal fixation (ORIF) is essential to restore the bony anatomy for subsequent THA, decreasing its complexity and improving component survival [12–14]. Conversely, others have postulated that initial ORIF increases the rate of infection, blood loss, and surgery time [6, 15]. Furthermore, there is no explicit evidence that ORIF improves the success rate of subsequent THA [16].

Additionally, patients with acetabular fractures are generally young and have posttraumatic osteoarthritis that results from a high activity level. A series reports high failure rates of subsequent THA, which have been attributed to younger age and increased activity [9, 11]. Therefore, in those patients, alternative bearing surfaces should reduce polyethylene wear and osteolysis that have been present in previous studies using traditional metal-on-polyethylene (MOP). Recently, modern ceramic-on-ceramic (COC) THA has demonstrated decreased risk of wear-induced osteolysis over MOP and then improved the long-term outcomes of THA [17, 18].

Therefore, the primary aim of the present study was to evaluate the influence of the mode of treatment of fracture, conservative treatment or ORIF, on the clinical outcomes of salvage THA. The secondary aim was to evaluate the long-term results associated with modern COC THA after failed acetabular fractures.

Methods

All patients who underwent THA for posttraumatic osteoarthritis or femoral head necrosis due to acetabular fractures during the period from January 1997 to January 2008 were eligible for inclusion in this study. Exclusion criteria were incomplete radiographic or clinical date and without adequate follow-up. Two patients (2 hips) had died of causes unrelated to surgery. Five patients (5 hips) were lost to follow-up. Thus, 33 remaining patients (33 hips) were available for review. Patient demographics and characteristics of the fractures are summarized in Table 1. This study was approved by our institutional review board.

Surgical technique and implants

Delayed THA was performed through a posterior approach in 25 hips, and a modified Hardinge approach in 8 hips. The acetabulum was prepared for routine primary THA. Retained hardware or heterotopic bone was not routinely removed unless it interfered with reaming and placement of the cup. Acetabular bone deficiency was classified based on American Academy of Orthopedic Surgeons (AAOS) classifications [19]. We adopted impaction bone grafting (IBG) combined with a cementless cup to address acetabular bone defects with segments of bone or morselized cancellous bone taken from the resected femoral head. Cementless acetabular fixation was used in all cases using a press-fit technique. If the initial press-fit fixation did

Table 1 Patient demographics and fracture features

Gender	
Male/female	21/12
Mean age (years)	45.1 ± 9.3 (range, 25–68)
Mean body mass index (kg/m^2)	23.5 ± 2.9 (range, 17.0–32.9)
Interval time between fracture and THA (month)	58 (range, 4–240)
Preoperative diagnosis	
Posttraumatic osteoarthritis	23
Femoral head necrosis	10
Fracture patterns	
Simple factures	
Posterior column	4
Posterior wall	7
Anterior column	2
Anterior wall	0
Transverse	3
Complex fractures	
Posterior wall + posterior column	3
Transverse + posterior wall	6
Both column	4
T-shaped	2
Anterior column + posterior hemitransverse	3
Fracture treatment	
ORIF	21
Non-ORIF	12

not provide sufficient cup stability, additional screw fixation was conducted. Joint articulation was either MOP or COC. MOP was used in 12 hips. A Synergy stem and Reflection acetabular cup (Smith & Nephew, USA) were used in six hips, a Self-Locking stem and SPH cup (Lima, Italy) was used in four hips, and a Bi-Metric stem and Universal cup (Biomet, USA) in two hips. COC was used in 21 hips, in which a C2 stem and "Sandwich" cup (Lima, Italy) was used in five hips, an F2L stem and "Sandwich" cup (Lima, Italy) in four hips, and an S-ROM stem and Duraloc cup (Depuy, USA) in 12 hips.

Perioperative regimen

Patients received antibiotic prophylaxis at 0.5 h before surgery and within the first 24 h postoperatively. Low-molecular-weight heparin was routinely administered for preventing thromboembolism. No patient received prophylaxis against heterotopic ossification. All patients were allowed to do quadriceps strengthening exercises and passive movements following surgery. Patients that had received a bone graft were instructed to restrict movement to touch-down weight-bearing for 6 weeks then gradually increase this to full weight-bearing thereafter.

Clinical and radiographic evaluation

Clinical and radiographic examinations were performed at 6 weeks, 6 months, 1 year, and annually thereafter. Hip function was assessed using the Harris Hip Score (HHS) [20]. All plain radiographs qualified for evaluation of biomechanical reconstruction are shown in Fig. 1. Linear polyethylene wear was measured using the method of Pollock et al. [21] using Digimizer software. Radiolucent lines and osteolysis were evaluated on postoperative serial radiographs according to the method of DeLee and Charnley [22] and Gruen et al. [23] for the acetabulum and femur, respectively. Bony ingrowth was described according to the criteria of Engh et al. [24]. Heterotopic ossification was classified according to the system of Brooker et al. [25].

Statistical methods

Statistical analyses were performed using SPSS v19.0 (SPSS, USA) statistical software. All data were expressed as mean ± standard deviation (SD) and were tested for equal variance using the Levene test. Categorical variables were evaluated using a chi-square test or Fisher's exact test for statistical significance. Continuous variables were assessed using a Student t test. The level of significance was set at $p < 0.05$. Survivorship analysis of reconstructions was assessed by the Kaplan–Meier. The endpoint was defined as a revision for any reason or definite radiographic signs of loosening.

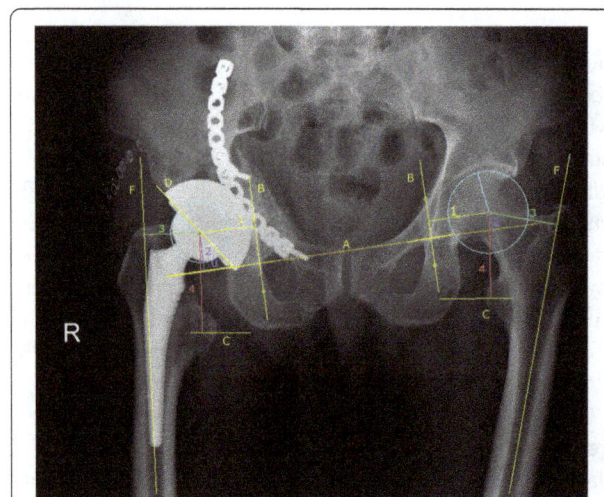

Fig. 1 Postoperative radiograph after THA with impacting bone grafting combined with a cementless cup. A, horizontal teardrop line; B, vertical teardrop line; C, midline lesser trochanter; D, a line along the lateral surface of the acetabular component; F, femoral shaft line. 1, horizontal hip center of rotation; 2, vertical hip center of rotation; 3, horizontal femoral offset; 4 vertical femoral offset; a, the angle between a line drawn between line A and line D

Results
Clinical outcomes

Mean follow-up time was 11.5 ± 3.0 years (range, 8–17 years) after primary THA. The mean duration between initial fracture and requirement for subsequent arthroplasty was not significantly different between the ORIF group and the non-ORIF group (52.8 months vs 62.4 months). Union was achieved in all fractures in the ORIF group, but four (33.3%) non-unions were in the non-ORIF group. For subsequent THA, the non-union fractures were treated with rigid internal fixation and bone grafting. In the ORIF group, the retained hardware was removed either in part or in its entirety in four patients (4/21) who had undergone prior ORIF of acetabular fractures. Six patients (6/21) in the ORIF group required acetabular reconstruction to address bony defects compared to seven patients (7/12) in the non-ORIF group, although the difference was not statistically significant ($p = 0.09$). The comparison revealed that longer surgery occurred in the ORIF group (189 min for ORIF vs 143 min for non-ORIF, $p = 0.02$) and greater blood loss (1289 ml for ORIF vs 750 ml for non-ORIF, $p < 0.01$). Differences in the average perioperative transfusion requirements were also found (6.6 units for ORIF vs 3.5 units for non-ORIF, $p < 0.01$) (Table 2).

Mean HHS improved across all patients from 44.0 ± 11.9 points (range, 27–58 points) preoperatively to 88.6 ± 5.1 points (range, 74–94 points) at the final follow-up. Excellent scores were observed in 24 hips, good in 7, and fair in 2. In the ORIF group, mean HHS increased from 45.9 ± 12.1 points (range, 27–58 points) to 89.0 ± 5.4 points (range, 74–94 points) ($p < 0.05$). In the non-ORIF patients, it improved from 40.8 ± 11.3 points (range, 29–58 points) to 87.9 ± 4.8 points (range, 79–94 points) ($p < 0.05$). However, difference in the mean HHS at final follow-up was not observed between the two groups ($p = 0.57$) (Table 2).

Radiographic results

Mean abduction angle was 33.8° ± 8.5° (range, 16–54°). At the final radiographic follow-up, surviving implants showed radiographic evidence of stable bony ingrowth (Fig. 2). All bone grafts united with the host bone, without any graft resorption observed. No acetabular component loosening was observed in either group. In the ORIF group, two acetabular revisions were performed due to infection and a ceramic liner fracture. In the non-ORIF group, one patient had ceramic liner fracture and underwent acetabular revision. Failure defined as revision of the acetabular component for any reason, the Kaplan–Meier survivorship of the prostheses was 88.9% (95% CI 76.9~100%). Moreover, overall survival rate was similar in both groups ($p = 0.85$): 89.3% in the ORIF group and 87.5% in the non-ORIF group (Fig. 3).

The impact of THA on biomechanical reconstruction parameters observed in the contralateral hip is shown in

Table 2 Perioperative data for ORIF and non-ORIF groups

Variable	ORIF group	Non-ORIF group	p value
Sex (M/F)	13/8	8/4	0.78
Age at THA (years)	44.9 ± 10.5	45.5 ± 7.2	0.86
Interval time between fracture and THA (months)	52.8 ± 12	62.4 ± 20	0.09
Bone defects	6	7	0.09
Fracture pattern			
Simple/complex	8/13	7/5	0.26
Harris hip score			
Preoperative	45.9 ± 12.1	40.8 ± 11.3	0.24
At last follow-up	89.0 ± 5.4	87.9 ± 4.8	0.57
Surgery duration (min)	189 ± 57	143 ± 32	0.02
Blood loss (ml)	1289 ± 429	750 ± 145	0.00
Perioperative transfusion requirements (u)	6.6	3.5	0.00

M male, *F* female

Mean ± SD

Table 3, although there were no significant differences between the non-ORIF and ORIF groups. Among the 33 patients, reconstructed hip center within 20 mm of vertical and horizontal symmetry happened in 27 patients compared with the contralateral hip, including 16 patients (7 non-ORIF vs 9 ORIF) with anatomical restoration and 11 patients (5 non-ORIF vs 6 ORIF) with a reconstructed hip center within 10–20 mm of vertical and horizontal symmetry. The remaining six patients, who were all in the ORIF group, had a reconstructed hip center more than 20 mm beyond vertical or horizontal symmetry, or both. Therefore, the rate of anatomical restoration was 58.3% (7/

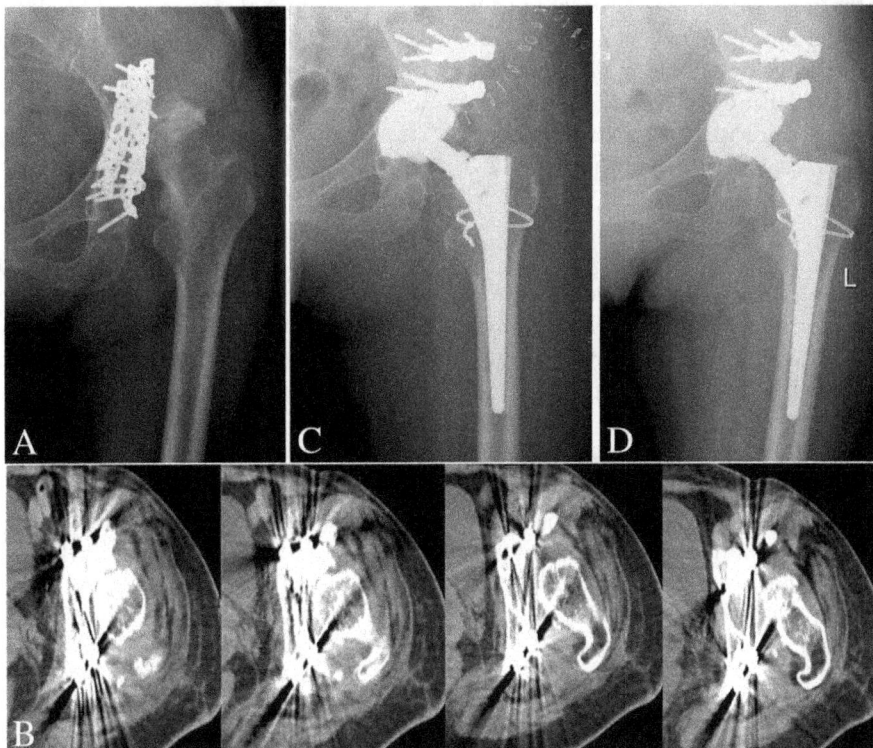

Fig. 2 Delayed total hip arthroplasty (THA) in a 51-year-old woman with posttraumatic arthritis secondary to acetabular fracture. **a** Preoperative radiograph. **b** Computed tomographic scans of the hip revealed the posterior acetabular wall defect. **c** Immediate postoperative X-ray after acetabular reconstruction with the structure bone graft combined with cementless cup. **d** A 15 years' follow-up X-ray showed the graft had completely united and no loosening or osteolysis around the acetabular or femoral component

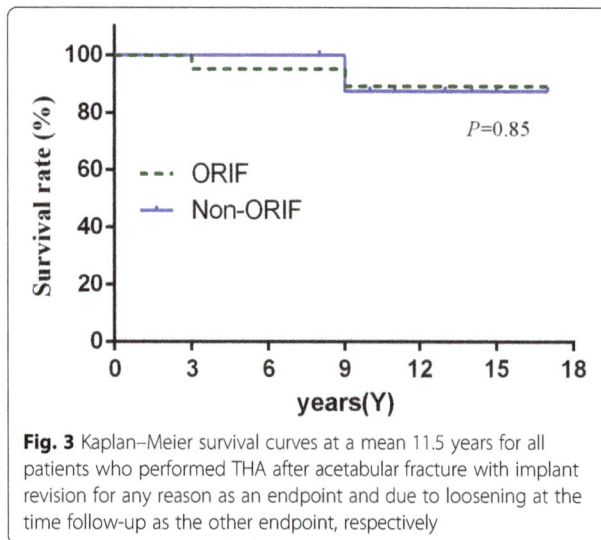

Fig. 3 Kaplan–Meier survival curves at a mean 11.5 years for all patients who performed THA after acetabular fracture with implant revision for any reason as an endpoint and due to loosening at the time follow-up as the other endpoint, respectively

12) in the non-ORIF group and 42.9% (9/21) in the ORIF group ($p = 0.12$). Anatomical restoration was not related to the method of fracture treatment ($r = 0.248$, $p = 0.163$).

Average rate of conventional linear polyethylene wear was 0.22 ± 0.05 mm/year with a mean of 11.5 years in the MOP group. At the final follow-up, linear wear of the polyethylene insert was measured > 0.2 mm/year in eight cases. Among them, six acetabular components formed partial radiolucent lines at the bone-implant interface, observed in zone I in four hips and in zone III in two hips. On the femoral side, two stems had radiolucent lines in Gruen zone 1. This had not affected acetabular or femoral component stability, and they had not been revised. In contrast, no radiolucent lines or osteolysis was observed in any patient in the COC group (Fig. 4).

Complications

Heterotopic ossification was observed in ten patients (seven in the ORIF group, three in the non-ORIF group). No heterotopic bone caused any adverse clinical effects. One posterior dislocation occurred in the ORIF group, which was successfully managed with closed reduction. The sciatic nerve was injured before THA in two patients in the ORIF group. No patient had new or progressive sciatic nerve symptoms after THA. Additionally, three revisions were performed (two ORIF group and one non-ORIF). One patient in the ORIF group underwent a successful two-stage

revision hip arthroplasty to control infection. Two "sandwich" liner fractures occurred in both ORIF and non-ORIF groups.

Discussion

When posttraumatic osteoarthritis develops secondary to acetabular fracture, THA is considered a reliable procedure to relieve pain and restore function [8, 26, 27]. Failed acetabular fractures after non-operative treatment often have bone defects, suffer non-union, or have residual pelvic deformity from malunion [11]. Similarly, following initial ORIF treatment, THA procedures not only faced the same difficulty as non-operatively treated fractures, but they also suffered problems related to previous surgery such as proliferative scar tissue, heterotopic bone formation, or obstructive hardware [6, 8, 9, 28]. In our study, we observed that the surgery duration and blood loss were greater in the ORIF group than in the non-ORIF group. However, no significant difference in average HHS was observed at the final follow-up between the two groups (ORIF group 89 vs non-ORIF 87.9, $p = 0.57$). In brief, performing a salvage THA following acetabular fracture is a challenging procedure. ORIF prior to THA resulted in more complex surgery which did not improve the final clinical outcome.

Acetabular bone defects and abnormal anatomy are contributing factors to the inferior THA outcomes experienced in the setting of previous acetabular fractures [7, 27]. Weber et al. [8] also demonstrated that large deficiencies in acetabular bone were associated with a poorer rate of long-term outcome after delayed THA. To restore bone stock and minimize acetabular deformity, various reconstruction techniques have been described to treat this issue effectively. IBG, a widely accepted technique for acetabular reconstruction after bone stock loss in revision THA, represents one option. Postoperative longevity of the acetabular component achieved from this technically demanding procedure is well documented in previous literature [29]. Based on this favorable experience, we reconstructed the acetabulum using the IBG technique with a cementless hemispherical cup in this study, obtaining sufficient host bone coverage and stability fixation (Fig. 2). Additionally, our results of THA in patients who were treated with ORIF for acetabular fractures demonstrated that ORIF did not reduce the incidence of bone defects compared with non-ORIF (6/21 vs 7/12, $p = 0.09$). Furthermore, the

Table 3 Biomechanical parameters on the operated hip compared to the native contralateral hip (unilateral hip arthroplasty). Data are presented as mean (SD, range)

Parameter	Non-ORIF ($n = 12$)	ORIF ($n = 21$)	p value
Horizontal hip center of rotation	+ 2.6 (± 0.59, − 7.9~10.3)	− 1.9 (± 8.3, − 20.6~12.2)	0.130
Vertical hip center of rotation	+ 5.2 (± 7.9, − 11.3~14.2)	+ 10.7(± 11.0, − 21.7~27.2)	0.134
Horizontal femoral offset	+ 1.4 (± 8.6, − 12.9~16.6)	+ 4.2(± 10.3, − 25.5~17.7)	0.29
Vertical femoral offset	+ 5.0 (± 12.9, − 19.4~24.2)	+ 9.1(± 7.8, − 13.2~25.0)	0.48

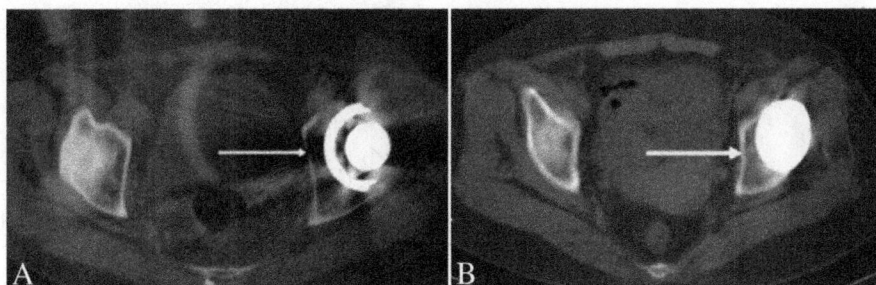

Fig. 4 a Local osteolysis around the acetabular was observed by computed tomography (CT) in the metal-on-polyethylene group. **b** No evidence of osteolysis around acetabular component was observed in the ceramic-on-ceramic group (white arrow)

incidence of anatomical restoration was 58.3% (7/12) in the non-ORIF group and 42.9% (9/21) in the ORIF group ($p = 0.12$). It was shown that anatomical restoration was not associated with fracture treatment ($r = 0.248$, $p = 0.163$). What is more, there was also no clear evidence that ORIF could improve the long-term outcomes of the subsequent THA. Ranawat et al. [16] also hypothesized that initial ORIF was not an essential procedure before THA and that anatomical restoration was not related to fracture treatment. Moreover, there was an increased risk of infection, peri-articular ossification, and scar tissue, and the presence of retained hardware increased the duration of surgery and blood loss [6, 28].

Ranawat et al. [16] reported that acetabular component survival rate was 97% with aseptic loosening and 79% with revision for any reason. Bellabarba et al. [13] also described a 10-year survival rate of 97% after uncemented acetabular reconstruction. In our study, we demonstrated a cementless acetabular component survival rate of 100% with loosening and 88.9% with revision for any reason, because of two "sandwich" ceramic liner fractures due to part design defects [30, 31]. After performing revision surgery, those two hips had well-fixed implants with no radiolucencies and had good clinical results in the follow-up study. Furthermore, acetabular component survival in both groups was similar regarding any reason at a mean follow-up of 11.5 years (Fig. 3). In brief, complex reconstruction in the non-ORIF group did not affect component survival and none of the hips were revised because of aseptic loosening.

Wear debris from conventional MOP can cause extensive osteolysis, threatening the long-term survival of cementless cups, especially in young patients [32]. Berry and Halasy [33] reported that 67% of revisions were associated with polyethylene wear and osteolysis. Roth et al. [26] reported that survivorship of the acetabular component declined from 87% at 10 years to 57% at 20 years for polyethylene wear or loosening. Similarly, our results revealed that 8 of 12 patients who underwent THA with conventional MOP had partial radiolucent lines at the bone-implant interface (Fig. 4). The most likely explanation for periprosthetic osteolysis in these patients is low patient age (average 45 years) combined with high activity level. Conversely, we did not observe osteolysis in any patient in the ceramic-on-ceramic group. Our previous study demonstrated that THAs using COC suffer significantly reduced wear and demonstrated improved component longevity [17]. On the basis of the data presented, therefore, one could speculate that optimization of long-term results with COC surfaces has the potential to solve the most common problems that result in revision surgery being required in these patients (aseptic loosening and osteolysis).

Our study may have some limitations. First, this was a retrospective study and not a prospective randomized study, which increased the possibility of selection bias. Secondly, the number of patients in the study was relatively small, and further studies involving more participants are anticipated. Finally, the acetabular components used in this study were not uniform and thus may compromise the robustness of the results.

Conclusion

In conclusion, Delayed THA with previous acetabular fractures is a challenging procedure. Our study found the initial fracture treatment does not influence the functional results and component survival of subsequent THA at long-term follow-up. Although acetabular osteolysis was observed in our patients, we believe that cementless THA with modern ceramic bearing surfaces will eliminate periprosthetic osteolysis and further improve long-term results.

Abbreviations
AAOS: American Academy of Orthopedic Surgeons; COC: Ceramic-on-ceramic; IBG: Impaction bone grafting; MOP: Metal-on-polyethylene; ORIF: Open reduction internal fixation; THA: Total hip arthroplasty

Funding
This study was supported by the Fundamental Research Funds for the Central Universities (JUSRP11865).

Authors' contributions

TW, XJZ, and JYS contributed to the study conception and design. JJZ and CW contributed to the acquisition of data. TW, JJZ, and CW contributed to the analysis and interpretation of data. TW drafted the manuscript, and XJZ and JYS revised it. All authors read and approved the final manuscript.

Competing interests

The authors declare that they have no competing interests.

References

1. Morison Z, et al. Total hip arthroplasty after acetabular fracture is associated with lower survivorship and more complications. Clin Orthop Relat Res. 2016;474(2):392–8.
2. Giannoudis PV, et al. Operative treatment of displaced fractures of the acetabulum - a meta-analysis. J Bone Joint Surg Br. 2005;87b(1):2–9.
3. Briffa N, et al. Outcomes of acetabular fracture fixation with ten years' follow-up. J Bone Joint Surg Br. 2011;93b(2):229–36.
4. Daurka JS, et al. Acetabular fractures in patients aged > 55 years a systematic review of the literature. Bone Joint J. 2014;96b(2):157–63.
5. Sierra RJ, et al. Acetabular fractures: the role of total hip replacement. Bone Joint J. 2013;95-B(11 Suppl A):11–6.
6. Makridis KG, et al. Total hip arthroplasty after acetabular fracture: incidence of complications, reoperation rates and functional outcomes: evidence today. J Arthroplast. 2014;29(10):1983–90.
7. Romness DW, Lewallen DG. Total hip arthroplasty after fracture of the acetabulum. Long-term results. J Bone Joint Surg Br. 1990;72(5):761–4.
8. Weber M, Berry DJ, Harmsen WS. Total hip arthroplasty after operative treatment of an acetabular fracture. J Bone Joint Surg Am. 1998; 80a(9):1295–305.
9. Jimenez ML, Tile M, Schenk RS. Total hip replacement after acetabular fracture. Orthop Clin North Am. 1997;28(3):435.
10. Mears DC, Velyvis JH. Primary total hip arthroplasty after acetabular fracture (Reprinted). J Bone Joint Surg Am. 2000;82a(9):1328–53.
11. Berry DJ. Total hip arthroplasty following acetabular fracture. Orthopedics. 1999;22(9):837–9.
12. Heeg M, Klasen HJ, Visser JD. Operative treatment for acetabular fractures. J Bone Joint Surg Br. 1990;72(3):383–6.
13. Bellabarba C, et al. Cementless acetabular reconstruction after acetabular fracture. J Bone Joint Surg Am. 2001;83-A(6):868–76.
14. Boraiah S, et al. Open reduction internal fixation and primary total hip arthroplasty of selected acetabular fractures. J Orthop Trauma. 2009;23(4):243–8.
15. Lai O, et al. Midterm results of uncemented acetabular reconstruction for posttraumatic arthritis secondary to acetabular fracture. J Arthroplast. 2011; 26(7):1008–13.
16. Ranawat A, et al. Total hip arthroplasty for posttraumatic arthritis after acetabular fracture. J Arthroplasty. 2009;24(5):759–67.
17. Wang T, et al. Ceramic-on-ceramic bearings total hip arthroplasty in young patients. Arthroplast Today. 2016;2(4):205–9.
18. Lewis PM, et al. Prospective randomized trial comparing alumina ceramic-on-ceramic with ceramic-on-conventional polyethylene bearings in total hip arthroplasty. J Arthroplast. 2010;25(3):392–7.
19. D'Antonio JA, et al. Classification and management of acetabular abnormalities in total hip arthroplasty. Clin Orthop Relat Res. 1989;243:126–37.
20. Harris WH. Traumatic arthritis of the hip after dislocation and acetabular fractures: treatment by mold arthroplasty. An end-result study using a new method of result evaluation. J Bone Joint Surg Am. 1969;51(4):737–55.
21. Pollock D, Sychterz CJ, Engh CA. A clinically practical method of manually assessing polyethylene liner thickness. J Bone Joint Surg Am. 2001;83-A(12):1803–9.
22. DeLee JG, Charnley J. Radiological demarcation of cemented sockets in total hip replacement. Clin Orthop Relat Res. 1976;121:20–32.
23. Gruen TA, McNeice GM, Amstutz HC. "Modes of failure" of cemented stem-type femoral components: a radiographic analysis of loosening. Clin Orthop Relat Res. 1979;141:17–27.
24. Engh CA, Bobyn JD, Glassman AH. Porous-coated hip replacement. The factors governing bone ingrowth, stress shielding, and clinical results. J Bone Joint Surg Br. 1987;69(1):45–55.
25. Brooker AF, et al. Ectopic ossification following total hip replacement. Incidence and a method of classification. J Bone Joint Surg Am. 1973; 55(8):1629–32.
26. von Roth P, et al. Total hip arthroplasty after operatively treated acetabular fracture: a concise follow-up, at a mean of twenty years, of a previous report. J Bone Joint Surg Am. 2015;97(4):288–91.
27. Schreurs BW, et al. Bone impaction grafting and a cemented cup after acetabular fracture at 3-18 years. Clin Orthop Relat Res. 2005;437:145–51.
28. Yuan BJ, Lewallen DG, Hanssen AD. Porous metal acetabular components have a low rate of mechanical failure in THA after operatively treated acetabular fracture. Clin Orthop Relat Res. 2015;473(2):536–42.
29. Iwase T, Ito T, Morita D. Massive bone defect compromises postoperative cup survivorship of acetabular revision hip arthroplasty with impaction bone grafting. J Arthroplasty. 2014;29(12):2424–9.
30. Kawano S, et al. Failure analysis of alumina on alumina total hip arthroplasty with a layered acetabular component: minimum ten-year follow-up study. J Arthroplasty. 2013;28(10):1822–7.
31. Wang T, et al. Mid term results of total hip arthroplasty using polyethylene-ceramic composite (Sandwich) liner. Indian J Orthop. 2016;50(1):10–5.
32. Dumbleton JH, Manley MT, Edidin AA. A literature review of the association between wear rate and osteolysis in total hip arthroplasty. J Arthroplasty. 2002;17(5):649–61.
33. Berry DJ, Halasy M. Uncemented acetabular components for arthritis after acetabular fracture. Clin Orthop Relat Res. 2002;405:164–7.

8

Plasma D-dimer is not useful in the prediction of deep vein thrombosis after total knee arthroplasty in patients using rivaroxaban for thromboprophylaxis

Cheng-Ta Wu[1], Bradley Chen[2], Jun-Wen Wang[1,3*], Shih-Hsiang Yen[1] and Chung-Cheng Huang[4]

Abstract

Background: Venous thromboembolism (VTE) is a serious complication following total joint replacement. The use of rivaroxaban, a highly selective and direct factor Xa inhibitor, has been used widely as a safe and efficacious way to prevent VTE after total joint replacements. However, little is known about the diagnostic efficacy of plasma D-dimer test on deep vein thrombosis (DVT) in patients using rivaroxaban for thromboprophylaxis. The study is aimed to investigate the trend and the diagnostic efficacy of D-dimer test on DVT in patients with primary total knee arthroplasty (TKA) using rivaroxaban for thromboprophylaxis.

Methods: Two hundred TKA patients using rivaroxaban postoperatively as chemical prophylaxis were reviewed. D-dimer levels were checked at 4 h after the surgery and on postoperative days 1 and 4. Venography was used to document the presence of DVT. The Mann-Whitney U test was used to detect the differences in the D-dimer levels at different time points in patients with and without DVT, followed by Bonferroni corrections for p values. Receiver operating characteristics (ROC) curves were constructed to determine the best cutoff values of the D-dimer test at each time point after the surgery.

Results: Twenty-nine of the 200 patients were found to have deep vein thrombosis by venography, resulting in an incidence of 14.5%. All patients with DVTs occurred in the distal calf veins, and only one patient was symptomatic. We found significant differences in D-dimer concentration between patients with and without DVT at postoperative day 4. The best cutoff value determined by receiver operating characteristics analysis was 3.8 mg/L at postoperative day 4, with an AUC equal to 63.5%, and a sensitivity, specificity, PPV, and NPV of 58.6, 76, 29.3, and 91.5%, respectively.

Conclusions: Rivaroxaban was effective on reducing DVT in patients undergoing TKA. Because all the DVTs occurred in the leg veins, decreased thrombus volume and size might result in poor accuracy of plasma D-dimer test in prediction or diagnosis of postoperative DVT.

Keywords: D-dimer, Total knee arthroplasty, Venous thromboembolism, Thromboprophylaxis, Rivaroxaban, Deep vein thrombosis

* Correspondence: wangjw@cgmh.org.tw
[1]Department of Orthopaedic Surgery, Kaohsiung Chang Gung Memorial Hospital, 123, Ta Pei Road, Niao Sung District, Kaohsiung, Taiwan, Republic of China
[3]College of Medicine, Chang Gung University, 123, Ta Pei Road, Niao Sung District, Kaohsiun0067, Taiwan, Republic of China
Full list of author information is available at the end of the article

Background

Venous thromboembolism (VTE) is a potentially serious complication following total joint replacement. The overall incidence of deep vein thrombosis (DVT) following total joint replacement in patients without thromboprophylaxis ranged around 40~70% in Western countries [1–3]. Similar prevalence has been reported in Asian populations [4–6]. While most of the patients were asymptomatic [7], propagation of the thrombi in the untreated patients could result in potential fatal outcome such as pulmonary embolism [8]. Early diagnosis of DVT is important in that timely pharmaceutical intervention with anticoagulants reduces the morbidity and mortality from VTE [9, 10]. However, accurate diagnosis of DVT remains challenging to clinical physician since the patients' symptoms and signs are unreliable. Venography and compressive ultrasonography are the two most often used modalities to diagnose the DVT. Nevertheless, certain limitations hamper their widespread application as screening tools. Despite of being considered the gold standard in the diagnosis of DVT in lower extremity [11], venography is a costly and invasive procedure carrying certain risk [3, 12]. On the other hand, the sensitivity of ultrasonography for distal and non-occlusive proximal DVT was reported to be less favorable and operator-dependent [12, 13].

As a plasma marker specific to endogenous fibrinolysis, D-dimer has been demonstrated to be sensitive and helpful in the diagnosis of DVT [6, 9, 14, 15]. D-dimer is the proteolytic end-product formed by the action of plasmin on cross-linked fibrin in the presence of calcium. Therefore, with only few exceptions, elevated D-dimer level is indicative of a process of fibrin formation and dissolution in ongoing thrombosis such as DVT [16]. It carries a neo-antigen that is different from the parent fibrinogen molecule. By means of detecting the neo-antigen with certain monoclonal antibodies, current commercially available assays are able to quantify the level of D-dimer in a simple and efficient way [15, 17]. In addition, measurement of D-dimer was reported to have the economic potential to spare the use of other expensive tests such as venography and ultrasonography [6]. Despite of its clinical and economic advantages, the diagnostic efficacy of D-dimer test remains controversial in patients undergoing total knee arthroplasty (TKA). Previous studies have shown that the test had a high negative predictive value to exclude the presence of DVT [10, 18]. However, high false-positive rate after major orthopedic surgery hampered its usefulness [9]. Several factors other than DVT such as surgical trauma itself and the use of pneumatic tourniquet could elevate D-dimer level [15, 16, 19]. This resulted in a questionable interpretation of D-dimer test for early detection of DVT after TKA. Some studies have shown a

correlation of elevated D-dimer test on postoperative days 4 or 7 after TKA with the occurrence of DVT [6, 9, 14]. However, most of the studies did not employ chemical thromboprophylaxis after the surgery. Niimi et al. reported the accuracy of D-dimer test to be less favorable in predicting DVT if fondaparinux, an injectable form of factor Xa inhibitor, was administered after TKA [20].

Rivaroxaban, one of the first licensed oral factor Xa inhibitors, has recently been used widely as a practical and efficacious way to prevent VTE after total joint replacements. Its influence for plasma D-dimer measurement on the diagnosis of postoperative DVT has not been investigated. The aim of this retrospective study is to investigate the trend and the diagnostic efficacy of D-dimer test on DVT in TKA patients using rivaroxaban for thromboprophylaxis.

Methods

Patients

Between August 2012 and April 2014, 294 eligible patients scheduled to undergo primary TKA for advanced osteoarthritis and postoperative venography for DVT screening were reviewed in retrospect. Patients were included in the analysis if they were (1) equal or older than 18 years of age, (2) undergoing unilateral primary TKA, and (3) documented with or without lower limb DVT after the surgery by ascending venography. Patients were excluded if they had (1) coagulopathy (such as hemophilia or thrombocytopenia); (2) significant liver disease; (3) severe renal impairment (creatinine clearance < 30 ml/min); (4) concomitant use of protease inhibitors of human immunodeficiency virus, or fibrinolytic agents that was contraindicated to the use of rivaroxaban; (5) prior surgery on the affected knee; (6) a history of thromboembolic disease requiring life-long anticoagulant therapy or anti-platelet drugs that could not be stopped before operation, and (7) no venographic report due to technical failure or refusal to receive the exam. As a result, 200 patients who fulfilled the criteria mentioned above were enrolled in the analysis. The study was conducted with a waiver of patient consent and approved by the Institution Review Board of our hospital.

Perioperative management and DVT prophylaxis

The demographics of the patients, including age, gender, body mass index (BMI), American Society of Anesthesiologists (ASA) grade, and types of anesthesia, were recorded. All patients completed routine preoperative work-up, including complete blood count, chemistry profiles, and coagulation profiles. Physical examination and preoperative D-dimer test precluded DVT before the surgery. All operations were performed under general or spinal anesthesia with a pneumatic tourniquet inflated to a pressure of 300 mmHg before the incision and released at the end of surgery after skin closure. The components of the TKA prostheses were all fixed with cemented technique. All patients received 10 mg of oral rivaroxaban (Xarelto, Bayer Shering Pharma AG, Wuppertal, Germany) once daily from postoperative day (POD) 1 to POD 14 according to the ACCP guideline for VTE prophylaxis in TKA patients [21]. No other modalities for VTE prophylaxis such as pneumatic compressive devices were used. Postoperative rehabilitation commenced from continuous passive motion of the knee after returning to the ward, followed by physical therapy for muscle strengthening and partial weight bearing ambulation with walker on the next day of the surgery. The hemovac was routinely removed on POD 2. The patients were allowed for hospital discharge if they were independent on ambulation with walker support and the operated knee joint reached a range of motion > 90°. All patients returned for follow-up at 2 weeks, 3 months, and 6 months after the surgery.

Laboratory data and venography
Preoperative data, including hemoglobin (Hb) level, prothrombin time, activated partial thromboplastin time, D-dimer level, and platelet count were collected. The Hb level was followed on POD 1, 2, and 4. The D-dimer levels were measured at 4 h after the end of the surgery, on POD 1 and POD 4. Total Hb loss was calculated by subtracting the lowest Hb level after operation from the preoperative Hb level based on the assumption that blood volume was normalized on POD 4. Total blood loss was calculated according to the method of Nadler et al. [22], which used the maximum postoperative reduction in Hb level adjusted for weight and height of the patient and the following formula: Total blood loss = (Total blood volume × [change in Hb level/preoperative Hb level]) × 1000 + volume transfused.

The measurement of plasma D-dimer level was performed with the INNOVANCE ® D-Dimer (Siemens Healthcare Diagnostics Products GmbH, Marburg, Germany) immunoturbidimetric assay, which used a monoclonal antibody (8D3) to detect and quantify only cross-linked D-dimer fragments.

Bilateral ascending venography of the legs was carried out on the next day after the last dose of rivaroxaban, or earlier if symptomatic, using the Rabinov and Paulin technique [23]. A positive diagnosis of DVT required the demonstration of filling defect signs in contrast-filled veins or cutoff signs of one or several deep veins (indirect signs of DVT) [14]. Computed tomographic angiography of the chest was performed if pulmonary embolism was suspected. All the radiographic images were interpreted by an independent radiologist (CCH).

Statistical analysis
Patients were divided into DVT and non-DVT groups based on the results of venography. Student's t test was used for comparison of continuous variables between the two groups in the distribution of demographic and baseline data (including age, BMI, total blood loss, and preoperative laboratory data). The χ2 test or Fisher exact test was used when analyzing the differences of dichotomous variables between the two groups (including gender, ASA score ≥ 3, types of anesthesia, and numbers of patients with blood transfusion). The results were expressed as the mean ± standard deviation.

The Mann-Whitney U test was used to detect the differences in the D-dimer levels at different time points in patients with and without DVT, followed by Bonferroni corrections for p values. Receiver operating characteristics (ROC) curves were constructed to determine the best cutoff values of the D-dimer test at each time point after the surgery. The sensitivity, specificity, and positive and negative predictive values of the D-dimer levels were calculated using the standard method of proportions. All tests were two-sided, and p < 0.05 was considered significant. All statistical comparisons were made using the Statistical Package for Social Sciences (SPSS) (version 22; SPSS Inc., Chicago, Illinois).

Results
The incidence of DVT
DVT was identified by venography in 29 of 200 patients with primary TKA resulting in an incidence of 14.5%. All 29 patients with DVTs occurred in the distal calf veins, and no patients developed proximal DVTs detected by venography. The distribution of thrombosis of the leg veins of the 29 patients was described (Table 1).

There was only one patient had leg edema and calf tenderness 1 month after the operation. Ascending venography revealed thrombosis over the peroneal vein of the operated leg. No pulmonary embolism or VTE-related complication occurred within 15 days following the surgery. There were no significant differences between DVT (+) and DVT (–) groups in terms of sex,

Table 1 Distribution of muscular, combined, and major leg vein DVT

	No. of patients	Percentage
Proximal DVT	0	0%
Distal DVT	29	
Isolated muscular branches	9	31%
Major leg veins	14	48%
Combined muscular and major leg veins	6	21%

Muscular branches included gastroneumus and soleus muscular veins; major leg veins included anterior and posterior tibial and peroneal veins

age, percentage of patients with ASA score ≥ 3, BMI, and types of anesthesia (Table 2).

D-dimer level and DVT

There were no significant differences in the pre-operative D-dimer concentrations between patients with postoperative DVT and without DVT (median, 0.5 mg/L vs. 0.5 mg/L, $p = 0.97$). In both groups, the levels of D-dimer rose markedly at 4 h immediately after the surgery ($p < 0.01$) and decreased gradually on POD1 and POD4 (Fig. 1). The plasma concentrations of D-dimer were found significantly higher in DVT (+) group than in DVT (−) group on POD4 (median, 4.0 mg/L vs. 3.3 mg/L, $p = 0.04$). The correlations of D-dimer levels and the occurrence of venographic DVT were shown in Table 3.

Diagnostic efficacy of D-dimer

Receiver operating characteristics (ROC) analyses of the D-dimer tests at each time point after the surgery were constructed (Fig. 2). The ROC curve obtained for various cutoff values of D-dimer levels at 4 h after the surgery determined a best cutoff value of 11.2 mg/L, yielding a sensitivity of 44.8%, specificity of 69.6%, PPV of 20%, and NPV of 88.1%. However, the area under the curve (AUC) was 54.7% and was statistically insignificant ($p = 0.42$). The best cutoff value at 1 day after the

surgery was 8.2 mg/L, and the AUC was equal to 58% ($p = 0.17$). The best cutoff value at 4 days after the surgery was 3.8 mg/L, with an AUC equal to 63.5% ($p = 0.02$), and a sensitivity, specificity, PPV, and NPV of 58.6, 76, 29.3, and 91.5%, respectively (Table 4).

Discussion

In this study, we have found a high peak value of D-dimer concentration at 4 h after surgery and decreased gradually on POD1 and POD4 in both DVT (+) and DVT (−) groups. Patients undergoing TKA sustained a higher incidence of postoperative DVT as compared with total hip arthroplasty (THA) owing to the use of tourniquet [24–26]. Prior venographic studies reported that the rates of DVT ranged from 30 to 57% for THA and from 40 to 84% for TKA in the absence of thromboprophylaxis [4, 5, 27]. A meta-analysis study also demonstrated that TKA patients managed with a tourniquet had higher risks of thromboembolic complications [28]. Inadequate exsanguination of the blood in the limb, stasis, and ischemia contribute to thrombosis formation [29]. Circulatory indices of thrombosis such as D-dimer values significantly increase immediately following deflation of the tourniquet after TKA [30]. It may decline 1 to 3 days postoperatively [31].

The usefulness of plasma D-dimer measurement in the prediction or diagnosis of postoperative DVT in asymptomatic patients after major orthopedic surgeries has been a controversial issue, as well as the cutoff value of the D-dimer level. Shiota et al. reported that over 10 mg/L of D-dimer concentration on POD7 indicated occurrence of DVT after lower limb arthroplasty [14]. Jiang et al. concluded that plasma D-dimer level was a useful screening test to exclude DVT after orthopedic surgery [32]. However, other authors reported the contradictory results [2, 33, 34]. The variability of timing of D-dimer measurement, selection of the patients, the diagnostic modalities of DVT, and with or without chemical anticoagulants postoperatively may result in the different conclusions.

The second finding of our study was that the D-dimer values were higher in DVT (+) group than DVT (−) group at 4 days after the surgery ($p = 0.04$). Similar finding was reported by Niimi et al. who found that D-dimer values were higher in patients with DVT than in patients without DVT on POD 7 ($p < 0.01$) when fondaparinux was used after THA and TKA [20]. They reported that the cutoff value of D-dimer at POD7 in patients treated with fondaparinux was 6.04 μg/ml, yielding a sensitivity of 85.7% and a poor specificity of 24.8%. They considered that the accuracy of D-dimer test for the diagnosis of DVT was decreased by the administration of fondaparinux. Mitani et al. also drew a conclusion that D-dimer concentration alone had limited value as a

Table 2 Comparison of demographic parameters of patients with and without DVT

Variables	DVT		p value
	Yes	No	
	(N = 29)	(N = 171)	
Male sex (F/M)	25/4	124/47	0.12
ASA score ≥ 3 [no./total no.(%)]	13/29(44.8%)	61/171(35.7%)	0.35
Age (years)	71.0 ± 6.9	69.0 ± 7.0	0.16
BMI (kg/m²)	26.5 ± 3.9	27.8 ± 3.5	0.07
Obesity (BMI ≥ 27, no.)	15	102	0.42
Pre-operative laboratory data			
Hemoglobin (g/dl)	12.6 ± 0.9	13.4 ± 1.1	< 0.01
Platelet count (10⁹cells/L)	249.2 ± 59.8	228.7 ± 55.1	0.27
PT INR	1.0 ± 0.04	1.0 ± 0.6	0.67
aPTT INR	1.0 ± 0.1	1.0 ± 0.1	0.28
Types of anesthesia (no.)			0.61
General anesthesia	25	139	
Spinal anesthesia	4	32	
Total blood loss (ml)	989.8 ± 300.3	1056.6 ± 335.7	0.32
Blood transfusion	0/29(0%)	8/171(4.7%)	0.61

All data are expressed as mean ± standard deviation
ASA American Society of Anesthesiologists, BMI Body mass index, INR International normalized ratio, PT Prothrombin time, aPTT Activated partial thromboplastin time

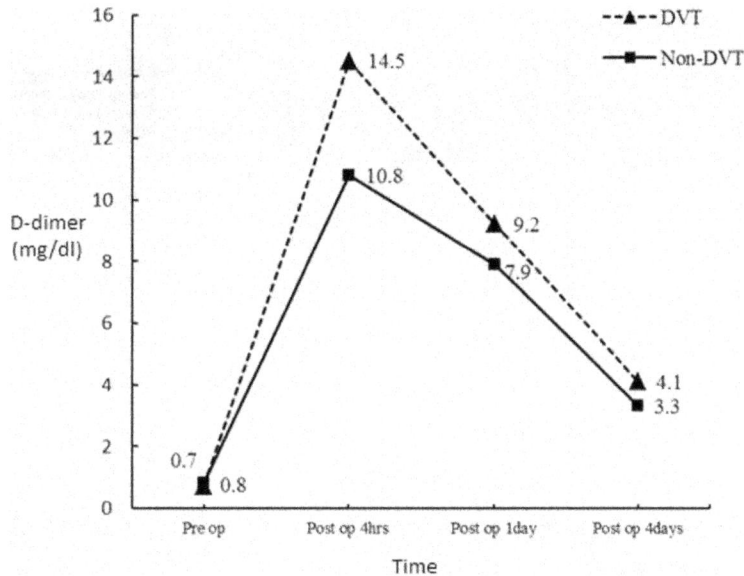

Fig. 1 Longitudinal changes of the D-dimer levels after TKA. The D-dimer levels reached a peak value at 4 h after the surgery and decreased gradually on POD1 and POD4 in both DVT (+) and DVT (–) groups. The D-dimer levels were significantly higher in patients with DVT than in patients without DVT on POD4

hemostatic marker for early detection of DVT after TKA [35]. In their study, administration of fondaparinux was employed for 14 days postoperatively for thromboprophylaxis, and all the patients with DVT were in calf veins and asymptomatic. Our study comprised 200 patients undergoing TKA with rivaroxaban for thromboprophylaxis. The results showed an incidence of 14.5% DVT (29/200). All DVTs were in the leg veins and asymptomatic except one patient. Although D-dimer values were significantly higher in DVT patients at POD4 ($p = 0.04$), the cutoff value (3.8 mg/L) has a low sensitivity (58.6%), specificity (76%), positive predictive value (29.3%), and borderline negative predictive value (91.5%). To keep low false-positive numbers, the cutoff value of D-dimer must have a negative predictive value approaching 100% [2, 15]. We consider a negative predictive value of 91.5% is not high enough to effectively exclude DVT. Furthermore, our results showed a wide

individual variation of D-dimer values on POD4 in DVT (+) group (1.66–9.81) as well as DVT (–) group (0.74–9.4). There were still some patients with positive venograms having low values of D-dimer. Therefore, the statistical difference in the D-dimer levels on POD4 might imply little clinical relevance. In this situation, there were no useful cutoff values to exclude DVT occurrence in these patients.

Another issue is the level of lower limb DVTs. Previous authors have demonstrated that plasma D-dimer test was useful to exclude proximal DVTs [36, 37]. Others reported its cost-effectiveness in the diagnosis of postoperative symptomatic DVTs [15]. On the opposite, the accuracy of D-dimer measurement for distal calf and asymptomatic thrombi was questionable [15, 33]. Therefore, D-dimers should be considered as a marker of larger intra- or extravascular fibrin formation after surgery [15]. Rivaroxaban has been shown to decrease the

Table 3 Correlations of D-dimer levels and DVT

Variables	DVT		p value[a]
	Yes	No	
	(N = 29)	(N = 171)	
Post-operative laboratory data:			
Pre-op D-dimer (mg/L)	0.5 (0.21–2.87)	0.5 (0.19–6.11)	0.97
Post-op 4 h D-dimer (mg/L)	9.2 (2.45–35.13)	8.5 (1.4–35)	0.56
Post-op day 1 D-dimer (mg/L)	8.2 (1.35–26.5)	5.6 (0.19–34.47)	0.26
Post-op day 4 D-dimer (mg/L)	4.0 (1.66–9.81)	3.3 (0.74–9.4)	0.04

The data are expressed as medians (min–max)
[a]The p values are expressed after Bonferroni corrections

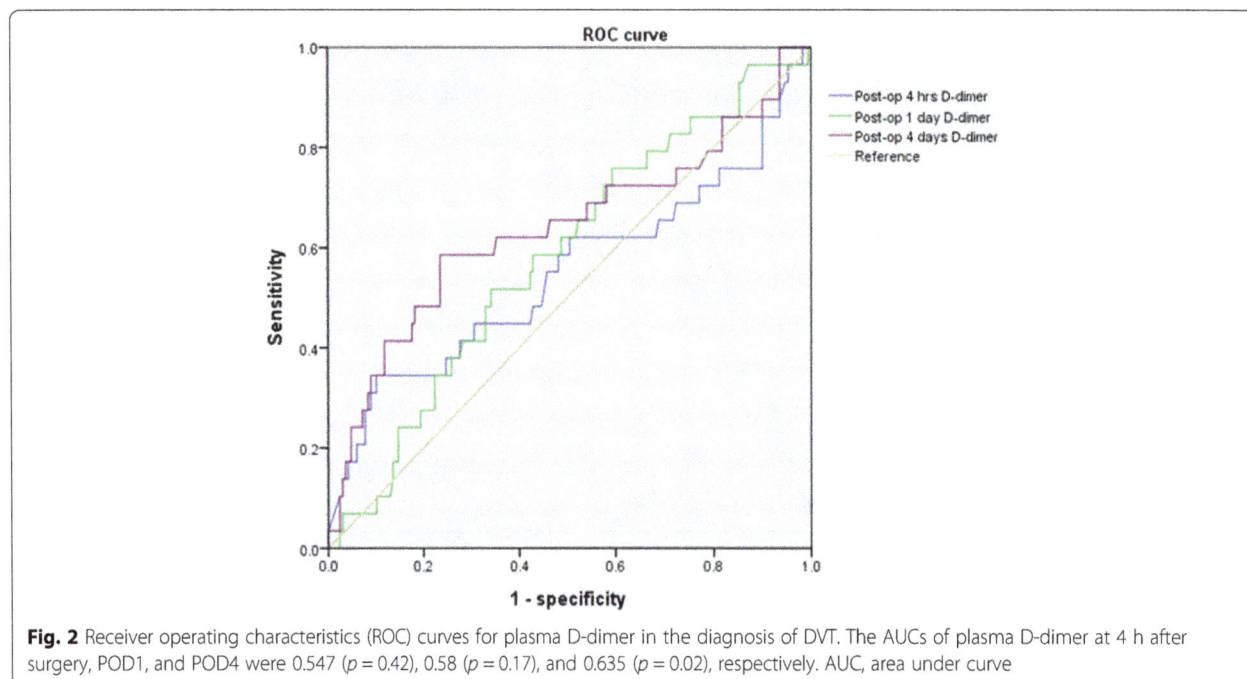

Fig. 2 Receiver operating characteristics (ROC) curves for plasma D-dimer in the diagnosis of DVT. The AUCs of plasma D-dimer at 4 h after surgery, POD1, and POD4 were 0.547 ($p = 0.42$), 0.58 ($p = 0.17$), and 0.635 ($p = 0.02$), respectively. AUC, area under curve

incidence of proximal DVTs after TKA [38]. Because of efficacy of oral anticoagulants, all 29 DVTs in our study were in the leg veins and asymptomatic except one. There were no proximal DVTs or pulmonary embolisms. The reduction of total thrombus volume and the amount of large emboli might result in poor accuracy of D-dimer tests in the prediction of postoperative DVT in the present study.

We recognized few limitations of this study. First, the number of the enrolled patients was small, and the lack of a control group limited our validation that rivaroxaban had an impact on postoperative D-dimer levels following TKA. In addition to being a highly selective and direct Factor Xa inhibitor, rivaroxaban was found to alter the fibrin network and increase porosities of the clot, resulting in a looser clot structure which became more susceptible to fibrinolysis [39]. These facts imply a more complex relationship between the anticoagulants and the hemostatic biomarkers. To the best of our knowledge, however, no study has focused on the influence of rivaroxaban on D-dimer test in the diagnosis of DVT before. Further investigations with larger sample size and a control group are needed. Second, this study was a retrospective review and no D-dimer test was conducted on the day when the ascending venography of both legs was performed. However, Bounameaux et al. has demonstrated that plasma D-dimer values did not differ between patients with or without DVT at the time of venography after TKA [33]. In that study, low-molecular-weight heparin was used for thromboprophylaxis. Third, most of the TKA patients followed a fast-track rehabilitation program and were discharged from the hospital averaged on POD4. While we noticed a significant correlation of D-dimer level on POD4 with the occurrence of DVT, we were unable to determine the longitudinal relationships between D-dimer concentrations with the development of DVT in the following course after discharge. That being said, the study still has its strengths. It is the first report focusing on the diagnostic efficacy of D-dimer test on DVT in TKA patients treated with rivaroxaban. All the patients in the study completed a 2-week chemical prophylaxis without undesirable complications. In addition, all the DVTs were documented by ascending venography.

Table 4 Cutoff values, sensitivity, specificity, and predictive values of D-dimer

D-dimer test	Best cutoff value (mg/L)	Sensitivity (%)	Specificity (%)	Positive (%) Predictive value	Negative (%)	AUC (%)	p value
Post-op 4 h	11.2	44.8	69.6	20.0	88.1	54.7	0.42
Post-op 1 day	8.2	51.7	64.9	20.0	88.8	58.0	0.17
Post-op 4 days	3.8	58.6	76.0	29.3	91.5	63.5	0.02

AUC area under curve

Conclusions
Our study showed that rivaroxaban was effective on reducing DVT in patients undergoing TKA. Because all the DVTs occurred in the leg veins, decreased thrombus volume and size might result in poor accuracy of plasma D-dimer test in prediction or diagnosis of postoperative DVT.

Abbreviations
ASA: American Society of Anesthesiologists; AUC: Area under curve; BMI: Body mass index; DVT: Deep vein thrombosis; NPV: Negative predictive value; POD: Postoperative day; PPV: Positive predictive value; ROC: Receiver Operating Characteristics; TKA: Total knee arthroplasty; VTE: Venous thromboembolism

Acknowledgements
The authors thanked Y.R. Yang and S.H. Ho for the data collection, management, and statistical counseling

Authors' contributions
CW, BC, and SY were responsible for the data analysis, interpretation. CW was a major contributor in writing the manuscript. JWW was responsible for the conception, design of the study, and revising the content. CCH was responsible for the radiological analysis and interpretation. All authors read and approved the final manuscript.

Competing interests
All authors declare that they have no competing interests.

Author details
[1]Department of Orthopaedic Surgery, Kaohsiung Chang Gung Memorial Hospital, 123, Ta Pei Road, Niao Sung District, Kaohsiung, Taiwan, Republic of China. [2]Institute of Public Health, National Yangming University, Taipei, Taiwan, Republic of China. [3]College of Medicine, Chang Gung University, 123, Ta Pei Road, Niao Sung District, Kaohsiun0067, Taiwan, Republic of China. [4]Department of Radiology, Kaohsiung Chang Gung Memorial Hospital, Kaohsiung, Taiwan, Republic of China.

References
1. Cordell-Smith JA, Williams SC, Harper WM, et al. Lower limb arthroplasty complicated by deep venous thrombosis. Prevalence and subjective outcome J Bone Joint Surg Br. 2004;86(1):99–101.
2. Dunn ID, Hui AC, Triffitt PD, et al. Plasma D-dimer as a marker for postoperative deep venous thrombosis. A study after total hip or knee arthroplasty. Thromb Haemost. 1994;72(5):663–5.
3. Wang CJ, Huang CC, Yu PC, et al. Diagnosis of deep venous thrombosis after total knee arthroplasty: a comparison of ultrasound and venography studies. Chang Gung Med J. 2004;27(1):16–21.
4. Dhillon KS, Askander A, Doraismay S. Postoperative deep-vein thrombosis in Asian patients is not a rarity: a prospective study of 88 patients with no prophylaxis. J Bone Joint Surg Br. 1996;78(3):427–30.
5. Kim YH, Kim JS. Incidence and natural history of deep-vein thrombosis after total knee arthroplasty. A prospective, randomised study J Bone Joint Surg Br. 2002;84(4):566–70.
6. Chen CJ, Wang CJ, Huang CC. The value of D-dimer in the detection of early deep-vein thrombosis after total knee arthroplasty in Asian patients: a cohort study. Thromb J. 2008;6:5.
7. Wang CJ, Wang JW, Weng LH, et al. Prevention of deep-vein thrombosis after total knee arthroplasty in Asian patients. Comparison of low-molecular-weight heparin and indomethacin. J Bone Joint Surg Am. 2004;86-a(1):136–40.
8. Maynard MJ, Sculco TP, Ghelman B. Progression and regression of deep vein thrombosis after total knee arthroplasty. Clin Orthop Relat Res. 1991; 273:125–30.
9. Sudo A, Wada H, Nobori T, et al. Cut-off values of D-dimer and soluble fibrin for prediction of deep vein thrombosis after orthopaedic surgery. Int J Hematol. 2009;89(5):572–6.
10. Nomura H, Wada H, Mizuno T, et al. Negative predictive value of D-dimer for diagnosis of venous thromboembolism. Int J Hematol. 2008;87(3):250–5.
11. Lensing AW, Buller HR, Prandoni P, et al. Contrast venography, the gold standard for the diagnosis of deep-vein thrombosis: improvement in observer agreement. Thromb Haemost. 1992;67(1):8–12.
12. Yoo MC, Cho YJ, Ghanem E, et al. Deep vein thrombosis after total hip arthroplasty in Korean patients and D-dimer as a screening tool. Arch Orthop Trauma Surg. 2009;129(7):887–94.
13. Barnes RW, Nix ML, Barnes CL, et al. Perioperative asymptomatic venous thrombosis: role of duplex scanning versus venography. J Vasc Surg. 1989; 9(2):251–60.
14. Shiota N, Sato T, Nishida K, et al. Changes in LPIA D-dimer levels after total hip or knee arthroplasty relevant to deep-vein thrombosis diagnosed by bilateral ascending venography. J Orthop Sci. 2002;7(4):444–50.
15. Crippa L, D'Angelo SV, Tomassini L, et al. The utility and cost-effectiveness of D-dimer measurements in the diagnosis of deep vein thrombosis. Haematologica. 1997;82(4):446–51.
16. Wada H, Sakuragawa N. Are fibrin-related markers useful for the diagnosis of thrombosis? Semin Thromb Hemost. 2008;34(1):33–8.
17. Niimi R, Hasegawa M, Sudo A, et al. Evaluation of soluble fibrin and D-dimer in the diagnosis of postoperative deep vein thrombosis. Biomarkers. 2010;15(2):149–57.
18. Wells PS, Anderson DR, Rodger M, et al. Evaluation of D-dimer in the diagnosis of suspected deep-vein thrombosis. N Engl J Med. 2003;349(13):1227–35.
19. Reikeras O, Clementsen T. Time course of thrombosis and fibrinolysis in total knee arthroplasty with tourniquet application. Local versus systemic activations. J Thromb Thrombolysis. 2009;28(4):425–8.
20. Niimi R, Hasegawa M, Shi DQ, et al. The influence of fondaparinux on the diagnosis of postoperative deep vein thrombosis by soluble fibrin and D-dimer. Thromb Res. 2012;130(5):759–64.
21. Falck-Ytter Y, Francis CW, Johanson NA, et al. Prevention of VTE in orthopedic surgery patients: Antithrombotic Therapy and Prevention of Thrombosis, 9th ed: American College of Chest Physicians Evidence-Based Clinical Practice Guidelines. Chest 2012;141(2 Suppl):e278S-e325S.
22. Nadler SB, Hidalgo JH, Bloch T. Prediction of blood volume in normal human adults. Surgery. 1962;51(2):224–32.
23. Rabinov K, Paulin S. Roentgen diagnosis of venous thrombosis in the leg. Arch Surg. 1972;104(2):134–44.
24. Hull R, Raskob G, Pineo G, et al. A comparison of subcutaneous low-molecular-weight heparin with warfarin sodium for prophylaxis against deep-vein thrombosis after hip or knee implantation. N Engl J Med. 1993; 329(19):1370–6.
25. McKenna R, Bachmann F, Kaushal SP, et al. Thromboembolic disease in patients undergoing total knee replacement. J Bone Joint Surg Am. 1976; 58(7):928–32.
26. Merli GJ. Update. Deep vein thrombosis and pulmonary embolism prophylaxis in orthopedic surgery. Med Clin North Am. 1993;77(2):397–411.
27. Cushner FD, Nett MP. Unanswered questions, unmet needs in venous thromboprophylaxis. Orthopedics. 2009;32(12 Suppl):62–6.
28. Tai TW, Lin CJ, Jou IM, et al. Tourniquet use in total knee arthroplasty: a meta-analysis. Knee Surg Sports Traumatol Arthrosc. 2011;19(7):1121–30.
29. Parmet JL, Horrow JC, Singer R, et al. Echogenic emboli upon tourniquet release during total knee arthroplasty: pulmonary hemodynamic changes and embolic composition. Anesth Analg. 1994;79(5):940–5.
30. Sharrock NE, Go G, Sculco TP, et al. Changes in circulatory indices of thrombosis and fibrinolysis during total knee arthroplasty performed under tourniquet. J Arthroplast. 1995;10(4):523–8.

31. Rafee A, Herlikar D, Gilbert R, et al. D-dimer in the diagnosis of deep vein thrombosis following total hip and knee replacement: a prospective study. Ann R Coll Surg Engl. 2008;90(2):123–6.

32. Jiang Y, Li J, Liu Y, et al. Risk factors for deep vein thrombosis after orthopedic surgery and the diagnostic value of D-dimer. Ann Vasc Surg. 2015;29(4):675–81.

33. Bounameaux H, Miron MJ, Blanchard J, et al. Measurement of plasma D-dimer is not useful in the prediction or diagnosis of postoperative deep vein thrombosis in patients undergoing total knee arthroplasty. Blood Coagul Fibrinolysis. 1998;9(8):749–52.

34. Jorgensen LN, Lind B, Hauch O, et al. Thrombin-antithrombin III-complex & fibrin degradation products in plasma: surgery and postoperative deep venous thrombosis. Thromb Res. 1990;59(1):69–76.

35. Mitani G, Takagaki T, Hamahashi K, et al. Associations between venous thromboembolism onset, D-dimer, and soluble fibrin monomer complex after total knee arthroplasty. J Orthop Surg Res. 2015;10:172.

36. Bongard O, Wicky J, Peter R, et al. D-dimer plasma measurement in patients undergoing major hip surgery: use in the prediction and diagnosis of postoperative proximal vein thrombosis. Thromb Res. 1994;74(5):487–93.

37. Wijns W, Daoud N, Droeshout I, et al. Evaluation of two D-dimer assays in the diagnosis of venous thromboembolism. Acta Clin Belg. 1998;53(4):270–4.

38. Lassen MR, Ageno W, Borris LC, et al. Rivaroxaban versus enoxaparin for thromboprophylaxis after total knee arthroplasty. N Engl J Med. 2008; 358(26):2776–86.

39. Varin R, Mirshahi S, Mirshahi P, et al. Whole blood clots are more resistant to lysis than plasma clots–greater efficacy of rivaroxaban. Thromb Res. 2013; 131(3):e100–9.

9

Clinical outcomes and repair integrity of arthroscopic rotator cuff repair using suture-bridge technique with or without medial tying: prospective comparative study

Kyung Cheon Kim[1], Hyun Dae Shin[2], Woo-Yong Lee[2]*(iD), Kyu-Woong Yeon[1] and Sun-Cheol Han[1]

Abstract

Background: There have been few studies comparing clinical and radiological outcomes between the conventional and knotless suture-bridge techniques. The purpose of this study was to evaluate and compare the functional outcomes and repair integrity of arthroscopic conventional and knotless suture-bridge technique for full-thickness rotator cuff tears.

Methods: We prospectively followed 100 consecutive patients (100 shoulders) with full-thickness rotator cuff tears treated with the arthroscopic conventional or knotless suture-bridge technique from October 2012 to July 2014. Enrolled patients returned for follow-up functional evaluations at 1 and 2 years after the operation. There were four outcome measures in this study: American Shoulder and Elbow Surgeons (ASES) scores, Shoulder Rating Scale of the University of California at Los Angeles (UCLA) scores, Constant scores, and visual analog scale (VAS) pain scores. Enrolled patients returned for follow-up magnetic resonance imaging or ultrasonography evaluation to confirm the integrity of the repaired cuff at 6 months post-operation (97% follow-up rate). Also, we investigated the preoperative cuff retraction of enrolled patients using preoperative MRI to find out correlation between the stage of cuff retraction and re-tear rate.

Results: At final follow-up, the average UCLA, ASES, Constant, and VAS scores had improved significantly to 32.5, 88.0, 80.4, and 1.3, respectively, in the conventional suture-bridge technique group and to 33.0, 89.7, 81.2, and 1.2, respectively, in the knotless suture-bridge technique group. The UCLA, ASES, Constant, and VAS scores improved in both groups after surgery (all $p < 0.001$), and there were no significant differences between the two groups at 2-year follow-up ($p = 0.292, 0.359, 0.709$, and 0.636, respectively). The re-tear rate of repaired rotator cuffs was 16.3% (8/49 shoulders) in the conventional suture-bridge technique group and 29.2% (14/48 shoulders) in the knotless suture-bridge technique group; this difference was not significant ($p = 0.131$). There were no significant differences between the re-tear rate of the two groups in the Patte stage I and II ($p = 0.358$ and 0.616).

Conclusions: The knotless suture-bridge technique showed comparable functional outcomes to those of conventional suture-bridge techniques in medium-to-large, full-thickness rotator cuff tears at short-term follow-up. The knotless suture-bridge technique had a higher re-tear rate compared with conventional suture-bridge technique, although the difference was not significant.

Keywords: Rotator cuff, Suture-bridge, Knotless, Medial knot tying

* Correspondence: studymachine@daum.net
[2]Department of Orthopedic Surgery, Regional Rheumatoid and Degenerative Arthritis Center, Chungnam National University Hospital, Chungnam National University School of Medicine, 266 Munwha-ro, Jung-gu, Daejeon 35015, South Korea
Full list of author information is available at the end of the article

Background

Rotator cuff tears (RCTs) comprise the majority of shoulder lesions in adult patients. The prevalence of RCTs among the general population is 22.1% and increases with age [1]. Despite widespread use, rotator cuff repair (RCR) surgeries do not always lead to clinically satisfactory outcomes; indeed, the failure rate of RCR is reportedly 40–50% [2–4]. Rotator cuff reattachment to the bone during RCR is a challenging clinical problem. To address this problem, surgical repair techniques have been continually developed over time in an attempt to reduce re-tear rates and improve functional outcomes. Recently, arthroscopic transosseous-equivalent suture-bridge RCR, namely, the suture-bridge technique (SBT), has been widely used to enhance healing at the site of tendon insertion of the repaired rotator cuff. This repair method involves insertion of a medial row with suture anchors that utilize mattress repairs [5–8]. However, techniques that employ a knotted medial row of anchors have been suspected to compromise vascular inflow to the healing tendon and increase the risk of type II failure (i.e., medial row failure), which is very difficult to treat [9–13]. More recently, knotless RCR techniques that involve application of knotless medial anchors, to improve vascular circulation and prevent type II failure, have been introduced [14–18].

Despite these innovations and documented benefits in a laboratory setting, postoperative clinical and radiological outcomes of newer SBTs, at short- to medium-term follow-up, have been equivocal [14, 18–20]. Moreover, few studies comparing clinical and radiological outcomes between the conventional and knotless SBT have been reported.

The purpose of this study was to evaluate and compare functional outcomes and repair integrity between arthroscopic conventional and knotless SBT for full-thickness RCTs.

Methods

Patient selection

We prospectively followed 100 consecutive patients (100 shoulders) with full-thickness RCTs treated with arthroscopic conventional or knotless SBT from October 2012 to July 2014 at our institute. A conventional SBT was used in the first 50 consecutive shoulders, and a knotless SBT was used in the next 50 consecutive shoulders (Table 1). We included full-thickness supraspinatus or infraspinatus tears 1–4 cm in length in the anterior-to-posterior dimension. We excluded patients with the following: (1) full-thickness RCTs smaller than 1 cm or larger than 4 cm in the anterior-to-posterior dimension, (2) a full-thickness subscapularis tear requiring concomitant repair, (3) neurological involvement, (4) revision operation, (5) operation after conversion of an advanced partial-thickness RCT to a full-thickness lesion,

Table 1 Demographic and surgical data of the two study groups

Variable	Conventional SBT	Knotless SBT	p value*
Number of patients	50	50	
Age at surgery, years	59.40 ± 7.45 (41–76)	59.90 ± 7.66 (47–74)	0.741
Gender, male	28 (56.0%)	24 (48.0%)	0.423
Affected shoulder, right	29 (58.0%)	34 (68.0%)	0.841
Duration of symptoms, months	5.86 ± 6.00 (1–36)	6.10 ± 9.05 (1–48)	0.876
Current smoker	9 (18.0%)	10 (20.0%)	0.532

Data are expressed as mean ± standard deviation (range) or number (percentage)
SBT Suture-bridge technique
*Paired t test; p < 0.05 denotes statistical significance

and (6) advanced arthritic changes in the glenohumeral joint. The demographic characteristics of the conventional and knotless SBT groups are listed in Table 1.

Surgical technique

All operations were performed by a single surgeon (first author) in the beach-chair position with the patient under general anesthesia. During conventional SBT, we used one or two Bio-Corkscrew suture anchors (4.5 or 5.5 mm according to the tear size; Arthrex, Naples, FL, USA), containing a suture eyelet and loaded with two No. 2 non-absorbable braided sutures, placed just lateral to the articular surface of the humeral head. The sutures perforated the tendon in a horizontal mattress stitch configuration, with an identical procedure then applied for the second medial anchor [5]. To establish the lateral row, suture bridge repair was achieved with two or three 4.5-mm knotless anchors (Bio-PushLock; Arthrex) that were fully inserted perpendicular to the cortical surface of the humerus, distal to the footprint anchor in conjunction with one suture from each medial anchor (Fig. 1).

For the knotless SBT, one or two of the same suture anchors were placed just lateral to the articular surface of the humeral head. In shoulders with a suture anchor inserted into the medial row, four suture limbs in the suture anchor were passed through the reduced tendon in an alternative configuration; a pilot hole for the 4.5-mm knotless anchors (Bio-PushLock; Arthrex) was prepared approximately 5–10 mm distal to the lateral edge of the greater tuberosity. Without tying the medial row, the same two suture limbs were linked to the knotless anchor, which was placed within the pilot hole. These steps were then repeated for a second knotless anchor. In shoulders with two suture anchors inserted into the medial row, four limbs from the sutures in the first suture anchor were passed through the tendon in an alternative configuration. Then, the second suture anchor was inserted and one suture was removed. After tying

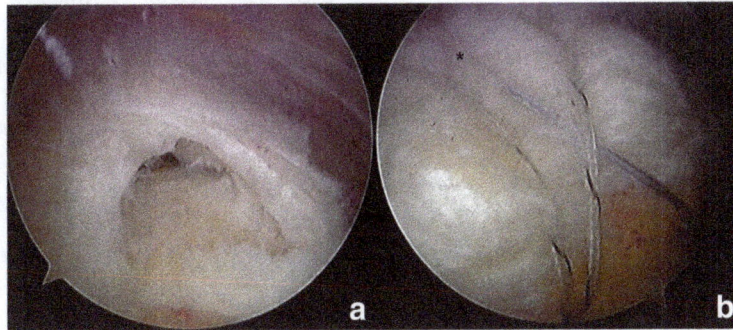

Fig. 1 a Arthroscopic view showing a rotator cuff tear involving the supraspinatus. **b** The arthroscopic view from the lateral portal shows complete repair of an rotator cuff tear using the knotless suture-bridge technique without medial tying (*)

the remaining suture twice to prevent sliding, two suture limbs were passed through the tendon in a mattress configuration. Without tying the medial row, the same two limbs, and one limb of the second anchor, were linked to the knotless anchor, which was placed within the pilot hole. These steps were again repeated for a second knotless anchor (Fig. 2).

The maximum anterior-to-posterior length of the RCTs was measured using a calibrated probe, introduced through the anterior or posterior portal while viewing the posterolateral or lateral portal under arthroscopic observation. The maximum medial-to-lateral length of the RCTs in oblique coronal images on preoperative T2-weighted magnetic resonance imaging (MRI) was estimated; because of the considerable variation in the medial-to-lateral length according to the position of the shoulder, we measured the tears on MRI instead of arthroscopy (Table 2). All of the measurements were performed by the first author. Important clinical differences between the conventional and knotless SBT groups are listed in Table 2.

Postoperative management

All patients received standardized pre- and perioperative care at a single hospital. The same treatment regimen

was prescribed to all patients, regardless of the repair status of the articular-side rotator cuff. Postoperatively, we recommended the use of a shoulder-immobilizing sling with an abduction pillow and provided instructions to maintain the shoulder at 30–40° internal rotation and 20° abduction. The patients performed gentle passive forward flexion exercises of the affected arm during the second postoperative week. The sling and abduction pillow were removed at 6 weeks postoperatively, and active mobilization was started. Active resistance-based muscle-strengthening exercises were started at 12 weeks postoperatively using Thera-Band equipment (HCM-Hygenic Corp., Batu Gajah, Malaysia). At 3–4 months after surgery, the patients were permitted to perform light activities, with sports participation and heavy labor being allowed after 6 months.

Clinical and radiological evaluation

Enrolled patients returned for a follow-up functional evaluation at 1 and 2 years after the operation. Clinical data were collected preoperatively and postoperatively at the 1- and 2-year follow-ups by two orthopedic surgeons. There were four outcome measures in this study: American Shoulder and Elbow Surgeons (ASES) scores, Shoulder Rating Scale of the University of California at

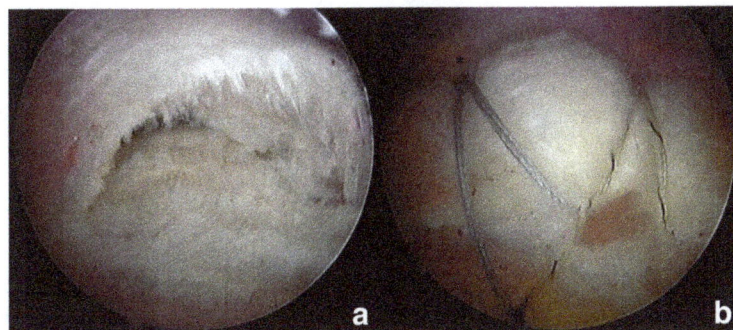

Fig. 2 a Arthroscopic view showing a rotator cuff tear involving the supraspinatus. **b** The arthroscopic view from the lateral portal shows complete repair of a rotator cuff tear using the conventional suture-bridge technique with medial tying (*)

Table 2 Clinical and surgical data of the two study groups

Variable	Conventional SBT	Knotless SBT	p value*
Total number of patients	50	50	
Clinical evaluation			
1-year follow-up	47 (94.0%)	48 (96.0%)	0.646
2-year follow-up	49 (98.0%)	47 (94.0%)	0.307
Postoperative radiologic evaluation	49 (98.0%)	48 (96.0%)	0.941
MRI	32	31	
US	17	17	
Tear size, mm			
Anterior-to-posterior	2.51 (1.6–4.0)	2.53 (1.5–3.9)	0.918
Medial-to-lateral	1.96 (0.8–3.5)	1.97 (0.5–3.5)	0.906
Cuff retraction (Patte stage)			0.188
Stage I	31 (63.3%)	23 (47.9%)	
Stage II	18 (36.7%)	25 (52.1%)	
Stage III	0	0	
Subacromial decompression	47 (94.0%)	47 (94.0%)	1.000
Biceps tenotomy	25 (50.0%)	25 (50.0%)	1.000

Data are expressed as mean (range) or number (percentage)
SBT suture-bridge technique, MRI magnetic resonance imaging, US ultrasonography
*Paired t test and χ^2 test; $p < 0.05$ denotes statistical significance

Los Angeles (UCLA) scores, Constant scores, and visual analog scale (VAS) pain scores. Active range of motion was measured by goniometry, while passive range of motion was not measured. The range of motion was measured with the patient in a standing position, and external rotation was assessed while the patient was standing with the arm in an adducted position.

Enrolled patients returned for follow-up MRI or ultrasonography (US) evaluation to confirm the integrity of the repaired cuff at 6 months post-operation (97% follow-up rate). One specialized musculoskeletal radiologist performed all follow-up US examinations using an IU-22 system (Philips Healthcare, Bothell, WA, USA). The MRI or US images were evaluated by an experienced radiologist. A recurrent tendon defect was diagnosed by US when a distinct hypoechoic or mixed hyper- and hypoechoic defect was visualized in both the transverse and longitudinal planes. A full-thickness re-tear was diagnosed when a focal defect was present in the rotator cuff, into which the deltoid muscle could be compressed with a probe to separate the torn tendon ends, or when the cuff retracted to such an extent that the torn ends could be distinctly visualized. MRI was used to classify the integrity of the tendon into one of two categories: (1) intact (sufficient thickness, Sugaya types I and II) or (2) insufficient/unhealed/re-torn [ranging from insufficient thickness (< 50% normal cuff thickness) to discontinuity, Sugaya types III–V] [21].

Also, we investigated the preoperative cuff retraction of enrolled patients returned for follow-up MRI or US evaluation using preoperative MRI to find out correlation between the stage of cuff retraction and re-tear rate. The degree of cuff retraction in the coronal plane of preoperative MRI was assessed by Patte classification: (1) stage I is a tear with minimal retraction, (2) stage II is a tear retracted medial to the humeral head footprint but not to the glenoid, and (3) stage III is a tear retracted to the level of the glenoid [22]. Important clinical differences between the groups are listed in Table 2.

Statistical analyses
According to a two-sided significance level of 0.05 and a power of 80%, we prospectively enrolled patients in this study. The sample size was calculated with consideration of each outcome measure, namely, the UCLA, ASES, Constant, and VAS scores. The sample size required to achieve an 80% power was 8, 10, 12, and 13 for the UCLA, ASES, Constant scores, and VAS, respectively. A minimum of 20 patients, which is the maximal sample size among the outcomes, was required to satisfy the conditions (the power of 80% and 20% maximum follow-up loss of patients). For the statistical analysis, the paired t test and χ^2 test were used to assess pre- and postoperative differences between the groups. The SPSS software package was used for all statistical analyses (ver. 12.0; SPSS Inc., Chicago, IL, USA) with the α level set at 0.05.

Results
Preoperatively, no significant differences were observed between the groups in the mean UCLA, ASES, Constant, or VAS scores ($p = 0.175$, 0.111, 0.432, and 0.890, respectively; Table 3). At 1-year follow-up, the average UCLA, ASES, Constant, and VAS scores had improved significantly to 31.1, 83.5, 72.1, and 1.9, respectively, in the conventional SBT group and to 31.7, 84.4, 73.9, and 1.4, respectively, in the knotless SBT group (Table 4). The UCLA, ASES, Constant, and VAS scores improved in both groups after surgery (all $p < 0.001$); however, there was no significant difference between the two

Table 3 Comparison of preoperative scores between the two study groups

Variable	Conventional SBT (50)	Knotless SBT (50)	p value*
UCLA	19.96 ± 4.30	18.46 ± 4.92	0.175
ASES	53.89 ± 15.15	51.43 ± 15.84	0.111
Constant	57.50 ± 13.15	57.98 ± 20.24	0.432
VAS	5.28 ± 1.88	5.79 ± 1.82	0.890

Numbers in parentheses are the numbers of patients in each group
Data are expressed as mean ± standard deviation
SBT suture-bridge technique, UCLA Shoulder Rating Scale of the University of California at Los Angeles, ASES American Shoulder and Elbow Surgeons score, VAS visual analog scale pain score
*Paired t test; $p < 0.05$ denotes statistical significance

Table 4 Comparison between the preoperative findings and postoperative clinical outcomes at 1-year follow-up

	Preoperative	1-year follow-up	p value*
UCLA			
Conventional SBT (47)	19.96 ± 4.41	31.09 ± 4.23	0.000
Knotless SBT (48)	18.46 ± 4.92	31.67 ± 2.83	0.000
ASES			
Conventional SBT (47)	52.95 ± 15.12	83.54 ± 15.26	0.000
Knotless SBT (48)	51.43 ± 15.84	84.42 ± 8.69	0.000
Constant			
Conventional SBT (47)	57.51 ± 13.51	72.06 ± 11.46	0.000
Knotless SBT (48)	57.98 ± 20.24	73.85 ± 10.87	0.000
VAS			
Conventional SBT (47)	5.30 ± 1.86	1.91 ± 2.05	0.000
Knotless SBT (48)	5.79 ± 1.82	1.94 ± 1.44	0.000

Numbers in parentheses are the numbers of patients in each group
Data are expressed as mean ± standard deviation
SBT suture-bridge technique, *UCLA* Shoulder Rating Scale of the University of California at Los Angeles, *ASES* American Shoulder and Elbow Surgeons score, *VAS* visual analog scale pain score
*Paired *t* test; *p* < 0.05 denotes statistical significance

Table 6 Comparison between the preoperative findings and postoperative clinical outcomes at 2-year follow-up

	Preoperative	2-year follow-up	p value*
UCLA			
Conventional SBT (49)	19.94 ± 4.34	32.51 ± 2.72	0.000
Knotless SBT (47)	18.38 ± 4.95	32.98 ± 1.42	0.000
ASES			
Conventional SBT (49)	53.67 ± 15.22	87.97 ± 10.68	0.000
Knotless SBT (47)	51.35 ± 16.00	89.70 ± 7.53	0.000
Constant			
Conventional SBT (49)	57.71 ± 13.20	80.37 ± 12.85	0.000
Knotless SBT (47)	57.91 ± 20.46	81.17 ± 7.61	0.000
VAS			
Conventional SBT (49)	5.29 ± 1.90	1.27 ± 1.22	0.000
Knotless SBT (47)	5.79 ± 1.84	1.15 ± 1.18	0.000

Numbers in parentheses are the numbers of patients in each group
Data are expressed as mean ± standard deviation
SBT suture-bridge technique, *UCLA* Shoulder Rating Scale of the University of California at Los Angeles, *ASES* American Shoulder and Elbow Surgeons score, *VAS* visual analog scale pain score
*Paired *t* test; *p* < 0.05 denotes statistical significance

groups at 1-year follow-up ($p = 0.434$, 0.733, 0.437, and 0.951, respectively; Table 5).

At final follow-up, the average UCLA, ASES, Constant, and VAS scores had improved significantly to 32.5, 88.0, 80.4, and 1.3, respectively, in the conventional SBT group and to 33.0, 89.7, 81.2, and 1.2, respectively, in the knotless SBT group (Table 6). The UCLA, ASES, Constant, and VAS scores improved in both groups after surgery (all $p < 0.001$), and there were no significant differences between the two groups at 2-year follow-up ($p = 0.292$, 0.359, 0.709, and 0.636, respectively; Table 7).

The re-tear rate of the repaired rotator cuffs was 16.3% (8/49 shoulders) in the conventional SBT group and 29.2% (14/48 shoulders) in the knotless SBT group; this difference was not significant ($p = 0.131$). Two types of re-tear patterns were identified in both the conventional and knotless SBT groups: (1) unhealed tendons [2/8 (25%) and 6/14 (42.9%), respectively; Fig. 3] and (2)

medially ruptured tendons with a healed footprint [6/8 (75%) and 8/14 (57.1%), respectively; Fig. 4]; different rate of re-tear pattern was statistically insignificant ($p = 0.402$). No intra- or perioperative complications were noted, and no patient showed neural injury, wound infection, or problems related to the suture anchor.

The re-tear rate was 22.2% (12/54 shoulders) in the Patte stage I and 23.3% (10/43 shoulders) in the stage II; this difference was not significant ($p = 1.000$). Also, the re-tear rate of the conventional SBT group was 16.1% (5/31 shoulders) in the stage I and 16.7% (3/18 shoulders) in the stage II; this difference was not significant ($p = 1.000$). The re-tear rate of the knotless SBT group was 30.4% (7/23 shoulders) in the stage I and 28.0% (7/25 shoulders) in the stage II; this difference was not significant ($p = 1.000$). And there were no significant differences between re-tear rate of the two groups in the Patte stage I and II ($p = 0.358$ and 0.616).

Table 5 Comparison of clinical outcomes between the two study groups at 1-year follow-up

	Conventional SBT (47)	Knotless SBT (48)	p value*
UCLA	31.09 ± 4.23	31.67 ± 2.83	0.434
ASES	83.54 ± 15.26	84.42 ± 8.69	0.733
Constant	72.06 ± 11.46	73.85 ± 10.87	0.437
VAS	1.91 ± 2.05	1.94 ± 1.44	0.951

Numbers in parentheses are the numbers of patients in each group
Data are expressed as mean ± standard deviation
SBT suture-bridge technique, *UCLA* Shoulder Rating Scale of the University of California at Los Angeles, *ASES* American Shoulder and Elbow Surgeons score, *VAS* visual analog scale pain score
*Paired *t* test; *p* < 0.05 denotes statistical significance

Table 7 Comparison of the clinical outcomes between the two groups at 2-year follow-up

	Conventional SBT (49)	Knotless SBT (47)	p value*
UCLA	32.51 ± 2.72	32.98 ± 1.42	0.292
ASES	87.97 ± 10.68	89.70 ± 7.53	0.359
Constant	80.37 ± 12.85	81.17 ± 7.61	0.709
VAS	1.27 ± 1.22	1.15 ± 1.18	0.636

Numbers in parentheses are the numbers of patients in each group
Data are expressed as mean ± standard deviation
SBT suture-bridge technique, *UCLA* Shoulder Rating Scale of the University of California at Los Angeles, *ASES* American Shoulder and Elbow Surgeons score, *VAS* visual analog scale pain score
*Paired *t* test; *p* < 0.05 denotes statistical significance

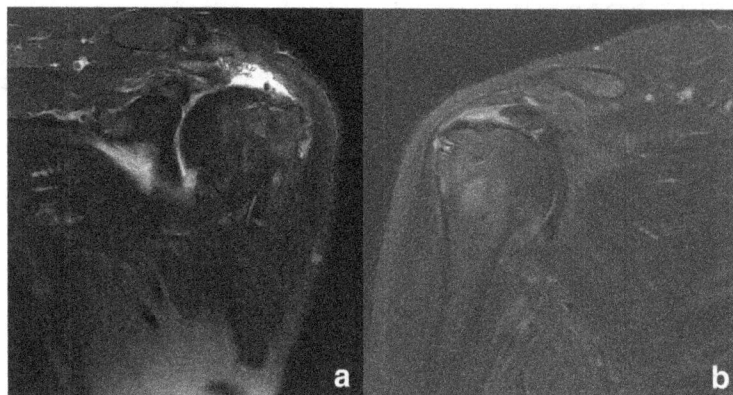

Fig. 3 Follow-up T2-weighted sagittal magnetic resonance imaging at 6 months post-operation shows an unhealed tendon of a repaired rotator cuff (type I re-tear). **a** Conventional suture-bridge technique. **b** Knotless suture-bridge technique

Discussion

This study evaluated the clinical and radiographic results of knot-tying and knotless SBTs for RCTs. We applied an SBT without knot-tying to reduce tension overload at the suture-tendon interface of the medial row and the likelihood of medial cuff failure. We hypothesized that the biological advantages inherent to the knotless SBT would result in a higher healing rate than that associated with the conventional knot-tying SBT.

Suture-bridge RCR was introduced to improve the biomechanical outcomes of RCR [5–7]. It is more convenient to fasten the compromised tendon to the footprint anchor firmly using the suture limbs of the medial suture knots. With the SBT, the mean pressurized contact area between the tendon and the tuberosity insertion footprint has proven superior to that of the conventional double-row technique [6–8]. The SBT also shows better ultimate-to-load failure outcomes and less gap formation than the double-row technique [6–8]. This biomechanical superiority of the SBT may contribute, at least in part, to the low rate of structural failure of repaired

cuffs. Moreover, double-row RCR, where each suture anchor is tied separately, is a technically demanding and time-consuming procedure [23].

In a study on medial rotator cuff failure after use of the arthroscopic double-row technique, Trantalis et al. [9] posited that the most likely causes of medial cuff failure were tension overload at the suture-tendon interface of the medial row, over-tensioning of the medial repair (resulting from an oblique and retrograde suture path), a relatively large hole in the rotator cuff caused by retrograde suture-passing instruments, and the effect of braided suture materials on their passage through the rotator cuff. In a study on medial rotator cuff failure after arthroscopic SBT, Cho et al. [12] suggested that the most likely causes of medial cuff failure were attempts to pass the tendon at the musculotendinous junction instead of at the tendon portion, which eventually renders the musculotendinous junction weak and vulnerable to re-tear, with an increased likelihood of strangulation, relatively rapid necrosis of the rotator cuff tendon at the medial row, and failure at the musculotendinous

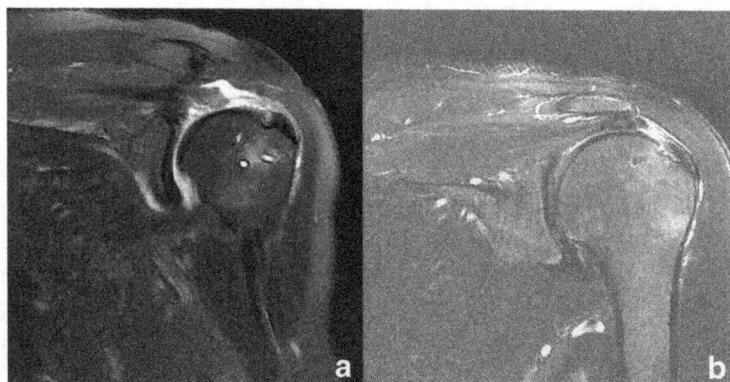

Fig. 4 Follow-up T2-weighted magnetic resonance imaging at 6 months post-operation shows medially ruptured tendons and a healed footprint of a repaired rotator cuff (type II re-tear). **a** Conventional suture-bridge technique. **b** Knotless suture-bridge technique

junction. To reduce the possibility of strangulation and relatively rapid necrosis of the rotator cuff tendon at the medial row, the type of knots used to secure the medial row, and the amount of tension used to tie them, should be considered carefully [14, 24].

Reducing unnecessary over-tension during RCT repair, developing new techniques that can distribute the load placed on the medial row may be important. Therefore, the knotless SBT may not only restore the footprint contact area of the rotator cuff, but may also reduce tension overload at the suture-tendon interface of the medial row [25, 26]. This may also reduce the likelihood of strangulation and relatively rapid necrosis of the rotator cuff tendon at the medial row [14]. As with arthroscopic double-row RCR, undue tension at the medial row due to use of conventional SBT may play a major role in repair failure [9]. This tension is usually concentrated at the medial row and is rarely exerted on the lateral row [9]. However, in knotless SBT, tension is usually concentrated at the lateral row and rarely at the medial row. Thus, pullout of the suture anchor at the lateral row after RCR may occur with the knotless SBT, particularly in patients with osteoporosis. Insufficient compression by the medial row suture limbs due to suture anchor pullout may compromise the healing of a repaired rotator cuff [27, 28].

The most frequently used portion of the Patte classification is retraction of the supraspinatus tendon in the coronal plane of MRI. The classification has been found to have moderate consent in assessing tear retraction in some reports [29, 30]. It has also been shown to have prognostic factor after RCR [31]. However, there were no significant differences of re-tear rate between Patte stage I and II. These results probably were due to confined tear size as inclusion criteria in this study, so that there was no RCT with Patte stage III. Also, there were no significant differences of re-tear rate between stages in each group. Therefore, there was no correlation between Patte stage and re-tear rate according to repair techniques.

This study had some limitations. First, although all of the US evaluations were performed by an experienced musculoskeletal radiologist, the technique remains examiner-dependent [32]. However, we did not perform the US examination ourselves to avoid surgeon bias [33]. Second, we could not evaluate preoperative muscle atrophy grades due to incomplete MRI data and the so-called Y-shaped view in some cases. Third, although there was no significant difference in the re-tear rate between groups, the likelihood of having a re-tear in the knotless SBT group was almost twice as high as in the conventional group. Therefore, this study might be under-powered to show this difference from the viewpoint of re-tear.

The study also had several strengths. First, the follow-up rate for the functional outcome and radiological evaluations was high (97%). Second, the study was prospective and enrolled homogeneous patients, with respect to tear size, who had full-thickness supraspinatus or infraspinatus tears 1–4 cm in length in the anterior-to-posterior dimension. Thus, the results can be considered reliable. Third, all of the operations were performed by the same surgeon.

Conclusions

The knotless SBT showed comparable functional outcomes to those of conventional SBT in medium-to-large, full-thickness RCTs at short-term follow-up. The knotless SBT had a higher re-tear rate compared with conventional SBT, although the difference was not significant.

Abbreviations
ASES: American Shoulder and Elbow Surgeons; MRI: Magnetic resonance imaging; RCR: Rotator cuff repair; RCT: Rotator cuff tear; SBT: Suture-bridge technique; UCLA: Shoulder Rating Scale of the University of California at Los Angeles; US: Ultrasonography; VAS: Visual analog scale

Authors' contributions
All authors made substantive intellectual contributions to this study to qualify as authors. KCK and WYL conceived of the study and contributed to the critical revision of the article for important intellectual content. HDS, KWY, and SCH collected the subjects' data. SCH performed the statistical analysis. An initial draft of the manuscript was written by KCK and WYL. All authors were involved in writing the manuscript. All authors read and approved the final manuscript.

Competing interests
The authors declare that they have no competing interests.

Author details
[1]Shoulder Center, Department of Orthopedic Surgery, TanTan Hospital, Daejeon, South Korea. [2]Department of Orthopedic Surgery, Regional Rheumatoid and Degenerative Arthritis Center, Chungnam National University Hospital, Chungnam National University School of Medicine, 266 Munwha-ro, Jung-gu, Daejeon 35015, South Korea.

References
1. Minagawa H, Yamamoto N, Abe H, Fukuda M, Seki N, Kikuchi K, et al. Prevalence of symptomatic and asymptomatic rotator cuff tears in the general population: from mass-screening in one village. J Orthop. 2013; 10(1):8–12.

2. Elia F, Azoulay V, Lebon J, Faraud A, Bonnevialle N, Mansat P. Clinical and anatomic results of surgical repair of chronic rotator cuff tears at ten-year minimum follow-up. Int Orthop. 2017;41(6):1219–26.

3. Heuberer PR, Smolen D, Pauzenberger L, Plachel F, Salem S, Laky B, et al. Longitudinal long-term magnetic resonance imaging and clinical follow-up after single-row arthroscopic rotator cuff repair: clinical superiority of structural tendon integrity. Am J Sports Med. 2017;45(6):1283–8.

4. Barnes LA, Kim HM, Caldwell JM, Buza J, Ahmad CS, Bigliani LU. Satisfaction, function and repair integrity after arthroscopic versus mini-open rotator cuff repair. Bone Joint J. 2017;99-B(2):245–9.

5. Park MC, ElAttrache NS, Ahmad CS, Tibone JE. "Transosseous-equivalent" rotator cuff repair technique. Arthroscopy. 2006;22(12):1360.e1–5.

6. Park MC, ElAttrache NS, Tibone JE, Ahmad CS, Jun BJ, Lee TQ. Part I: footprint contact characteristics for a transosseous-equivalent rotator cuff repair technique compared with a double row repair technique. J Shoulder Elb Surg. 2007;16(4):461–8.

7. Park MC, Tibone JE, ElAttrache NS, Ahmad CS, Jun BJ, Lee TQ. Part II: biomechanical assessment for a footprintrestoring transosseous-equivalent rotator cuff repair technique compared with a double-row repair technique. J Shoulder Elb Surg. 2007;16(4):469–76.

8. Quigley RJ, Gupta A, Oh JH, Chung KC, McGarry MH, Gupta R, et al. Biomechanical comparison of single-row, double-row, and transosseous-equivalent repair techniques after healing in an animal rotator cuff tear model. J Orthop Res. 2013;31(8):1254–60.

9. Trantalis JN, Boorman RS, Pletsch K, Lo IK. Medial rotator cuff failure after arthroscopic double-row rotator cuff repair. Arthroscopy. 2008;24(6):727–31.

10. Yamakado K, Katsuo S, Mizuno K, Arakawa H, Hayashi S. Medial-row failure after arthroscopic double-row rotator cuff repair. Arthroscopy. 2010;26(3):430–5.

11. Wang VM, Wang FC, McNickle AG, Friel NA, Yanke AB, Chubinskaya S, et al. Medial versus lateral supraspinatus tendon properties: implications for double-row rotator cuff repair. Am J Sports Med. 2010;38(12):2456–63.

12. Cho NS, Lee BG, Rhee YG. Arthroscopic rotator cuff repair using a suture bridge technique: is the repair integrity actually maintained? Am J Sports Med. 2011;39(10):2108–16.

13. Kim YK, Moon SH, Cho SH. Treatment outcomes of single- versus double-row repair for larger than medium-sized rotator cuff tears: the effect of preoperative remnant tendon length. Am J Sports Med. 2013;41(10):2270–7.

14. Rhee YG, Cho NS, Parke CS. Arthroscopic rotator cuff repair using modified Mason-Allen medial row stitch: knotless versus knot-tying suture bridge technique. Am J Sports Med. 2012;40(11):2440–7.

15. Vaishnav S, Millett PJ. Arthroscopic rotator cuff repair: scientific rationale, surgical technique, and early clinical and functional results of a knotless self-reinforcing double-row rotator cuff repair system. J Shoulder Elb Surg. 2010;19(2):83–90.

16. Barber FA, Drew OR. A biomechanical comparison of tendon-bone interface motion and cyclic loading between single-row, triple-loaded cuff repairs and double-row, suture-tape cuff repairs using biocomposite anchors. Arthroscopy. 2012;28(9):1197–205.

17. Burkhart SS, Adams CR, Burkhart SS, Schoolfield JD. A biomechanical comparison of 2 techniques of footprint reconstruction for rotator cuff repair: the SwiveLock-FiberChain construct versus standard double-row repair. Arthroscopy. 2009;25(3):274–81.

18. Millett PJ, Espinoza C, Horan MP, Ho CP, Warth RJ, Dornan GJ, et al. Predictors of outcomes after arthroscopic transosseous equivalent rotator cuff repair in 155 cases: a propensity score weighted analysis of knotted and knotless self-reinforcing repair techniques at a minimum of 2 years. Arch Orthop Trauma Surg. 2017;137(10):1399–408.

19. Boyer P, Bouthors C, Delcourt T, Stewart O, Hamida F, Mylle G, et al. Arthroscopic double-row cuff repair with suture-bridging: a structural and functional comparison of two techniques. Knee Surg Sports Traumatol Arthrosc. 2015;23(2):478–86.

20. Hug K, Gerhardt C, Hanevald H, Scheibel M. Arthroscopic knotless-anchor rotator cuff repair: a clinical and radiological evaluation. Knee Surg Sports Traumatol Arthrosc. 2015;23(9):2628–34.

21. Sugaya H, Maeda K, Matsuki K, Moriishi J. Functional and structural outcome after arthroscopic full-thickness rotator cuff repair: single-row versus dual-row fixation. Arthroscopy. 2005;21(11):1307–16.

22. Patte D. Classification of rotator cuff lesions. Clin Orthop Relat Res. 1990;254:81–6.

23. Kim KC, Rhee KJ, Shin HD, Kim YM. A modified suture-bridge technique for a marginal dog-ear deformity caused during rotator cuff repair. Arthroscopy. 2007;23(5):562.e1–4.

24. Virk MS, Bruce B, Hussey KE, Thomas JM, Luthringer TA, Shewman EF, et al. Biomechanical performance of medial row suture placement relative to the musculotendinous junction in transosseous equivalent suture bridge double-row rotator cuff repair. Arthroscopy. 2017;33(2):242–50.

25. Kim KC, Shin HD, Cha SM, Park JY. Comparisons of retear patterns for 3 arthroscopic rotator cuff repair methods. Am J Sports Med. 2014;42(3):558–65.

26. Ide J, Karasugi T, Okamoto N, Taniwaki T, Oka K, Mizuta H. Functional and structural comparisons of the arthroscopic knotless double-row suture bridge and single-row repair for anterosuperior rotator cuff tears. J Shoulder Elb Surg. 2015;24(10):1544–54.

27. Kummer F, Hergan DJ, Thut DC, Pahk B, Jazrawi LM. Suture loosening and its effect on tendon fixation in knotless double-row rotator cuff repairs. Arthroscopy. 2011;27(11):1478–84.

28. Leek BT, Robertson C, Mahar A, Pedowitz RA. Comparison of mechanical stability in double-row rotator cuff repairs between a knotless transtendon construct versus the addition of medial knots. Arthroscopy. 2010;26(Suppl 9):S127–33.

29. Kuhn JE, Dunn WR, Ma B, Wright RW, Jones G, Spencer EE, et al. Interobserver agreement in the classification of rotator cuff tears. Am J Sports Med. 2007;35(3):437–41.

30. Spencer EE Jr, Dunn WR, Wright RW, Wolf BR, Spindler KP, McCarty E, et al. Interobserver agreement in the classification of rotator cuff tears using magnetic resonance imaging. Am J Sports Med. 2008;36(1):99–103.

31. Gladstone JN, Bishop JY, Lo IK, Flatow EL. Fatty infiltration and atrophy of the rotator cuff do not improve after rotator cuff repair and correlate with poor functional outcome. Am J Sports Med. 2007;35(5):719–28.

32. Park JY, Siti HT, Keum JS, Moon SG, Oh KS. Does an arthroscopic suture bridge technique maintain repair integrity? A serial evaluation by ultrasonography. Clin Orthop Relat Res. 2010;468(6):1578–87.

33. Lafosse L, Brozska R, Toussaint B, Gobezie R. The outcome and structural integrity of arthroscopic rotator cuff repair with use of the double-row suture anchor technique. J Bone Joint Surg Am. 2007;89(7):1533–41.

Dynamic hip kinematics during squatting before and after total hip arthroplasty

Keisuke Komiyama[1], Satoshi Hamai[1*] ⓘ, Daisuke Hara[1], Satoru Ikebe[3], Hidehiko Higaki[2], Kensei Yoshimoto[1], Kyohei Shiomoto[1], Hirotaka Gondo[2], Yifeng Wang[2] and Yasuharu Nakashima[1]

Abstract

Background: The difference in in vivo kinematics before and after total hip arthroplasty (THA) for the same subjects and the clearance between the liner and neck during squatting have been unclear. The purpose of the present study was to clarify (1) the changes in the in vivo kinematics between prosthetic hips and osteoarthritis hips of the same subjects and (2) the extent of the liner-to-neck clearance during squatting under weight-bearing conditions.

Methods: This study consisted of 10 patients who underwent unilateral THA for symptomatic osteoarthritis. Using a flat-panel X-ray detector, we obtained continuous radiographs during squatting. We analyzed the hip joint's movements using three-dimensional-to-two-dimensional model-to-image registration techniques. We also quantified the minimum distance at maximum flexion and extension, and the minimum angle at maximum flexion between the liner and stem neck.

Results: The maximum hip flexion angles post-THA (80.7° [range, 69.4–98.6°]) changed significantly compared with the pre-THA values (71.7° [range, 55.2°–91.2°]). The pelvic tilt angle (posterior +, anterior–) at the maximum hip flexion post-THA (10.4° [range, – 6.7° to 26.9°]) was significantly smaller than that at pre-THA (16.6° [range, – 3° to 40.3°]). The minimum anterior and posterior liner-to-neck distances averaged 10.9 and 8.0 mm, respectively, which was a significant difference. The minimum liner-to-neck angle at maximum flexion averaged 34.7° (range, 20.7°–46.3°). No liner-to-neck contact occurred in any of the hips.

Conclusion: THA increased the range of hip joint motion and the pelvis tilted anteriorly more after than before THA, with sufficient liner-to-neck clearance during squatting. These data may be beneficial for advising patients after THA regarding postoperative activity restrictions in daily life.

Keywords: Kinematics, Range of motion, Squatting, Total hip arthroplasty, 3D-to-2D model-to-image registration techniques

Background

Total hip arthroplasty (THA) is the best surgical procedure for patients with end-stage osteoarthritis (OA) of the hip joint and is highly effective in relieving pain and improving function [1–3]. The clinical success of THA allows patients to resume their activities of daily living easily, and this includes squatting motions [4]. In Non-Western cultures, squatting is one of the fundamental activities of daily living and requires deep ranges of motion in flexion [5, 6]. Due to such requirements for

deep flexibility of the prosthetic hip, there are concerns for impingement and dislocation after THA. Therefore, the knowledge of the in vivo kinematics of the prosthetic hip associated with squatting and the clearance between the liner and neck (liner-to-neck clearance) could be beneficial for advising for patients after THA regarding postoperative activity restrictions in daily life.

Accurate evaluations of kinematics under weight-bearing conditions have been achieved using three-dimensional (3D)-to-two-dimensional (2D) model-to-image registration techniques [7–9]. Recently, these techniques have been applied to the kinematic analyses of hips affected by OA and subsequent THA procedures [10, 11]. We previously reported that, with respect to squatting, patients with OA

* Correspondence: hamachan@ortho.med.kyushu-u.ac.jp
[1]Department of Orthopedic Surgery, Graduate School of Medical Sciences, Kyushu University, 3-1-1 Maidashi, Higashi-ku, Fukuoka 812-8582, Japan
Full list of author information is available at the end of the article

were unable to deeply flex their femurs due to limited range of motion (ROM) of the hip joints. Additionally, patients with OA tilted their pelvis more posteriorly to maintain a deeply flexed posture than did healthy subjects [10]. In prosthetic hips, Koyanagi et al. revealed that the mean maximum hip flexion ROM was 86.2 °, which is smaller than the mean maximum hip flexion angle of 95.4 ° in normal native hips [5, 12]. However, to the best of our knowledge, no previous report has demonstrated the changes in in vivo 3D kinematics during squatting pre- and post-THA for the same subjects using the accurate 3D-to-2D model-to-image registration techniques.

The purpose of the present study was to clarify (1) the changes in the in vivo kinematics between prosthetic hips and OA hips of the same subjects and (2) the extent of the liner-to-neck clearance during squatting under weight-bearing conditions.

Methods

Patients

The protocol in the current study was approved by our institutional review board. All patients provided informed consent to participate in this study. Between August 2012 and October 2015, 177 patients with 200 hips underwent primary cementless THA by two senior surgeons (Y.N. and S.H.). Among the original 177 patients, 10 of them (10 hips) met all the inclusion criteria, which were (1) unilateral THA for symptomatic OA (2) no previous surgery of the ipsilateral hip, (3) no previous surgery of the spine or other joints, (4) obtaining the informed consent prior to THA, and (5) ability to squat safely without assistance before and after THA. Demographic data of the patients are shown in Table 1. There were 6 women and 4 men with a mean age at the time of THA of 65 ± 8 years (range, 55–84 years). The mean height was 156 ± 7 cm (range, 148–168 cm), and the mean body mass index (BMI) was 23 ± 4 kg/m^2 (range, 18–31 kg/m^2). According to the Kellgren-Lawrence

scale, 2 hips were classified as grade III and 8 hips were classified as grade IV. [13] The pre- and post-THA mean Harris hip scores were 48 ± 7 (range, 40–57) and 95 ± 3 (range, 91–99), respectively. The mean post-THA follow-up was 43 ± 11 months (range, 23–59 months). No patient had a history of any complication after THA.

Surgical procedures and implants

All operations were performed through a posterolateral approach with repair of the posterior soft tissue [14]. The combined anteversion technique was adopted to cope with the wide range of femoral anteversion of hip dysplasia at our institution. The cup was placed according to stem anteversion so that combined anteversion ranged from 40° to 60° [15]. A cementless hemispherical press-fit cup, straight metaphyseal fit stem, and high cross-linked ultra-high molecular weight polyethylene liner (AMS and PerFix HA; Aeonian; Kyocera, Kyoto, Japan) were used [16, 17]. All femoral heads were alumina ceramic, and the head sizes were 32 mm in 9 cases and 26 mm in 1 case. There are two types of rims in the Aeonian liner, one is a 15 ° elevated rim (elevated rim liner) to prevent dislocation of the femoral head, and the other is not elevated (flat liner). Four hips used the elevated rim liners, and 6 hips used the flat liner, respectively. When using the elevated rim liner, we recorded the location on the cup where the top of the rim was placed.

The orientations of the acetabular cup and stem were measured using the postoperative computed tomography (CT) data. The cup inclination was measured as the angle of abduction using the inter-tear-drop line as the baseline (radiographic inclination). The cup anteversion was measured as the angle of anteversion in the sagittal plane (operative anteversion). Femoral anteversion was measured as the angle of anteversion between the prosthetic femoral neck and transepicondylar axis [18].

Table 1 Demographic data

Patient no.	1	2	3	4	5	6	7	8	9	10
Sex	Male	Male	Female	Female	Male	Female	Female	Female	Female	Male
Diagnosis	OA	DDH	DDH	DDH	OA	DDH	DDH	DDH	DDH	OA
Age at THA (years old)	61	65	56	60	55	70	68	63	68	84
Affected side	Right	Left	Left	Left	Right	Right	Left	Right	Right	Left
Height (cm)	155	161	161	148	168	153	148	152	149	163
Body weight (kg)	73	63	46	46	70	44	40	55	64	65
BMI (kg/m^2)	30.5	24.3	17.7	21	24.7	18.8	18.3	24	28.5	24.5
Preoperative HHS	51	53	44	51	40	57	45	41	40	56
Postoperative HHS	97	98	91	91	91	98	94	99	97	95
Follow-up period (months)	59	47	49	38	49	36	36	23	48	48

OA osteoarthritis, *DDH* developmental dysplasia of the hip, *THA* total hip arthroplasty, *BMI* body mass index, *HHS* Harris hip score

Kinematic analysis

We essentially followed the method in accordance with previous reports, and we partially referenced the kinematics data regarding pre-THA [10, 19]. The 3D positions and orientations of the pelvis, acetabular cup, femur, and femoral stem during squatting were determined using 3D-to-2D model-to-image registration techniques. Continuous radiographic images were used to survey squatting movements using a flat-panel X-ray detector (Ultimax-I, Toshiba, Tochigi, Japan) with the following parameters: image area of 420 mm × 420 mm, resolution of 0.274 mm × 0.274 mm/pixel, and frame rate of 3.5 frames/s (Fig. 1). Each subject routinely underwent CT (Aquilion, Toshiba, Tochigi, Japan) with a 512 × 512 image matrix, a 0.35 × 0.35 pixel dim, and 1-mm-slice thicknesses from the superior edge of the pelvis to just below the knee joint line. Anatomical coordinate systems of the pelvis and femur were embedded in each bone model derived from CT data according to our previous study [10, 19]. Computer simulation was performed to generate virtual, digitally reconstructed radiographs in which the light source and the projected plane parameters were set to be identical to the actual radiographic imaging conditions. Each model silhouette was matched with the actual silhouette by translating and rotating the 3D model to minimize the number of unmatched pixels between the silhouettes. The orientation of the femur relative to the pelvis: hip movements, was determined using the Cardan/Euler angle system in x-y-z order (flexion/extension, adduction/abduction, internal/external rotation). The maximum errors associated with tracking the position of the femur/stem relative to the pelvis/acetabular cup were 0.36/0.43 mm, 0.37/0.48 mm, and 0.48 °/0.52 °, respectively, for in-plane translation, out-of-plane translation, and rotation, respectively [10, 19].

Regarding the liner-to-neck clearance, we quantified the minimum distance at maximum flexion and extension and the angle at maximum flexion between the liner and stem neck using a computer-aided design software program ([CATIA V5]; Dassault Systemes, Vélizy-Villacoublay, France) (Fig. 2) [19, 20].

Statistical analysis

All data are expressed as mean ± standard deviation (SD) and were tested for normality using the Shapiro-Wilk test. To compare hip kinematics before and after THA in the same patient, normally distributed variables were evaluated using the paired t test. Non-normally distributed variables were evaluated using the independent Wilcoxon signed-rank test. Statistical significance was defined as a P value $< .05$. The statistical analyses were performed using JMP Software (Version 11; SAS Institute, Cary, NC, USA).

Results

Orientation of the components

The mean cup inclination and mean cup anteversion were 39.1 ± 5.4° (range, 30.1°–48.0°) and 18.5 ± 12.0° (range, 4.3°–40.0°), respectively. The mean stem anteversion was 31.7 ± 6.8° (range, 22.0°–42.1°), and the mean combined anteversion was 50.3 ± 9.3° (range, 36.9°–67.5°) (Table 2).

Kinematics of the hip joint

The maximum hip flexion angles were determined during squatting at 10% of the squat ascent cycle pre-THA, and at 15% of the squat ascent cycle post-THA,

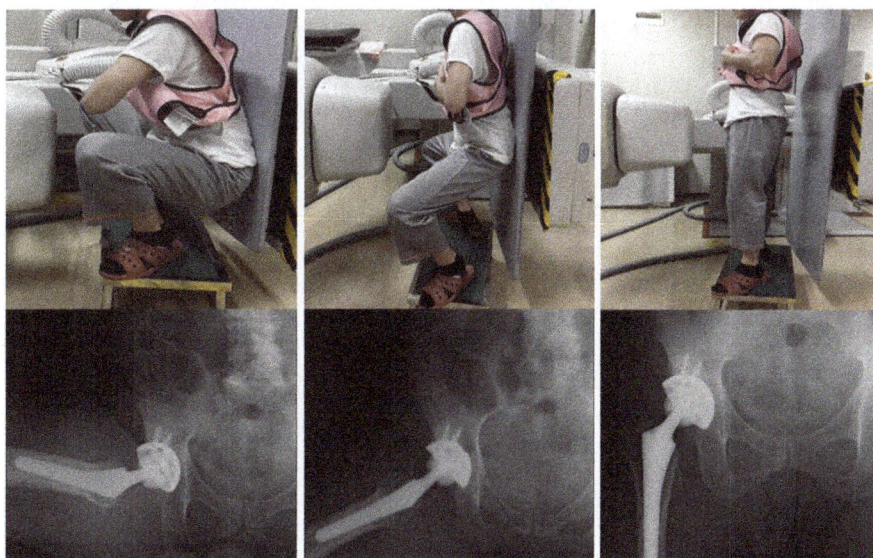

Fig. 1 The hip motions during squatting were captured as continuous X-ray images using a flat panel X-ray detector. Patients before and after total hip arthroplasty stood from a squat position with their heel down

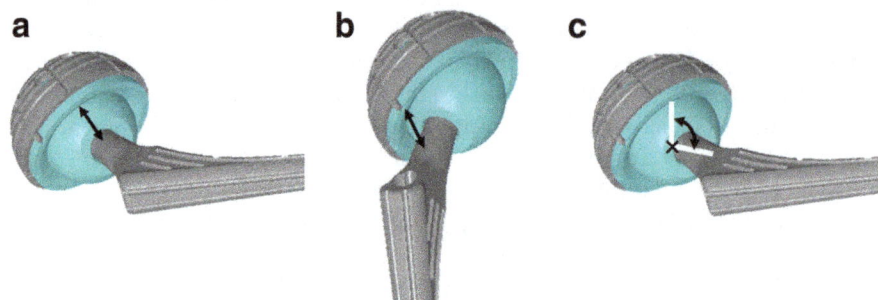

Fig. 2 The minimum distance at maximum flexion (**a**) at maximum extension (**b**), and the angle at maximum flexion (**c**) between the liner and stem neck

respectively (Fig. 3). The kinematics data of each patient are shown in Table 3. The maximum femoral and hip flexion angles post-THA (94.9 ± 6.8° [range, 85.4°–104.6°] and 80.7 ± 10.0° [range, 69.4°–98.6°], respectively) changed significantly (P = .013 and P = .005, respectively) compared with the pre-THA values (86.2 ± 7.3° [range, 70.9°–94.3°] and 71.7 ± 11.9° [range, 55.2°–91.2°], respectively) (Figs. 3 and 4). In the squatting position, the pelvis tilted backward and gradually tilted forward with standing. The pelvic tilt angle (posterior +, anterior–) at the maximum hip flexion post-THA (10.4 ± 10.4° [range, – 6.7° to 26.9°] was significantly (P = .0463) smaller than that at pre-THA (16.6 ± 13.3° [range, – 3° to 40.3°]) (Fig. 5).

Liner-to-neck clearance

The liner-to-neck clearance data for the each patient are shown in Table 3. The minimum anterior and posterior liner-to-neck distances averaged 10.9 ± 2.2 mm (range, 7.3–14.8 mm) and 8.0 ± 2.4 mm (range, 3.6–11.2 mm), respectively, and the difference was significant (P = .0143). The minimum liner-to-neck angle at maximum flexion averaged 34.7 ± 7.3° (range, 20.7–46.3°). No liner-to-neck contact occurred in any of the hips during squatting.

Discussion

To our knowledge, no previous reports have demonstrated the changes in in vivo hip kinematics during

squatting pre- and post-THA for the same subjects using accurate 3D-to-2D model-to-image registration techniques. The current study elucidated the dynamic hip kinematics during squatting before and after THA and quantified the liner-to-neck clearance. The maximum hip flexion significantly changed from 72° pre-THA to 81° post-THA, and the pelvic tilt angle at the maximum hip flexion post-THA was 10° , which was significantly smaller than the 17° measurement pre-THA. The anterior and posterior liner-to-neck distances averaged 11 and 8 mm, respectively, and the differences were significant. The mean minimum liner-to-neck angle was 35°, and there was no liner-to-neck contact during squatting in any of the hips.

A previous study found that patients with OA were not able to flex their femurs deeply due to limited ROM of the hip joints during squatting. They also tend to tilt their pelvises more posteriorly to maintain a deeply flexed posture than did healthy subjects [10]. The present study revealed that the maximum hip flexion was improved by approximately 9°. The pelvic tilt at the maximum hip flexion post-THA was significantly inclined and measured approximately 7° more anteriorly than pre-THA for the same subjects. We found that THA increased the range of the femoral and hip joint motions during squatting, and the compensation to maintain deeply flexed postures was reduced. Sagittal pelvic mobility is integral in flexing the torso to maintain

Table 2 Component data

Patient no.	1	2	3	4	5	6	7	8	9	10
Cup size (mm)	52	50	48	46	52	48	48	48	50	54
Head size (mm)	32	32	32	26	32	32	32	32	32	32
Polyethylene liner	Flat	Flat	Flat	Flat	Elevated	Elevated	Flat	Flat	Elevated	Elevated
Cup inclination (°)	36.6	42	30.1	44	41.2	37.1	34.1	42.4	48	35.2
Cup anteversion (°)	4.3	16	11	10.1	26.8	5	24	35.3	38	14.9
Stem anteversion (°)	34.8	37	38.1	34	26.4	42.1	28.1	32.2	22.6	22
Combined anteversion (°)	39.1	53	49.1	44.1	53.2	47.1	52	67.5	60.6	36.9

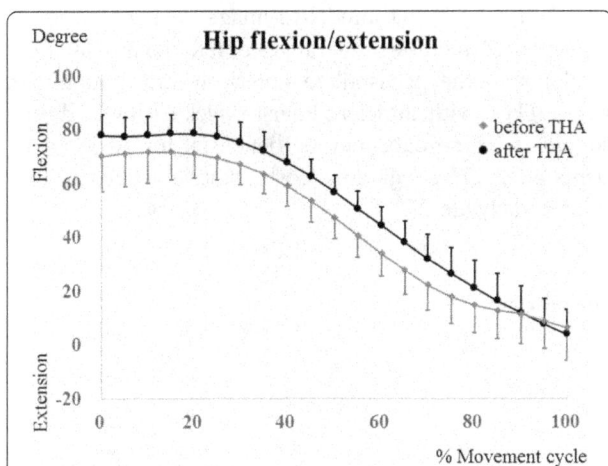

Fig. 3 The hip flexion/extension angles during squatting in patients before total hip arthroplasty (THA) (gray lines) and patients after THA (black lines). Error bars show standard deviation

balance and to allow the large hip flexion angles that are essential for deep squats [21].

It has been reported that approximately 95 to 102° of maximum hip flexion occurs during squatting in healthy subjects [5, 22]. Our study showed that the maximum hip flexion significantly changed from 72° pre-THA to 81° post-THA. Although THA provided increased ROM in patients with OA, prosthetic hips were not able to recover the kinematics to the level of healthy hips. Catelli et al. reported that joint kinematics of the pelvis and hip do not return to the level of healthy hips after THA during squatting and dual-mobility implant combined with the poorer functional scores [23]. A limited

range of hip flexion persisted even after THA, which might have affected postoperative functional outcomes during activities of daily living, especially those requiring deeply flexed postures.

Specific postures might include potential risks of prosthetic impingement and could cause postoperative dislocation, and polyethylene wear after THA [24, 25]. However, we found only a few reports which quantified the liner-to-neck distances while squatting. In our study, the anterior and posterior liner-to-neck distances averaged 11 and 8 mm, respectively, and the differences were significant. Furthermore, the minimum liner-to-neck angle at maximum flexion was 21°. Koyanagi et al. reported that the minimum angle leading up to theoretical prosthetic impingement was more than 10° [12]. Based on the analysis, we concluded that the liner-to-neck clearance during squatting after THA was sufficient in these patients.

There are several limitations in the present study. First, the number of patients in this study was small. A larger sample size with a wider variation in component position might result in greater statistical reliability and reveal correlation between implant positioning and minimum liner-to-neck clearance; this topic needs further clarification. Second, kinematic processing of radiographic measurements imparts a risk of radiation exposure. However, we believe that this represents an important data-driven approach to provide feedback on the activities of daily living specific advice for each patient. Third, this study examined only a single component design. Although the design is similar to that of many others that are currently available, the results could differ. Fourth, the sequential motions during

Table 3 Patient kinematic data

Patient No.	1	2	3	4	5	6	7	8	9	10
Maximum hip flexion (°)										
Pre-THA	59.5	73.1	67.2	83.5	73.3	70.7	59.4	84.3	91.2	55.2
Post-THA	75.6	73.3	71.6	90.5	81.3	87.5	71.2	87.6	98.6	69.4
Maximum femoral flexion (°)										
Pre-THA	77.2	92.9	85.8	93.8	87	86.9	87.2	85.5	94.3	70.9
Post-THA	96.5	92.1	91.7	102.1	86	92.1	104.6	85.4	103.1	95.1
Pelvic tilt at maximum hip flexion (°)										
Pre-THA	40.3	20.6	15.5	8.1	− 3	18.9	31.2	2.5	7.6	23.9
Post-THA	20.3	15.4	16.7	4.2	3.5	3.8	17.6	− 6.7	2.3	26.9
Liner-to-neck clearance										
the minimum anterior distance (mm)	10	9.5	11.4	8.2	11.2	12.4	12.4	12.1	14.8	7.3
the minimum posterior distance (mm)	10.1	7	9.9	8.9	11.2	7.3	10.1	5.8	6	3.6
the minimum angle at maximum hip flexion (°)	30.6	32.6	35.2	31.8	31	34.9	44	40.1	46.3	20.7

THA total hip arthroplasty
The pelvic tilt (posterior +, anterior −) angles

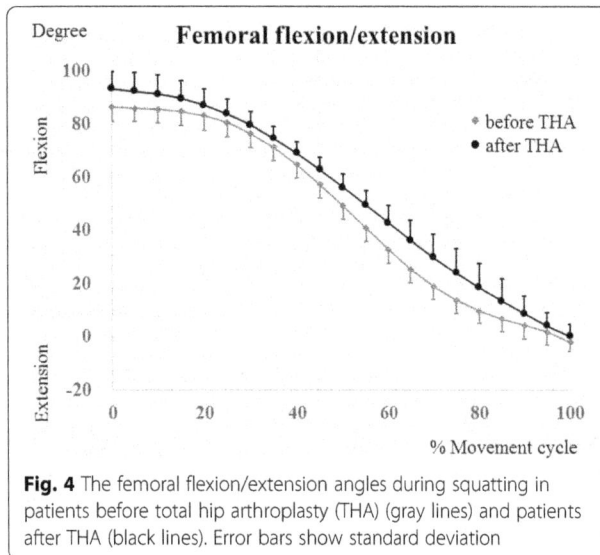

Fig. 4 The femoral flexion/extension angles during squatting in patients before total hip arthroplasty (THA) (gray lines) and patients after THA (black lines). Error bars show standard deviation

using the 3D-to-2D model-to-image registration techniques. THA increased the ranges of femoral and hip joint motion and the pelvis tilted anteriorly more after than before THA, with sufficient liner-to-neck clearance during squatting. These data may be beneficial for advising patients after THA regarding postoperative activity restrictions in daily life.

Abbreviations
2D: Two-dimensional; 3D: Three-dimensional; BMI: Body mass index; CT: Computed tomography; DDH: Developmental dysplasia of the hip; FOV: Field of view; HHS: Harris hip score; OA: Osteoarthritis; ROM: Range of motion; SD: Standard deviation; THA: Total hip arthroplasty

Funding
This study was supported by JSPS KAKENHI Grant No. 15K10450 and 25870499, grant from the Japan Orthopaedics and Traumatology Foundation, Inc. (No. 263), and grant from the Nakatomi Foundation.

squatting were collected into twice, because even the large flat-panel X-ray detector that was used in this study provided a limited field of view (FOV). It might be necessary that the development of fluoroscopy is expected to achieve quite a large FOV. Finally, the patients included in this study were all Japanese with lower BMI compared to the Caucasian average. The patients with a BMI ≥ 30 kg/m^2 could show different kinematic data with limited maximum hip flexion angle.

Conclusion
We quantified the change in hip kinematics before and after THA and the liner-to-neck clearance while squatting

Authors' contributions
KK, SH, DH, SI, HH, and YN contributed to the conception and design of the study. KK, SH, DH, KY, and KS performed acquisition of data. KK, SH, DH, SI, HH, HG, and YW conducted data analysis, and KK, SH, and YN contributed to data interpretation and preparation of the manuscript. All authors read and approved the final version of the manuscript.

Competing interests
The authors declare that they have no competing interests.

Author details
[1]Department of Orthopedic Surgery, Graduate School of Medical Sciences, Kyushu University, 3-1-1 Maidashi, Higashi-ku, Fukuoka 812-8582, Japan. [2]Department of Life Science, Faculty of Life Science, Kyushu Sangyo University, 2-3-1 Matsugadai, Higashi-ku, Fukuoka 813-0004, Japan. [3]Department of Creative Engineering, National Institute of Technology, Kitakyushu College, 5-20-1 Shii, Kokuraminami-ku, Kitakyushu, Fukuoka 802-0985, Japan.

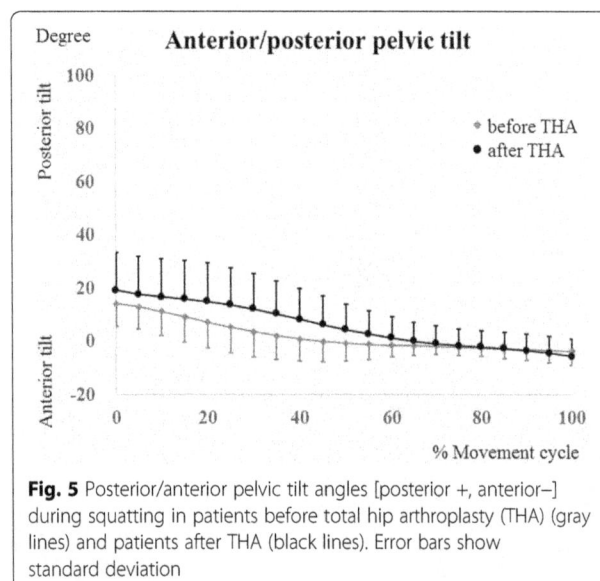

Fig. 5 Posterior/anterior pelvic tilt angles [posterior +, anterior−] during squatting in patients before total hip arthroplasty (THA) (gray lines) and patients after THA (black lines). Error bars show standard deviation

References
1. Learmonth ID, Young C, Rorabeck C. The operation of the century: total hip replacement. Lancet. 2007;370(9597):1508–19.
2. Chang RW, Pellisier JM, Hazen GB. A cost-effectiveness analysis of total hip arthroplasty for osteoarthritis of the hip. JAMA. 1996;275(11):858–65.
3. Jacobsen S, Sonne-Holm S, Soballe K, Gebuhr P, Lund B. Hip dysplasia and osteoarthrosis: a survey of 4151 subjects from the osteoarthrosis substudy of the Copenhagen City Heart Study. Acta Orthop. 2005;76(2):149–58.
4. Rissanen P, Aro S, Slatis P, Sintonen H, Paavolainen P. Health and quality of life before and after hip or knee arthroplasty. J Arthroplast. 1995;10(2):169–75.
5. Hemmerich A, Brown H, Smith S, Marthandam SS, Wyss UP. Hip, knee, and ankle kinematics of high range of motion activities of daily living. J Orthop Res. 2006;24(4):770–81.
6. Tang H, Du H, Tang Q, Yang D, Shao H, Zhou Y. Chinese patients' satisfaction with total hip arthroplasty: what is important and dissatisfactory? J Arthroplast. 2014;29(12):2245–50.
7. Komistek RD, Dennis DA, Mahfouz M. In vivo fluoroscopic analysis of the normal human knee. Clin Orthop Relat Res. 2003;410:69–81.

8. Hamai S, Moro-oka TA, Miura H, Shimoto T, Higaki H, Fregly BJ, Iwamoto Y, Banks SA. Knee kinematics in medial osteoarthritis during in vivo weight-bearing activities. J Orthop Res. 2009;27(12):1555–61.

9. Ishimaru M, Shiraishi Y, Ikebe S, Higaki H, Hino K, Onishi Y, Miura H. Three-dimensional motion analysis of the patellar component in total knee arthroplasty by the image matching method using image correlations. J Orthop Res. 2014;32(5):619–26.

10. Hara D, Nakashima Y, Hamai S, Higaki H, Ikebe S, Shimoto T, Yoshimoto K, Iwamoto Y. Dynamic hip kinematics in patients with hip osteoarthritis during weight-bearing activities. Clin Biomech. 2016;32:150–6.

11. Tsai T-Y, Li J-S, Wang S, Lin H, Malchau H, Li G, Rubash H, Kwon Y-M. A novel dual fluoroscopic imaging method for determination of THA kinematics: in-vitro and in-vivo study. J Biomech. 2013;46(7):1300–4.

12. Koyanagi J, Sakai T, Yamazaki T, Watanabe T, Akiyama K, Sugano N, Yoshikawa H, Sugamoto K. In vivo kinematic analysis of squatting after total hip arthroplasty. Clin Biomech. 2011;26(5):477–83.

13. Kellgren JH, Lawrence JS. Radiological assessment of osteo-arthrosis. Ann Rheum Dis. 1957;16(4):494–502.

14. Pellicci PM, Bostrom M, Poss R. Posterior approach to total hip replacement using enhanced posterior soft tissue repair. Clin Orthop Relat Res. 1998;355:224–8.

15. Nakashima Y, Hirata M, Akiyama M, Itokawa T, Yamamoto T, Motomura G, Ohishi M, Hamai S, Iwamoto Y. Combined anteversion technique reduced the dislocation in cementless total hip arthroplasty. Int Orthop. 2014;38(1):27–32.

16. Sato T, Nakashima Y, Akiyama M, Yamamoto T, Mawatari T, Itokawa T, Ohishi M, Motomura G, Hirata M, Iwamoto Y. Wear resistant performance of highly cross-linked and annealed ultra-high molecular weight polyethylene against ceramic heads in total hip arthroplasty. J Orthop Res. 2012;30(12):2031–7.

17. Nakashima Y, Sato T, Yamamoto T, Motomura G, Ohishi M, Hamai S, Akiyama M, Hirata M, Hara D, Iwamoto Y. Results at a minimum of 10 years of follow-up for AMS and PerFix HA-coated cementless total hip arthroplasty: impact of cross-linked polyethylene on implant longevity. J Orthop Sci. 2013;18(6):962–8.

18. Yoshioka Y, Siu D, Cooke TD. The anatomy and functional axes of the femur. J Bone Joint Surg Am. 1987;69(6):873–80.

19. Hara D, Nakashima Y, Hamai S, Higaki H, Ikebe S, Shimoto T, Yoshimoto K, Iwamoto Y. Dynamic hip kinematics during the golf swing after total hip arthroplasty. Am J Sports Med. 2016;44(7):1801–9.

20. Yoshimoto K, Hamai S, Higaki H, Gondoh H, Nakashima Y. Visualization of a cam-type femoroacetabular impingement while squatting using image-matching techniques: a case report. Skelet Radiol. 2017;46(9):1277–82.

21. Lamontagne M, Kennedy MJ, Beaule PE. The effect of cam FAI on hip and pelvic motion during maximum squat. Clin Orthop Relat Res. 2009;467(3):645–50.

22. Hara D, Nakashima Y, Hamai S, Higaki H, Ikebe S, Shimoto T, Hirata M, Kanazawa M, Kohno Y, Iwamoto Y. Kinematic analysis of healthy hips during weight-bearing activities by 3D-to-2D model-to-image registration technique. Biomed Res Int. 2014;2014:457573.

23. Catelli DS, Kowalski E, Beaule PE, Lamontagne M. Does the dual-mobility hip prosthesis produce better joint kinematics during extreme hip flexion task? J Arthroplast. 2017;32(10):3206–12.

24. Shon WY, Baldini T, Peterson MG, Wright TM, Salvati EA. Impingement in total hip arthroplasty a study of retrieved acetabular components. J Arthroplasty. 2005;20(4):427–35.

25. Marchetti E, Krantz N, Berton C, Bocquet D, Fouilleron N, Migaud H, Girard J. Component impingement in total hip arthroplasty: frequency and risk factors. A continuous retrieval analysis series of 416 cup. Orthop Traumatol Surg Res. 2011;97(2):127–33.

11

Comparison of suprapatellar and infrapatellar intramedullary nailing for tibial shaft fractures: a systematic review and meta-analysis

Liqing Yang*, Yuefeng Sun and Ge Li

Abstract

Background: Optimal surgical approach for tibial shaft fractures remains controversial. We perform a meta-analysis from randomized controlled trials (RCTs) to compare the clinical efficacy and prognosis between infrapatellar and suprapatellar intramedullary nail in the treatment of tibial shaft fractures.

Methods: PubMed, OVID, Embase, ScienceDirect, and Web of Science were searched up to December 2017 for comparative RCTs involving infrapatellar and suprapatellar intramedullary nail in the treatment of tibial shaft fractures. Primary outcomes were blood loss, visual analog scale (VAS) score, range of motion, Lysholm knee scores, and fluoroscopy times. Secondary outcomes were length of hospital stay and postoperative complications. We assessed statistical heterogeneity for each outcome with the use of a standard χ^2 test and the I^2 statistic. The meta-analysis was undertaken using Stata 14.0.

Results: Four RCTs involving 293 participants were included in our study. The present meta-analysis indicated that there were significant differences between infrapatellar and suprapatellar intramedullary nail regarding the total blood loss, VAS scores, Lysholm knee scores, and fluoroscopy times.

Conclusion: Suprapatellar intramedullary nailing could significantly reduce total blood loss, postoperative knee pain, and fluoroscopy times compared to infrapatellar approach. Additionally, it was associated with an improved Lysholm knee scores. High-quality RCTs were still required for further investigation.

Keywords: Tibial shaft fractures, Infrapatellar, Suprapatellar, Intramedullary nail, Meta-analysis

Background

Tibial shaft fracture is common and comprises about 2% of workload in all fractures in adult [1, 2]. The intramedullary nail (IMN) fixation is reported to be a successful surgical procedure for the treatment of tibial shaft fracture and shows improved outcome in functional recovery [3]. The traditional infrapatellar is the common surgical approach to insert an IMN for the tibial shaft fracture. However, this approach requires a flexed knee and makes it difficult to use correctly in proximal third tibial shaft fractures, because the quadriceps muscle forces the proximal fragment into extension, resulting in deformities of angulation and fragment displacement [4]. Additionally, chronic postoperative knee pain is one of the most frequent complications after IMN insertion; the incidence was reported varying from 10 to 80% [5, 6].

The semiextended approach for tibial IMN insertion was first introduced in 2000 and then was modified into suprapatellar approach [7]. It has more simple access to entry point at proximal tibia, facilitates fracture reduction, and avoids patellar

* Correspondence: yanglq@sj-hospital.org
Department of orthopedics, Shengjing Hospital of China Medical University, Shenyang 110004, China

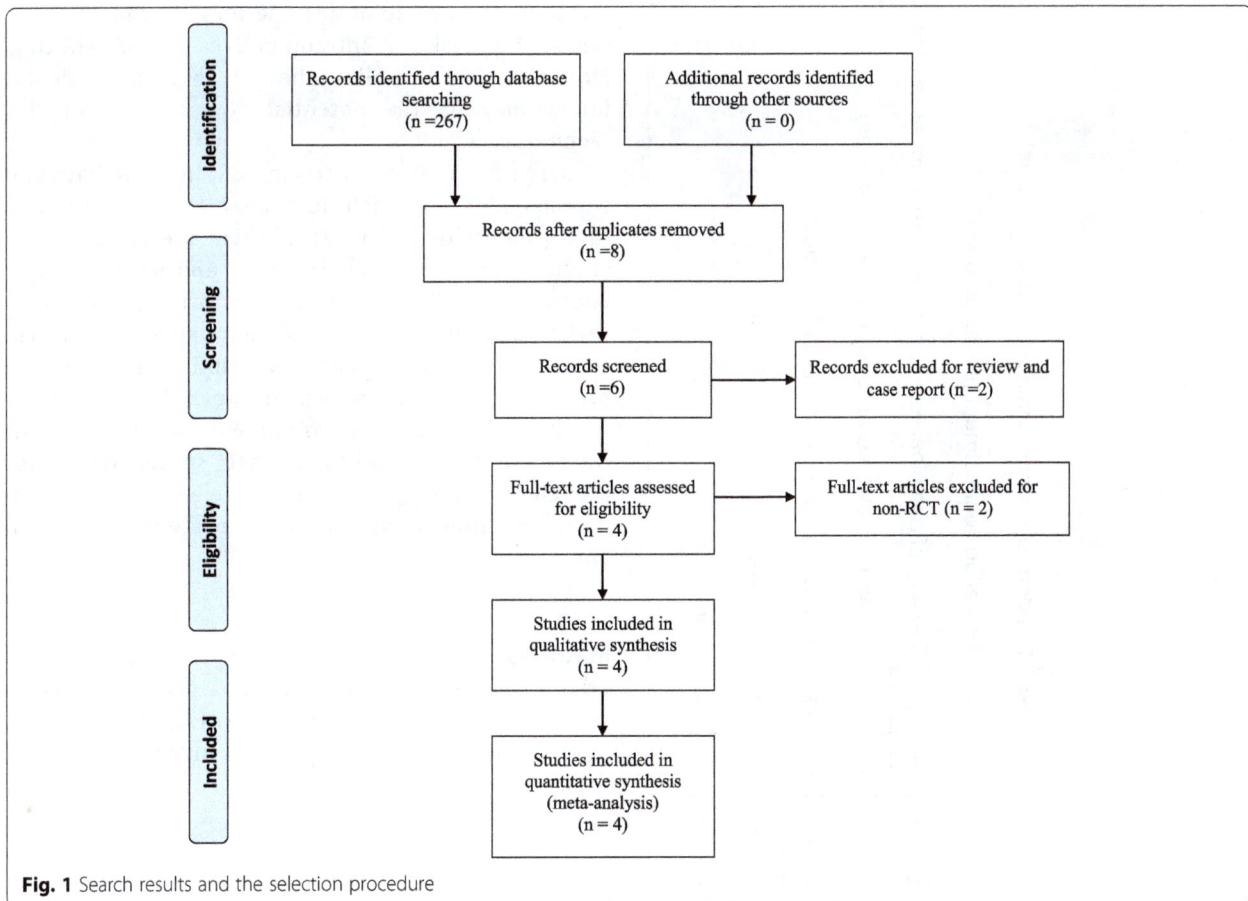

Fig. 1 Search results and the selection procedure

Table 1 Trial characteristics

Author	Study design	Location	Sample size (IP/SP)	Mean age (IP/SP)	Female patient (IP/SP)	Type of fractures	IP group	SP group	Follow-up
Chan, 2015	RCT	USA	14/11	43/40	4/5	Open tibial shaft fractures: 3 Closed tibial shaft fractures: 22	Infrapatellar tibial nail insertion	Suprapatellar tibial nail insertion	16 months
Zhe, 2016	RCT	China	30/38	46/42	4/3	Open tibial shaft fractures: 8 Closed tibial shaft fractures: 60	Infrapatellar intramedullary nailing	Suprapatellar intramedullary nailing	6 months
Sun, 2016	RCT	China	81/81	47/46	16/15	Open tibial shaft fractures: 21 Closed tibial shaft fractures: 141	Infrapatellar intramedullary nailing	Suprapatellar intramedullary nailing	24 months
Sreekumar, 2017	RCT	India	17/21	44/42	9/8	Open tibial shaft fractures: 5 Closed tibial shaft fractures: 33	Infrapatellar tibial nail	Suprapatellar tibial nail	12 months

IP infrapatellar, *SP* suprapatellar, *RCT* randomized controlled trial

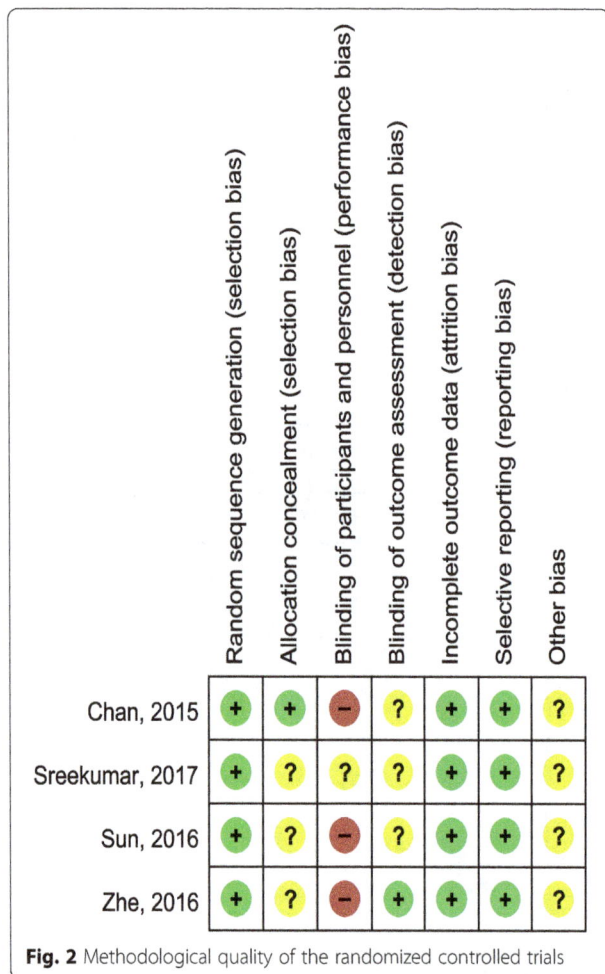

Fig. 2 Methodological quality of the randomized controlled trials

disorder of knee joint [8]. Besides, it can also decrease the risk of intraoperative second shifting. However, some studies showed that intraarticular injury may be the potential complication of this technique.

Currently, the comparison of infrapatellar and suprapatellar approach for tibial IMN insertion is rarely reported, and most of them are retrospective studies. The optional surgical approach remains controversial. Therefore, we perform a systematic review and meta-analysis of randomized controlled trials (RCTs) to compare the clinical efficacy and prognosis between classical infrapatellar and suprapatellar IMN in the treatment of tibial shaft fractures. We hypothesize that suprapatellar approach is superior to infrapatellar approach in terms of functional outcome, postoperative pain, and complications.

Methods

Ethical approval for this study was deemed unnecessary because it was a review of existing literature and did not involve any handling of individual patient's data.

Search methodology

Two reviewers independently searched PubMed, OVID, Embase, ScienceDirect, and Web of Science. All databases were searched up to December 2017, without restrictions on publication date and language. The terms were used to search the databases: "tibia shaft fracture," "intramedullary nail," "infrapatellar," and "suprapatellar." Search terms were combined using the Boolean operators "AND" or "OR." Reference lists of relevant articles were manually searched to identify additional trials.

tendon. Additionally, the extended position of the lower limb allows for easier fluoroscopic imaging [4]. Zhan et al. reported that suprapatellar approach may be effective in reducing the incidence of postoperative knee pain and prevent degenerative

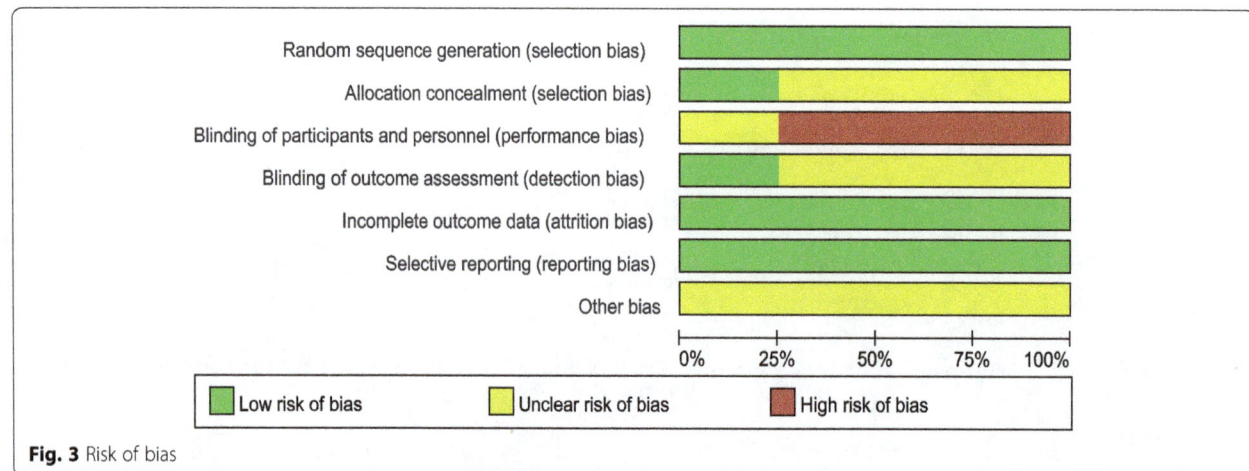

Fig. 3 Risk of bias

Inclusion and exclusion criteria

Studies were considered eligible when they met following criteria: (1) published clinical RCTs; (2) patients with tibial shaft fracture, intervention groups received infrapatellar approach IMN, and control groups received suprapatellar approach IMN; and (3) studies with at least one of the following outcomes: blood loss, visual analog score (VAS), range of motion, Lysholm knee scores, fluoroscopy times, length of hospital stay, and postoperative complications. Studies would be excluded from present meta-analysis for incomplete data, case reports, conference abstract, or review articles.

Study selection

Two investigators independently selected articles according to the criteria described above. The full text was scanned to determine whether articles fit the inclusion criteria. We resolved disagreements by discussion until a consensus was search. If no consensus was reached, a third investigator was consulted.

Data extraction

Two investigators independently extracted the data from the eligible studies that met the inclusion criteria. A double-check procedure was performed to test the accuracy of the extracted data. The information extracted from the studies were as follows: first author names, publishing year, study design, sample size, age, gender, intervention of each groups, duration of follow-up, and outcome measures. Primary outcomes were blood loss, visual analog scale (VAS) score, range of motion, Lysholm knee scores, and fluoroscopy times. Secondary outcomes were length of hospital stay and postoperative complications. Corresponding authors were consulted to obtain incomplete outcome data.

Data analysis

We performed all meta-analysis using the Stata 14.0 software. For continuous outcomes, the number of patients, means, and standard deviations were pooled to a weighted mean difference (WMD) and a 95% confidence interval (CI). For dichotomous outcomes, the risk difference (RD) and the 95% CI were assessed. The assessment for statistical heterogeneity

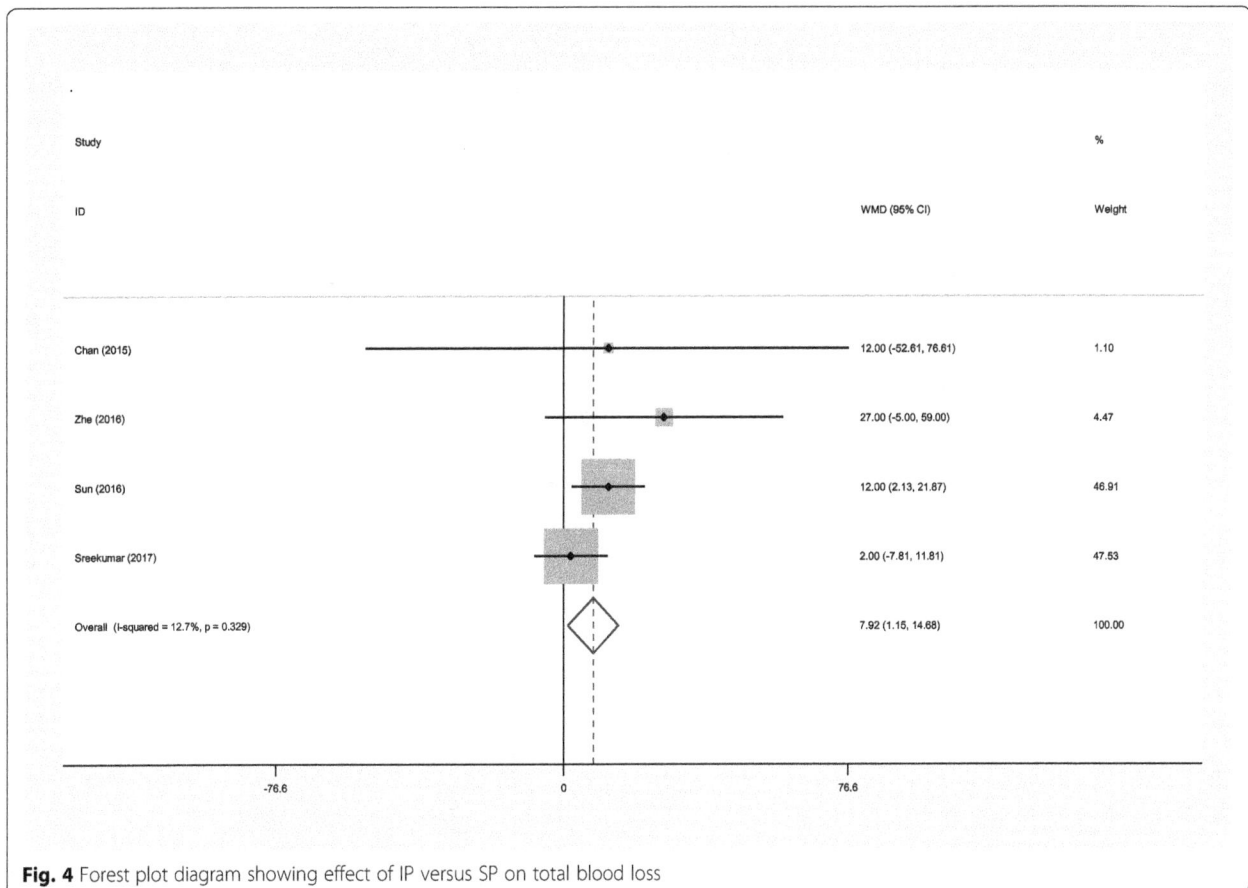

Fig. 4 Forest plot diagram showing effect of IP versus SP on total blood loss

was calculated using the chi-square and I-square tests. A fixed-effects model was used when $I^2 < 50\%$ and $P > 0.05$; otherwise, the random-effects model was adopted.

Quality assessment

A quality assessment of each RCT was performed according to the Cochrane Handbook for Systematic Reviews of Interventions. Two authors independently evaluated the risk of bias of the included RCTs based on the following items: random sequence generation, allocation concealment, blinding, incomplete outcome data, selective reporting, and other sources of bias. The evidence grade was assessed using the guidelines of the GRADE (Grading of Recommendations, Assessment, Development, and Evaluation) working group including the following items: risk of bias, inconsistency, indirectness, imprecision, and publication bias. The recommendation level of evidence was classified into the following categories: (1) high, which means that further research is unlikely to change confidence in the effect estimate; (2) moderate, which means that further research is likely to significantly change confidence in the effect estimate but may change the estimate; (3) low, which means that further research is likely to significantly change confidence in the effect estimate and to change the estimate; and (4) very low, which means that any effect estimate is uncertain. GRADE pro version 3.6 software is used for the evidence synthesis.

Results
Search result

A total of 267 studies related to IMN and tibial shaft fractures were reviewed. After reading the titles and abstracts, 263 studies were excluded from the present meta-analysis. Four RCTs [9–12] which published between 2015 and 2017 eventually satisfied the eligibility criteria for this study. There were 142 participants in the experimental groups and 151 patients in the control groups. The search process was proceeded as presented in Fig. 1.

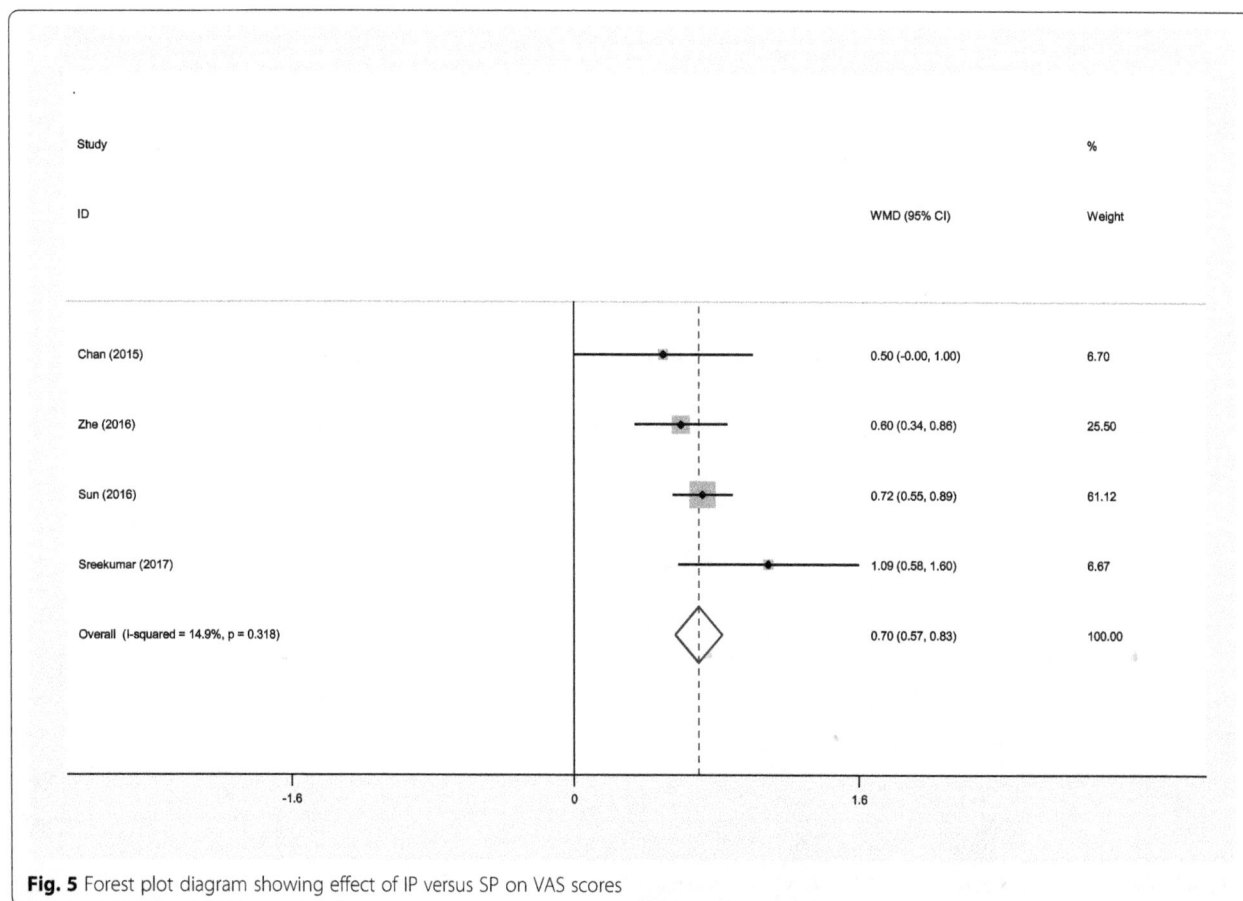

Fig. 5 Forest plot diagram showing effect of IP versus SP on VAS scores

Study characteristics

All of the included studies were RCTs. There were two RCTs performed in China and one each in the USA and India. All RCTs had defined eligibility criteria. The sample size ranged from 25 to 162 and average age ranged from 40 to 47 years old. In these studies, the experimental groups received infrapatellar approach IMN for tibial shaft fractures and the control groups received suprapatellar approach IMN. Duration of follow-up ranged from 6 to 16 months. The characteristics of the included studies are shown in Table 1.

Risk of bias

Seven aspects of the RCTs related to the risk of bias were assessed, following the instructions in the Cochrane Handbook for Systematic Reviews of Interventions (Fig. 2). Randomization was performed in all RCTs and all of them mentioned that the list of random numbers were generated from a computer. Only one [9] article used sealed envelopes for allocation concealment. None RCTs reported double blinding to the surgeons and participants. One study [10] showed that assessor was blinded. Low risk of bias due to incomplete outcome data and selective outcome reporting were detected. Judgments regarding each risk of bias item were presented as percentages across all the included RCTs in Fig. 3.

Outcome analysis

Total blood loss

All RCTs reported the total blood loss following IMN fixation. No statistical heterogeneity was observed in our study ($\chi^2 = 3.44$, df = 3, $I^2 = 12.7\%$, $P = 0.329$); therefore, a fixed-effects model was applied. There was significant difference between the infrapatellar groups and suprapatellar groups regarding the total blood loss (WMD = 7.92, 95% CI 1.15 to 14.68, $P = 0.022$; Fig. 4).

VAS scores

All RCTs showed the postoperative VAS scores at the first follow-up after IMN fixation. There was no significant heterogeneity ($\chi^2 = 3.52$, df = 3, $I^2 = 14.9\%$, $P = 0.318$); therefore, a fixed-effects model was adopted. The result of meta-analysis indicated that suprapatellar groups was associated with a significant

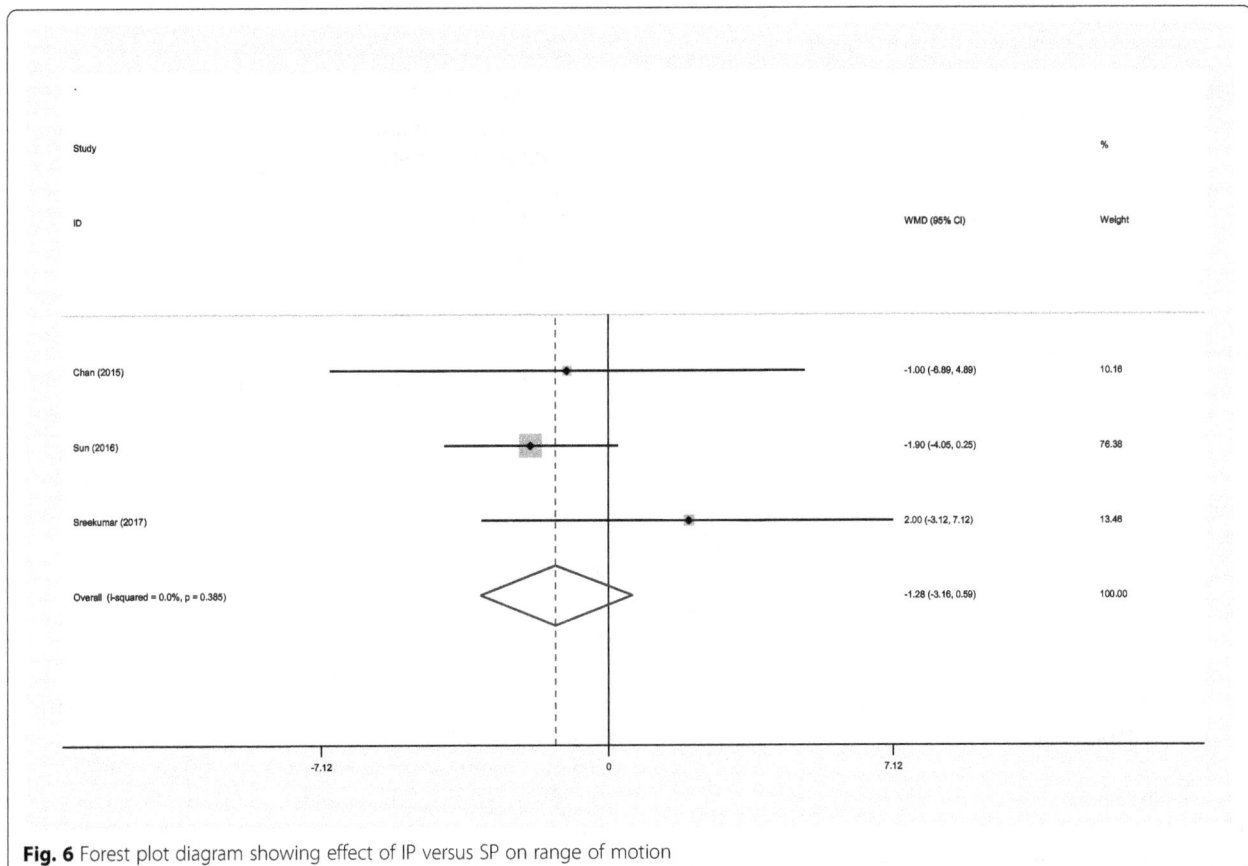

Study ID		WMD (95% CI)	% Weight
Chan (2015)		-1.00 (-6.89, 4.89)	10.16
Sun (2016)		-1.90 (-4.05, 0.25)	76.38
Sreekumar (2017)		2.00 (-3.12, 7.12)	13.46
Overall (I-squared = 0.0%, p = 0.385)		-1.28 (-3.16, 0.59)	100.00

Fig. 6 Forest plot diagram showing effect of IP versus SP on range of motion

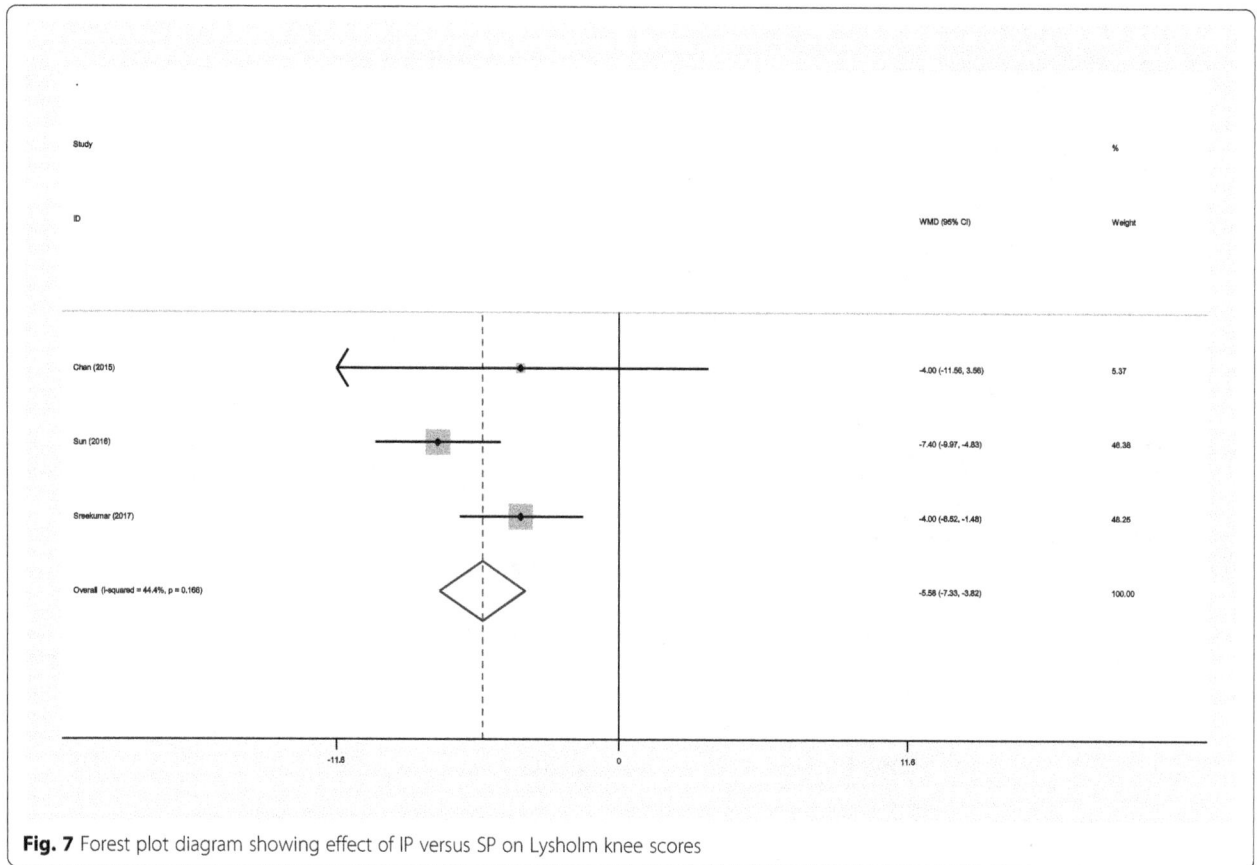

Fig. 7 Forest plot diagram showing effect of IP versus SP on Lysholm knee scores

reduction in the VAS scores (WMD = 0.70, 95% CI 0.570 to 0.83, P = 0.000; Fig. 5).

Range of motion

Three RCTs provided the outcome of range of motion after IMN fixation. There was no significant heterogeneity (χ^2 = 1.91, df = 2, I^2 = 0%, P = 0.385) and a fixed-effects model was used. The pooled results demonstrated that there was no significant difference between two groups regarding the range of motion (WMD = – 1.28, 95% CI – 3.16 to 0.59, P = 0.180; Fig. 6).

Lysholm knee scores

Lysholm knee scores were reported in three RCTs. There was no significant heterogeneity (χ^2 = 3.60, df = 2, I^2 = 44.4%, P = 0.166), and a fixed-effects model was used. The present meta-analysis revealed that there was significant difference between two groups in terms of Lysholm knee scores (WMD = – 5.58, 95% CI – 7.33 to – 3.83, P = 0.000; Fig. 7).

Fluoroscopy times

Two RCTs showed the fluoroscopy times during surgery. Significant statistical heterogeneity was found

(χ^2 = 5.46, df = 1, I^2 = 81.7%, P = 0.019), and a random-effects model was applied. There was significant difference between groups regarding the total fluoroscopy times (WMD = 26.70, 95% CI 3.15 to 50.25, P = 0.026; Fig. 8).

Length of hospital stay

Three RCTs showed the length of hospital stay. A fixed-effects model was adopted because no significant heterogeneity was found (χ^2 = 0.21, df = 2, I^2 = 0%, P = 0.901). There was no significant difference between the two groups in terms of length of hospital stay (WMD = – 0.05, 95% CI – 0.33 to 0.23, P = 0.713; Fig. 9).

Postoperative complications

Three RCTs reported the postoperative complications including nonunion or delayed union. A fixed-effects model was adopted (χ^2 = 3.25, df = 5, I^2 = 0%, P = 0.662). There was no significant difference between groups regarding the incidence of the postoperative complications (RD = 0.01, 95% CI – 0.03 to 0.04, P = 0.755; Fig. 10).

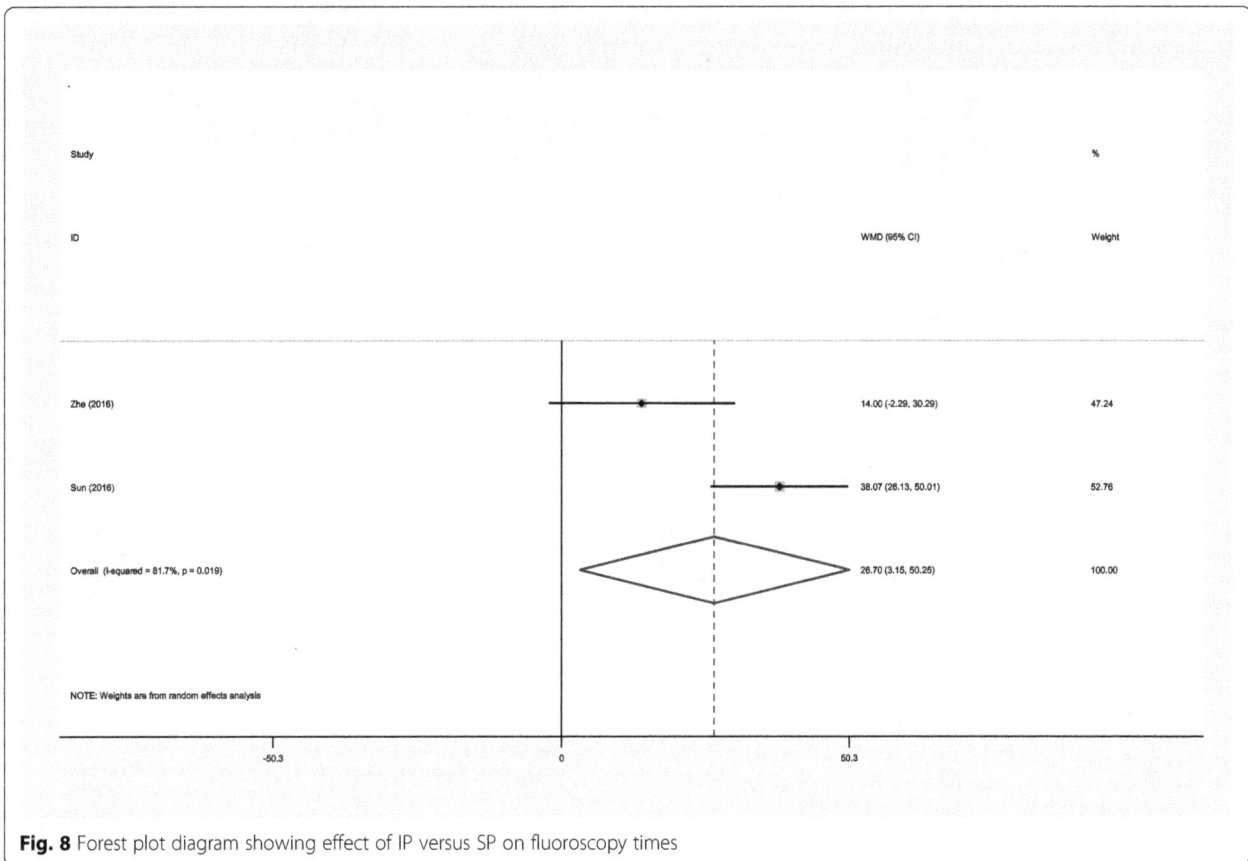

Fig. 8 Forest plot diagram showing effect of IP versus SP on fluoroscopy times

Evidence level and recommendation strengths

Quality of evidence was evaluated by the GRADE system. The evidence quality for each outcome was moderate to high. Therefore, we agreed that the overall evidence quality was moderate, which means that further research is likely to significantly change confidence in the effect estimate but may change the estimate (Table 2).

Publication bias

Publication bias was assessed by a funnel plot diagram. The funnel plot diagrams of total blood loss and VAS scores were symmetrical, indicating a low risk of publication bias (Figs. 11 and 12).

Discussion

To the best of our knowledge, it was the first meta-analysis from RCTs to compare the clinical and functional outcomes of the knee joint after infrapatellar versus suprapatellar tibial nail insertion. The most important finding of the present meta-analysis was that suprapatellar approach of IMN was associated with a significant reduction in total blood, VAS scores, and fluoroscopy times compared with infrapatellar approach. Additionally, there were significant differences between groups regarding the Lysholm knee scores. However, there was no evidence that suprapatellar approach was associated with a lower incidence of joint degeneration of the patellofemoral joint. Further research was still required. The overall evidence quality was moderate, which means that further research is likely to significantly change confidence in the effect estimate but may change the estimate.

Tibial shaft fractures were common in long bone and were usually caused by high-energy trauma such as traffic accidents and falling from a height [13, 14]. The IMN was considered the gold standard for the treatment of tibial shaft fractures with advantages of preferred stable fixation and less damage to vascularity and soft tissue [15]. Suprapatellar did not injure the tendon and was considered popular surgical approach [16]. Additionally, suprapatellar IMN could insert nail with knee extended and avoid the risk of infrapatellar nerve damage. Reducing perioperative blood loss was an important issue which may promote recovery and

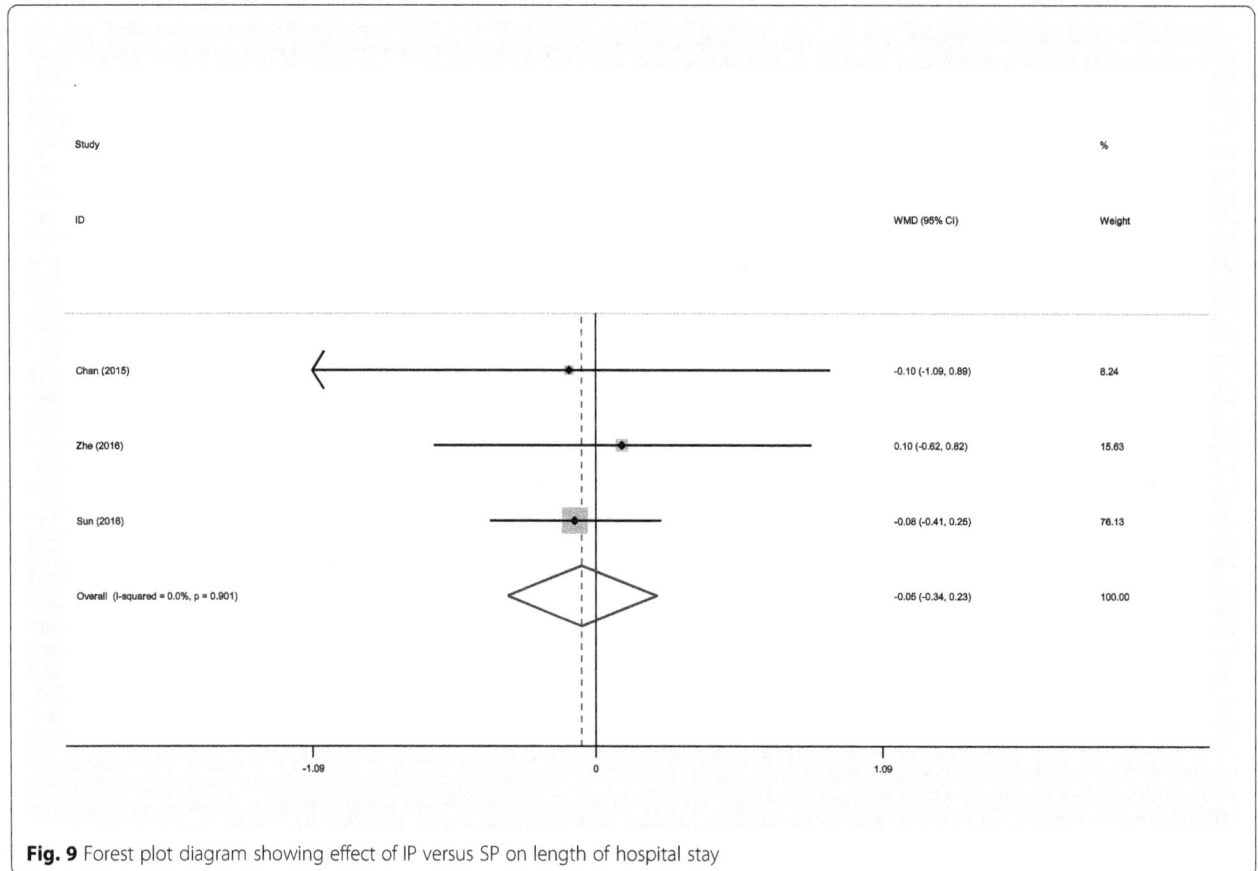

Fig. 9 Forest plot diagram showing effect of IP versus SP on length of hospital stay

decrease the transfusion requirements. Few RCTs reported the total blood loss between various surgical approaches in tibial shaft fractures. The present meta-analysis revealed that suprapatellar approach was associated with a significant reduction of total blood loss.

Effective pain management may improve patients' satisfaction and decrease postoperative complications. Postoperative pain following intramedullary nailing surgery was the major concern, and patients often complained of moderate to severe pain [17, 18]. It may be caused by the injury of the knee structure and nerve. Besides, surgical stress response which included inflammatory components also induced postoperative pain. Leliveld and Verhofstad [19] reported that 38% patients who underwent infrapatellar incision had complication of chronic knee pain and the incidence of iatrogenic damage to the infrapatellar nerve after IMN was high and lasting. Injury to this nerve appeared to be associated with postoperative knee pain. The suprapatellar approach was performed by an incision which was proximal to the patella, and the intramedullary nail passed through trochlear groove. Theoretically, there was no risk of injury to the patellar tendon and the infrapatellar nerve. Courtney et al. [20] reported that the infrapatellar nerve could be well protected with suprapatellar approach. Gaines et al. [21] showed that there was a higher risk of articular structure damage with infrapatellar approach than with suprapatellar approach; however, there was no significant statistical difference. Based on the current controversy, we performed this meta-analysis from published RCTs and indicated that there was a lower incidence of knee pain with suprapatellar approach compared to infrapatellar insertion.

Decreased range of motion after IMN was an undesirable outcome and was well documented in studies and was varied [22]. Multiple factors may affect the range of motion such as the damage to the vascularity and soft tissue. However, different surgical approach for tibial shaft fractures remains controversial. Leliveld and Verhofstad [19] reported that knee range of motion was equivalent to the unaffected side with infrapatellar tibial IMN on long-term follow-up. Though Chan et al. [9] showed an improved range of motion with suprapatellar

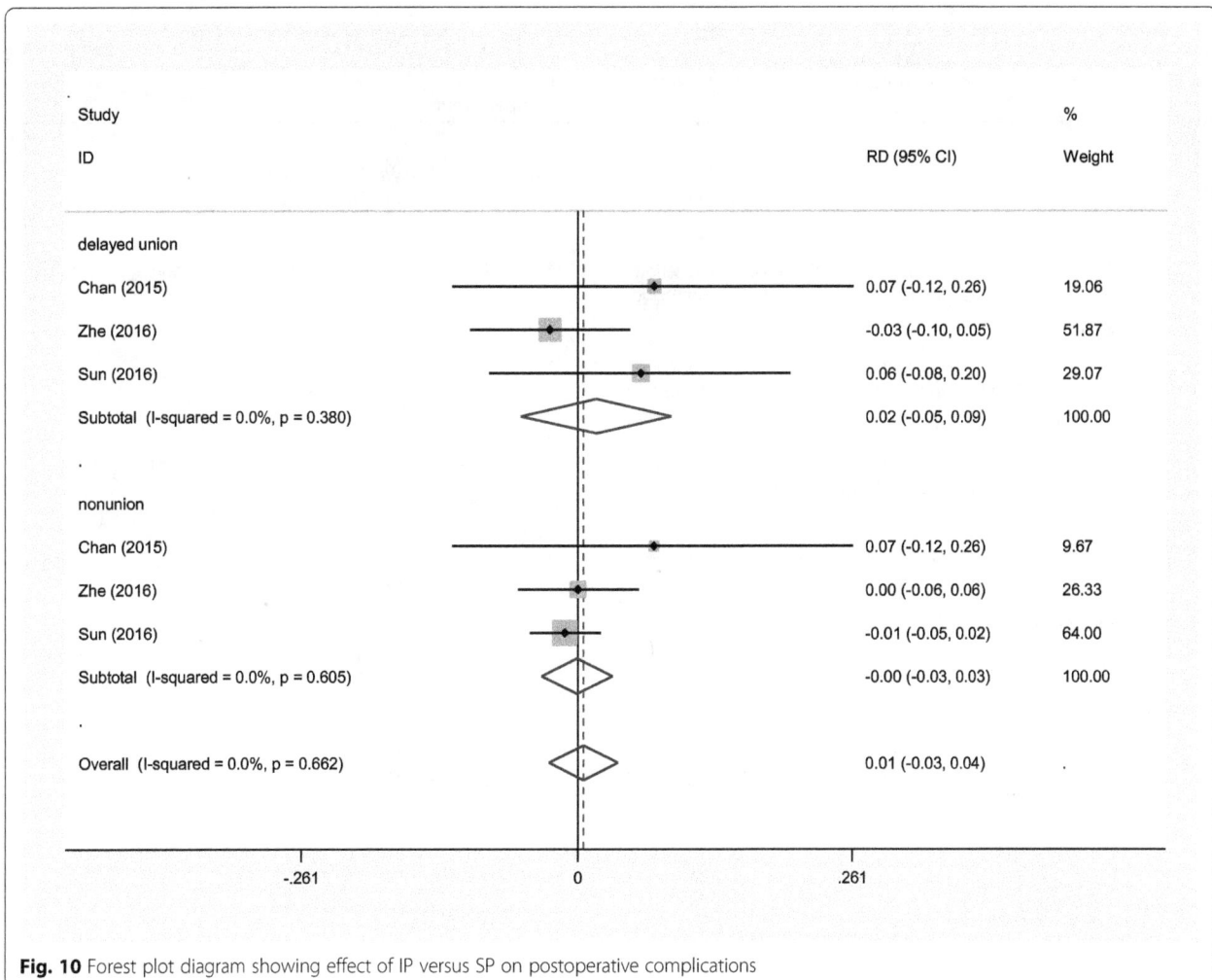

Fig. 10 Forest plot diagram showing effect of IP versus SP on postoperative complications

approach compared with infrapatellar approach, there was no significant difference. Our study observed no significant statistical difference. Long-term follow-up was required.

Lysholm et al. [23] published their first knee scoring scale in 1982. It was a questionnaire that contained eight items about the function and symptom of knee, which described a validated evaluation of patient activities of daily living. It has been widely used in various types of knee fractures. Song et al. [24] showed that there was a closely relationship between Lysholm knee scores and knee pain in patients undergoing tibial IMN. Our study indicated that there was an improved Lysholm knee scores in suprapatellar groups compared with infrapatellar groups. Fluoroscopy time was significantly shorter in suprapatellar groups. The infrapatellar position made it difficult to perform a fluoroscopy during the surgical procedure. Capturing the orthogonal view of tibia was much easier with knee in semi-extended position, and this position may simplify the reduction of the fracture [25].

Several potential limitations of the present meta-analysis should be noted: (1) only four RCTs were included in our study, and the sample sizes were small; thus, it may result in overestimating the outcomes; (2) methodological weakness existed in all RCTs which may influence the results; (3) due to the limited studies, we failed to perform a subgroup analyses to investigate the other factors, such as gender, age, body mass index, and fracture type; thus, we could not determine the source of heterogeneity; (4) short-term follow-ups may lead to an underestimation of complications; and (5) all included RCTs were English and Chinese publications; thus, publication bias was unavoidable.

Conclusion

Suprapatellar intramedullary nailing could significantly reduce total blood loss, postoperative knee pain, and

Table 2 The GRADE evidence quality

No. of studies	Design	Limitations	Inconsistency	Indirectness	Imprecision	IP groups	SP groups	Effect	Quality	Importance
Quality assessment						No. of patients		Effect	Quality	Importance
Total blood loss										
4	RCT	Serious limitations	No serious inconsistency	No serious indirectness	No serious imprecision	142	151	WMD = 7.92, 95% CI 1.15 to 14.68	High	Critical
VAS scores										
4	RCT	Serious limitations	No serious inconsistency	No serious indirectness	No serious imprecision	142	151	WMD = 0.70, 95% CI 0.570 to 0.83	High	Critical
Range of motion										
3	RCT	Serious limitations	No serious inconsistency	No serious indirectness	No serious imprecision	112	113	WMD = − 1.28, 95% CI − 3.16 to 0.59	High	Critical
Lysholm knee scores										
3	RCT	Serious limitations	No serious inconsistency	No serious indirectness	No serious imprecision	112	113	WMD = − 5.58, 95% CI − 7.33 to − 3.83	High	Critical
Fluoroscopy times										
2	RCT	Serious limitations	Serious inconsistency	No serious indirectness	No serious imprecision	111	119	WMD = 26.70, 95% CI 3.15 to 50.25	Moderate	Critical
Length of hospital stay										
3	RCT	Serious limitations	No serious inconsistency	No serious indirectness	No serious imprecision	125	130	WMD = − 0.05, 95% CI − 0.33 to 0.23	High	Critical
Postoperative complications										
3	RCT	Serious limitations	No serious inconsistency	No serious indirectness	No serious imprecision	125	130	RD = 0.01, 95% CI − 0.03 to 0.04	High	Critical

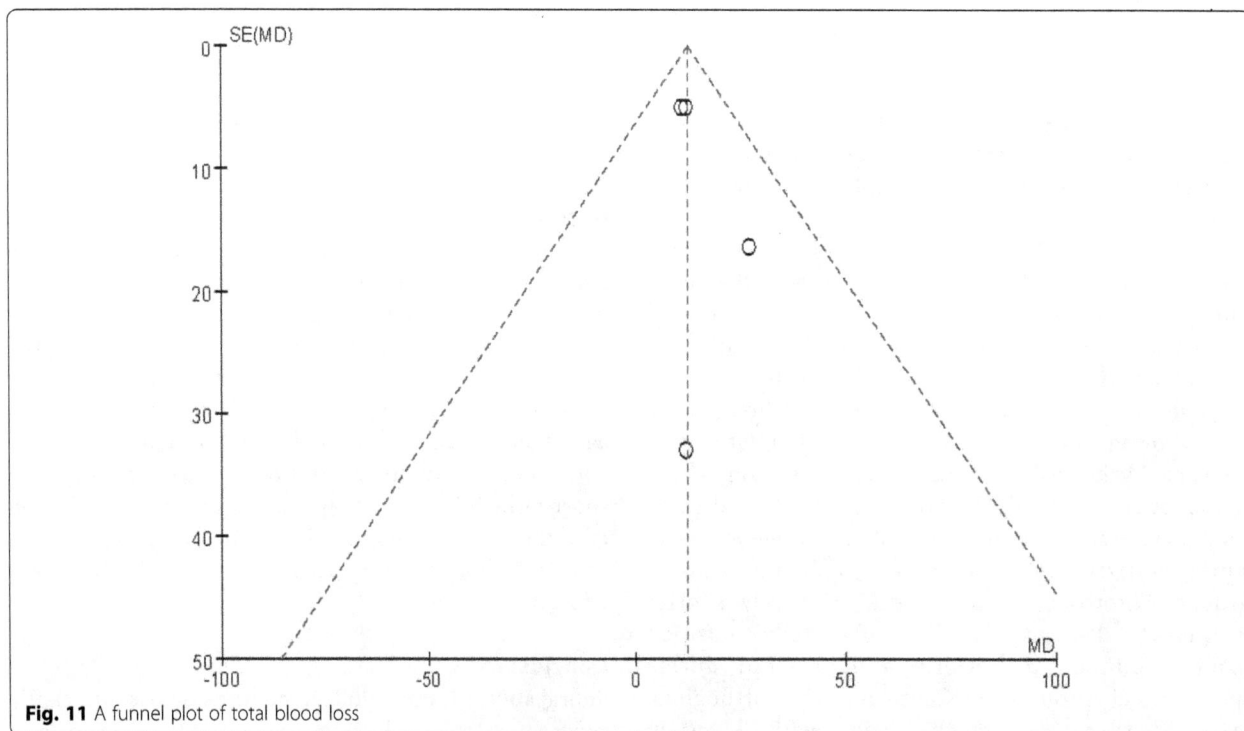

Fig. 11 A funnel plot of total blood loss

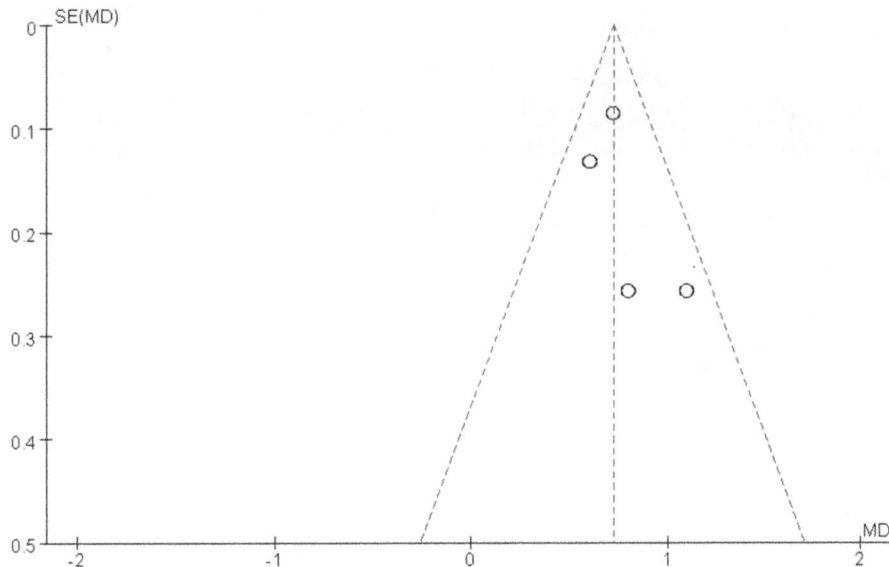

Fig. 12 A funnel plot of VAS scores

fluoroscopy times compared to infrapatellar approach. Additionally, it was associated with an improved Lysholm knee scores. High-quality RCTs were still required for further investigation.

Abbreviations
IMN: Intramedullary nail; RCT: Randomized controlled trials; VAS: Visual analog score

Authors' contributions
LY contributed to the data collections and wrote the manuscript. YS and GL studied the design. All authors read and approved the final manuscript.

Competing interests
The authors declare that they have no competing interests.

References
1. Larsen P, Lund H, Laessoe U, Graven-Nielsen T, Rasmussen S. Restrictions in quality of life after intramedullary nailing of tibial shaft fracture: a retrospective follow-up study of 223 cases. J Orthop Trauma. 2014;28(9): 507–12.
2. Court-Brown CM, Caesar B. Epidemiology of adult fractures: a review. Injury. 2006;37(8):691–7.
3. Ahmad N, Khan MS, Afridi SA, Afridi SA, Awan AS, Afridi SK, Sultan S, Saifullah K, Lodhi FS. Efficacy and safety of interlocked intramedullary nailing for open fracture shaft of tibia. Journal of Ayub Medical College, Abbottabad : JAMC. 2016;28(2):341–4.
4. Zelle BA, Boni G. Safe surgical technique: intramedullary nail fixation of tibial shaft fractures. Patient safety in surgery. 2015;9:40.
5. Lefaivre KA, Guy P, Chan H, Blachut PA. Long-term follow-up of tibial shaft fractures treated with intramedullary nailing. J Orthop Trauma. 2008;22(8): 525–9.
6. Toivanen JA, Vaisto O, Kannus P, Latvala K, Honkonen SE, Jarvinen MJ. Anterior knee pain after intramedullary nailing of fractures of the tibial shaft. A prospective, randomized study comparing two different nail-insertion techniques. J Bone Joint Surg Am. 2002;84-A(4):580–5.
7. Hernigou P, Cohen D. Proximal entry for intramedullary nailing of the tibia. The risk of unrecognised articular damage. The Journal of bone and joint surgery British volume. 2000;82(1):33–41.
8. Zhendong H, Li J, Hu Z, Orthopedics T. Comparison of therapeutic effects of suprapatellar approach and infrapatellar approach intramedullary nail for tibial shaft fractures. J Pract Orthop. 2017;23(9):794–7
9. Chan DS, Serrano-Riera R, Griffing R, Steverson B, Infante A, Watson D, Sagi HC, Sanders RW. Suprapatellar versus infrapatellar tibial nail insertion: a prospective randomized control pilot study. J Orthop Trauma. 2016;30(3): 130–4.
10. Wang Z, Li S, Wang X, Tang X. Supra-patellar versus infra-patellar intramedullary nailing in treatment of tibial shaft fractures. Chin J Orthop Trauma. 2016;18(4):283–9.
11. Sun Q, Nie X, Gong J, Wu J, Li R, Ge W, Cai M. The outcome comparison of the suprapatellar approach and infrapatellar approach for tibia intramedullary nailing. Int Orthop. 2016;40(12):2611–7.
12. Sreekumar K, Sreekumar K. Suprapatellar versus infrapatellar tibial nail insertion: a prospective randomized control pilot study. J Evid Based Healthc. 2017;4(45):2765–8.
13. Guruprasad Y, Chauhan DS. Tibial shaft fracture following graft harvestment for nasal augmentation. National journal of maxillofacial surgery. 2012;3(2): 239–41.
14. Anandasivam NS, Russo GS, Swallow MS, Basques BA, Samuel AM, Ondeck NT, Chung SH, Fischer JM, Bohl DD, Grauer JN. Tibial shaft fracture: a large-scale study defining the injured population and associated injuries. Journal of clinical orthopaedics and trauma. 2017;8(3):225–31.
15. Bode G, Strohm PC, Sudkamp NP, Hammer TO. Tibial shaft fractures—management and treatment options. A review of the current literature. Acta Chir Orthop Traumatol Cechoslov. 2012;79(6):499–505.
16. Morandi M, Banka T, Gaiarsa GP, Guthrie ST, Khalil J, Hoegler J, Lindeque BG. Intramedullary nailing of tibial fractures: review of surgical techniques and description of a percutaneous lateral suprapatellar approach. Orthopedics. 2010;33(3):172–9.

17. Song SY, Chang HG, Byun JC, Kim TY. Anterior knee pain after tibial intramedullary nailing using a medial paratendinous approach. J Orthop Trauma. 2012;26(3):172–7.

18. Jang Y, Kempton LB, TO MK, Sorkin AT. Insertion-related pain with intramedullary nailing. Injury. 2017;48(Suppl 1):S18–21.

19. Leliveld MS, Verhofstad MH. Injury to the infrapatellar branch of the saphenous nerve, a possible cause for anterior knee pain after tibial nailing? Injury. 2012;43(6):779–83.

20. Courtney PM, Boniello A, Donegan D, Ahn J, Mehta S. Functional knee outcomes in infrapatellar and suprapatellar tibial nailing: does approach matter? Am J Orthop. 2015;44(12):E513–6.

21. Gaines RJ, Rockwood J, Garland J, Ellingson C, Demaio M. Comparison of insertional trauma between suprapatellar and infrapatellar portals for tibial nailing. Orthopedics. 2013;36(9):e1155–8.

22. Keating JF, O'Brien PI, Blachut PA, Meek RN, Broekhuyse HM. Reamed interlocking intramedullary nailing of open fractures of the tibia. Clin Orthop Relat Res. 1997;338:182–91.

23. Lysholm J, Gillquist J. Evaluation of knee ligament surgery results with special emphasis on use of a scoring scale. Am J Sports Med. 1982;10(3):150–4.

24. Song SY, Chang HG, Byun JC. Anterior knee pain after tibial IMN using a medial paratendinous approach. J Orthop Trauma. 2012;26:172–7.

25. Brink O. Suprapatellar nailing of tibial fractures: surgical hints. Current orthopaedic practice. 2016;27(1):107–12.

12

Modified triple pelvic osteotomy for adult symptomatic acetabular dysplasia: clinical and radiographic results at midterm follow-up

Jiajun Wu[1], Yang Yang[2], Xiuhui Wang[1], Xiaoxiao Zhou[1*] and Changqing Zhang[3*]

Abstract

Background: Acetabular dysplasia is the most common cause of secondary arthritis of the hip joint. Achieving maximum restoration of the acetabular coverage and medialization of the femoral head remains difficult with the original Steel triple pelvic osteotomy for acetabular dysplasia in children and adults. This study intended to answer the following questions: (1) Are the midterm functional results of our modified procedure favorable, particularly in relation to Harris scores? and (2) On the basis of the Tönnis grade, does this procedure has a different effect on radiographic parameters and functional results at midterm follow-up?

Methods: This study included 26 consecutive adult patients with symptomatic acetabular dysplasia (28 hips) who underwent modified triple pelvic osteotomy through two incisions between July 2005 and June 2012. According to the preoperative Tönnis grade, the patients were divided into T0 (Tönnis grade 0), T1 (Tönnis grade 1), and T2 (Tönnis grade 2) groups. Wiberg center-edge (CE) angle, Sharp acetabular angle, lateralization, and Harris scores were analyzed to assess the radiographic and clinical outcomes.

Results: The mean CE angle (28.43° [± 3.58°], $p < 0.05$), Sharp acetabular angle (36.39° [± 3.26°], $p < 0.05$), lateralization (16.82 mm [± 3.10 mm], $p < 0.05$), and Harris scores (89.07 [± 4.97], $p < 0.05$) at the last follow-up significantly improved compared to those preoperatively. Multiple comparisons of radiographic outcomes among the three groups indicated no significant difference ($p < 0.05$). Harris scores in group T2 were significantly lower than those in groups T0 ($p < 0.05$) and T1 ($p < 0.05$). No major complication was observed.

Conclusions: Our modified triple pelvic osteotomy for adult symptomatic acetabular dysplasia with early-stage osteoarthritis could lead to excellent radiographic outcomes, good clinical results, and lower complication rates.

Keywords: Modified triple pelvic osteotomy, Symptomatic acetabular dysplasia, Tönnis grade, Harris score, Radiographic outcomes

* Correspondence: zhouxx1493@126.com; Drzhangchangqing@163.com
Jiajun Wu and Yang Yang are co-first authors.
[1]Department of Orthopedics, Zhoupu Hospital Affiliated to Shanghai
University of Medicine & Health Sciences, No. 1500 Zhouyuan Road, Pudong
New Area, Shanghai 201318, China
[3]Department of Orthopedics, Shanghai Sixth People's Hospital Affiliated to
Shanghai Jiao Tong University, No. 600 Yishan Road, Xuhui District, Shanghai
201306, China
Full list of author information is available at the end of the article

Background

Acetabular dysplasia with a poorly developed acetabulum and insufficient femoral head coverage is the most common cause of secondary arthritis of the hip joint [1]. The Steel triple pelvic osteotomy for acetabular dysplasia has become widely used in either children or adults to restore hip joint biomechanical properties, relieve hip joint symptoms, and alter osteoarthritis development since Steel described it in 1973 [2]. The major drawback with the original Steel triple pelvic osteotomy is the difficulty in achieving maximum restoration of the acetabular coverage and medialization of the femoral head, resulting in an unpredictable prognosis [3–7]. Various modified triple pelvic osteotomies as a treatment for adult acetabular dysplasia have been developed with the intent of achieving favorable clinical results [8–12].

This study aimed to review our series of patients treated with modified triple pelvic osteotomy for adult acetabular dysplasia and describe a variation in this procedure. The following questions were raised: (1) What are the midterm functional results of this procedure, particularly in relation to Harris scores? and (2) On the basis of the Tönnis grade, does this procedure have a different effect on radiographic parameters and functional results at midterm follow-up?

Methods

Patients

This study included 28 consecutive patients aged > 18 years (30 hips) who had symptomatic acetabular dysplasia on standard pelvic radiography accompanied by early-stage osteoarthritis and underwent modified triple pelvic osteotomy at our institution between July 2005 and June 2012. Patients with acetabular dysplasia secondary to Down syndrome, inflammatory arthritis, Legg–Calvé–Perthes disease, neuromuscular conditions, and associated severe arthritis were excluded. One patient who was lost to follow-up and another who lacked complete radiographic data were excluded. Finally, 26 patients (28 hips) were included in this study. This study was approved by the institutional review board of Shanghai Sixth People's Hospital, and informed consent was obtained from all patients.

Methods
Surgical technique

Step 1: Exposure and osteotomy The procedure was performed through two incisions, with all patients under general anesthesia and in the supine position. The first incision (approximately 10 cm) was created along the anterior superior iliac crest to expose the iliac crest; the iliacus and gluteal muscles were bluntly detached to expose the greater sciatic notch. A jigsaw was placed through the greater sciatic notch using a customized tangential clamp, and iliac wing osteotomy was then performed. The second incision (approximately 5 cm) was created on the medial surface of the proximal thigh, located in the middle third of the medial thighs and parallel to the inguen through the space between the adductor brevis and adductor longus muscles; osteotomy of the ischial and pubic rami was completed (Fig. 1).

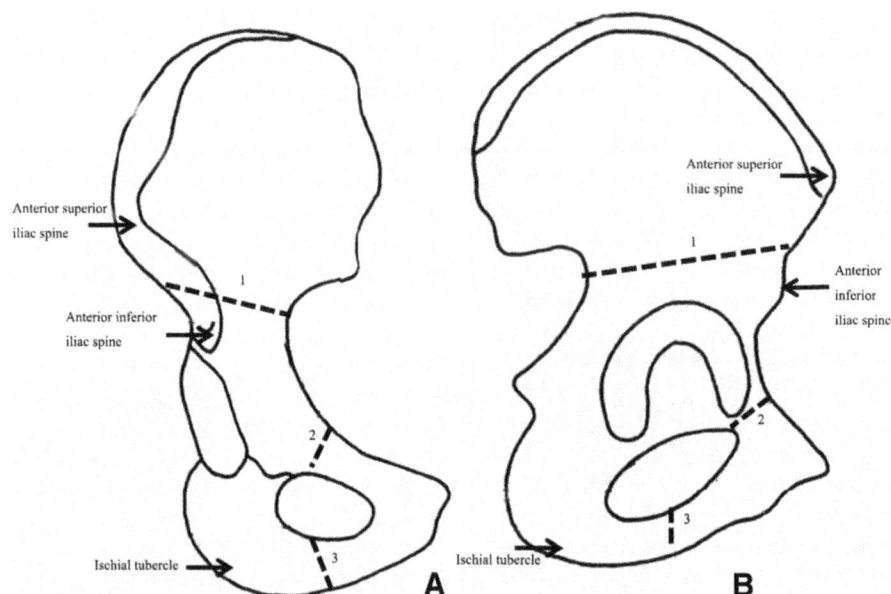

Fig. 1 Diagram showing the **a** anteroposterior and **b** lateral views of the surgical technique. 1, iliac osteotomy; 2, pubic osteotomy; and 3, ischial osteotomy

Step 2: Restoration and fixation After completing the three osteotomies, the acetabulum was mobilized to provide improved anterior and lateral coverage of the femoral head, which required rotation and traction of the limb under radiographic monitoring. Two 3.5-mm K-wires were inserted into the iliac osteotomy gap above the iliac wing, and a pre-bent locking reconstruction plate (DePuy Orthopaedics, Inc., Warsaw, IN, USA) was also used to fix the osteotomy fragments. Moreover, allograft (cortical–cancellous blocks; Osteorad Biological Materials Co., Taiyuan, China) was placed on the iliac osteotomy sites. Finally, the correction of CE angle and Sharp acetabular angle was estimated using the anteroposterior pelvic radiograph after the fixation with C-arm fluoroscopy.

Step 3: Closing and rehabilitation A negative pressure drainage tube was placed into the first incision prior to its closure. After the surgery, no immobilization and traction were required. Three days later, patients were instructed to perform hip and knee flexion exercises. At 3 months after surgery, all patients were encouraged to ambulate using crutches with 25 to 35% of their body weight for 2 weeks and subsequently walk without crutches. K-wires and plates were removed at 1–2 years after surgery; all patients were followed up once annually using standard pelvic radiography and Harris scoring system at the outpatient department.

Methods of assessment

All surgeries were performed by the senior author (CQZ). All standard anteroposterior pelvic radiographs before surgery and at the last follow-up were assessed by one author (JJW) who was blinded to the patient clinical status, and Harris hip scores were also analyzed (YY). Radiographic parameters included the Tönnis grade [13] used to evaluate osteoarthritic changes, Wiberg center-edge (CE) angle [14] used to determine the coverage of the anterior and middle/posterior areas of the femoral head, Sharp acetabular angle [15] used to determine the slopes of the anterior and middle/posterior portions of the acetabulum, and lateralization of the femoral head [16], which represents the distance from the medial edge of the femoral head to the ilioischial line (Fig. 2). According to preoperative Tönnis grade, patients were divided into group T0 (Tönnis grade 0), group T1 (Tönnis grade 1), and group T2 (Tönnis grade 2).

Statistical analysis

Statistical analyses were performed using SPSS version 23 (IBM Corp., Armonk, NY, USA). Paired t test and chi-squared test were used to compare numeric variables and Tönnis grades, respectively, before the

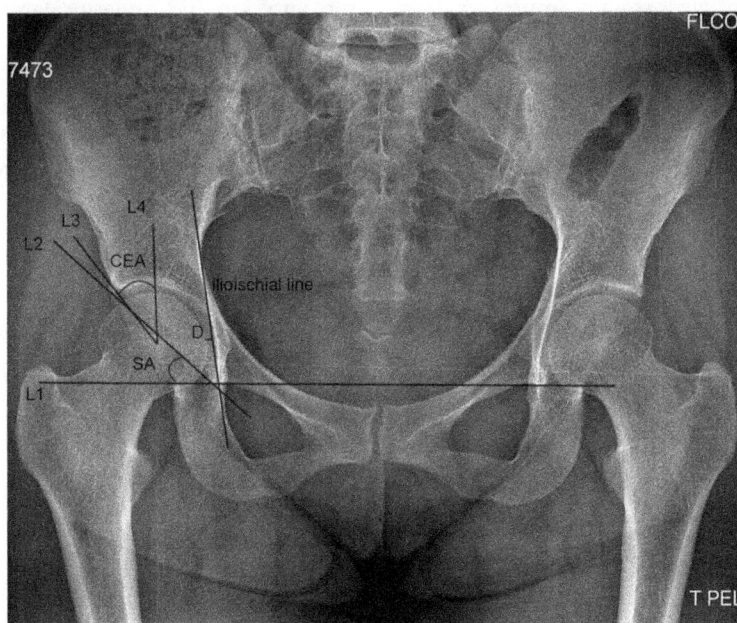

Fig. 2 Diagram showing the radiographic parameters measured. L1 is the trans-teardrop line. L2 is the line between the teardrop and the acetabular edge. L3 is the line connecting the femoral head center and the acetabular edge. L4 is the vertical line at the femoral head center. The ilioischial line is the line connecting the lateral borders of the greater sciatic notch and obturator foramen. Sharp acetabular (SA) angle is the angle between L1 and L2, whereas center-edge angle (CEA) is the angle between L3 and L4. D is the distance between the medial femoral head and ilioischial line, which represents lateralization

surgery and at the last follow-up in all patients. Multiple comparisons among the three groups were performed by least significant difference; $p < 0.05$ was considered statistically significant. Continuous variables were presented as mean ± standard deviation.

Results

The mean age at surgery in all patients was 36.29 years (± 9.78) (range, 19–49) (Table 1), whereas that in groups T0, T1, and T2 was 31.08 (± 9.88) (range, 19–47), 37.30 (± 8.50) (range, 21–45), and 45.00 years (± 3.63) (range, 39–49), respectively (Table 2). Multiple comparisons among the three groups indicated that the mean age at surgery in group T2 was significantly higher than that in group T0 ($p < 0.05$) (Table 2). The right, left, and both sides were affected in 14, 10, and 2 patients, respectively. Their chief complaints were pain and limp. Patients were followed up for a mean of 8.93 years (± 1.94) (range, 6–13) (Table 1); in all patients, radiographic parameters significantly improved at the last follow-up compared with those preoperatively, with a 23.75° increase in CE angle, 16.18° decrease in Sharp acetabular angle, and 1.39 mm decrease in lateralization ($p < 0.05$) (Table 3). Multiple comparisons of radiographic outcomes among the three groups showed no significant difference at the last follow-up (Table 4). Further, there was no statistically significant difference in operative time and estimated operative blood loss in all groups ($p > 0.05$) (Table 1).

The Harris scores in all patients improved from 73.71 (± 4.95) preoperatively to 89.07 (± 4.97) at the last follow-up, with variation in values being 15.36 ($p < 0.05$) (Table 3). Multiple comparisons showed significantly lower Harris scores in group T2 than in groups T0 and T1 at the last follow-up ($p < 0.05$) (Table 5).

No significant change in Tönnis grades preoperatively and at the last follow-up was observed ($p > 0.05$) (Table 6). Of the 28 hips, 12, 10, and 6 preoperatively had Tönnis grades 0, 1, and 2, respectively; more advanced osteoarthritis was not observed. In contrast, at the last follow-up, 13, 8, and 7 hips had Tönnis grades 0, 1, and 2, respectively, with no hip with Tönnis grade 3 or more advanced osteoarthritis having been

Table 1 General data of all patients

Item	Values	Range
Gender (male/female)	7/19	
Operative side (left/right)	12/16	
Age at surgery (years)	36.29 ± 9.78	19–49
Operation time (min)	102.50 ± 23.15	60–150
Estimated operative blood loss (ml)	805 ± 241.12	470–1350
Follow-up period (years)	8.93 ± 1.94	6–13

Table 2 General data of the three groups

Tönnis grade	Age (range, years)	Operative time (min)	Estimated operative blood loss (ml)
Group T0	31.08 ± 9.88 (19–47)	98.75 ± 17.21	801.67 ± 263.09
Group T1	37.30 ± 8.50 (21–45)	98.00 ± 24.29	842.00 ± 272.06
Group T2	45.00 ± 3.63[a] (39–49)	117.50 ± 28.94	750.00 ± 148.46

[a]T2 vs. T0, $p = 0.003$. All values are expressed as mean ± standard deviation. Differences are considered significant at $p < 0.05$

observed. The Tönnis grade changed from grades 0 to 1 and from grades 1 to 2 in two hips.

No nonunion at the iliac osteotomy site, lower extremity palsy, discrepancy in leg length longer than 2 cm, dislocation or posterior subluxation of the hip joint, deep wound infection, or deep vein thrombosis occurred. A superficial wound infection in the iliac region was treated in three patients by changing the dressings. No major complication was observed in the present study.

Discussion

The relationship between the degree of radiographically detected dysplasia and development of osteoarthritis of the hip joint has been confirmed [17–19]. Acetabular dysplasia is generally characterized by a shallow acetabulum and malposition of the femoral head, leading to insufficient femoral head coverage on the anterior and superior lateral side. Thus, a small contact area between the femoral head and acetabulum increases the contact stress, resulting in sharply increased hip joint reaction forces beyond the cartilage stress threshold, which leads to cartilage deterioration and osteoarthritis of the hip joint [20].

The Steel triple pelvic osteotomy [2] was developed to increase the femoral head surface burdened by stress and medialize the femoral head by redistributing the increased contract stress from the ilium to the pubic and ischial rami, making the reorientation of the acetabulum possible. Several studies showed that the original Steel triple pelvic osteotomy [3, 6] or

Table 3 Preoperative and last follow-up results of radiographic parameters and Harris scores in 28 hips

Item	Before operation	Last follow-up	Improvement	p value
CE angle (°)	4.68 ± 3.99	28.43 ± 3.58	23.75	< 0.001
Sharp angle (°)	52.57 ± 5.73	36.39 ± 3.26	16.18	< 0.001
Lateralization (mm)	18.21 ± 4.89	16.82 ± 3.10	1.39	< 0.05
Harris score	73.71 ± 4.95	89.07 ± 4.97	15.36	< 0.001

All values are expressed as mean ± standard deviation. Differences are considered significant at $p < 0.05$

Table 4 Radiographic parameters of the three groups at different follow-up periods

Tönnis grade	CE angle (pre)	CE angle (last)	Sharp acetabular angle (pre)	Sharp acetabular angle (last)	Lateralization (pre)	Lateralization (last)
Group T0	4.33 ± 4.16	28.50 ± 4.17	50.58 ± 4.38	36.25 ± 3.31	16.83 ± 5.52	15.83 ± 3.71
Group T1	5.80 ± 4.66	27.90 ± 3.73	53.10 ± 5.36	35.70 ± 3.13	19.60 ± 3.84	17.30 ± 2.06
Group T2	3.50 ± 2.07	29.17 ± 2.23	55.67 ± 7.87	37.83 ± 3.49	18.67 ± 5.20	18.00 ± 3.10

CE, center edge; pre, preoperative; last, last follow-up. All values are expressed as mean ± standard deviation. Differences are considered significant at $p < 0.05$

modified triple pelvic osteotomy [8, 10, 11] not only improved radiographic parameters but also relieved pain, led to satisfactory clinical results, and could retard osteoarthritis development in adults. However, owing to restrictions on strong ligamentous attachments in the original Steel triple pelvic osteotomy, it is difficult to achieve optimum coverage and medialization of the femoral head. The use of relatively nonrigid implants can result in nonunion and rehabilitation delay, and using three incisions makes the procedure complex. A posterior approach for ischial ramus osteotomy can pose a risk of sciatic nerve injury. The outcomes were unsatisfactory and suboptimal [21].

In our study, the mean CE angle improved by 23.75°, the mean Sharp acetabular angle decreased by 16.18°, and the lateralization increased by 1.39 mm at the last follow-up compared to those before surgery, suggesting that our new modified triple pelvic osteotomy not only results in better restoration of the normal anatomical characteristics of the acetabulum but also offers precise reorientation and stable fixation of the osteotomy site, achieving a satisfactory clinical outcome (Fig. 3).

Compared with the original Steel triple pelvic osteotomy, our simple modified anteromedial longitudinal approach at the proximal thigh could simultaneously expose both the pubic and ischial rami without involving the sciatic nerve; moreover, it was easier to achieve optimum coverage and medialization of the femoral head. The use of locking reconstruction plate and pins for fixation of the osteotomy site could lead to a rigid fixation of osteotomy fragments, maintain hip joint stability, promote early postoperative rehabilitation [8], and prevent nonunion of osteotomy fragments compared with the use of pins only, such as in the original Steel triple pelvic osteotomy.

However, attention should be paid to the risk of injury to the femoral nerves and vessels. Moreover, our modified procedure simplified the surgical procedures without the need for intraoperative postural changes and could allow for the achievement of the goal of fast learning.

Triple pelvic osteotomy performed in younger patients with or without early-stage osteoarthritis is believed to result in almost normal orientation of the acetabulum and prevent or delay osteoarthritis development [9, 22]. To date, there are few studies in the literature that compared the clinical and radiographic results of patients with different osteoarthritis grades. In this study, our series of patients with Tönnis grade 0 or 1 had significantly improved clinical results compared with those with Tönnis grade 2 at different follow-up periods; it has been shown that patients with advanced osteoarthritis are more likely to have an unfavorable clinical outcome, which may imply that triple pelvic osteotomy is more suitable for patients with low-grade osteoarthritis than for patients with advanced osteoarthritis.

The limitations of the present study include its retrospective design, relatively small number of patients, and inherent difficulties in retrieving complete data. Moreover, radiographic measurements may vary from one observer to another, introducing a significant uncontrolled variable. In this study, no hip procedures were converted to total hip arthroplasty at a mean follow-up of 8.93 years, which was considered a relatively short follow-up period. The long-term clinical results of the procedure remain unknown, and further studies with longer follow-up periods are required to clarify this. However, we believe that our data provided evidence that our modified triple pelvic osteotomy can effectively delay the progression and exacerbation of symptomatic acetabular dysplasia.

Table 5 Harris scores preoperatively and at the last follow-up

Tönnis grade	Before operation	Last follow-up
Group T0	76.42 ± 4.89	91.75 ± 3.67
Group T1	72.60 ± 4.33	89.70 ± 3.86
Group T2	70.17 ± 3.31[a]	82.67 ± 3.08[b]

[a]Preoperatively—T2 vs. T0, $p = 0.009$; [b]At the last follow-up—T2 vs. T0, $p = 0.001$; T2 vs. T1, $p = 0.001$. All values are expressed as mean ± standard deviation. Differences are considered significant at $p < 0.05$

Table 6 Tönnis grades for 28 hips preoperatively and at the last follow-up

Tönnis grade	Before operation, n (%)	Last follow-up, n (%)
Group T0	12 (42.86)	13 (46.43)
Group T1	10 (35.71)	8 (28.57)
Group T2	6 (21.43)	7 (25.00)

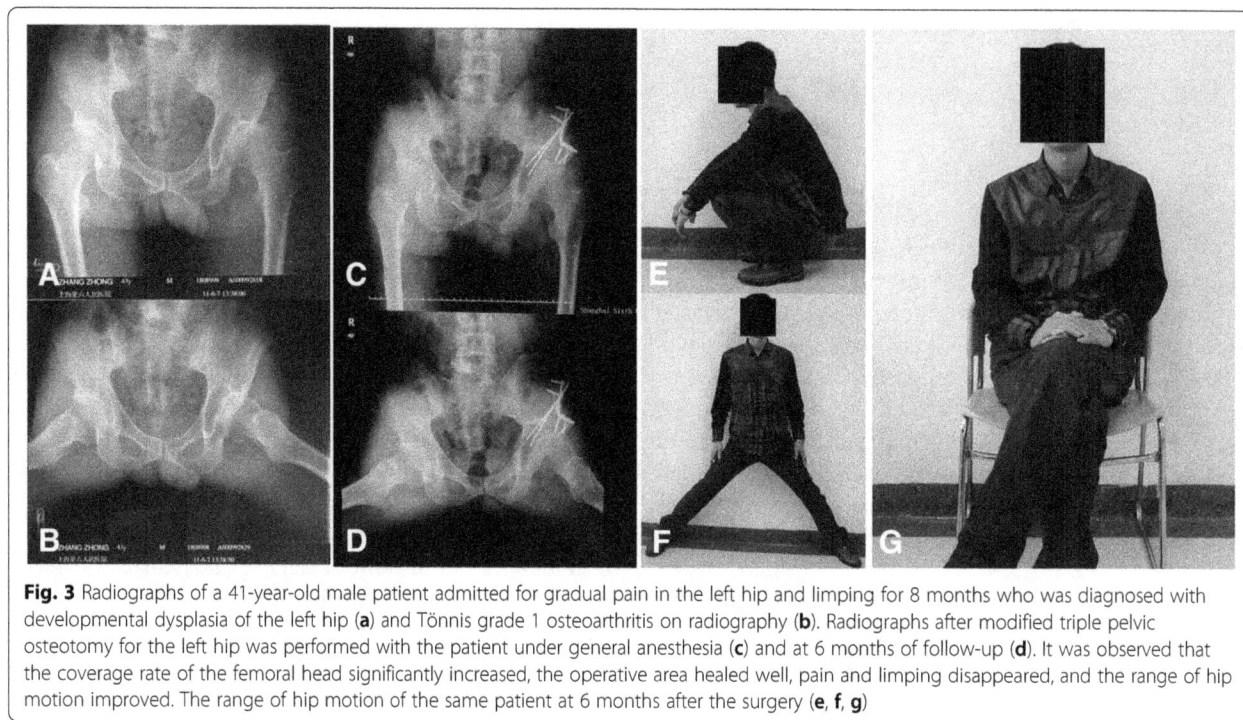

Fig. 3 Radiographs of a 41-year-old male patient admitted for gradual pain in the left hip and limping for 8 months who was diagnosed with developmental dysplasia of the left hip (**a**) and Tönnis grade 1 osteoarthritis on radiography (**b**). Radiographs after modified triple pelvic osteotomy for the left hip was performed with the patient under general anesthesia (**c**) and at 6 months of follow-up (**d**). It was observed that the coverage rate of the femoral head significantly increased, the operative area healed well, pain and limping disappeared, and the range of hip motion improved. The range of hip motion of the same patient at 6 months after the surgery (**e, f, g**)

Conclusion

The performance of our modified triple pelvic osteotomy technique as a treatment for adult symptomatic acetabular dysplasia led to good clinical results, excellent radiographic outcomes, and lower complication rates. Younger patients with symptomatic acetabular dysplasia and low-grade osteoarthritis are more likely to have better clinical results. Long-term follow-up is necessary to determine the outcome of this modified procedure.

Abbreviation
CE: Center-edge

Acknowledgements
We would like to thank Editage [www.editage.cn] for the English language editing.

Funding
This work was sponsored by the Natural Science Foundation of Shanghai (16ZR1431600), Pudong New Area Science and Technology Development Foundation (PKJ2016-Y40), Seed Fund of Shanghai University of Medicine & Health Sciences (HMSF-17-21-029), Projects of Medical and Health Technology Program in Zhejiang Province (2018PY079), Fund for the Key Subject Construction of Sanitary System of Shanghai Pudong New District (PWZxq2017-12), Special Fund for Scientific and Technological Development of Pudong Health and Family Planning Commission (PW2016A-21), and Fund for the Most Important Discipline Construction of Zhoupu Hospital of Shanghai Pudong New District (ZP-XK-2015a-2).

Authors' contributions
JJW and CQZ contributed to the experiment conception and design. JJW contributed to the radiographic measurements and assessments. YY contributed to the postoperative clinical assessments and data analysis. JJW, XHW, YY, and XXZ contributed to the writing of the manuscript. All authors read and approved the final manuscript.

Competing interests
The authors declare that they have no competing interests.

Author details
[1]Department of Orthopedics, Zhoupu Hospital Affiliated to Shanghai University of Medicine & Health Sciences, No. 1500 Zhouyuan Road, Pudong New Area, Shanghai 201318, China. [2]Department of Orthopedics, Taizhou Hospital Affiliated to Wenzhou Medical University, Zhejiang, China. [3]Department of Orthopedics, Shanghai Sixth People's Hospital Affiliated to Shanghai Jiao Tong University, No. 600 Yishan Road, Xuhui District, Shanghai 201306, China.

References
1. Jacobsen S. Adult hip dysplasia and osteoarthritis. Studies in radiology and clinical epidemiology. Acta Orthop Suppl. 2006;77:1–37.
2. Steel HH. Triple osteotomy of the innominate bone. J Bone Joint Surg Am. 1973;55:343–50.
3. Steel HH. Triple osteotomy of the innominate bone. A procedure to accomplish coverage of the dislocated or subluxated femoral head in the older patient. Clin Orthop Relat Res. 1977;122:116–27.

4. Dungl P, Rejholec M, Chomiak J, Grill F. The role of triple pelvic osteotomy in therapy of residual hip dysplasia and sequel of AVN: long-term experience. Hip Int. 2007;17(Suppl 5):S51–64.

5. van Hellemondt GG, Sonneveld H, Schreuder MH, Kooijman MA, de Kleuver M. Triple osteotomy of the pelvis for acetabular dysplasia: results at a mean follow-up of 15 years. J Bone Joint Surg Br. 2005;87:911–5.

6. de Kleuver M, Kooijman MA, Pavlov PW, Veth RP. Triple osteotomy of the pelvis for acetabular dysplasia: results at 8 to 15 years. J Bone Joint Surg Br. 1997;79:225–9.

7. Liddell AR, Prosser G. Radiographic and clinical analysis of pelvic triple osteotomy for adult hip dysplasia. J Orthop Surg Res. 2013;8:17.

8. Lipton GE, Bowen JR. A new modified technique of triple osteotomy of the innominate bone for acetabular dysplasia. Clin Orthop Relat Res. 2005;434:78–85.

9. Tönnis D, Behrens K, Tscharani F. A modified technique of the triple pelvic osteotomy: early results. J Pediatr Orthop. 1981;1:241–9.

10. Rahimi H, Kachooei AR, Hallaj-Moghaddam M, Gharedaghi M, Mirkazemi M, Shahpari O, et al. A modified triple pelvic osteotomy for the treatment of hip hypoplasia. Arch Bone Joint Surg. 2013;1:31–4.

11. Li YC, Wu KW, Huang SC, Wang TM, Kuo KN. Modified triple innominate osteotomy for acetabular dysplasia: for better femoral head medialization and coverage. J Pediatr Orthop B. 2012;21:193–9.

12. Eren A, Omeroglu H, Guven M, Ugutmen E, Altintas F. Incomplete triple pelvic osteotomy for the surgical treatment of dysplasia of the hip in adolescents and adults. J Bone Joint Surg Br. 2005;87:790–5.

13. Tönnis D. Congenital dysplasia and dislocation of the hip in children and adults. Berlin: Springer-Verlag; 1987.

14. Wiberg G. Studies on dysplastic acetabula and congenital subluxation of the hip joint: with special reference to the complication of osteoarthritis. Acta Chir Scand. 1939;83:53–68.

15. Sharp IK. Acetabular dysplasia: the acetabular angle. Bone Joint J. 1961;43:268–72.

16. Clohisy JC, Carlisle JC, Beaule PE, Kim YJ, Trousdale RT, Sierra RJ, et al. A systematic approach to the plain radiographic evaluation of the young adult hip. J Bone Joint Surg Am. 2008;90(Suppl 4):47–66.

17. Hsin J, Saluja R, Eilert RE, Wiedel JD. Evaluation of the biomechanics of the hip following a triple osteotomy of the innominate bone. J Bone Joint Surg Am. 1996;78:855–62.

18. McCarthy JC, Lee JA. Acetabular dysplasia: a paradigm of arthroscopic examination of chondral injuries. Clin Orthop Relat Res. 2002;405:122–8.

19. Jacobsen S, Sonne-Holm S, Soballe K, Gebuhr P, Lund B. Hip dysplasia and osteoarthrosis: a survey of 4151 subjects from the osteoarthrosis substudy of the Copenhagen city heart study. Acta Orthop. 2005;76:149–58.

20. Vukasinovic Z, Spasovski D, Kralj-Iglic V, Marinkovic-Eric J, Seslija I, Zivkovic Z, et al. Impact of triple pelvic osteotomy on contact stress pressure distribution in the hip joint. Int Orthop. 2013;37:95–8.

21. de Kleuver M, Kooijman MA, Kauer JM, Kooijman HM, Alferink C. Pelvic osteotomies: anatomic pitfalls at the ischium. A cadaver study. Arch Orthop Trauma Surg. 1998;117:376–8.

22. Baki ME, Abdioglu A, Aydin H, Kerimoglu S, Bak C. Triple pelvic osteotomy for the treatment of symptomatic acetabular dysplasia in adolescents and adults : a review of 42 hips. Acta Orthop Belg. 2016;82:699–704.

13

Biomechanics of common fixation devices for first tarsometatarsal joint fusion—a comparative study with synthetic bones

Rene Burchard[1,2,3]* ⓘ, Robin Massa[2], Christian Soost[4], Wolfgang Richter[5], Gerhard Dietrich[5], Arne Ohrndorf[5], Hans-Jürgen Christ[5], Claus-Peter Fritzen[5], Jan Adriaan Graw[6,7] and Jan Schmitt[8]

Abstract

Background: Hallux valgus disease is a common deformity of the forefoot. There are currently more than 100 surgical approaches for operative treatment. Because hypermobility of the first tarsometatarsal joint is considered to be causal for hallux valgus disease, fusion of the tarsometatarsal joint is an upcoming surgical procedure. Despite the development of new and increasingly stable fixation devices like different locking plates, malunion rates have been reported in 5 to 15% of cases.

Methods: Biomechanical comparison of three commonly used fixation devices (a dorsal locking plate, a plantar locking plate, and an intramedullary fixation device) was performed by weight-bearing simulation tests on synthetic bones. Initial compression force and stiffness during simulation of postoperative weight-bearing were analysed.

Results: Fixation of the first tarsometatarsal joint with the plantar plate combination demonstrated a higher stiffness compared to fixation with the intramedullary implant or the medial locking plate. The intramedullary device provided the highest initial compression force. Failure was detected in the following ranking: (1) the angle-stable intramedullary fixation device, (2) the medial located plate, and (3) the plantar locking plate.

Conclusion: The intramedullary device demonstrated the highest initial compression force of the three tested implants. The plantar locking plate showed the best overall stability during weight-bearing simulation. Further clinical research is necessary to analyse if the intramedullary fixation device needs a longer period of non-weight-bearing to reach a better non-union rate compared to the plantar locking plate.

Keywords: Lapidus fusion, Angle stable, Locking plate, Intramedullary fixation device, Hallux valgus

Background

Hallux valgus disease is a very common deformity of the forefoot and was first described by Carl Hueter in 1870 [1, 2]. It is defined by a lateral deviation of the great toe and a medial deviation of the first metatarsal bone [1].

While non-operative treatment only reduces symptoms like pain and inflammation but cannot improve the deformity of the bone, operative treatment is much more common. However, there are more than 100 surgical

approaches for treatment of hallux valgus disease. There have been attempts to develop treatment algorithms based on the degrees of deviation of the first metatarsal bone and including co-variables such as joint degeneration or incongruity [3, 4].

Hypermobility of the first tarsometatarsal joint is considered to be causal for hallux valgus disease [1]. Therefore, fusion of the first tarsometatarsal joint is an upcoming surgical procedure in the treatment of hallux valgus deformity [5]. In the past, the so-called Lapidus procedure, as a combined fusion of the first tarsometatarsal joint and the medial and intermediate cuneiform bones, often performed as a classical fixation with two crossed screws, has been described as a standard

---
* Correspondence: rene.burchard@uni-wh.de
[1]Department of Health, University of Witten/Herdecke, Witten, Germany
[2]Department of Trauma and Orthopaedic Surgery, Kreisklinikum Siegen, Weidenauer Str. 76, 57076 Siegen, Germany
Full list of author information is available at the end of the article

technique by many authors [6, 7]. Based on the Lapidus procedure, modified techniques with an isolated fusion of the first tarsometatarsal joint were developed [8–10]. Progressive developments of new fixation devices such as newly designed locking plates make early weight-bearing and a more comfortable postoperative treatment possible [11]. However, malunion rates between 5 and 15% have been reported [12]. Therefore, one might assume that locking implants will replace the screw procedures to avoid longer postoperative immobilisation periods and lower malunion rates [11]. In addition, high initial compression forces between bone fragments are a predictor for a good consolidation between the fragments in procedures such as osteosyntheses, osteotomies, and arthrodeses [13]. New developments in hardware design and implant techniques combined with the patients' expectations for a fast recovery and return to normal life have triggered recent research for the best implant device and surgical procedure. Many research groups have compared various hardware solutions such as crossed screws, dorsal and plantar locking plates, and intramedullary locking devices in cadaver or synthetic bone studies [12, 14–16]. Nevertheless, the actual literature shows heterogeneous results referring to recent fixation concepts in this field of foot surgery.

However, all surgical procedures to fix the tarsometatarsal joint in hallux valgus disease should provide a minimal non-union rate with a maximum of postoperative comfort and safety for the patient. Therefore, the aim of this study was to investigate, if common and innovative surgical approaches using a medial locking plate, a plantar locking plate, or an intramedullary locking device differ in their initial capacity of compression of the osteosynthesis. In addition, to detect a postinterventional loss of stability including a bone-implant-combination failure, weight-bearing in a healing shoe was simulated and stability of the osteosynthesis was compared among groups.

Methods
Experimental set-up
Nine ($n = 9$) composite synthetic bone pairs (First Metatarsal Model 3423 and Cuneiform Model 3421-1, Sawbones Europe AB, Malmö, Sweden) were analysed. Synthetic bones are considered to have similar structural and mechanical properties like natural bones. A potential bias associated with different bone shapes, bone qualities, or bone sizes when using cadaveric specimens is eliminated by using synthetic bone [17, 18].

A typical arthrodesis of the first tarsometatarsal joint with a tangential cut of articular sides was performed, and a pressure sensor (FlexiForce® Load/Force Sensor, Tekscan, South Boston, USA) was inserted into the fusion gap between the first metatarsal and the cuneiform synthetic bone before fixation of the implant. A special

sawing template was used to guarantee that all osteotomies were performed with a repetitious accuracy (Fig. 1a). Three bone-implant-combinations were tested, and experiments were run in triplicates. The same surgeon, certified by the German Society for Foot Surgery, performed each osteosynthesis. After arthrodesis, the cuneiform bone was fixed rigidly in a specially designed mounting device, which was constructed to guide a cyclic sinusoidal testing simulation. Tests were performed in the versatile material testing system MTS 810® (MTS Systems GmbH, Berlin, Germany) with tensile loads to simulate the stress due to the walking process. The forces are measured with an additional load cell (ME KD24S, ME-Meßsysteme GmbH, Hennigsdorf, Germany). A laser (M5L/10®, MEL Mikroelektronik GmbH, Eching, Germany), attached at the mounting device with the fixed cuneiform bone, measured the motion between the cuneiform and the first metatarsal

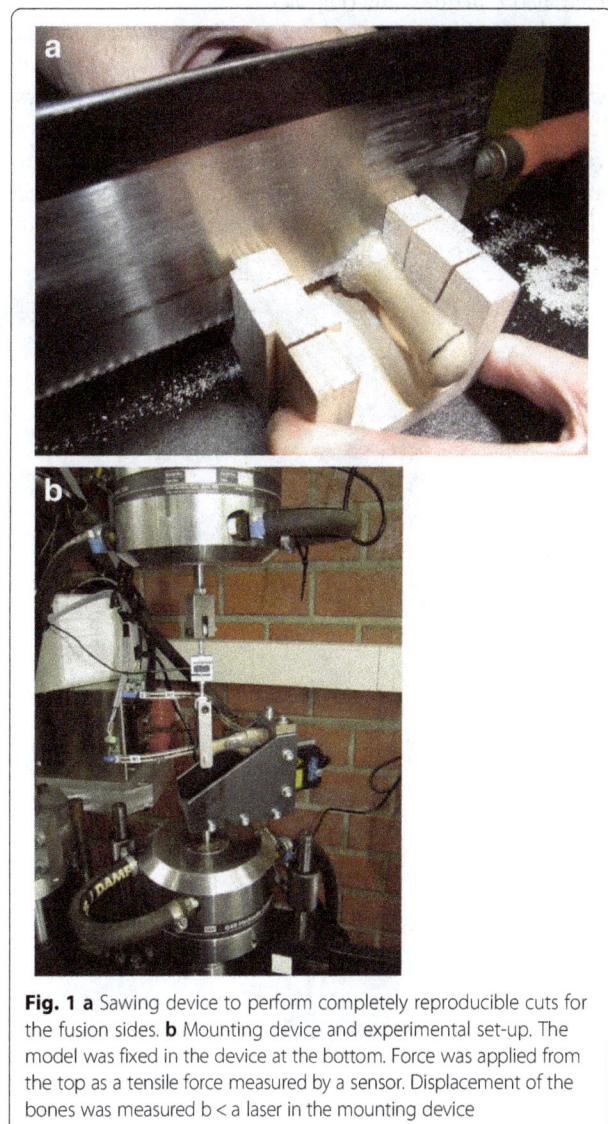

Fig. 1 a Sawing device to perform completely reproducible cuts for the fusion sides. **b** Mounting device and experimental set-up. The model was fixed in the device at the bottom. Force was applied from the top as a tensile force measured by a sensor. Displacement of the bones was measured b < a laser in the mounting device

bone (Fig. 1b). Data were recorded by the digital controller MTS Star II® (MTS Systems GmbH, Berlin, Germany) and a HBM Spider8 data acquisition system (HBM GmbH, Darmstadt, Germany).

Implants

Two different extramedullary locking plates and one intramedullary locking fixation device were compared with each other:

PEDUS L Plantar Lapidus Plate® (Axomed GmbH, Freiburg, Germany): a titanium plantar locking plate with four holes for 2.7-mm angle-stable cortical screws, 39 mm long. Two proximal screws and two distal screws were inserted bicortically. In addition, a 4.0-mm cannulated crossed screw of the same manufacturer was used. The screw was inserted from the dorsal and distal side of the first metatarsal bone in direction to the plantar and proximal side of the cuneiform bone. The plate was fixed at the plantar side (Fig. 2a).

Double bridge plate® (Königsee Implantate GmbH, Allendorf, Germany): a titanium H-shaped locking plate with four holes for 2.7-mm angle-stable cortical screws, 22 mm long. Two proximal screws and two distal screws were inserted bicortically. In addition, a 4.0-mm cannulated crossed screw of the same manufacturer was used. The screw was inserted from the dorsal and distal side of the first metatarsal bone in direction to the plantar and proximal side of the cuneiform bone. The plate was fixed at the plantar side (Fig. 2b).

IOFix® (Extremity Medicals, Parsippany, USA): an angle-stable intramedullary fixation device with a two-part construct of a 5.0-mm-thick and 40-mm-long lag screw and a 8.0-mm-thick and 25-mm-long X-Post®. The X-Post® was implanted into the first metatarsal bone from the dorsal to the plantar side. Implantation was bicortically with a 1-cm bone bridge to the arthrodesis side. The lag screw was applied in a 60° angle into the cuneiform bone through the plantar cortex (Fig. 2c).

Testing protocols

The following protocols were performed: a measurement of the initial compression forces in the arthrodesis gap (I), a non-destructive sinusoidal load test (II), and a load-to-failure test (III). In each protocol, force was applied directing from the plantar to the dorsal surface in a 90° angle to the ground to simulate standing and walking. The sinusoidal load test was used to simulate a postoperative patient, partially weight bearing in a healing shoe. After a preload of 10 N, cyclic loads between 5 and 50 N were applied sinusoidally with a frequency of 0.5 Hz and 5000 cycles. Then, stiffness of the fusion at the initial phase and at the end phase was compared by

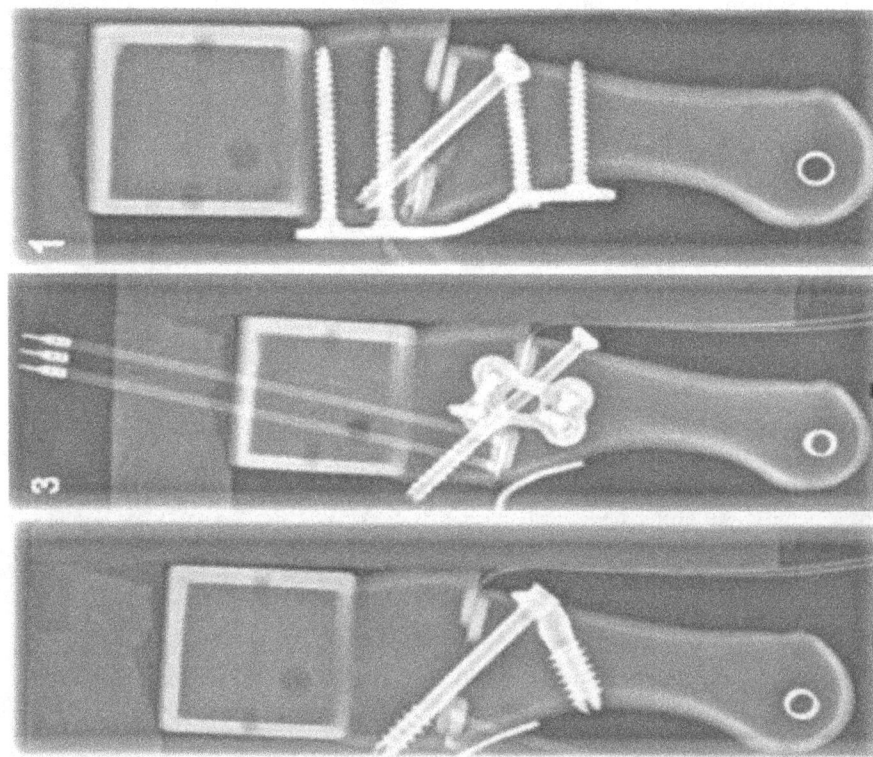

Fig. 2 X-ray images of the three models. **a** Plantar locking plat with crossed screw, **b** medial locking plate with crossed screw, and **c** the intramedullary angle-stable implant

measurements of displacement of the bones with a laser. After the continuous load test, the load-to-failure test was performed. All of the three synthetic bones, each one of them with a different implant for osteosynthesis (see above), were loaded until fracturing.

Statistics

Statistical analysis was performed with statistical software package SPSS® Version 24 (IBM, Armonk, North Castle, New York, USA). Compression forces were compared using one-way analysis of variance (ANOVA) followed by post hoc tests with Bonferroni correction for multiple testing. The non-destructive loadings were compared using ANOVA with repeated measures followed by post hoc tests with Bonferroni correction. The repeated measures are an initial test of displacement, a stress phase, and the final test of displacement. For the load-to-failure test, Kaplan-Meier curves were generated from survival data of the implants and groups were compared using log-rank test, the Tarone-Ware

test, and the modified Wilcoxon test. A P value of less than 0.05 was considered significant.

Results

Test protocol I

Compression of bone fragments is a known promoter of consolidation. Therefore, compression forces between the different synthetic bones were measured after the osteosynthesis was performed. The highest initial compression force was provided by the IOFix® implant (131 ± 55 N), followed by the medial locking plate (87 ± 51 N) and the plantar plate (3 ± 1 N,) (Fig. 3a). The low initial compression force values for the plantar plate construct where measured as recently as the second locking screw was applied beyond the arthrodesis gap (Fig. 3b). The initial compression force provided by IOFix® implant differed from the force provided by the PEDUS-L® ($P = 0.033$). Taken together, these data suggest that the IOFix® device provided the highest compression force.

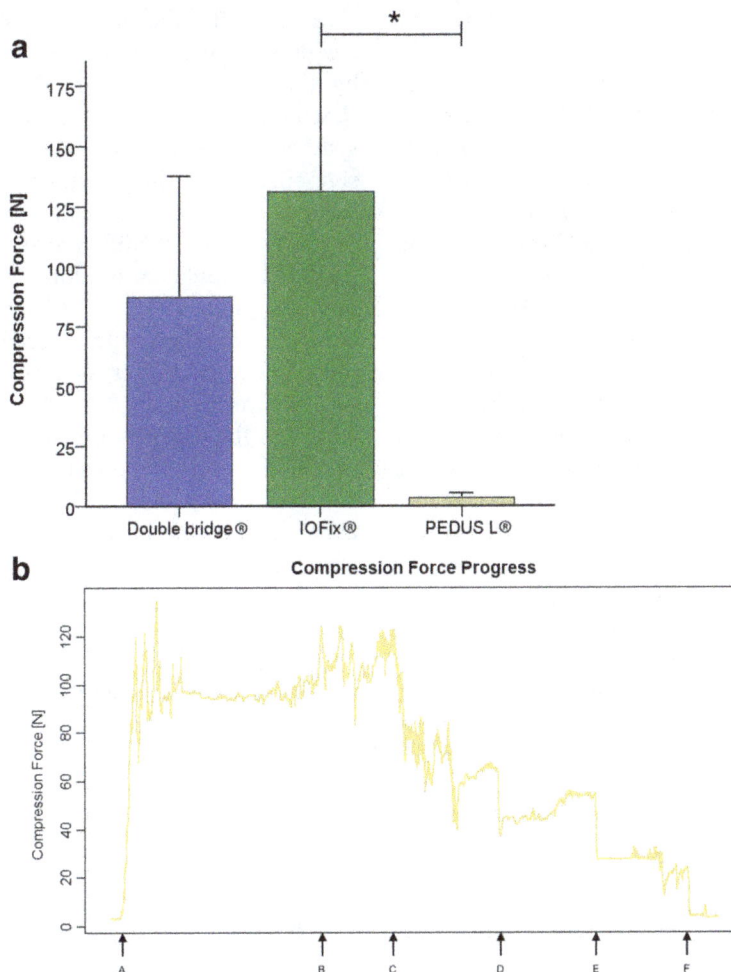

Fig. 3 a Initial compression forces measured directly after osteosynthesis in newton. Differences between the groups were significant over all (*$P = 0.033$, corrected by Bonferroni). **b** Compression force progress for the plantar locking plate. Points of the steps of osteosynthesis were documented at the x-axis

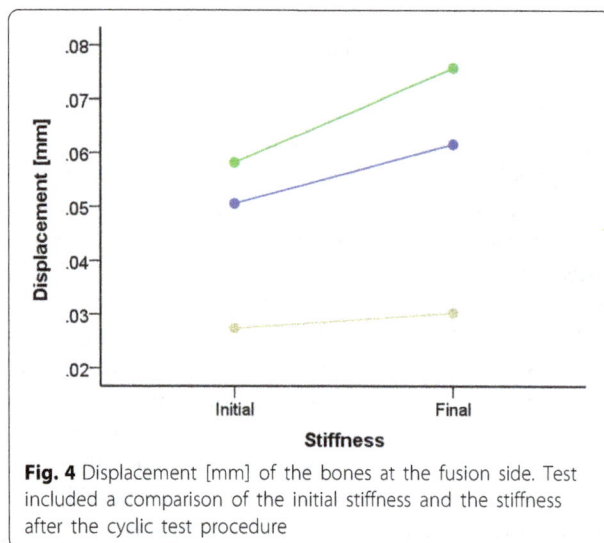

Fig. 4 Displacement [mm] of the bones at the fusion side. Test included a comparison of the initial stiffness and the stiffness after the cyclic test procedure

Test protocol II

The second test protocol was performed to analyse the stability of the osteosynthesis while simulating weight-bearing in a healing shoe. Differences between the initial and the final displacement of the synthetic bones and differences between the three bone-implant-combinations were analysed (Fig. 4): while the IOFix® combination and the Double bridge plate® combination showed significant loosening after the 5000 cycles, the PEDUS L Plantar Lapidus Plate® combination demonstrated rigid conditions after the test (Table 1). The stiffness provided by the IOFix® combination did not differ compared to the stiffness provided by the Double bridge plate® combination (*P* = 0.143). Furthermore, the stiffness provided by the PEDUS L Plantar Lapidus Plate® combination was superior compared to both of the other fixation methods (vs. Double bridge plate® *P* ≤ =0.000, vs. IOFix® *P* ≤ 0.000). Taken together, fixation with the plantar plate combination demonstrated a higher stiffness after the non-destructive sinusoidal load test compared to fixation with the IOFix® implant or the medial locking plate.

Test protocol III

The load-to-failure test was performed for all nine bone-implant-combination models to test the stability of the different implant devices until fracture of the bone. Failure was recognised in the following ranking: (1) the angle-stable intramedullary IOFix® fixation device (173 ± 8 N), (2) the medial located Double bridge plate® (324 ± 24 N), and (3) the PEDUS L Plantar Lapidus Plate® (377 ± 41 N, Fig. 5).

Discussion

The aim of this study was to compare actual implants for the fusion of the first tarsometatarsal joint in hallux surgery. Initial compression force and stiffness during postoperative weight-bearing was examined. The intramedullary device (IOFix®) demonstrated the highest initial compression force among the three tested implants. The plantar locking plate showed the best overall stability during cyclic weight-bearing simulation and had the lowest interfragmentary diastase.

Many study groups use cadaver specimens for implant research [12, 15, 16]. Cadaver specimens offer conditions similar to an in vivo setting (ligaments, periosteum, bone mineral density). In contrast, synthetic bones offer identical bone shapes and densities for all study samples and therefore provide an exact and reproducible experimental setting [17, 18].

The basic experimental set-up of this study was chosen based on the work of Roth and coworkers [12]. While Roth and colleagues used a distance-controlled method of force application and measurements, the present study was performed in a frequency-controlled set-up with a value recalculation by the intercept theorem. Using the latter method, measurements of the fusion gap between the two synthetic bones become more accurate because side-effects like plastic strains of the bone or of the fixation in the mounting device are eliminated.

Comparisons of different fixation devices for the modified Lapidus procedure were also performed in previous studies [12, 14–16]. Knutsen and colleagues compared fixations with crossed screws, a dorsal locking plate without a crossed screw, and the IOFix® device with each other [14]. They found a higher failure load for the IOFix® compared to the crossed screw procedure and the dorsal locking plate fixation. In contrast to the approach reported by Knutsen and colleagues, in the current study, a compression screw was inserted in every implant group to evaluate the initial compression force. Roth and colleagues found a greater stability of the fixated bone using a plantar locking plate compared to the IOFix® [12]. Furthermore, Klos and colleagues confirmed an advantage of a plantar orientation of implants when they compared fixation with a medial locking plate with crossed screws and in another study a plantar against a dorsomedial locking plate [15, 16]. Similar to those findings, in the current study, the plantar locking plate

Table 1 Displacement between the cuneiform and the metatarsal bones before and after performing the test protocol II in millimetre

	IOFix® mean (SD)	Double bridge plate® mean (SD)	Pedus L Plate® mean (SD)
Initial displacement	0.058 ± 0.005	0.051 ± 0.003	0.027 ± 0.005
Final displacement	0.076 ± 0.017	0.062 ± 0.002	0.030 ± 0.007

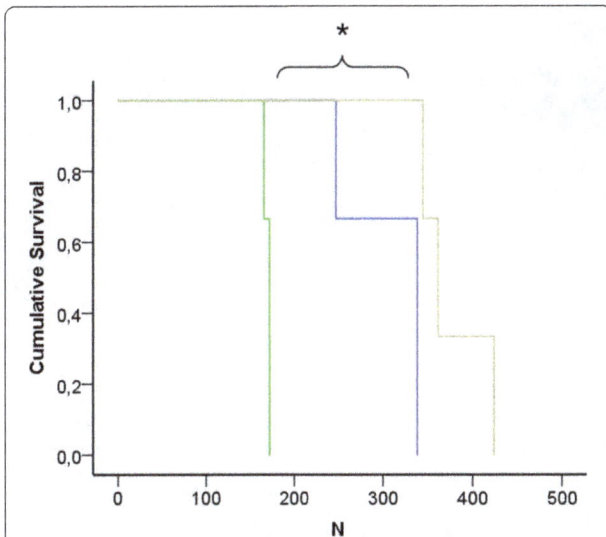

Fig. 5 Cumulative survival of the three implant model groups related to the force due to failure in newton. The intramedullary implant showed the earliest failure, followed by the medial locking plate and the plantar locking plate (*log-rank test $P = 0.002$, Tarone-Ware test $P = 0.005$, and the modified Wilcoxon test $P = 0.003$)

showed the highest stability (Fig. 4) and the highest failure load (Fig. 5).

Interestingly, there was a complete loss of compression after the locking plate was applied. The high rigidity of the PEDUS L® Plate, which is able to override the initial compression by the crossed screw, might explain this effect. However, this compression loss was not seen when the Double bridge plate® was used. Because the thicker plate design could be responsible for this finding, further research should address which types of locking plates are able to override the compression of a screw. These devices might be sufficient to fix the bone fragments with a forceps rendering a screw unnecessary. The intramedullary IOFix® device showed the earliest failure and the lowest stability during test protocol II. Therefore, advantages like a small incision and fast technique have to be balanced against outcome-relevant parameters such as failure rate and stability. Further research should be performed to investigate if a longer postoperative immobilisation or the use of an additional, second intramedullary device could improve implant stability. In summary, choosing the right implant for arthrodesis of the first tarsometatarsal joint has to remain an individual decision for every surgical case. Whether the use a rigid plantar plate with high stability is associated with a decreased non-union rate should be addressed in future research.

Conclusion

The modified Lapidus procedure is a common treatment of medial deviation of the first metatarsal bone in hallux

valgus disease. Modern fixation devices provide a higher stability and earlier weight-bearing than crossed screws. The intramedullary device (IOFix®) demonstrated the highest initial compression force of the three tested implants. The plantar locking plate showed the best overall stability during cyclic weight-bearing simulation and had the lowest interfragmentary diastase. Further research with clinical data is necessary to study if the IOFix® needs a longer period of non-weight-bearing to reach a better non-union rate compared to locking plates and if compression screws are unnecessary in addition to locking plates.

Abbreviation
SD: Standard deviation

Acknowledgements
Dr. Graw is a participant in the BIH-Charité Clinician Scientist Program funded by the Charité—Universitätsmedizin Berlin and the Berlin Institute of Health.

Funding
This study has been funded by Gesellschaft für Prävention und Rehabilitation im Sport e.V.

Authors' contributions
RB and RM conceived and designed the experiments. RB, RM, GD, AO, HJC, WR, and CPF performed the experiments. RB, RM, CS, JAG, and JS analysed the data. CS performed the statistical analysis. RB, RM, JAG, and JS wrote the paper. All authors read and approved the final version of the manuscript.

Competing interests
The authors declare that they have no competing interests.

Author details
[1]Department of Health, University of Witten/Herdecke, Witten, Germany. [2]Department of Trauma and Orthopaedic Surgery, Kreisklinikum Siegen, Weidenauer Str. 76, 57076 Siegen, Germany. [3]School of Science and Technology, University of Siegen, Siegen, Germany. [4]Department of Statistics an Econometrics, University of Siegen, Kohlbettstr, 15, 57072 Siegen, Germany. [5]Department of Mechanical Engineering, University of Siegen, Paul-Bonatz-Str. 9-11, 57076 Siegen, Germany. [6]Department of Anesthesiology and Operative Intensive Care Medicine, Charité—Universitätsmedizin Berlin, Campus Virchow-Klinikum, Augustenburger Platz 1, 13353 Berlin, Germany. [7]Berlin Institute of Health, Berlin, Germany. [8]Department of Orthopaedics and Trauma Surgery, Lahn-Dill-Kliniken Wetzlar, Forsthausstraße 1, 35578 Wetzlar, Germany.

References
1. Durman DC. Metatarsus primus varus and hallux valgus. AMA Arch Surg. 1957;74(1):128–35.
2. Hueter C. Klinik der Gelenkkrankheiten mit Einschluss der Orthopädie. Leipzig: Vogel; 1870.

3. Fraissler L, Konrads C, Hoberg M, Rudert M, Walcher M. Treatment of hallux valgus deformity. EFORT Open Rev. 2016;1(8):295–302.

4. Sharma J, Aydogan U. Algorithm for severe hallux valgus associated with metatarsus adductus. Foot Ankle Int. 2015;36(12):1499–503.

5. Cottom JM, Vora AM. Fixation of lapidus arthrodesis with a plantar interfragmentary screw and medial locking plate: a report of 88 cases. J Foot Ankle Surg. 2013;52(4):465–9.

6. Klaue K, Hansen ST, Masquelet AC. Clinical, quantitative assessment of first tarsometatarsal mobility in the sagittal plane and its relation to hallux valgus deformity. Foot Ankle Int. 1994;15(1):9–13.

7. Baravarian B, Briskin GB, Burns P. Lapidus bunionectomy: arthrodesis of the first metatarsocunieform joint. Clin Podiatr Med Surg. 2004;21(1):97–111.

8. Lapidus PW. Operative correction of the metatarsus primus varus in hallux valgus. Surg Gynecol Ostet. 1934;58:183–91.

9. Easley ME, Trnka HJ. Current concepts review: hallux valgus part II: operative treatment. Foot Ankle Int. 2007;28(6):748–58.

10. Coughlin MJ. Hallux valgus. J Bone Joint Surg Am. 1996;78(6):932–66.

11. Coughlin MJ, Mann RA. In: Coughlin MJ, Mann RA, Saltzman CL, editors. Hallux valgus. 8th ed. Philadelphia: Elsevier; 2007. p. 181–363.

12. Roth KE, Peters J, Schmidtmann I, Maus U, Stephan D, Augat P. Intraosseous fixation compared to plantar plate fixation for first metatarsocuneiform arthrodesis: a cadaveric biomechanical analysis. Foot Ankle Int. 2014;35(11): 1209–16.

13. Perren SM. Physical and biological aspects of fracture healing with special reference to internal fixation. Clin Orthop Relat Res. 1979;138:175–96.

14. Knutsen AR, Fleming JF, Ebramzadeh E, Ho NC, Warganich T, Harris TG, Sangiorgio SN. Biomechanical comparison of fixation devices for first metatarsocuneiform joint arthrodesis. Foot Ankle Spec. 2017;10(4):322–8.

15. Klos K, Gueorguiev B, Mückley T, Fröber R, Hofmann GO, Schwieger K, Windolf M. Stability of medial locking plate and compression screw versus two crossed screws for lapidus arthrodesis. Foot Ankle Int. 2010;31(2):158–63.

16. Klos K, Simons P, Hajduk AS, Hoffmeier KL, Gras F, Fröber R, Hofmann GO, Mückley T. Plantar versus dorsomedial locked plating for Lapidus arthrodesis: a biomechanical comparison. Foot Ankle Int. 2011;32(11):1081–5.

17. Cristofolini L, Viceconti M. Mechanical validation of whole bone composite tibia models. J Biomech. 2000;33(3):279–88.

18. Heiner AD, Brown TD. Structural properties of a new design of composite replicate femurs and tibias. J Biomech. 2001;34(6):773–81.

14

Early versus late intramedullary nailing for traumatic femur fracture management: meta-analysis

Ayman El-Menyar[1,2,3]* ⓘ, Mohammed Muneer[4], David Samson[1], Hassan Al-Thani[5], Ahmad Alobaidi[6], Paul Mussleman[7] and Rifat Latifi[8]

Abstract

Introduction: There is no consensus yet on the impact of timing of femur fracture (FF) internal fixation on the patient outcomes. This meta-analysis was conducted to evaluate the contemporary data in patients with traumatic FF undergoing intramedullary nail fixation (IMN).

Methods: English language literature was searched with publication limits set from 1994 to 2016 using PubMed, Scopus, MEDLINE (OVID), EMBASE (OVID), Web of Science, and Cochrane Central Register of Controlled Trials (CENTRAL). Studies included randomized controlled trials (RCTs), prospective observational or retrospective cohort studies, and case-control studies comparing early versus late femoral shaft fractures IMN fixation. Variable times were used across studies to distinguish between early and late IMN, but 24 h was the most frequently used cutoff. The quality assessment of the reviewed studies was performed with two instruments. Observational studies were assessed with the Newcastle-Ottawa Quality Assessment Scale. RCTs were assessed with the Cochrane Risk of Bias Tool.

Results: We have searched 1151 references. Screening of titles and abstracts eliminated 1098 references. We retrieved 53 articles for full-text screening, 15 of which met study eligibility criteria.

Conclusions: This meta-analysis addresses the utility of IMN in patients with FF based on the current evidence; however, the modality and timing to intervene remain controversial. While we find large pooled effects in favor of early IMN, for reasons discussed, we have little confidence in the effect estimate. Moreover, the available data do not fill all the gaps in this regard; therefore, a tailored algorithm for management of FF would be of value especially in polytrauma patients.

Keywords: Meta-analysis, Intramedullary nailing, Femur fracture, Quality assessment, Orthopedic, Trauma

Background

Traumatic femur fracture (FF) continues to be associated with a considerable rate of morbidity and mortality [1]. However, these unfavorable outcomes could be contributed to several factors such as patient age and stability, mechanism of injury, comorbidities, associated injuries, and the time and approach of the management. Diaphyseal FF is mostly result of high-energy trauma and its incidence ranges from 9.9 to 12 for every 100,000 persons/year [2, 3]. Prior data showed that the average patient age is 25 years and around 60% of injuries occur in men. The considerable energy required to cause many of these fractures often provokes injuries in other structures, above all is the ipsilateral hip and knee and they often go undiagnosed [2–4].

The treatment of choice for diaphyseal FF is internal fixation with intramedullary nail (IMN) stabilization; it achieves correct alignment and high rate of bone healing with low complications rate and early limb mobility [5–7]. However, the optimal timing for internal fixation remains controversial [8–13].

* Correspondence: aymanco65@yahoo.com
[1]Department of Surgery Clinical Research Unit, Westchester Medical Center Health Network, Valhalla, New York, USA
[2]Trauma Surgery, Clinical Research, Hamad General Hospital, Doha, Qatar
Full list of author information is available at the end of the article

The concept of early stabilization of long bone fractures including FF was established many years ago. It was suggested to provide early total care for patients of polytrauma associated with head injury. This approach was aiming to have lesser pulmonary complications and reduced length of hospital stay [14–17]. However, it was recently accepted to perform a minimal intervention surgery (i.e., damage control approach) that temporarily fixes FF until the patient general condition allows definitive management. There is no consensus regarding the effect of early versus late fixation of FF on the clinical outcomes. We conducted this meta-analysis with extensive statistical assessment to evaluate the contemporary data in patients with traumatic FF undergoing early versus late IMN, in different clinical settings. We sought to explore the literatures to know whether the concurrent meta-analysis able to fill the gaps in the nailing management of FF.

Methodology
Search strategy and registration
English language literature was searched with publication limits set from 01 June 1994 to 31 June 2016 in the following scholarly databases: PubMed, Scopus, MEDLINE (OVID), EMBASE (OVID), Web of Science, and Cochrane Central Register of Controlled Trials (CENTRAL). Additionally, searches were conducted in the gray literature in order to retrieve relevant unpublished scholarly materials.

Focused terms (subject headings, synonyms, etc.) utilized in the searches were reflective of the broad terms of "intramedullary nailing," "femur fracture," and "shaft." This study was registered it in the PROSPERO registry (CRD 42017057866). This report follows the Preferred Reporting Items for Systematic Reviews and Meta-Analyses (PRISMA) statement [18].

Study types
Studies included randomized controlled trials (RCTs), prospective observational or retrospective cohort studies, and case-control studies comparing early versus late femoral shaft fractures IMN fixation. Variable times were used across studies to distinguish between early and late IMN, but 24 h was the most frequently used cutoff.

Participant types
We included studies with adult patients, any sex, and with no restriction on inclusion of ethnicities or patients with co-morbidities.

Data extraction and management
Data were extracted by a single reviewer, confirmed by two other reviewers, and entered into EndNote. Information included authorship, publication year, methodology

of the study, population, intervention, timing of the surgery, and relevant outcome measures.

Inclusion criteria
Included traumatic patients with femur shaft fractures that were treated by reamed antegrade IMN, all patients below 70 years and above 14 years and single and bilateral femur fractures are both included.

Exclusion criteria
Included patients below 14 years or above 70 years, patients with trochanteric, neck, or distal FF, treated FF by temporal external fixation followed by definitive IMN, patients died within 24 h of admission, and pathological FFs.

Outcomes
Both clinical outcomes and surrogates were included, i.e., mortality, length of hospital stay, ICU length stay, any complications, bed sore, wound infection, sepsis, organ failure, all pulmonary complications, acute respiratory distress syndrome (ARDS), pneumonia, deep vein thrombosis (DVT), pulmonary embolism, and fat embolism .

Study quality assessment
The quality assessment of the reviewed studies was performed with two instruments. Observational studies were assessed with the Newcastle-Ottawa Quality Assessment Scale [19]. Randomized controlled trials were assessed with the Cochrane Risk of Bias Tool [20].

Statistical analysis
Unadjusted odds ratios (ORs) were extracted from individual studies. When articles also reported ORs adjusted for confounders, the magnitude of confounding was computed as the difference between the unadjusted OR and the adjusted OR divided by the unadjusted OR, expressed as a percentage. Meta-analyses were carried out using the inverse variance weighted random effects method. Heterogeneity was assessed with the Q statistic and I^2. Forest plots contain individual study ORs and 95% confidence intervals (CIs), along with pooled ORs which were considered statistically significant if the 95% confidence interval (CI) excluded the null value of 1.0, equivalent to a p value < 0.05. Funnel plots were produced as a graphic technique to assess potential publication bias. Egger's regression tests of publication bias were also conducted and were considered significant if the p value for slope was < 0.05. Meta-analytic forest plots and funnel plots were produced with Review Manager 5.3 (Cochrane Collaboration, Copenhagen, Denmark). Tests for publication bias were performed with STATA 9.2 (StataCorp, College Station, TX).

Results

Study selection

Search of PubMed, EMBASE, and Cochrane Central Register of Controlled trials identified 1151 references. Screening of titles and abstracts eliminated 1098 references. We retrieved 53 articles for full-text screening, 15 of which met study eligibility criteria (Fig. 1).

Study quality assessment

Two studies were RCTs, and 13 were retrospective cohort studies. All cohort studies earned favorable (star) ratings on these items: (1) representativeness of the exposed (early IMN) cohort; (2) selection of the non-exposed (late IMN) cohort; (3) ascertainment of exposure; (4) assessment of outcome; (5) sufficient length of follow-up and adequacy of follow-up of cohorts. No cohort study clearly stated whether participants were free of the outcomes of interest at the start of the study. Only two cohort studies [21, 22] addressed comparability of cohorts on the basis of the design or analysis, earning two stars. Harvin et al. [21] conducted multivariable logistic regression modeling in which IMN performed < 24 h or was not adjusted for injury severity

score (ISS) and revised trauma score (RTS). Morshed et al. [22] constructed a marginal structural model using inverse probability of treatment-weighting and adjustment for 10 potential confounding variables. Another cohort study [23] described use of multivariate regression analysis to control for age, ISS, and type and severity of associated injuries; however, the article did not report adjusted OR estimates and is thus rated unfavorably on comparability of cohorts.

Of the two RCTs, the trial by Pape et al. [24] was generally rated more favorably. This study was rated as low risk of bias on these items: selection bias–random sequence generation; selection bias–allocation concealment; attrition bias–incomplete outcome data; and reporting bias–selective reporting. Despite favorable ratings for selection bias, this study observed several statistically significant differences on baseline characteristics and used multivariable regression models that controlled for ISS and RTS. This trial was rated as high risk of bias for detection bias—blinding of outcome assessment and was rated as unclear bias on performance bias—blinding of participants and personnel. Pape adjusted for ISS, RTS, and head injury severity in their analyses. At

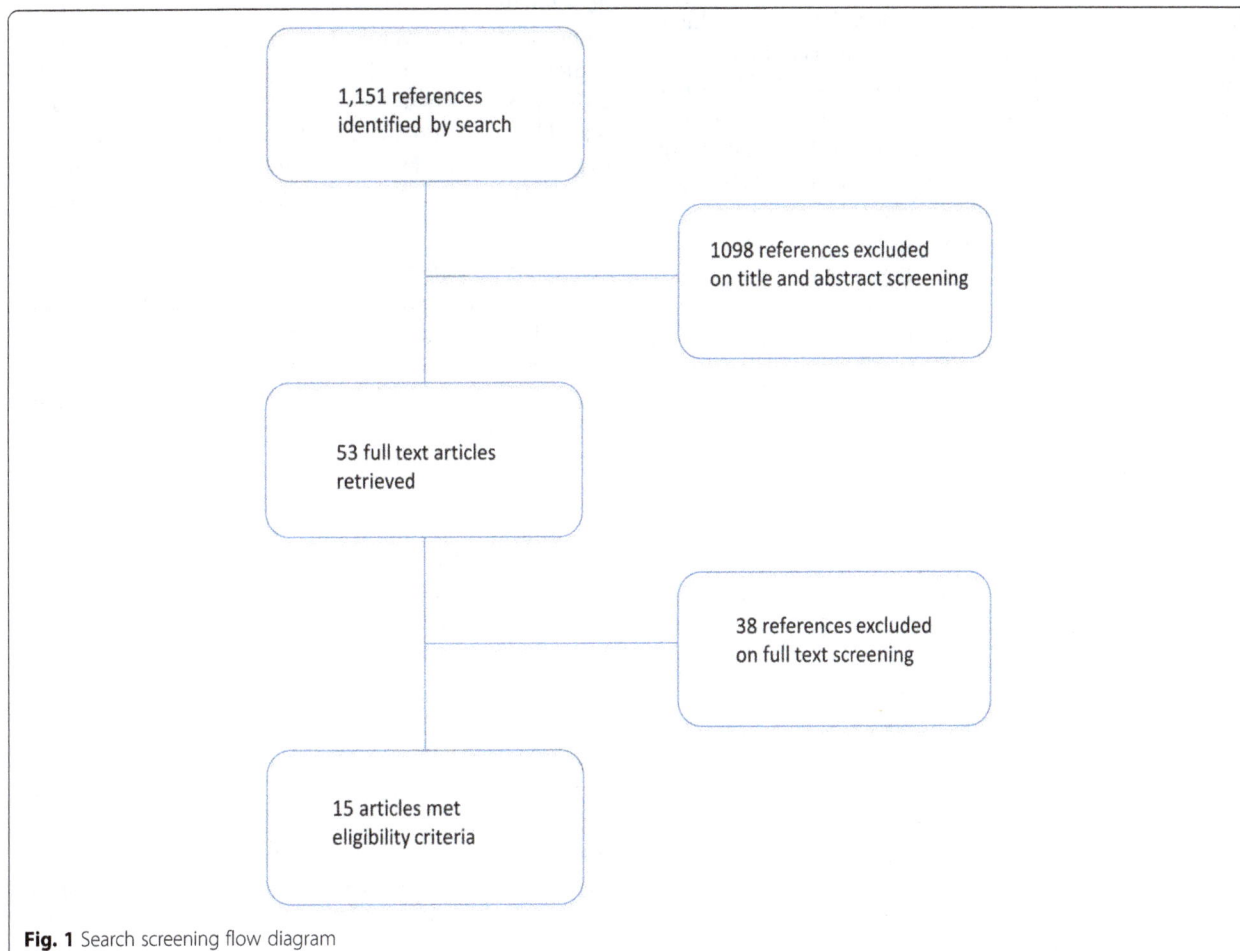

Fig. 1 Search screening flow diagram

baseline, early IMN and late IMN groups differed significantly on these variables, in addition to the new injury severity score (NISS), and abbreviated injury scale (AIS) head. The RCT by Bone et al. [25] was rated as high risk for performance bias and detection bias and low risk for attrition bias and reporting bias. It was rated as unclear bias for both selection bias items.

All complications

Two retrospective cohort studies reported results on any and all complications [23, 30]. Neither study addressed comparability of groups in design or analysis. A high degree of statistical heterogeneity was observed (I^2 = 98%). The summary estimate of odds of any complication between early and late IMN was not statistically significant (pooled OR = 1.28, 95% CI 0.08, 20.84).

Pulmonary complications

One RCT and four retrospective cohort studies contributed to this meta-analysis [21, 24, 25–27]. The RCT was rated as high risk of selection bias. One of the cohort studies addressed comparability in the analysis [21], but only the unadjusted data are included in this meta-analysis. Of the four studies that reported the composite outcome, pulmonary complications, all included both pneumonia and pulmonary embolism in the outcome definition. Nahm et al. also included ARDS. Charash et al. [26] added fat embolism, while Bone et al. [25] added abnormal blood gas levels. These five studies collectively enrolled 2180 patients. No statistical heterogeneity was observed (I^2 = 0%). Early IMN was associated with a lower odds of pulmonary complications, compared with late IMN (pooled OR = 0.20, 95% CI 0.15, 0.28). The study by Harvin et al. [21] reported both an unadjusted OR and an adjusted OR. The magnitude of confounding was calculated as – 64.6%, moving the point estimate from 0.26 to 0.43; statistical adjustment yielded a weaker association between early IMN and pulmonary complications (Fig. 2).

Acute respiratory distress syndrome

Two RCTs and 8 retrospective cohort studies reported on ARDS [1, 22, 24–31]. Only the RCT by Pape et al. [22] reported adjusted estimates of the OR, but the meta-analysis includes only the unadjusted OR from this study. No other studies attempted to control for confounding either by design or analysis. The aggregate number of patients in these 10 studies is 2924. No statistical heterogeneity was observed (I^2 = 0%). Early IMN was associated with a lower odds of ARDS, compared with late IMN (pooled OR = 0.39, 95% CI 0.26, 0.57). Pape et al. [22] presented both unadjusted and adjusted ORs. The magnitude of confounding was – 20.0%, enough to null the impact of early IMN: the unadjusted

OR, used in pooling, was 0.85, whereas the adjusted OR was 1.02.

Pneumonia

One RCT and six retrospective cohort studies presented data on the incidence of pneumonia [22, 24–27, 29, 30]. The Pape et al. [22] RCT provided the OR adjusted for ISS and RTS; however, only the unadjusted OR is included in this meta-analysis. Together, these 7 studies included 2238 patients. There was a low degree of statistical heterogeneity among these studies (I^2 = 31%). Early IMN was associated with a lower odds of pneumonia, compared with late IMN (pooled OR = 0.37, 95% CI 0.26, 0.54). By comparing unadjusted and adjusted ORs, the RCT in this set of studies showed a very large magnitude of confounding: – 186.9%. By controlling for two confounding variables the point estimate OR value changed from 0.48 to 1.39. Adjustment changed not only the magnitude of the association, but also reversed the direction.

Fat embolism

One RCT and three retrospective cohort studies gave data for the occurrence of fat embolism [25, 26, 29, 32]. None of the observational studies adjusted for potential confounders. The total of participants across studies was 1570. No statistical heterogeneity was observed (I^2 = 0%). There was no statistically significant association between timing of IMN and odds of fat embolism. The pooled OR was 0.64 and the 95% CI was 0.26 to 1.62.

Pulmonary embolism

One RCT and four retrospective studies reported data for pulmonary embolism [24–27, 29], but there were zero events in both early and late groups in one study, making estimation of the OR impossible, so that study [27] was excluded. No observational study adjusted the OR for confounders. Summed across studies, the total number of patients was 1867. No statistical heterogeneity was observed (I^2 = 0%). There was no statistically significant association between timing of IMN and odds of pulmonary embolism. The pooled OR was 0.71 and the 95% CI was 0.21 to 2.39.

Deep vein thrombosis

Two retrospective cohort studies provided evidence on DVT risk [21, 24]. The Harvin et al. study [21] was controlled for ISS and RTS. A total of 678 patients participated in these studies. Statistical heterogeneity among these studies is low (I^2 = 11%). Compared with late IMN, early IMN is associated with a statistically significant reduction in the odds of DVT (pooled OR = 0.39, 95% CI 0.21, 0.71) (Fig. 3).

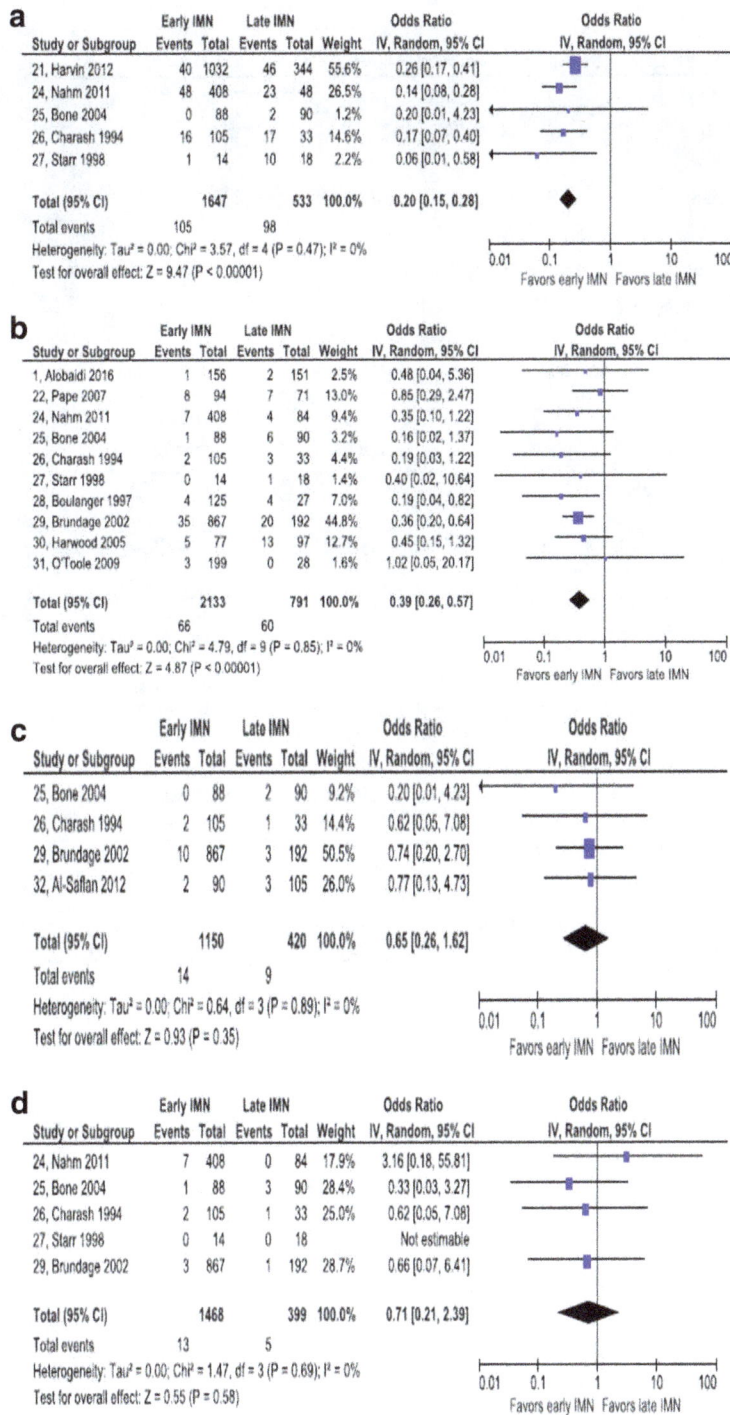

Fig. 2 Forest plot of pulmonary complications. **a** Pulmonary complications. **b** Acute respiratory distress syndrome. **c** Fat embolism. **d** Pneumonia

Multiorgan failure

One RCT and two retrospective cohort studies collected data on multiorgan failure [22, 24, 30]. The RCT adjusted for ISS and RTS. The aggregate number of patients in these two studies was 831. There was a minor degree of statistical heterogeneity ($I^2 = 30\%$). There was a statistically significant association between timing of IMN and multiorgan failure: pooled OR = 0.38, 95% CI 0.16, 0.90. The magnitude of confounding in the RCT was − 11.6%, enough to change a weak nonsignificant effect favoring early IMN to a weak nonsignificant effect favoring late IMN.

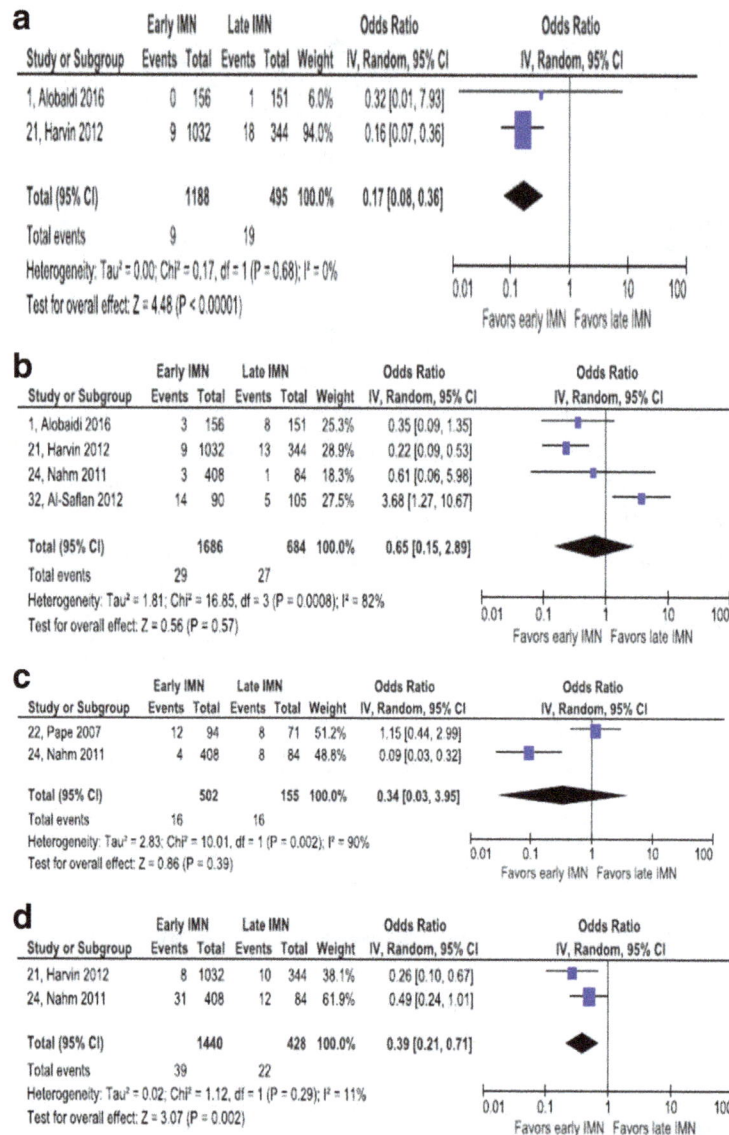

Fig. 3 Forest plot of cutaneous, infectious, and vascular complications. **a** Decubitus ulcer. **b** Wound infection. **c** Deep vein thrombosis. **d** Pulmonary embolism

Wound infection

Four retrospective cohort studies reported on wound infection. None addressed confounding in the analysis [1, 21, 24, 32]. A total of 2370 patients were included in these four studies. Considerable statistical heterogeneity was observed in this set of studies (I^2 = 82%). There was no statistically significant association between timing of IMN and wound infection: pooled OR = 0.65, 95% CI 0.15, 2.89.

Sepsis

One RCT and one retrospective cohort study reported on the risk of sepsis after IMN [22, 24]. The retrospective cohort study did not report outcomes adjusted for potential confounding, while the RCT did report

adjusted outcome measures. The magnitude of confounding in the RCT was – 13.9%, indicating a slightly stronger estimate of an effect favoring late IMN after adjustment. A high degree of statistical heterogeneity among these two studies was observed (I^2 = 90%). The pooled OR (0.34) did not reach statistical significance (95% CI 0.03, 3.95).

Decubitus ulcer

Two retrospective cohort studies addressed the incidence of decubitus ulcers [1, 21]. Neither addressed confounding in the analysis. Between these two studies, 1683 patients were enrolled. No statistical heterogeneity was observed (I^2 = 0%). There was a statistically significant association between early IMN and reduced odds of decubitus ulcer occurrence: OR = 0.17, 95% CI 0.08, 0.36.

Mortality

Eleven retrospective cohort studies included data on mortality [1, 21, 23, 24, 26, 27, 29–31, 33, 34]. None reported ORs adjusted for confounders. The total number of patients was 8600. There was a moderate degree of

statistical heterogeneity among these studies (I^2 = 51%). The association between early IMN and reduced mortality achieved statistical significance: OR = 0.46, 95% CI 0.26, 0.82 (Fig. 4).

Discussion

In general, the timing of surgical management in trauma patients should attain maximum benefit of surgery and

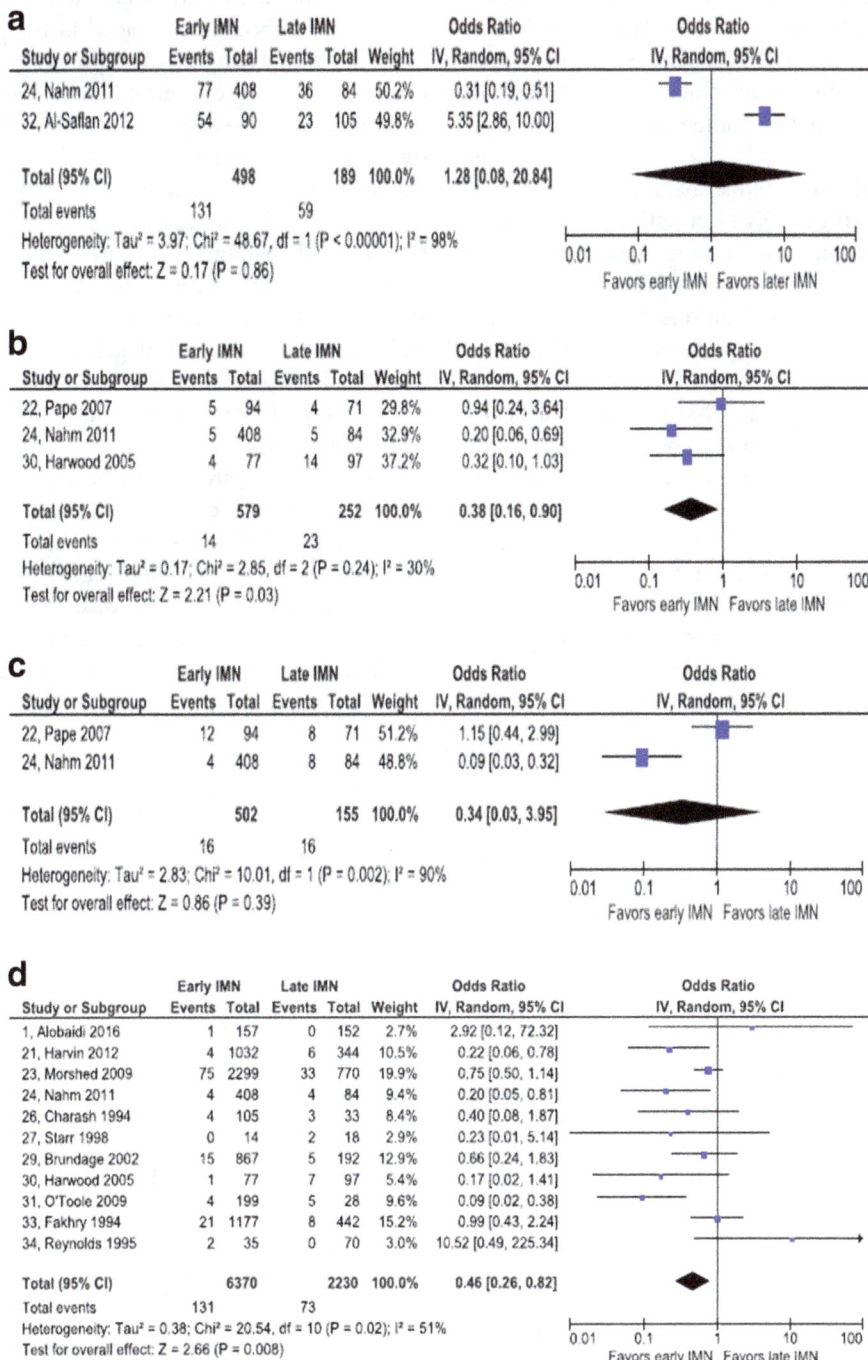

Fig. 4 Forest plot of other complications. **a** Any complications. **b** Sepsis. **c** Multiorgan failure. **d** Mortality

minimum or nil complications. Time to intervene in orthopedic surgery has ultimate prognostic impact; however, the optimum timing is still debatable in traumatic FF [35]. In long bone and pelvic fracture, it has been shown that early surgical fixation is associated with better cardiac function and pulmonary performance, respectively [36, 37]. Of note, FF is often a high-energy injury and also might have associated thoracic [17, 25] or head injuries [15, 38–40]. Moreover, internal fixation with IMN has physiologic consequences; therefore, a lot of considerations and a particular algorithm should be in the decision-makers mind [15]. Figure 5 shows a proposed algorithm for the management of FF (shaft) in adult patients based on the contemporary evidence in the literature.

In 2016, Liu et al. published a meta-analysis that addressed the impact of early IMN in patients with severe chest trauma; however, the authors have done their search up to the year 2011 only [41]. The present meta-analysis sheds more light on this debate (early versus late IMN in FF patients) in different clinical settings up to the mid of 2016.

Among the outcomes of IMN that were pooled in the present analysis, we found statistically significant results for any pulmonary complication, ARDS, pneumonia, decubitus ulcers, multiorgan failure, DVT, and mortality, while results were not statistically significant for pulmonary embolism, fat embolism, wound infection, sepsis, and any complication.

For pulmonary injury, it was reported that early IMN fixation of femoral shaft fractures could contribute to an additional respiratory damage and may trigger ARDS in the presence of chest injury, particularly in borderline patients [24]. However, we found that early IMN has lower odds of pulmonary complications, ARDS, and pneumonia than late IMN fixation. Therefore, in some studies, it was suggested that pulmonary complications could be related to the chest injury itself rather than the methods of FF fixation in polytrauma patients [16, 24]. However, reamed nailing performed within the initial 24 h was found to have a potentially negative effect on the lung and should be avoided in the presence of chest trauma. Pape et al. [42, 43] reported a sustained inflammatory response only after intramedullary femoral instrumentation that was done within the first 24 h. In such high-risk trauma patients, it is thought that the damage control orthopedic surgery approach is a wise option to avoid such complications. Weninger et al. [44] evaluated 45 patients with severe thoracic trauma and FF stabilized with unreamed IMN within the first 24 h and found that the rates of ARDS, multiorgan failure, and mortality were not negatively influenced by early unreamed IMN. The patients' general condition also has its own word for the method and outcome after IMN in polytrauma cases.

This meta-analysis did not show a significant association between the time of IMN and the occurrence of pulmonary embolism. However, Gray et al. [45] found that IMN resulted in a significantly high initial pulmonary embolic load; but there was no detectable effect on the coagulation profile, pulmonary inflammation, or mortality over the first 24 h after injury. In one study,

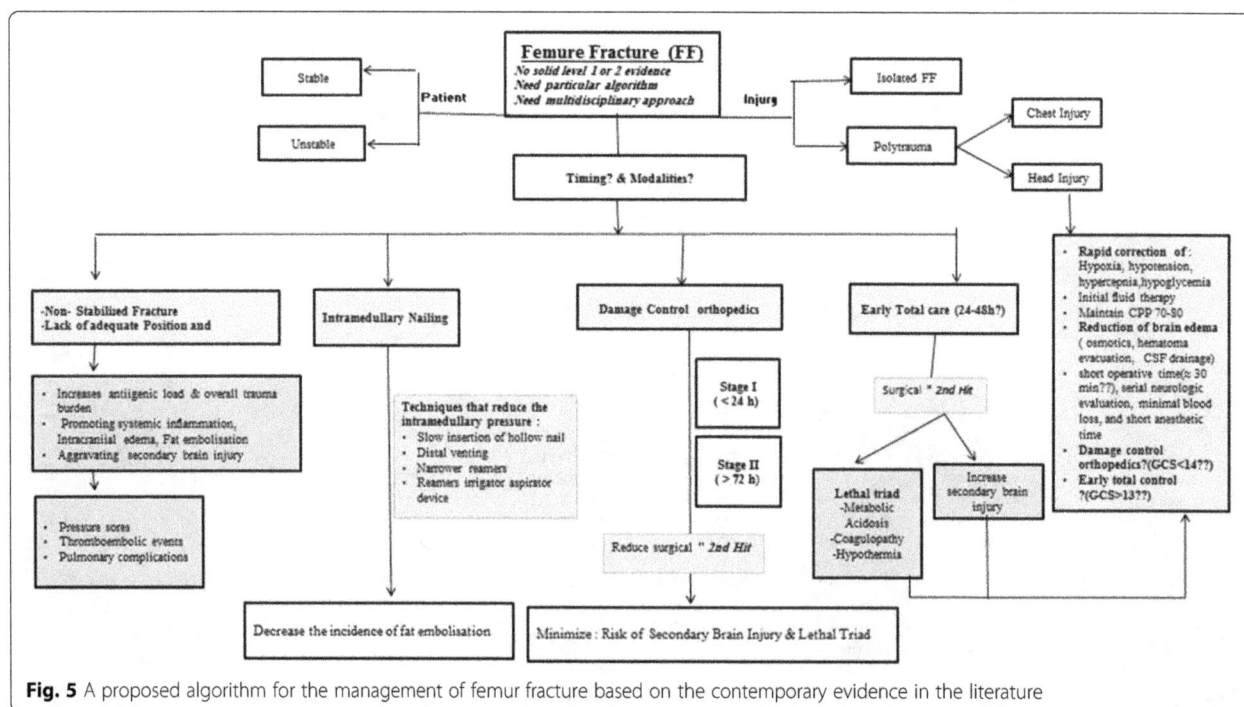

Fig. 5 A proposed algorithm for the management of femur fracture based on the contemporary evidence in the literature

Brundage et al. [29] reported 17 (1.2%) cases with fat embolism (13 in the operative and 4 in non-operative group) with no significant association between its occurrence and the time of IMN. Also they reported five cases of pulmonary embolism (all were in the operative group and 4 of them were associated with high ISS). A prior meta-analysis of six studies founds no difference in the incidence of venous thromboembolism between early and late IMN groups [35].We could not find any information reading the use of DVT prophylaxis in the entire analyzed studies.

The relationship between early fracture and the risk of fat embolism has been addressed in few studies [46–49]. In one study, due to increased medullary canal pressure during nailing process, fat extravasation into the lung vasculature has been shown during reaming by intraoperative transesophageal echocardiogram [47]. There are some approaches like slow insertion of hollow nails, distal venting, narrower reamers, and reamer irrigator aspirator devices have been shown to reduce this intramedullary pressure [50, 51].

In our meta-analysis, patients who had early IMN were significantly associated with fewer decubitus ulcers. However, wound infection was shown to have no association with the timing of IMN. Early IMN allows patients earlier rehabilitation and mobility. Therefore, the risk to develop to decubitus ulcer is less.

There is an ongoing debate regarding the optimal temporal approach for surgical stabilization in patients with concomitant head injuries. During the first 24 h post injury, intramedullary fracture fixation, may reduce the patient's mean arterial pressure and cerebral perfusion pressure and lead to secondary brain insults and deterioration of the neurologic state [10, 52, 53].

There is a lack of prospectively randomized trials that focus on the temporal approach of fracture fixation in multiple trauma patients with concomitant head injury [10, 13].

Jaicks et al. [39] reported on 33 patients with closed head injury (AIS score > 2) that required operative fracture fixation. They found a higher rate of intraoperative hypotension (62%) and hypoxia (11%) in the early stabilized fracture cases with a worse neurologic outcome. It has been reported that intraoperative hypotension or hypoxia explained the lower discharge GCS score in patients who underwent early fracture fixation in patients with concomitant head injuries [39, 52].

Advocates of delayed surgical management of femoral fractures in patients with concomitant head injury maintain the high risk of secondary brain insult if the aggressive treatment of fractures interferes with resuscitation or neurosurgical monitoring [10, 13]. Moreover, Townsend et al. reviewed 61 patients with moderate-to-severe blunt head injury and FF who were divided into four groups based on the timing of the orthopedic surgical correction [52]. The investigators found a significantly higher risk of intraoperative hypotension (68%) in patients who underwent definitive fracture fixation within the first 2 h of admission in comparison to 8% if fracture fixation was delayed more than 24 h. In the current meta-analysis, there were eight studies that described the management of FF in patients with head injury, of which only four studies reported the severity of head injury (head AIS > 2) [25, 31, 33, 54].

Prior reports showed that short operative time (≈ 30 min), serial neurologic evaluation, minimal blood loss, and short anesthetic time (i.e., damage control approach) are important factors to minimize secondary brain injury [15].

The present analysis shows that early IMN is associated with less mortality rate which goes in line with most of the studies; however, the association between timing of IMN and multiorgan failure was not significant.

Limitations

In this meta-analysis, Newcastle-Ottawa Quality Assessment Scale was used to assess the methodologic quality of observational studies. Included cohort studies were rated favorably on most items. The exceptions were the selection bias item regarding demonstration that the outcome of interest was not present at the start of the study and comparability of cohorts on the basis of the design or analysis. None of the 16 cohort studies was favorable on the former and only two studies reported attempts to control for confounding in statistical analysis. The lack of control for potential confounding is a major flaw in this evidence base. In the few instances in which studies reported both unadjusted ORs and adjusted ORs, it is possible to quantify the magnitude of confounding present. Across four outcomes, adjustment nearly always resulted in moving the point estimate away from the more favorable unadjusted estimate. Thus, adjustment tended to lead to weaker estimates of association and in one case led to an estimate characterized by the opposite direction of association.

The GRADE system for assessing the strength of a body of evidence recommends starting with a level of low evidence when it is based primarily on observational studies [55]. GRADE also recommends reducing strength to very low when observational studies fail to take confounding into account in the analysis. While this meta-analysis finds large pooled effects favoring early IMN, for reasons discussed, we have little confidence in the effect estimate. So far, it seems that the available meta-analyses would not fully answer or fill the gaps in the current clinical practice.

Conclusions

This meta-analysis addresses the utility of IMN in patients with FF based on the current evidence; however, the modality and timing to intervene remain controversial. While we find large pooled effects in favor of early IMN, for reasons discussed, we have little confidence in the effect estimate. Moreover, the available data do not fill all the gaps in this regard; therefore, a tailored algorithm for management of FF would be of value especially in polytrauma patients.

Abbreviations

ARDS: Acute respiratory distress syndrome; DVT: Deep vein thrombosis; FF: Femur fracture; IMN: Intramedullary nailing; ISS: Injury severity scoring; RTS: Revised trauma scoring

Acknowledgements

We thank research office staff at HMC and Westchester Medical Center, NY. This study will be presented in part at the 13th Annual Academic Surgical Congress to be held 30 January–1 February 2018 in Jacksonville, FL.

Authors' contributions

AE is involved in the study design, search and data collection, analysis and interpretation, and writing of the manuscript. MM is involved in the study design, search and data collection, analysis and interpretation, and writing of the manuscript. DS is involved in the search, statistical analysis, and writing of the manuscript. HA is involved in the study design, data interpretation, and writing of the manuscript. AA helped in the study design and writing of the manuscript. PM contributed to the study design, search and data collection. RL is involved in the study design, data interpretation, and writing of the manuscript. All authors have read and approved the final submitted manuscript.

Competing interests

The authors declare that they have no competing interests.

Author details

[1]Department of Surgery Clinical Research Unit, Westchester Medical Center Health Network, Valhalla, New York, USA. [2]Trauma Surgery, Clinical Research, Hamad General Hospital, Doha, Qatar. [3]Clinical Medicine, Weill Cornell Medical School, Doha, Qatar. [4]Department of Surgery, Hamad General Hospital, Doha, Qatar. [5]Department of Surgery, Trauma and Vascular Surgery, Hamad General Hospital, Doha, Qatar. [6]Department of Surgery, Orthopedic Surgery, Al Wakrah Hospital, Doha, Qatar. [7]Distributed eLibrary, Weill Cornell Medical School, Doha, Qatar. [8]Department of Surgery, Westchester Medical Center Health Network and New York Medical College, Valhalla, New York, USA.

References

1. Alobaidi AS, Al-Hassani A, El-Menyar A, et al. Early and late intramedullary nailing of femur fracture: a single center experience. Int J Crit Illn Inj Sci. 2016;6(3):143–7.
2. Salminen ST, Pihlajamaki HK, Avikainen VJ, Bostman ON. Population based epidemiologic and morphologic study of femoral shaft fractures. Clin Orthop Relat Res. 2000;372:241–9.
3. Regel G, Lobenhoffer P, Grotz M, Pape HC, Lehmann U, Tscherne H. Treatment results of patients with multiple trauma: an analysis of 3406 cases treated between 1972 and 1991 at a german level I trauma center. J Trauma. 1995;38:70–8.
4. Bengner U, Ekbon T, Johnell O, Nilsson DE. Incidence of femur and tibial shaft fractures, epidemiology 1950-1983 in Malmo Sweden. Acta Orthop Scand. 1994;61:251–4.
5. Arneson TJ, Malton LJ III, Lewallen DG, O'Fallon WN. Epidemilogy of diaphyseal and distal femoral fractures in Rochester Minnesota, 1965-1984. Clin Orthop Relat Res. 1988;234:188–94.
6. Brumback RJ, Virkus WW. Intramedullary nailing of the femur: reamed versus nonreamed. J Am Acad Orthop Surg. 2000;8:83–90.
7. Bucholz RW, Jones A. Fractures of the shaft of the femur. J Bone Joint Surg Am. 1991;73-A:1561–6.
8. Wolinsky P, Tejwani N, Richmond JH, Kj K, Egol K, Stephen DJG. Controversies in intramedullary nailing of femoral shaft fractures. AAOS Instruct Course Lect. 2002;51:291–303.
9. JO A, Luber K, Park T. The effect of femoral nailing on cerebral perfusion pressure in head-injured patients. J Trauma. 2003;54(6):1166–70.
10. Flierl MA, Stoneback JW, Beauchamp KM, et al. Femur shaft fracture fixation in head-injured patients: when is the right time? J Orthop Trauma. 2010;24(2):107–14.
11. Nahm NJ, Vallier HA. Timing of definitive treatment of femoral shaft fractures in patients with multiple injuries: a systematic review of randomized and nonrandomized trials. J Trauma Acute Care Surg. 2012;73(5):1046–63.
12. M B, Guyatt GH, Khera V, Kulkarni AV, Sprague S, Schemitsch EH. Operative management of lower extremity fractures in patients with head injuries. Clin Orthop Relat Res. 2003;407:187–98.
13. Nau T, Kutscha-Lissberg F, Muellner T, Koenig F, Vecsei V. Effects of a femoral shaft fracture on multiply injured patients with a head injury. World J Surg. 2003;27(3):365–9. Epub 2003 Feb 27
14. Lhowe DW, Hansen ST. Immediate nailing of open fractures of the femoral shaft. J Bone Joint Surg Am. 1988;70:812–20.
15. Scalea TM, Boswell SA, Scott JD, Mitchell KA, Kramer ME, Pollak AN. External fixation as a bridge to intramedullary nailing for patients with multiple injuries and with femoral fractures: damage control orthopedics. J Trauma. 2000;48:613–23.
16. Bone LB, Johnson KD, Weigelt J, Scheinberg R. Early versus delayed stabilization of femoral fractures. A prospective randomized study. J Bone Joint Surg Am. 1989;71:336–40.
17. Behrman SW, Fabian TC, Kudsk KA, Taylor JC. Improved outcome with femur fractures: early vs. delayed fixation. J Trauma. 1990;30:792–7.
18. Moher D, Liberati A, Tetzlaff J, Altman DG. Preferred reporting items for systematic reviews and meta-analyses: the PRISMA statement. BMJ. 2009;339:b2535. pmid:19622551
19. Wells GA, Shea B, O'Connell D, et al. The Newcastle-Ottawa Scale (NOS) for assessing the quality of nonrandomised studies in meta-analyses. Available from: http://www.ohri.ca/programs/clinical_epidemiology/oxford.htm (Accessed 17 Oct 2016).
20. Higgins JPT, Altman DG, Sterne, JAC (editors). Chapter 8: Assessing risk of bias in included studies. In: Higgins JPT, Green S (editors). Cochrane handbook for systematic reviews of interventions. The Cochrane Collaboration, 2011. Version 5.1.0 [updated March 2011]. Available from http://handbook-5-1.cochrane.org/chapter_8/8_assessing_risk_of_bias_in_included_studies.htm.
21. Harvin JA, Harvin WH, Camp E, Caga-Anan Z, Burgess AR, Wade CE, et al. Early femur fracture fixation is associated with a reduction in pulmonary complications and hospital charges: a decade of experience with 1,376 diaphyseal femur fractures. J Trauma Acute Care Surg. 2012;73(6):1442–8.
22. Pape HC, Rixen D, Morley J, et al. EPOFF Study Group. Impact of the method of initial stabilization for femoral shaft fractures in patients with multiple injuries at risk for complications (borderline patients). Ann Surg. 2007;246(3):491–9. discussion 499–501
23. Morshed S, Miclau T 3rd, Bembom O, Cohen M, Knudson MM, Colford JM Jr. Delayed internal fixation of femoral shaft fracture reduces mortality among patients with multisystem trauma. J Bone Joint Surg Am. 2009;91:3–13.
24. Nahm NJ, Como JJ, Wilber JH, Vallier HA. Early appropriate care: definitive stabilization of femoral fractures within 24 hours of injury is safe in most patients with multiple injuries. J Trauma. 2011;71:175–85.

25. Bone LB, Johnson KD, Weigelt J, Scheinberg R. Early versus delayed stabilization of femoral fractures: a prospective randomized study. Clin Orthop Relat Res. 2004;422:11–6.

26. Charash WE, Fabian TC, Croce MA. Delayed surgical fixation of femur fractures is a risk factor for pulmonary failure independent of thoracic trauma. J Trauma. 1994;37(4):667–72.

27. Starr AJ, Hunt JL, Chason DP, Reinert CM, Walker J. Treatment of femur fracture with associated head injury. J Orthop Trauma. 1998;12(1):38–45.

28. Boulanger BR, Stephen D, Brenneman FD. Thoracic trauma and early intramedullary nailing of femur fractures: are we doing harm? J Trauma. 1997;43(1):24–8.

29. Brundage SI, McGhan R, Jurkovich GJ, Mack CD, Maier RV. Timing of femur fracture fixation: effect on outcome in patients with thoracic and head injuries. J Trauma. 2002;52(2):299–307.

30. Harwood PJ, Giannoudis PV, van Griensven M, Krettek C, Pape HC. Alterations in the systemic inflammatory response after early total care and damage control procedures for femoral shaft fracture in severely injured patients. J Trauma. 2005;58(3):446–52. discussion452–4

31. O'Toole RV, O'Brien M, Scalea TM, Habashi N, Pollak AN, Turen CH. Resuscitation before stabilization of femoral fractures limits acute respiratory distress syndrome in patients with multiple traumatic injuries despite low use of damage control orthopedics. J Trauma. 2009;67(5):1013–21.

32. Al-Saflan MA, Azam MQ, Sadat-Ali M. Are we prepared for orthopedic trauma surgery outside normal working hours? A retrospective analysis. Ulus Travma Acil Cerrahi Derg. 2012;18(4):328–32. https://doi.org/10.5505/tjtes.2012.82084.

33. Fakhry SM, Rutledge R, Dahners LE, Kessler D. Incidence, management, and outcome of femoral shaft fracture: a statewide population-based analysis of 2805 adult patients in a rural state. J Trauma. 1994;37(2):255–60. discussion 260-1

34. Reynolds MA, Richardson JD, Spain DA, Seligson D, Wilson MA, Miller FB. Is the timing of fracture fixation important for the patient with multiple trauma? Ann Surg. 1995;222(4):470–8. discussion 478-81

35. Gandhi RR, Overton TL, Haut ER, et al. Optimal timing of femur fracture stabilization in polytrauma patients: a practice management guideline from the eastern Association for the Surgery of trauma. J Trauma Acute Care Surg. 2014;77(5):787–95.

36. Lozman J, Deno DC, Feustel PJ, et al. Pulmonary and cardiovascular consequences of immediate fixation or conservative management of long-bone fractures. Arch Surg. 1986;121:992–9.

37. Goldstein A, Phillips T, Sclafani SJA, et al. Early open reduction and internal fixation of the disrupted pelvic ring. J Trauma. 1986;26:325–33.

38. Scalea TM, Scott JD, Brumback RJ, et al. Early fracture fixation may be "just fine" after head injury: no difference in central nervous system outcomes. J Trauma. 1999;46:839–46.

39. Jaicks RR, Cohn SM, Moller BA. Early fracture fixation may be deleterious after head injury. J Trauma. 1997;42:1–6.

40. Poole GV, Miller JD, Agnew SG, et al. Lower extremity fracture fixation in head-injured patients. J Trauma. 1992;32:654–9.

41. Liu XY, Jiang M, Yi CL, Bai XJ, Hak DJ. Early intramedullary nailing for femoral fractures in patients with severe thoracic trauma: a systemic review and meta-analysis. Chin J Traumatol. 2016;19(3):160–3.

42. Pape HC. Primary intramedullary femur fixation in multiple trauma patients with associated lung contusion-a cause of posttraumatic ARDS? J Trauma. 1993;34(4):540–7.

43. Pape HC, Grimme K, Van Griensven M, et al. EPOFF Study Group. Impact of intramedullary instrumentation versus damage control for femoral fractures on immunoinflammatory parameters: prospective randomized analysis by the EPOFF Study Group. J Trauma. 2003;55(1):7–13.

44. Weninger P, Figl M, Spitaler R, Mauritz W, Hertz H. Early unreamed intramedullary nailing of femoral fractures is safe in patients with severe thoracic trauma. J Trauma. 2007;62(3):692–6.

45. Gray AC, White TO, Clutton E, Christie J, Hawes BD, Robinson CM. The stress response to bilateral femoral fractures: a comparison of primary intramedullary nailing and external fixation. J Orthop Trauma. 2009;23:90–9.

46. Talucci RC, Manning J, Lampard S, et al. Early intramedullary of femoral shaft fractures: a cause of fat embolism syndrome. Am J Surg. 1983;146:107–11.

47. Manning JB, Bach AW, Herman CM, et al. Fat release after femur nailing in the dog. J Trauma. 1983;23:322–6.

48. Turchin DC, Anderson GI, Schemitsch EH. Pulmonary and systemic fat embolization following medullary canal pressurization. Trans OrthopRes Soc. 1982;20:252–6.

49. Pell AC. The detection of fat embolism by transesophageal echocardiography during reamed intramedullary nailing. A study of 24 patients with femoral and tibial fractures. JBJS Br. 1993;75(6):921–5.

50. Pape HC. Timing of fixation of major fractures in blunt polytrauma: role of conventional indicators in clinical decision making. J Orthop Trauma. 2005; 19(8):551–62.

51. Müller C. Effect of flexible drive diameter and reamer design on the increase of pressure in the medullary cavity during reaming. Injury. 1993; 24(Suppl 3):40–7.

52. Townsend RN, Lheureau T, Protech J, Riemer B, Simon D. Timing fracture repair in patients with severe brain injury (Glasgow Coma Scale score <9). J Trauma. 1998;44(6):977–82. discussion 982–3

53. Stahel PF, Ertel W, Heyde CE. Traumatic brain injury: impact on timing and modality of fracture care [in German]. Orthopade. 2005;34:852–64.

54. Tuttle MS, Smith WR, Williams AE, et al. Safety and efficacy of damage control external fixation versus early definitive stabilization for femoral shaft fractures in the multiple-injured patient. J Trauma. 2009;67(3):602–5.

55. Guyatt GH, Oxman AD, Vist G, et al. GRADE guidelines: 4. Rating the quality of evidence–study limitations (risk of bias). J Clin Epidemiol. 2011;64(4):407–15.

15

Comparison of early complications between the use of a cannulated screw locking plate and multiple cancellous screws in the treatment of displaced intracapsular hip fractures in young adults: a randomized controlled clinical trial

Zhiqiang Wang, Yi Yin, Qingshan Li, Guanjun Sun, Xu Peng, Hua Yin and Yongjie Ye[*]

Abstract

Background: The incidence of early postoperative complications of displaced intracapsular hip fractures is high. The purpose of this study was to compare the early postoperative complications and assess the incidence of femoral neck shortening on using a newly designed proximal femoral cannulated screw locking plate (CSLP) versus multiple cancellous screws (MCS) in the treatment of displaced intracapsular hip fractures in young adults.

Methods: Sixty-eight young adult patients with displaced intracapsular hip fractures were randomly assigned to either the CSLP group or the MCS group and treated routinely by internal fixation with either the CSLP or the MCS. Harris Hip Score, nonunion, failure of fixation, overall complications, and femoral neck shortening were recorded and compared.

Results: Two patients (5.88%) in the CSLP group and eight (23.53%) in the MCS group had postoperative nonunion ($P < 0.05$). There was one case (2.94%) of fixation failure in the CSLP group and three cases (8.82%) in the MCS group ($P > 0.05$). Three patients (8.82%) in the CSLP group and 11 (32.35%) in the MCS group had overall complications ($P < 0.05$). Mean femoral neck shortening was 5.10 mm in the vertical plane and 5.11 mm in the horizontal plane in the CSLP group and 11.14 mm in the vertical plane and 10.51 mm in the horizontal plane in the MCS group. Severe femoral neck shortening (≥ 10 mm) did not occur in either the vertical or the horizontal plane in any patient of the CSLP group but occurred in 10 patients (28.57%) in the vertical plane and in 8 (22.86%) patients in the horizontal plane in the MCS group.

Conclusions: Compared with MCS, the use of CSLP in the treatment of displaced intracapsular hip fractures in young adults can reduce the rates of postoperative nonunion and overall complications and minimize femoral neck shortening.

Keywords: Intracapsular hip fracture, Shortening, Complication

* Correspondence: 38262773@qq.com
Department of Orthopaedics Surgery, Suining Central Hospital, Suining
629000, Sichuan, China

Background

Displaced intracapsular hip fractures in young adults are generally caused by high-energy trauma. Along with a severely damaged blood supply, there is a high risk of postoperative nonunion and femoral head avascular necrosis [1–3]. Various options exist for internal fixation of the hip, including a sliding hip screw/side plate device and multiple cannulated parallel lag screws [4]. However, even with the use of these treatment methods, the incidence of early postoperative complications such as nonunion and failure of fixation is high [5–7].

The use of multiple cancellous screws (MCS) can lead to dynamic compression at the fracture site during axial loading, resulting in a shortened femoral neck. A shortened femoral neck or an offset can cause abductor muscle weakness as a result of a decreased lever arm as well as overall limb shortening, which has been shown to be associated with significantly lower Physical Functioning and Role Physical SF-36 subscores [8–10]. The use of MCS has also been shown to correlate with a decreased quality of life [8], which may be not acceptable in active young adults.

A recent study [11] has shown that compared to three other kinds of internal fixation devices, cannulated screws, DHS, and dynamic condylar screw (DCS), fixed-angle proximal femoral locking plate (PFLP) has the best biomechanical properties, with the highest axial stiffness. However, there are few successful reports focusing on this method in the treatment of displaced femoral neck fractures in young adults.

Since February 2009, we have been using a newly designed fixed-angle device—a cannulated screw locking plate (CSLP, Xiamen Double Engine Medical Material Co. Ltd)—in the treatment of displaced intracapsular hip fractures in young adults (Garden type III–IV, OTA 31-B2.3 or 31-B3) (Fig. 1). We conducted a randomized controlled study in order to compare postoperative complications and femoral neck shortening on use of the CSLP versus MCS. Historical literature dealing with this question is sparse and this is to our knowledge the first attempt at comparing femoral neck shortening after use of a fixed-angle device versus the conventional fixation method.

We hypothesized that the use of the CSLP in the treatment of displaced intracapsular hip fractures in young adults could reduce the rates of early postoperative nonunion and failure of fixation. In addition, we presumed that the use of the CSLP would minimize postoperative shortening.

Methods

Approval for the study was obtained from our Institutional Review Board. Each patient provided written informed consent, agreeing to participate in this study. A total of 180 patients with intracapsular hip fractures who were hospitalized in our department between February

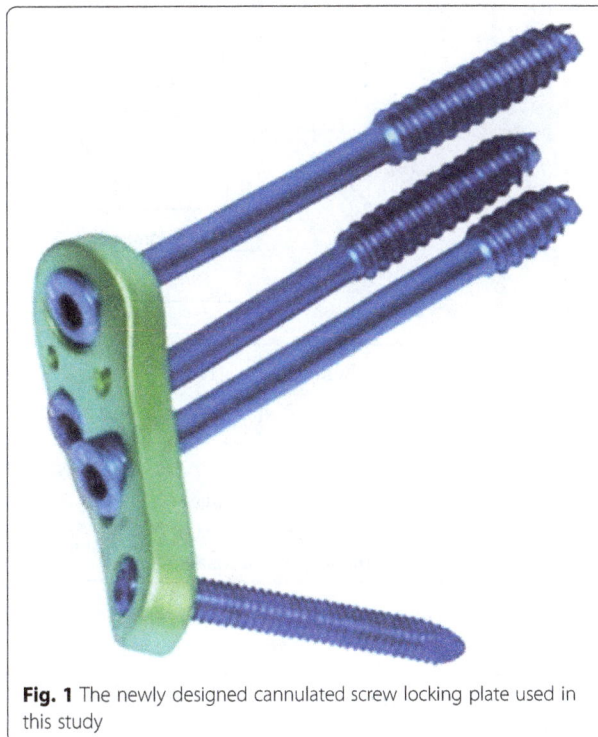

Fig. 1 The newly designed cannulated screw locking plate used in this study

2009 and December 2017 were enrolled in the study (Fig. 2). The inclusion criteria were (1) age between 18 and 50 years, (2) intracapsular hip fractures resulting from high-energy injuries (e.g., traffic accidents, falls, and sports injuries), (3) recent intracapsular hip fractures (less than < 48 h), (4) displaced intracapsular hip fractures (Garden type III–IV, OTA 31-B2.3 or 31-B3), and (5) surgical approaches of closed or open reduction and internal fixation. The exclusion criteria were (1) pathological or old fractures (injury time > 3 weeks) or undisplaced intracapsular hip fractures (Garden type I–II), (2) severe blood and immune system diseases, (3) severe multiple traumas or a previous history of ipsilateral hip or femur surgery, (4) conditions such as osteoarthritis and post-dysplastic deformities, and (5) follow-up time of less than 1 year. Patients with osteonecrosis, secondary displacement (nonunion), or reoperation were included in the study even if their follow-up time was less than 1 year. Eighty-two patients were randomly assigned to either the CSLP group or the MCS group. Randomization was performed using identical, sealed, opaque envelopes. Patients were treated routinely by internal fixation with either the CSLP or MCS. In both patient groups, surgeries were performed by two experienced orthopedic surgeons (Y.J.Y., Y.Y.). The postoperative Harris Hip Score, postoperative complications, and femoral neck shortening were compared between the two groups.

Patients in both groups were given either general or regional anesthesia while in a supine position on the

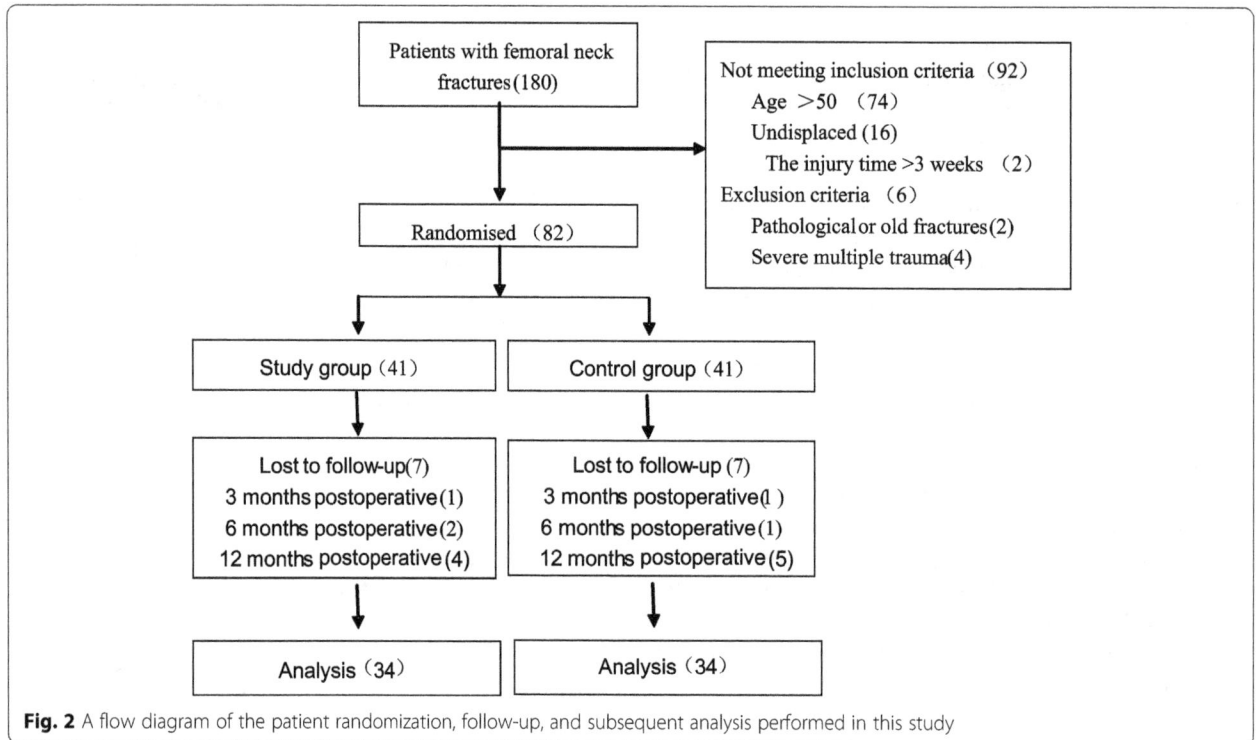

Fig. 2 A flow diagram of the patient randomization, follow-up, and subsequent analysis performed in this study

fracture table with the affected hip elevated by an angle of 10–15°. The traction bed was used for closed reduction, and anteroposterior and lateral radiographs of the femoral neck were obtained using the C-arm X-ray machine. Garden's alignment index was adopted to evaluate the effectiveness of closed reduction. Reduction was considered acceptable if the angle between the femoral medial cortex and the central axis of the compression trabeculae in medial femoral head was 160–180° on the anteroposterior radiograph and 180° on the lateral radiograph and if there was a maximum difference of 20° in Garden's alignment index on the lateral radiograph before and after reduction. Otherwise, the effectiveness of the closed reduction was not considered ideal, and internal fixation was considered essential after open reduction. A Watson-Jones approach [12] was used, and the fracture was opened by performing an inverted T-shaped incision in the capsule. A Kirschner wire was used to manipulate the head of the femur.

For the patients in the CSLP group, a 5–8-cm downward longitudinal incision was made from the greater trochanter of the femur. The iliotibial band and the vastus lateralis muscle were incised and 4–5 cm of bone surface under the greater trochanter was exposed. Next, the guide wire was drilled into the inferior portion of the femoral neck, and the position of the guide wire in the femoral neck was confirmed under fluoroscopy. The Kirschner wire was placed on a CSLP, and two other guide wires were drilled into the femoral neck. The

hollow drill was placed into the drill hole of the guide wire. Locking cannulated screws of appropriate length were selected and tightened. The stabilizing screw was finally secured at the bottom of the locking plate. During the operation, the split gaskets were initially fixed onto the locking holes, and the screws were tightened to enable compression of the fracture ends. The gaskets were removed to lock the screws before a stabilizing screw was finally placed into the distal end of the steel plate. Theoretically, the three screws should be arranged in an inverted triangle in the femoral neck and the average distance from the screw tip to the femur head apex should be 5–10 mm (Fig. 3).

For patients in the MCS group, a 4–6-cm longitudinal incision was made below the greater trochanter of the femur. The iliotibial band and the vastus lateralis muscle were incised, and the lateral surface of the femur below the greater trochanter was exposed. A 3.2-mm guide wire was placed on the skin in front of the femoral neck in order to draw it close to the inferior-medial cortex of the femoral neck. Another guide wire was drilled into the femoral head from the midpoint of the lateral femoral cortical bone (parallel to the front guide wire), so that the tip of the guide wire was located behind the femoral head, and the anteversion angle was maintained within 10°. A second guide wire was then drilled in slightly above it. A third guide wire was drilled from the base of the greater trochanter, along the tensile trabecular bone, passing through the femoral neck and

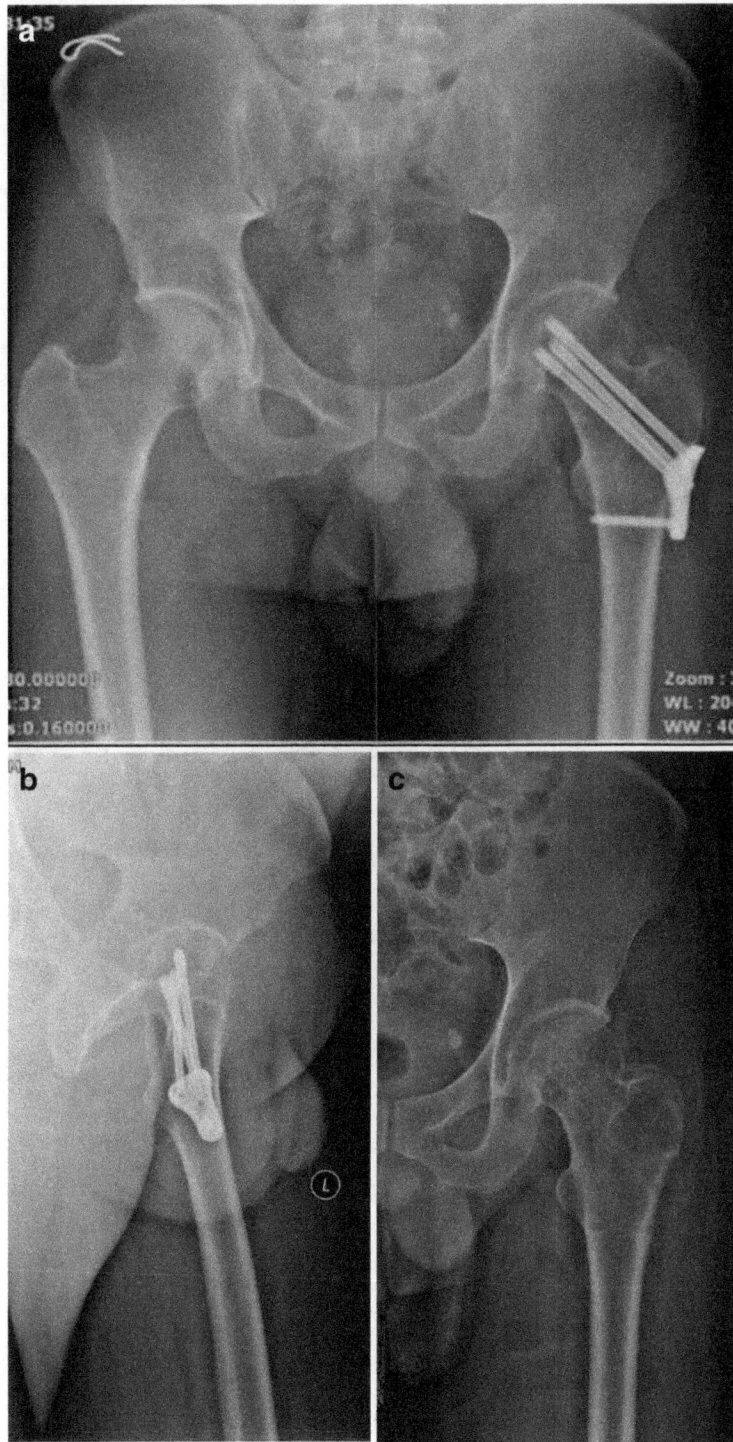

Fig. 3 Anteroposterior view of pelvic (**a**) and lateral radiograph of the femoral neck (**b**) after closed reduction and internal fixation with the cannulated screw locking plate. Anteroposterior view of the hip after internal fixation was removed (**c**)

penetrating into the femoral head. The anteversion angle was maintained within 5° such that the guide wire was located at the more anterior part of the femoral head. The desired length of each cannulated screw was measured and the guide wire was pulled after drilling into the 7.3-mm length of the corresponding half-threaded cannulated screw. The surgeons chose to fix femoral neck fractures with screws in an inverted triangle with the depth of the cannulated screws reaching an area 3 mm under the femoral head cartilage (Fig. 4).

Regular follow-ups were performed at 6 weeks, 3 months, 6 months, and 1 year after surgery. On clinical evaluation at the latest follow-up, pain and limitation of movement were recorded. The Harris Hip Score [13] was calculated to evaluate hip function. On radiological [14, 15] or CT scan [15, 16] evaluation, the degree of union, loss of fracture alignment, and position of implant were observed. Femoral neck shortening was measured on digital radiographs using Adobe Photoshop CS 6 (Adobe Systems Inc., CA, USA), as described previously [17, 18]. The fractured hip on the most recent anteroposterior radiograph was compared with the contralateral hip on radiographs taken at the time of the injury. The uninjured side was outlined, overlapped over the fractured side, and adjusted for differences in size. Femoral neck shortening was assessed in the horizontal (abductor moment arm shortening) and vertical (femur length decrease) plane. Known diameters of screws were used to correct for differences in radiograph magnification.

Statistical analysis

Statistical analysis was performed using SPSS version 17.0 (SPSS Inc., Chicago, IL, USA). Continuous data are expressed as mean ± standard deviation. The t test for two independent samples was used to analyze normally distributed data. The rank-sum test was used for data

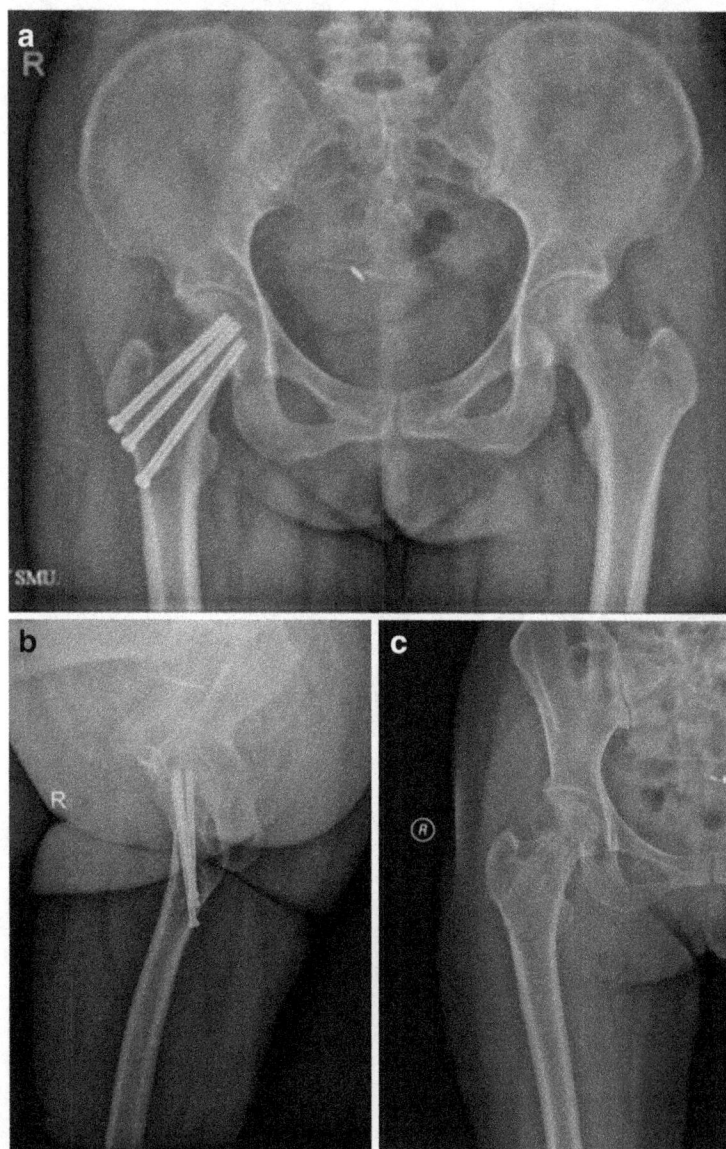

Fig. 4 Anteroposterior view of pelvic (**a**) and lateral radiograph of the femoral neck (**b**) after closed reduction and internal fixation with three cannulated screws. Anteroposterior view of the hip after internal fixation was removed (**c**)

with heterogeneity of variance and non-normal distribution. Categorical data were compared using the χ^2 test or the Fisher exact probability method if the theoretical frequency was less than 1. A P value of < 0.05 was considered statistically significant. The overall postoperative complication rate was defined as the sum of the individual rates of nonunion and fixation failure.

Results

Table 1 shows the baseline preoperative data, including gender, age, cause of injury, fracture type, Harris Hip Scores, and time from diagnosis to surgery. Patients in the CSLP group had a mean age of 45.12 ± 5.38 years, whereas those in the MCS group had a mean age of 46.02 ± 6.23 years. The CSLP group included 55.88% of female patients and 44.12% of male patients, whereas the MCS group had 47.06% of female patients and 52.94% of male patients. The mean Harris Hip Score was 12.20 ± 2.18 in the CSLP group and 13.98 ± 2.16 in the MCS group. The mean time from diagnosis to surgery was 31.62 ± 6.79 h in the CSLP group and 32.84 ± 5.12 h in the MCS group. There were no statistically significant differences in Garden classification and OTA classification between the two groups of patients ($P > 0.05$). The causes of injuries varied between the two groups of patients. Traffic accidents were the main cause of injury (47.06%) in the CSLP group, whereas falls were the main cause of injury in the MCS group (52.94%).

Table 1 Preoperative clinical data

	CSLP group (%)	MCS group	χ^2/t value	P value
Gender				
Male	15 (44.12)	18 (52.94)	0.54	0.51
Female	19 (55.88)	16 (47.06)		
Age (years)	45.12 ± 5.38	46.02 ± 6.23	− 0.54	0.97
Harris Hip Score	12.20 ± 2.18	13.98 ± 2.16	− 0.392	0.427
Causes of injuries				
Sport injuries	12 (35.29)	10 (29.41%)	4.76	0.03
Traffic accidents	16 (47.06%)	6 (17.65%)		
Falls	6 (17.65%)	18 (52.94%)		
Garden classification				
Type III	23 (67.65%)	21 (61.76%)	0.2576	0.6118
Type IV	11 (32.35%)	13 (38.23%)	0.2576	0.6118
OTA classification				
OTA 31-B2.3	11 (32.35)	9 (26.47)	0.2833	0.5945
OTA 31-B3.1	8 (23.53)	10 (29.41)	0.3022	0.5825
OTA 31-B3.2	9 (26.47)	8 (23.53)	0.0784	0.7794
OTA 31-B3.3	6 (17.65)	7 (20.59)	0.0951	0.7578
Time from diagnosis				
To surgery (hours)	31.62 ± 6.79	32.84 ± 5.12	− 0.72	0.528

Postoperative results
CSLP group
The mean follow-up period was 21.7 ± 4.66 months. All but two patients underwent closed reduction and internal fixation, and the mean Garden's alignment index was $169.71 \pm 4.66°$ on the anteroposterior position and $171.87 \pm 5.46°$ on the lateral position. The mean Harris Hip Scores of healed patients that were revised were 59.04 ± 4.13, 78.81 ± 3.43, 90.47 ± 5.79, and 92.63 ± 5.55 at 6 weeks, 3 months, 6 months, and 1 year after surgery, respectively (Fig. 5). During the follow-up period, postoperative nonunion occurred in two patients (5.88%) and one case underwent fixation failure. Three patients (8.82%) underwent total hip arthroplasty. Mean femoral neck shortening is 5.10 mm in the vertical plane and 5.11 mm in the horizontal plane. The rates of no/mild and moderate decrease were 70.58% and 29.41% in the vertical plane and 76.47% and 23.53% in the horizontal plane. Severe decrease femoral neck shortening (10 mm or greater) did not occur in any patient both in the vertical and horizontal plane in this group (Fig. 6).

MCS group
The mean follow-up period was 24.8 ± 5.78 months. Two patients underwent open reduction after failure of closed reduction. The mean Garden's alignment index was $170.59 \pm 4.69°$ on the anteroposterior position and $171.93 \pm 5.62°$ on the lateral position. The mean Harris Hip Scores of healed patients were 58.32 ± 5.26, 77.63 ± 3.34, 89.87 ± 4.24, and 89.74 ± 5.33 at 6 weeks, 3 months, 6 months, and 1 year after surgery, respectively (Fig. 5). During the follow-up period, postoperative nonunion occurred in eight patients (23.53%) and three patients (8.82%) developed fixation failure including screw withdrawal accompanied by displacement and angulation of the fracture site and withdrawal of cannulated screws without displacement and angulation of the fracture site. Nine patients (26.47%) underwent total hip arthroplasty in the second phase. Two patients (5.71%) received conservative treatment after removal of the internal fixation and ultimately achieved bone healing. Shortening of the femoral neck is common in this group. Mean decrease is 11.14 mm in the vertical plane and 10.51 mm in the horizontal plane. The rates of no/mild and moderate femoral neck shortening were 35.29% and 35.29% in the vertical plane and 44.12% and 32.35% in the horizontal plane. Severe femoral neck shortening occurred in 10 patients (29.41%) in the vertical plane and 8 (23.52%) patients in the horizontal plane (Fig. 6).

There were statistically significant differences in the rates of postoperative nonunion ($P = 0.0399$), shortening of the femoral neck ($P < 0.001$), and overall complications ($P = 0.0164$) between the two groups of patients during the follow-up period. There were no statistically

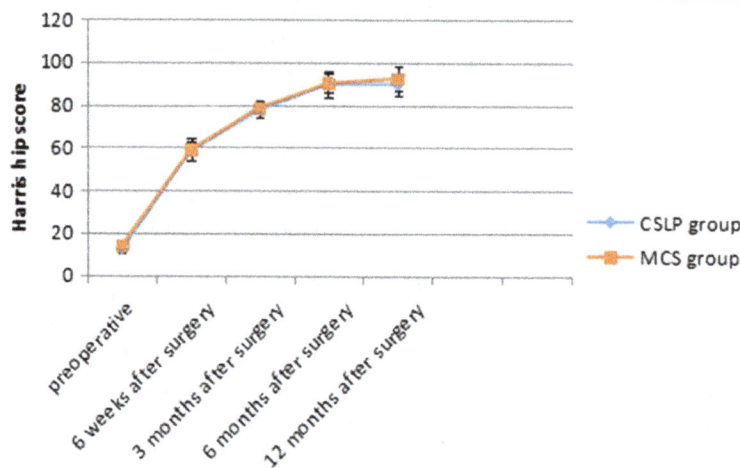

Fig. 5 This figure illustrates the Harris Hip Scores for both groups from the preoperative to the postoperative periods. Note the increasing trend in postoperative scores for both groups

significant differences in Harris Hip Score and fixation failure between the two groups of patients ($P > 0.05$) (Table 2).

Discussion

Although various implants have been developed for internal fixation with open or closed reduction of femoral neck fractures, predicting healing of the femoral neck by stable fixation without shortening continues to be challenging.

In our study, although the rates of fixation failure are lower in the CSLP group (2.94%) than in the MCS group (8.82%), the difference was not statistically significant. It is possible that the CSLP is a device with a fixed angle, where the placement directions and the spacing intervals of screws are fixed and cannot be adjusted. If the diameter of the femoral neck is smaller, the screws can penetrate through the bone cortex, resulting in fixation failure. However, the rates of nonunion were 5.88% in the CSLP group and 23.53% in the MCS group. Overall complications occurred in three patients (8.82%) treated with CSLP and in 11 patients (32.35%) treated with MCS. These differences were statistically significant. We assume that the major reason for the poorer results in the MCS group was insufficient mechanical stability. Because of the lack of support on the medial side behind the femoral neck and in cases where the outer cortex was unable to withstand a certain torque, multiple-screw fixation would not be ideal. Another limitation of the MCS technique is the inability to control rotation [19]. As a fixed-angle device, the CSLP consists of a small proximal femoral locking plate and four cannulated screws. The plate can provide effective support, the three screws are arranged

in an inverted triangle in the femoral neck to guarantee stability, the bolt-plate locking design could help avoid loosening and withdrawal of the cannulated screws, and the other screw can be used to fix the femoral shaft, effectively preventing the rotation of the screw plate after surgery and strengthening internal fixation. The design may explain why the CSLP is superior to MCS. Biomechanical experiments have showed that, compared with MCS, a fixed-angle device can increase resistance to shear forces and reduce micromotion [11], which seems to impair the healing process. However, the CSLP itself has no longitudinal pressurization effect. If pressurization is needed initially intraoperatively, the split gaskets must be fixed onto the locking holes, and the screws are tightened so that the fracture sites are compressed. The gaskets are then removed to lock the screws and achieve the effect of compression locking. In fact, it is not clear whether dynamic compression is necessary or whether the compression achieved during fixation is sufficient. One randomized controlled trial [20] reported higher failure rates for displaced femoral neck fractures when sliding hip screws were used in a dynamic compression mode compared to static locking (33% vs. 18%).

To the best of our knowledge, there are only a few published reports on the use of a proximal femoral locking plate in the treatment of intracapsular hip fractures (Table 3). To effectively compare our treatment results with previously published results on the treatment of displaced femoral neck fractures, we used similar statistical methods for analysis. Parker et al. [21] reported a nonunion rate of 7% in 46 patients who were treated with reduction and Targon Femoral Neck Hip Screw internal fixation for displaced fractures. However, that study was conducted in an elderly cohort with a

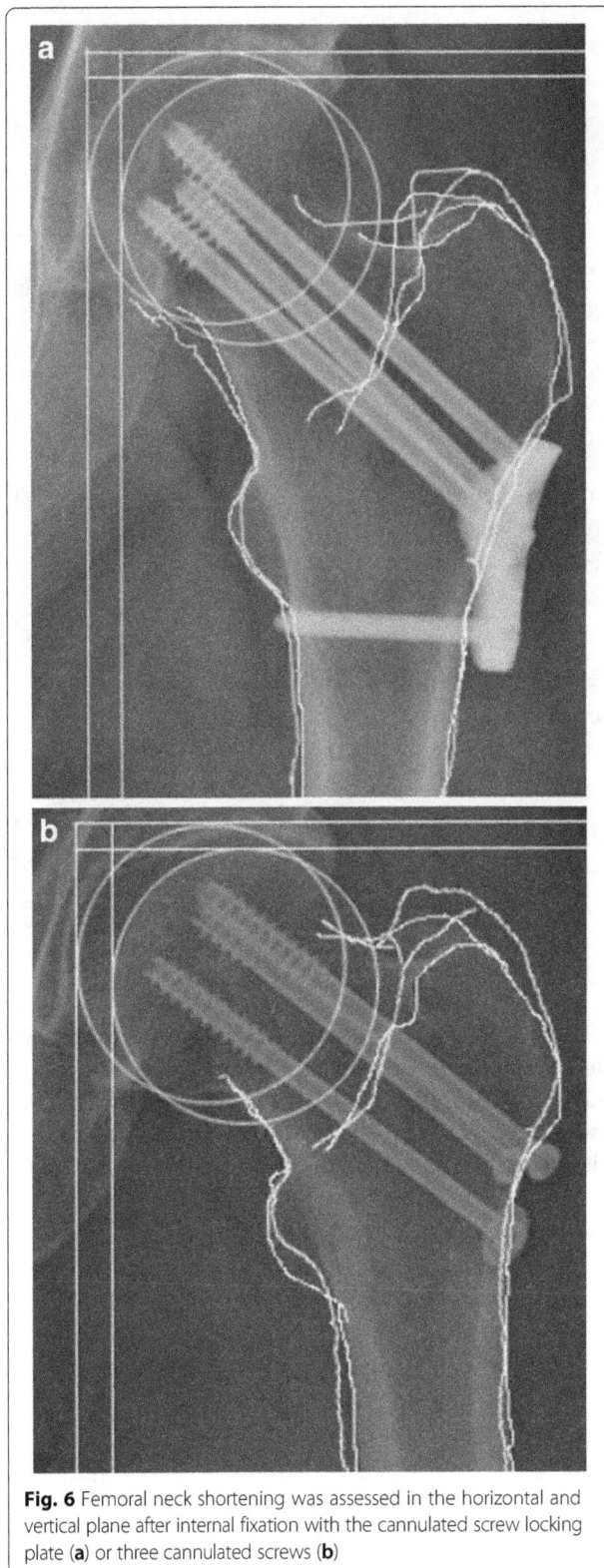

Fig. 6 Femoral neck shortening was assessed in the horizontal and vertical plane after internal fixation with the cannulated screw locking plate (**a**) or three cannulated screws (**b**)

nonunion rates of 3.2% and 46.8%, respectively. Although the conclusion is consistent with ours, that study too was not a randomized controlled study but used a historical control instead. Ismail et al. performed a cross-sectional study of six displaced fractures in patients aged 17–55 years who were treated with Cloverleaf Locking Plate Fixation. The nonunion rate was reported to be 0%. Although the results were promising, only six cases of displaced fractures were analyzed. Additionally, the procedure employed was not minimally invasive, because the plate is much longer than the plate we used. Lin et al. [23] reported a nonunion rate of 7% in patients aged 21-65 years treated for displaced intracapsular hip fractures with a proximal femoral locking plate with cannulated screws, identical to the device used in our study. The nonunion rate was similar to that in our study. However, the previous study had no control group. On comparing our results with previously published results, the nonunion rate in the CSLP group in our study was lower than that in the study by Parker and higher than that in the other studies. In a recent report, Berkes et al. [24] described their experience with the Posterolateral Femoral Locking Plate, reporting a 63.6% rate of catastrophic failure in displaced fractures. They concluded that this device was not appropriate for intracapsular femoral fractures. The reason for the difference in results among the studies is not fully understood. It could be related to implant design, patient selection, follow-up time, injury-operation interval, quality of reduction, position of the internal fixation, and percentage of open reductions.

There is a consensus that shortening of the femoral neck is common after screw fixation of femoral neck fractures [10]. Data for femoral neck fractures treated with multiple cannulated screws indicate a shortening rate of 27 to 31% [8]. In light of this, we assess the incidence of femoral neck shortening quantitatively and qualitatively on using CSLP versus MCS in the treatment of displaced intracapsular hip fractures in young adults. In our study, the mean decrease was 5.10 mm in the vertical plane and 5.11 mm in the horizontal plane. Severe femoral neck shortening (≥ 10 mm) did not occur in any patient in either the vertical or the horizontal plane in the CSLP group. However, in the MCS group, the mean decrease was 11.14 mm in the vertical plane and 10.51 mm in the horizontal plane. Severe femoral neck shortening occurred in 10 patients (29.41%) in the vertical plane and in 8 patients (23.53%) in the horizontal plane. This implies that the CSLP also acts as a length-stable implant; locking of the screw to the side plate could prevent additional femoral neck shortening. However, MCS cannot provide enough resistance to shortening as it is based only

mean patient age of 75 years and had neither a control group nor randomization. Thein et al. [22] compared Targon FN and MCS in a clinical study and noted

Table 2 Postoperative results

	CSLP group (n = 34)	MCS group (n = 34)	x^2 value/t value/z value	P value
Follow-up period (month)	21.7 ± 4.66	24.8 ± 5.78	− 2.710	0.009
Garden's alignment index				
Anteroposterior (degree)	169.71 ± 4.66	170.59 ± 4.69	− 0.253	0.801
Lateral (degree)	171.87 ± 5.46	171.93 ± 5.62	1.262	0.211
Harris Hip Score				
6 weeks after surgery	59.04 ± 4.13	58.32 ± 5.26	0.651	0.651
3 months after surgery	78.81 ± 3.43	77.63 ± 3.34	1.462	0.148
6 months after surgery	90.47 ± 5.79	89.87 ± 4.24	0.591	0.556
1 year after surgery	92.63 ± 5.55	89.74 ± 5.33	1.709	0.092
Femoral neck shortening				
In the vertical plane				
Mean decrease (mm)	5.10 ± 1.90	11.14 ± 2.78	− 11.13	< 0.0001
No/mild (0–4.9)	24 (70.58%)	12 (35.29%)	− 6.11[※]	
Moderate (5–9.9)	10 (29.41%)	12 (35.29%)		< 0.0001
Severe (10 or greater)	0	10 (29.41%)		
In the horizontal plane				
Mean decrease (mm)	5.11 ± 1.90	10.51 ± 2.78	− 10.61	0.000
No/mild (0–4.9)	26 (76.47%)	15 (44.12%)		
Moderate (5–9.9)	8 (23.53%)	11 (32.35%)	− 5.74[※]	< 0.0001
Severe (10 or greater)	0	8 (23.53%)		
Nonunion (%)	2 (5.88%)	8 (23.53%)	4.22	0.0399[★]
Failure of fixation (%)[#]	1 (2.94%)	3 (8.82%)		0.6135[★]
Overall complications (%)[&]	3 (8.82%)	11 (32.35%)	5.757	0.0164[★]

[※]Rank sum test
[★]Fisher's exact test
[&]Overall complications = nonunion + failure of fixation

on the friction of the bone/unthreaded portion of the screw interface [25].

We are aware of several limitations of this study. The trial was conducted at a single center and the sample size is small. Although the patients were randomized, double blinding was not performed. We did not compare time to heal between the two groups due to the limited follow-up time points. Furthermore, the 1- to 2-year follow-up is needed to visualize the shape of the femur after healing and

Table 3 A comparative literature summary of the common postoperative complications for femoral neck fractures

Author	Year	N of patients[☆]	Age (year)	Internal fixation	Follow-up (month)	Nonunion (%)	Fixation failure	Overall complications (%)	Control group	Study style
Lin D	2011	29	47 (21–65)	LPCS[①]	43	2 (7)	–	4 (14)	No	Prospective
Thein R	2014	31	50.9 ± 16.0	Targon FN[②]	17	1 (3.2)	–	4 (12.9)	Historical control	Prospective
Parker MJ	2009	46	75 (42–103)	Targon FN[②]	≥ 12	7 (15.2)	–	9 (19.6)	No	Prospective
Berkes MB	2012	11	71.7 ± 13.7	PLFLP[③]	23	–	7 (63.6)	8 (72.7)	Case-control	Retrospective
Ismail HD	2012	6	17–55	CLPF[④]	≥ 12	0	–	–	No	Cross-sectional study
Wang ZQ	2015	34	45.12 ± 5.38	CSLP[⑤]	21.7	2 (5.88)	1 (2.94)	3 (8.82)	Randomized controlled	Prospective

[☆]Only included those patients with displaced intracapsular hip fractures
[①]LPCS, proximal femoral locking plate with cannulated screws
[②]Targon FN, the Targon Femoral Neck Hip Screw
[③]PLFLP, the Posterolateral Femoral Locking Plate
[④]CLPF, Cloverleaf Locking Plate Fixation
[⑤]CSLP, proximal femoral cannulated screw locking plate

how the constructs held up after full weight-bear in the further study.

Conclusion

Our study demonstrated that the use of the CSLP in the treatment of displaced intracapsular hip fractures in young adults can reduce the rates of postoperative nonunion, overall complications, and femoral neck shortening. Evaluation of long-term results will require larger sample sizes and a longer follow-up period.

Abbreviations

CSLP: Cannulated screw locking plate; DCS: Dynamic condylar screw; MCS: Multiple cancellous screws; PFLP: Proximal femoral locking plate

Authors' contributions

YJY and ZQW carried out the entire procedure including the literature search and data extraction. QSL performed the statistical analysis, drafted the manuscript, and revised the submitted manuscript. GJS and HY conceived of the study, coordinated and participated in the entire process of drafting, and revised the manuscript. YY and XP contributed to the statistical analysis and revision of the manuscript. All authors have contributed significantly. All authors read and approved the final manuscript.

Competing interests

The authors declare that they have no competing interests.

References

1. Haidukewych GJ, Rothwell WS, Jacofsky DJ, Torchia ME, Berry DJ. Operative treatment of femoral neck fractures in patients between the ages of fifteen and fifty years. J Bone Joint Surg Am. 2004;86-A:1711–6.
2. Liporace F, Gaines R, Collinge C, Haidukewych GJ. Results of internal fixation of Pauwels type-3 vertical femoral neck fractures. J Bone Joint Surg Am. 2008;90:1654–9.
3. Davidovitch RI, Jordan CJ, Egol KA, Vrahas MS. Challenges in the treatment of femoral neck fractures in the nonelderly adult. J Trauma. 2010;68:236–42.
4. Parker MJ, Blundell C. Choice of implant for internal fixation of femoral neck fractures. Meta-analysis of 25 randomised trials including 4,925 patients. Acta Orthop Scand. 1998;69:138–43.
5. Swiontkowski MF. Intracapsular fractures of the hip. J Bone Joint Surg Am. 1994;76:129–38.
6. Estrada LS, Volgas DA, Stannard JP, Alonso JE. Fixation failure in femoral neck fractures. Clin Orthop Relat Res. 2002;(399):110–8.
7. Lowe JA, Crist BD, Bhandari M, Ferguson TA. Optimal treatment of femoral neck fractures according to patient's physiologic age: an evidence-based review. Orthop Clin North Am. 2010;41:157–66.
8. Tidermark J, Ponzer S, Svensson O, Söderqvist A, Törnkvist H. Internal fixation compared with total hip replacement for displaced femoral neck fractures in the elderly. A randomised, controlled trial. J Bone Joint Surg Br. 2003;85:380–8.
9. Charles MN, Bourne RB, Davey JR, Greenwald AS, Morrey BF, Rorabeck CH. Soft-tissue balancing of the hip: the role of femoral offset restoration. Instr Course Lect. 2005;54:131–41.
10. Zlowodzki M, Jonsson A, Paulke R, Kregor PJ, Bhandari M. Shortening after femoral neck fracture fixation: is there a solution? Clin Orthop Relat Res. 2007;461:213–8.
11. Aminian A, Gao F, Fedoriw WW, Zhang LQ, Kalainov DM, Merk BR. Vertically oriented femoral neck fractures: mechanical analysis of four fixation techniques. J Orthop Trauma. 2007;21:544–8.
12. Nakai T, Liu N, Fudo K, Mohri T, Kakiuchi M. Early complications of primary total hip arthroplasty in the supine position with a modified Watson-Jones anterolateral approach. J Orthop. 2014;11:166–9.
13. Harris WH. Traumatic arthritis of the hip after dislocation and acetabular fractures: treatment by mold arthroplasty. An end-result study using a new method of result evaluation. J Bone Joint Surg Am. 1969;51:737–55.
14. Milgram JW. Nonunion and pseudarthrosis of fracture healing. A histopathologic study of 95 human specimens. Clin Orthop Relat Res. 1991; (268):203–13.
15. Assiotis A, Sachinis NP, Chalidis BE. Pulsed electromagnetic fields for the treatment of tibial delayed unions and nonunions. A prospective clinical study and review of the literature. J Orthop Surg Res. 2012;7:24.
16. Dickson K, Katzman S, Delgado E, Contreras D. Delayed unions and nonunions of open tibial fractures. Correlation with arteriography results. Clin Orthop Relat Res. 1994;(302):189–93.
17. Zlowodzki M, Ayieni O, Petrisor BA, Bhandari M. Femoral neck shortening after fracture fixation with multiple cancellous screws: incidence and effect on function. J Trauma. 2008;64:163–9.
18. Zlowodzki M, Brink O, Switzer J, Wingerter S, Woodall J Jr, Petrisor BA, et al. The effect of shortening and varus collapse of the femoral neck on function after fixation of intracapsular fracture of the hip: a multi-centre cohort study. J Bone Joint Surg Br. 2008;90:1487–94.
19. Ly TV, Swiontkowski MF. Management of femoral neck fractures in young adults. Indian J Orthop. 2008;42:3–12.
20. Frandsen PA, Andersen PE Jr, Christoffersen H, Thomsen PB. Osteosynthesis of femoral neck fracture. The sliding-screw-plate with or without compression. Acta Orthop Scand. 1984;55:620–3.
21. Parker MJ, Stedtfeld HW. Internal fixation of intracapsular hip fractures with a dynamic locking plate: initial experience and results for 83 patients treated with a new implant. Injury. 2010;41:348–51.
22. Thein R, Herman A, Kedem P, Chechik A, Shazar N. Osteosynthesis of unstable intracapsular femoral neck fracture by dynamic locking plate or screw fixation: early results. J Orthop Trauma. 2014;28:70–6.
23. Lin D, Lian K, Ding Z, Zhai W, Hong J. Proximal femoral locking plate with cannulated screws for the treatment of femoral neck fractures. Orthopedics. 2012;35:e1–5.
24. Berkes MB, Little MT, Lazaro LE, Cymerman RM, Helfet DL, Lorich DG. Catastrophic failure after open reduction internal fixation of femoral neck fractures with a novel locking plate implant. J Orthop Trauma. 2012;26: e170–6.
25. Alves T, Neal JW, Weinhold PS, Dahners LE. Biomechanical comparison of 3 possible fixation strategies to resist femoral neck shortening after fracture. Orthopedics. 2010;33(4):233.

16

Treatment of simple bone cysts using endoscopic curettage: a case series analysis

Hisaki Aiba[1], Masaaki Kobayashi[1,5*], Yuko Waguri-Nagaya[2], Hideyuki Goto[1], Jun Mizutani[3], Satoshi Yamada[1], Hideki Okamoto[1], Masahiro Nozaki[1], Hiroto Mitsui[3], Shinji Miwa[1], Makoto Kobayashi[1], Kojiro Endo[1], Shiro Saito[1], Taeko Goto[4] and Takanobu Otsuka[1]

Abstract

Background: Endoscopic curettage is considered applicable for the treatment of simple bone cysts with the expectation that it might be less invasive than open curettage. In this study, we investigated the efficacy of endoscopic curettage for the treatment of simple bone cysts. The goal was to investigate the incidence of cyst recurrence and bone healing after endoscopic curettage. Moreover, complications and functionality at the final follow-up were evaluated.

Methods: From 2003 to 2014, 37 patients with simple bone cysts underwent endoscopic curettage. Twenty-four were male and 13 were female, with a mean age of 14.7 years. Endoscopic curettage was performed with the support of an arthroscope via 7–8 mm holes penetrated by cannulated drills with a small incision. The cysts underwent curettage using angled curettes, rongeurs, and an electrical shaver until the normal bone was observed in the medullary cavity. To investigate the bone healing after endoscopic curettage, we evaluated the consolidation of the cyst at the final evaluation (Modified Neer Classification) and the time to solid union after operation, which was defined as the sufficient thickness of the cortical bone to prevent fracture and allow physical activities.

Results: Recurrence occurred in seven patients (18.9%). A log-rank analysis revealed that contact with the physis was associated with recurrence ($p = 0.006$). Among 31 patients (83.7%), the consolidation of cyst was considered healed at the final X-ray follow-up period, and in these patients, the mean time taken for solid union of cortical bone thinning was 4. 0 months (standard deviation, 2.4). With regard to major complications of endoscopic curettage, a transient radial nerve palsy and two postoperative fractures occurred. The former problem was managed conservatively and the latter problems by transient internal fixation; these problems were managed without any further complications. All patients had a good postoperative function.

Conclusions: Endoscopic curettage might be a useful alternative as it is a minimally invasive procedure for the treatment of simple bone cysts. Considering the relatively smaller size of this study, further investigation should be necessary for deducing the reliable conclusion.

Keywords: Endoscopy, Endoscopic curettage, Simple bone cysts, Recurrence, Minimally invasive procedure

* Correspondence: mkoba@med.nagoya-cu.ac.jp
[1]Department of Orthopedic Surgery, Nagoya City University Graduate School of Medical Sciences, 1, Kawasumi, Mizuho-cho, Mizuho-ku, Nagoya 467-8601, Japan
[5]Department of Orthopedic Surgery, Ogaki Municipal Hospital, 4-86 Minaminokawa-cho, Ogaki 503-8502, Japan
Full list of author information is available at the end of the article

Background

Simple bone cysts (SBCs) are benign bone tumors that arise mainly at the proximal humerus, femur, or calcaneus [1]. The cystic cavity is filled with serous or serosanguineous fluid and lined by thin fibrovascular connective tissue membrane. The etiology of this lesion has been enigmatic; however, obstruction from venous outflow might be one of the reasons that a cystic cavity fills with fluid. Moreover, the disturbance in growth at the epiphysial plate was considered the cause of cystic cavity [2]. Usually, these cysts weaken the cortex, predisposing the bone to pathologic fracture [3]. SBCs are most commonly found in adolescent from birth to 20 years of age [4].

Although there still have not been a study with a high level of evidence and comparison among each treatment is difficult, many methods of treatment have been introduced, including observation [5], steroid injections [6], curettage with or without bone grafting [7], or insertion of a cannulated pin/screw [8, 9]. Each management method has pros and cons. The observation method requires a relatively longer time for consolidation of the cystic cavity and prolonged restriction of activity to prevent pathologic fractures [10]. Steroid injection is a non-operative treatment and was proven to be superior to bone marrow injection in the randomized controlled trial, but it sometimes required multiple procedures because of low healing rate [11]. The open curettage with or without bone grafting is still the cornerstone for treatment and superior to steroid injection in terms of healing rate as demonstrated in the retrospective comparative study performed by Sung et al. [3]. However, this technique is too aggressive with occasional postoperative complications and recurrence after surgery sometimes occurs. Decompression of cystic cavity by making holes using multiple drilling [12] or insertion of a cannulated pin or screw conforms the etiology of the SBC. However, there are still lacking evidence and soft tissue damage to access the bone surface that cannot be ignored. Moreover, inserted pins can sometimes be dislodged from the cannulated bone, which leads to irritation of tissues surrounding the pin [8, 9].

However, eventual healing of SBC is assured in many cases; some patients require multiple attempts to deal with a recurrence; thus, minimal invasiveness per treatment is especially desired. Here, we introduce endoscopic curettage (ESC) for SBC with the expectation that this procedure will have lower invasiveness and relatively higher success rate compared to other traditional procedures and elaborate on our surgical and clinical outcomes with this treatment approach.

Methods

Patient characteristics

From 2003 to 2014, we extracted the data of 40 patients histologically diagnosed as having SBCs. The analyses of their specimens were conducted at the Division of Pathology of Nagoya City University. Among these patients, three patients aged over 30 years were excluded from the analysis because the etiology of older patients might be different [2, 13]. Finally, a total of 24 male and 13 female patients, with a mean age of 14.7 (standard deviation [SD], 6.3) years, were included in the study. The tumors were located in 29 tubular bones (18 humeri, 8 femurs, 2 radii, and 1 tibia), 2 flat bones (pelvises), and 6 short bones (calcanei). All patients were monitored for at least 6 months after solid union and the consolidation of bone (Modified Neer Classification A–B [described in postoperative evaluation section]). In cases in which the cyst did not consolidate over time (Modified Neer Classification C–D), follow-up periods were extended to at least 3 years after the operation. The mean follow-up period was 33.8 (SD 26.1) months.

Surgical procedure

All surgical procedures were conducted or supervised by MK. The localization of the tumor was identified with an image intensifier, and marks were drawn on the skin along the edge of the tumor. The number of portals needed depended on the size of the tumor and location.

The surgical procedure was performed with the aid of an inflatable tourniquet. In cases in which the tourniquet was not applicable (e.g., tumors located in the proximal humerus, pelvis, or proximal femur), epinephrine (equivalent to 3.3 mg/L) was added into the irrigation fluid to control the blood loss.

After making an approximately 1-cm incision in the skin, the soft tissue was bluntly dissected until reaching the bone surface. The cortical bone was pierced with a 2.0-mm Kirschner wire, and intraosseous fluid was obtained through the pierced bone and observed for its color and properties (Figs. 1a, b). The small bone hole was enlarged using step-up cannulated drills up to 7 or 8 mm (Figs. 1c and 2a). Subsequently, the second portal was made in the same fashion, and if necessary, a third or fourth one was made. An arthroscope (usually 4 mm in diameter, or 2.7 mm in the case of cysts in a small bone) was inserted into the cavity of the cyst to observe the inside of the cyst.

Under endoscopic visualization, the surgical instruments, including arthroscopic curette (Fig. 2b) or forceps (Fig. 2c), were inserted through the portal at various angles (Fig. 1d). The arthroscope and surgical instruments were exchanged to ensure complete observation of the cavity. The cystic lesion was thoroughly removed until the normal bone was seen in the medullary cavity (Fig. 1e, f). In cases with multiple compartments in the cavity, the septa are resected using shavers. By opening the separated compartments, reduction of internal pressure of each cyst is achieved. The blind area in the vicinity of the endoscope portals was carefully observed.

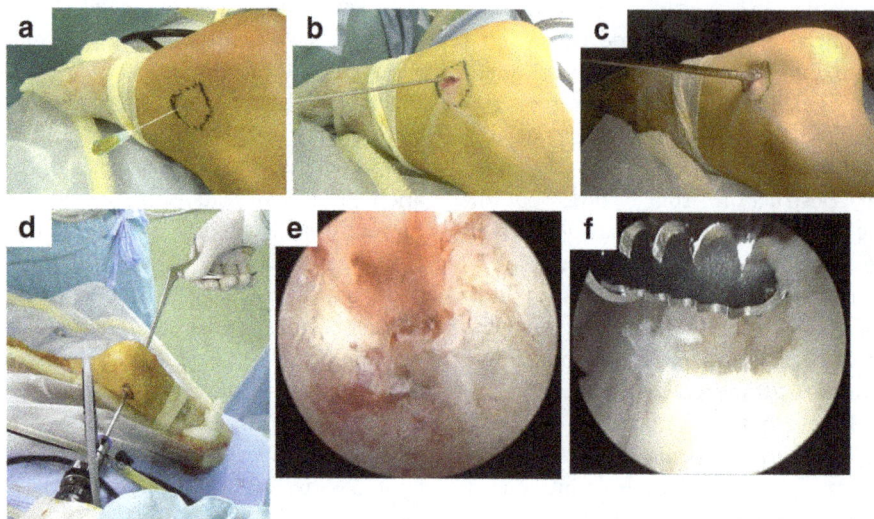

Fig. 1 The intraoperative findings were obtained during surgery for simple bone cyst in the right calcaneus. Collection of intracavity fluid (**a**). Penetration of bone with Kirschner wire (**b**). Step-wise cannulation of the small hole (**c**). Surgical maneuver (**d**). Intracavity findings before curettage (**e**). Normal cortical bone after complete curettage (**f**)

In the postoperative periods, the patients with lower limb lesions were limited to bearing half of their weight by using a crutch for 1 month, followed by 1 month of two-thirds partial weight bearing with a crutch, and full weight bearing only after 3 months if bone healing was confirmed. On the other hand, the patients with upper limb or non-weight-bearing bone cysts had no limitations of any activities, except for contact sports, until solid union.

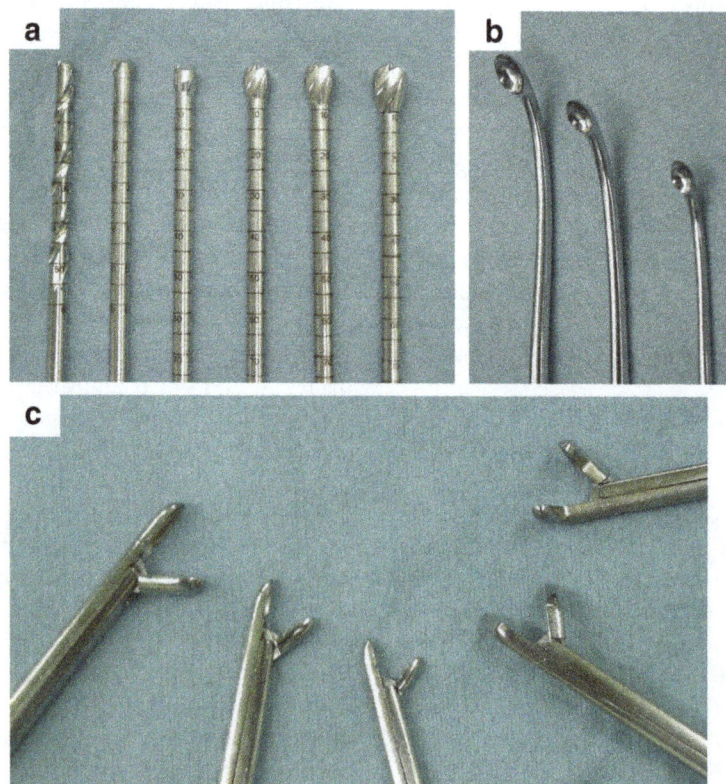

Fig. 2 Surgical instruments. Step-up cannulated drills (**a**). Variously angled curettes (**b**). Angled forceps (**c**)

Postoperative evaluation

Complication rate and functionality (assessed in terms of the Musculoskeletal Tumor Society Score) were evaluated after treatment [14]. As for the bone healing after ESC, we evaluated solid union, which was defined by the method of Hou et al. [15]: "the cortical wall thickness was sufficient to prevent further fracture and allowed unrestricted physical activity." Moreover, the consolidation of the cyst at the final evaluation was assessed according to the Modified Neer Classification [13] (Table 1), by an orthopedic surgeon and radiologist with independent of patients' information.

Statistical analysis

Kaplan-Meier analysis and the log-rank test were used to determine the association between recurrence and patient variables. Radiographical images (Modified Neer Classification) at the final assessment were evaluated independently and cross-checked by an orthopedic surgeon (HA) and radiologist (TG) who were both blinded to all other patient information. The kappa value was then calculated. For the statistical analysis of the categorical data, the chi-square analysis was used. A p value < 0.05 was considered significant. All values were presented either as mean ± standard deviation or median with range, depending on the distribution. All statistical analyses were conducted using SPSS version 24 (IBM, Chicago, IL).

Results

ESCs were performed from 2.5 portals on average (4 portals in 3 cases; 3 portals in 11 cases; 2 portals in 23 cases). The number of portals depended on the length of the lesion to ensure an appropriate working space for curettage and better viewing area. The median operative time was 88.8 (range, 42.0 to 186.0) min. The median volume of intraoperative bleeding, estimated from the total amount of irrigation fluid, was 21.7 ml (range, almost zero to 205.0 ml). Typical cases of SBC treated with ESC are shown in Figs. 3 and 4.

Table 1 Modified Neer Classification [13]

Classification	Description	Details
A	Healed	Cyst filled with new bone with small radiolucent area (< 1 cm)
B	Healed with a defect	Radiolucent area (< 50% diameter) with enough cortical thickness
C	Persistent cyst	Radiolucent area (≧ 50% diameter) with thin cortical rim
D	Recurrent cyst	Cyst reappears in the obliterated area or increased residual radiolucent area

Recurrence after ESC

During follow-up, recurrence occurred in seven patients (18.9%), at a median of 17.5 months (range, 7.8 to 28.8 months) after surgery. Among patients with recurrent cysts ($n = 7$), four patients underwent ESC again, and thereafter, the cystic lesions were well managed; two patients requested open curettage and artificial bone graft (OSferion®, Olympus Co., Tokyo, Japan); and one patient without any symptoms was observed. From the log-rank analysis, recurrence was associated with continuity of the cyst to the physis ($p = 0.006$, Table 2).

Healing after ESC

A total of 31 patients (83.7%) were categorized as healed (class A or B), and of these patients, the mean time of healing after the operation was 4.0 (SD 2.4) months. The kappa value was substantial (0.64, $p = 0.002$) between the two observers. The residue of the cyst was associated with ages under 10 years ($p = 0.034$, chi-square analysis). Despite there being no significant difference, cyst residue did not occur in patients with the cyst located in the calcaneus ($p = 0.239$; chi-square analysis of calcaneus to other bones).

Complications and function after ESC

All patients had an excellent function after ESC. With regard to minor complications in the humerus, two patients retained a slight deformity, without any symptoms, that was related to the dislocation of the pathological fracture before their first visit. Transient radial nerve palsy occurred for a patient with a large cystic lesion across the shaft of the humerus, probably due to iatrogenic blunt compression of the radial nerve during the ESC. Six months later, the palsy had spontaneously recovered without any deficit. Moreover, two postoperative fractures occurred (Fig. 5) and required temporal internal fixation (for 6 and 13 months).

Discussion

Although the etiology of a unicameral bone cyst has not been fully elucidated, conventional treatments have been to decompress the intraosseous pressure; irrigate the cyst to decrease any bone-destroying enzymes, such as prostaglandin-E2 or gelatinase [16]; remove the cyst membrane; and stimulate the bone healing process [15].

Historically, the percutaneous injection of steroids and aspiration of the fluid in the cavity were first reported by Scaglietti et al. [17]. Although this procedure is not highly invasive, multiple injections are required, and the recurrence rate is high. In 1986, Campanacci et al. [18] reported that 32% of patients with bone cyst had a recurrence or no change after the first treatment. Chang et al. [19] reported that 49% of patients of bone cyst required subsequent injections of steroids, and 44% of patients who had a second

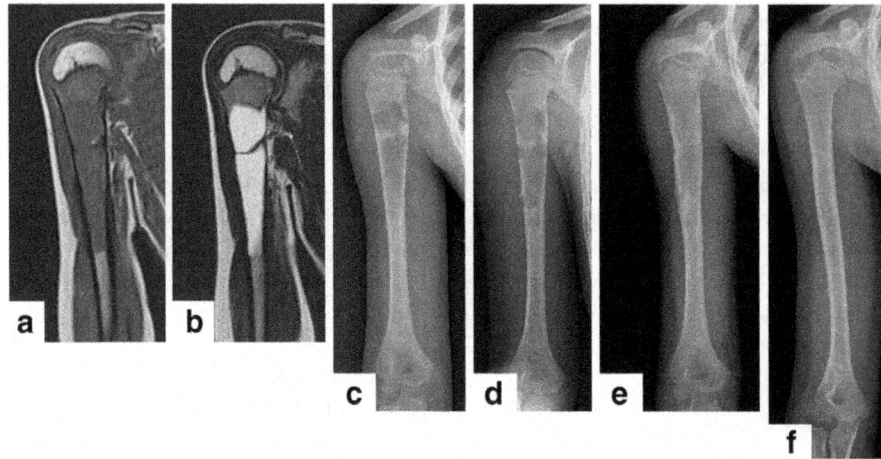

Fig. 3 The typical case of simple bone cyst in the right humerus treated with endoscopic curettage. A 6-year-old boy bruised his shoulder (**a** T1-weighted magnetic resonance [MRI]; **b** T2-weighted MRI; **c** X-ray). After 6 months of conservative therapy, the patient underwent endoscopic curettage via three portals (**d** postoperative image). Three months after the procedure, healing was confirmed with a callus around the portals and consolidation in the cavity (**e** solid union). Three years later, the bone was remodeled without any residual tumor or angular deformity (**f** class A)

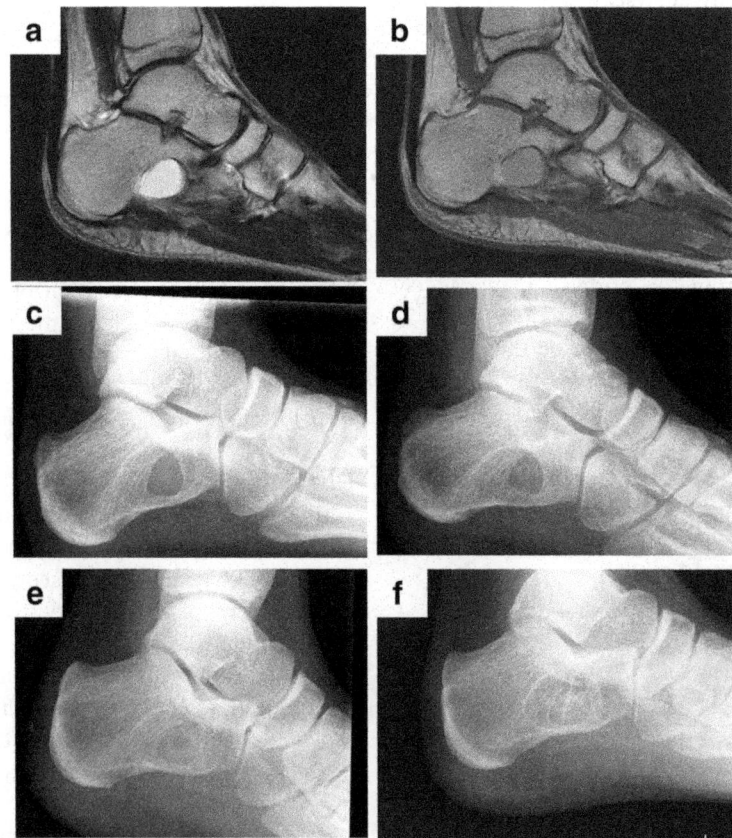

Fig. 4 Typical case of simple bone cyst in the calcaneus treated with endoscopic curettage. An 8-year-old boy experienced heel pain without an apparent cause (**a** T1-weighted MRI; **b** T2-weighted MRI; **c** X-ray). Endoscopic curettage C was performed via two portals (**d** postoperative image). After 3 months, healing was confirmed with consolidation of the cyst (**e**), and the cavity was completely filled with new bone 6 years after the operation (**f**, class A)

Table 2 Association between variables and recurrence

Variables	Number of cases (N = 37)	Recurrence	p value; chi-square analysis
Age, year			0.103
< 10	7	3	
≧ 10	30	4	
Sex			0.567
Male	24	4	
Female	13	3	
Location*			0.285
Tubular bone	29	6	
Flat bone	2	1	
Short bone	6	0	
Contact with physis			0.006
Yes	12	4	
No	25	3	
Maximum length of tumor			0.471
≧ 50 mm	14	2	
< 50 mm	23	5	

*Comparison for pooled over strata

injection ended up with failure. In 2007, Wright et al. reported the result of steroid injection therapy by randomized control trial with a comparison to autologous bone marrow injection, revealing the superiority of steroid injection. The healing rate of steroid injection cohort was 42%, and the subsequent fracture rate occurred in 11 cases per 38 patients [11].

Open curettage of the bone cyst with bone grafting, including autograft, allograft, or hydroxyapatite bone substitute, increases the healing rate after surgery. This treatment is simple and easy to learn, but some authors do not recommend it as the initial treatment [3] due to concerns of donor-site infection, iatrogenic fracture, or growth plate injury. Neer et al. reported the outcomes of open curettage and bone grafting with comparison to conservative therapy (immobilization after pathological fracture) for SBC and reported its superiority in terms of healing rate (77 vs 4%, open curettage vs conservative therapy, respectively) and subsequent fracture rate (2.4 vs 80%, respectively) [13]. In 1986, Campanacci et al. reported the outcomes about the bone curettage with bone grafting for a large number of cases (n = 178), and the healing rate was 68% [18]. Recently, Sung et al. reported in their retrospective comparative study, the outcomes including treatment failure (defined clinically as a subsequent pathologic fracture or need for retreatment to prevent pathologic fracture) and complications. After curettage and bone grafting, 64% of the patients

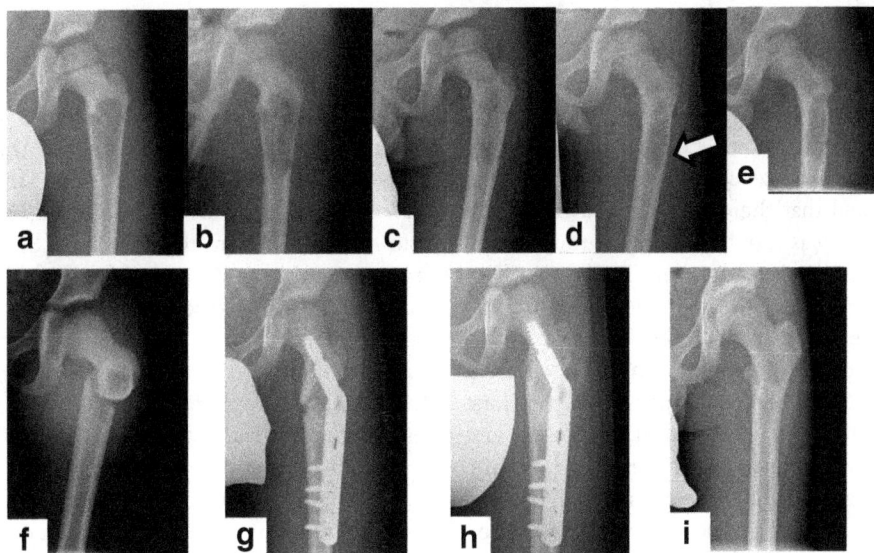

Fig. 5 Recurrence and pathologic fracture after second endoscopic curettage. A 5-year-old boy had left coxalgia; from the X-ray image (**a**), simple bone cyst was suspected. The first endoscopic curettage was performed via two portals (**b**). After 2 months, bone healing had begun with cortical enlargement and consolidation of cancellous bone (**c**). However, approximately 1 year after the endoscopic curettage, the cystic lesion (white arrow) had become prominent and recurrence was suspected (**d**). A second endoscopic curettage was performed (**e**). After discharge with a crutch, the patient fell, and a subtrochanteric fracture was identified (**f**). Open reduction and internal fixation with a compression hip screw (Ti-VFx II tube plate®, Zimmer Biomet, Warsaw, USA) and artificial bone grafting (OSferion®, OLYMPUS) were performed (**g**), and after 6 months, bone union was confirmed (**h**) and the implants removed. Three years after the first endoscopic curettage, no recurrence or complications had occurred (**i**)

experienced treatment failure and 21% complained about pain [3].

Given that the optimal treatment for SBC has remained questionable, a meta-analysis integrated 62 articles with a total of 3217 patients with SBC [1]. According to the review, the failure rate—defined as recurrence or persistence of cyst—was 23.9% (overall), with a rate of 61.1% for conservative treatment, 23.2% for curettage with autograft, and 28.5% for methylprednisolone acetate injection. This indicated that the recurrence of 18.9% after ESC in this study was at least not lower compared to that in other studies. However, there may be many factors that influence the results; thus, the comparison of the results between this work and previous studies is difficult. In other words, selection of treatment must be based on various factors, including invasiveness, reproducibility, recurrence rate, and comorbidities.

ESC for benign bone tumors, including SBCs, enchondromas, and aneurysmal bone cysts, has been performed in our institution since the early 1990s [20–22]. We have reported favorable outcomes for patients with enchondromas treated with ESC between 1992 and 2016, with a recurrence rate of 3.3% among 120 patients and a mean time for bone healing of 2.9 months without postoperative contracture [20]. Until now, the report about ESC for SBC was limited, except for the lesion arising from the calcaneus. A pilot study comparing open versus endoscopic curettage and bone grafting was conducted by Yildirim et al. in 2011 [23]. This study included 26 patients, who were equally assigned into two groups. They reported similar healing rates (92.3 and 100% for open curettage and ESC with bone grafting, respectively), and direct visualization and less soft tissue damage were the advantages of this technique. Nishimura et al. also reported a comparative study of the result of ESC with calcium phosphate cement for the calcaneus lesion, which revealed that there was no recurrence and time to sports activity was rapid in the ESC group [24].

Despite the several case reports about ESC for SBC in the tubular bone [25–27], there had never been reports of ESC in a relatively large case series. We have determined that arthroscopy provides an accurate assessment of tumor resection via direct examination of the bone marrow cavity for the complete removal of the cyst and is less invasive compared to the other methods. Likewise, Choi et al. [27] reported the outcomes of endoscopic curettage for various benign bone tumors. They stated that the small number of incisions (two incisions in most cases) had many advantages, such as less bleeding and less damage to the adjacent soft tissue and bone. Furthermore, blind drilling or excessive curettage, which could lead to intraoperative fracture or brittleness of the treated bone, can be avoided [28]. However, we should note that the learning curve or skill of the surgeon might

affect the outcomes of ESC; in other words, surgeons must have an experience in both arthroscopic surgery and treatment of bone tumor. Thus, standardization of this treatment for every institution might be difficult, but we believe that ESC can be applied for many treatments, apart from SBC.

Regarding recurrence after surgery, we reported that the risk factor for the recurrence was the attachment to physis. This is probably related to the activity of SBC; the cyst separated from the physis is considered latent [29]. In addition, other reports documented that the recurrence is more likely in patients younger than 10 years old [13, 29] and larger cysts are at a higher risk of recurrence [30, 31]. Moreover, multilocular cysts are more likely to recur [18, 32] as curettage may leave some areas behind. In our series, we performed complete resections of the septa of the multilocular cysts, which can prevent the recurrence of these lesions.

In this study, some major complications of surgery occurred in four patients. One patient had transient nerve palsy, probably caused by iatrogenic blunt compression of the nerve during the procedure around the radial groove. To minimize the complications with ESC, thorough planning before the operation to determine the location of the access ports is needed to avoid neurovascular structures. Additionally, two patients had postoperative fractures early in the study period. Because the strength of the bone might be transiently weakened after curettage of the cavity, careful observation and rigid prohibition of weight bearing are necessary until considerable bone formation, especially in cases in which the cyst was located in the lower extremities. Considering the previous reviews about postoperative fractures with incidence rates of 0–20% for open curettage and 0–30% for steroid injection [33], the fracture rate is within the range of the previous study. However, the prediction of postoperative fracture is not easy because many factors influenced bone strength. Ahn and Park noted from the analysis of SBC and aneurysmal bone cysts that destruction of > 85% of the length of the cortex in the transverse plane on both anteroposterior and lateral views was a risk factor for pathological fracture [34]. Furthermore, Nakamura et al. reported that cyst wall thickness, with a cutoff value of 0.5 mm, was an important risk factor for pathological fractures [35]. However, the specificity of each threshold was not very high. In addition to the length or cyst wall thickness, we deemed that a high lesion/cortex ratio (the ratio between the maximum width of the lesion to the bone [36] and the cyst located in the lower extremity or trochanteric area should be carefully considered if ESC is planned.

This study had several limitations. First, to evaluate the outcomes of this treatment more precisely, comparison with other treatments should have been performed. Second, the sample size was limited; thus, the power of this study is not strong. Finally, validation of the duration of follow-up was another concern in this study. Teoh also reported that the time to recurrence was variable, ranging from 2 to 27 months after surgery [29]. In this study, all patients were monitored for at least 6 months after bone consolidation (Modified Neer Classification A–B). This is because, once the cystic cavity was fully consolidated, recurrence was unusual. However, three of our patients showed late recurrences (22–29 months after the operation). Clinically, these cases of recurrence involved persistent cysts (Modified Neer Classification C). Therefore, if bone healing was delayed, an extension of the follow-up period would be necessary. However, because of the slow-growing nature of the latent residual cysts, the exact determination of recurrence using plain radiography was sometimes difficult; therefore, clinicians sometimes had difficulty in determining when follow-up could be discontinued.

Conclusions
We have reported a relatively large case series of SBC treated with ESC. ESC might be a useful alternative as it is a minimally invasive procedure for the treatment of simple bone cysts. Considering the relatively smaller size of this study, further investigation should be necessary for deducing the reliable conclusion.

Abbreviations
ESC: Endoscopic curettage; SBC: Simple bone cyst; SD: Standard deviation

Acknowledgements
We thank the staff of the Division of Pathology of Nagoya City University Hospital for the evaluation of the histological specimens.

Authors' contributions
HA contributed to the software, validation, visualization, formal analysis, data curation, and original draft. MsK is the main surgeon and contributed to the conceptualization, methodology, and supervision. YWN, HG, and HO are surgeons and contributed to the supervision. JM and SY contributed to the supervision and data curation. MN is a surgeon and contributed to the conceptualization and methodology. HM and MkK is a surgeon. SM contributed to the review and editing. KE and SS contributed to the data curation. TG contributed to the radiological assessment. TO contributed to the review and editing, project administration,and conceptualization. All authors read and approved the final manuscript.

Competing interests
The authors declare that they have no competing interests.

Author details
[1]Department of Orthopedic Surgery, Nagoya City University Graduate School of Medical Sciences, 1, Kawasumi, Mizuho-cho, Mizuho-ku, Nagoya 467-8601, Japan. [2]Department of Joint Surgery for Rheumatic Diseases, Nagoya City University Graduate School of Medical Sciences, 1, Kawasumi, Mizuho-cho, Mizuho-ku, Nagoya 467-8601, Japan. [3]Department of Rehabilitation Medicine, Nagoya City University Graduate School of Medical Sciences, 1, Kawasumi, Mizuho-cho, Mizuho-ku, Nagoya 467-8601, Japan. [4]Department of Radiology, Nagoya City University Graduate School of Medical Sciences, 1, Kawasumi, Mizuho-cho, Mizuho-ku, Nagoya 467-8601, Japan. [5]Department of Orthopedic Surgery, Ogaki Municipal Hospital, 4-86 Minaminokawa-cho, Ogaki 503-8502, Japan.

References
1. Kadhim M, Thacker M, Kadhim A, Holmes L Jr. Treatment of unicameral bone cyst: systematic review and meta analysis. J Child Orthop. 2014;8:171–91. https://doi.org/10.1007/s11832-014-0566-3.
2. Abdel-Wanis ME, Tsuchiya H. Simple bone cyst is not a single entity: point of view based on a literature review. Med Hypotheses. 2002 Jan;58(1):87–91.
3. Sung AD, Anderson ME, Zurakowski D, Hornicek FJ, Gebhardt MC. Unicameral bone cyst: a retrospective study of three surgical treatments. Clin Orthop Relat Res. 2008;466:2519–26. https://doi.org/10.1007/s11999-008-0407-0.
4. Mascard E, Gomez-Brouchet A, Lambot K. Bone cysts: unicameral and aneurysmal bone cyst. Orthop Traumatol Surg Res. 2015;101(1 Suppl):S119–27. https://doi.org/10.1016/j.otsr.2014.06.031. Epub 2015 Jan 8
5. Pogoda P, Priemel M, Linhart W, Stork A, Adam G, Windolf J, et al. Clinical relevance of calcaneal bone cysts: a study of 50 cysts in 47 patients. Clin Orthop Relat Res. 2004;424:202–10.
6. Glaser DL, Dormans JP, Stanton RP, Davidson RS. Surgical management of calcaneal unicameral bone cysts. Clin Orthop Relat Res. 1999;360:231–7.
7. Moreau G, Letts M. Unicameral bone cyst of the calcaneus in children. J Pediatr Orthop. 1994;14:101–4.
8. Tsuchiya H, Abdel-Wanis ME, Uehara K, Tomita K, Takagi Y, Yasutake H. Cannulation of simple bone cysts. J Bone Joint Surg Br. 2002;84:245–8.
9. Shirai T, Tsuchiya H, Terauchi R, Tsuchida S, Mizoshiri N, Ikoma K, et al. Treatment of a simple bone cyst using a cannulated hydroxyapatite pin. Medicine (Baltimore). 2015;94:e1027. https://doi.org/10.1097/MD.0000000000001027.
10. Mylle J, Burssens A, Fabry G. Simple bone cysts. A review of 59 cases with special reference to their treatment. Arch Orthop Trauma Surg. 1992;111(6):297–300.
11. Wright JG, Yandow S, Donaldson S, Marley L, Simple Bone Cyst Trial Group. A randomized clinical trial comparing intralesional bone marrow and steroid injections for simple bone cysts. J Bone Joint Surg Am. 2008 Apr; 90(4):722–30. https://doi.org/10.2106/JBJS.G.00620.
12. Chigira M, Maehara S, Arita S, Udagawa E. The aetiology and treatment of simple bone cysts. J Bone Joint Surg Br. 1983;65(5):633–7.
13. Neer CS, Francis KC, Marcove RC, Terz J, Carbonara PN. Treatment of unicameral bone cyst. A follow-up study of one hundred seventy-five cases. J Bone Joint Surg Am. 1966;48:731–45.
14. Enneking WF, Dunham W, Gebhardt MC, Malawar M, Pritchard DJ. A system for the functional evaluation of reconstructive procedures after surgical treatment of tumors of the musculoskeletal system. Clin Orthop Relat Res. 1993;286:241–6.
15. Hou HY, Wu K, Wang CT, Chang SM, Lin WH, Yang RS. Treatment of unicameral bone cyst: a comparative study of selected techniques. J Bone Joint Surg Am. 2010;92:855–62. https://doi.org/10.2106/JBJS.I.00607.
16. Komiya S, Minamitani K, Sasaguri Y, Hashimoto S, Morimatsu M, Inoue A. Simple bone cyst. Treatment by trepanation and studies on bone resorptive factors in cyst fluid with a theory of its pathogenesis. Clin Orthop Relat Res. 1993:287, 204–11.
17. Scaglietti O, Marchetti PG, Bartolozzi P. Final results obtained in the treatment of bone cysts with methylprednisolone acetate (depo-medrol) and a discussion of results achieved in other bone lesions. Clin Orthop Relat Res. 1982;165:33–42.
18. Campanacci M, Capanna R, Picci P. Unicameral and aneurysmal bone cysts. Clin Orthop Relat Res. 1986;204:25–36.
19. Chang CH, Stanton RP, Glutting J. Unicameral bone cysts treated by injection of bone marrow or methylprednisolone. J Bone Joint Surg Br. 2002;84:407–12.

20. Okamoto H, Kobayashi M, Sekiya I, Shinzi M, Endo K, Otsuka T. Surgery for enchondroma on the fingers—endoscopic curettage. The Central Japan Journal of Orthopaedic Surgery & Traumatology. 2017;60:53–4. [in Japanese]
21. Otsuka T, Kobayashi M, Yonezawa M, Kamiyama F, Matsushita Y, Matsui N. The treatment of enchondromas in the hand by endoscopic curettage without bone grafting. Arthroscopy. 2002;18:430–5.
22. Sekiya I, Matsui N, Otsuka T, Kobayashi M, Tsuchiya D. The treatment of enchondromas in the hand by endoscopic curettage without bone grafting. J Hand Surg (Br). 1997;22:230–4.
23. Yildirim C, Akmaz I, Sahin O, Keklikci K. Simple calcaneal bone cysts: a pilot study comparing open versus endoscopic curettage and grafting. J Bone Joint Surg Br. 2011 Dec;93(12):1626–31. https://doi.org/10.1302/0301-620X.93B12.27315.
24. Nishimura A, Matsumine A, Kato K, Aasanuma K, Nakamura T, Fukuda A, Sudo A. Endoscopic versus open surgery for calcaneal bone cysts: a preliminary report. J Foot Ankle Surg. 2016;55(4):782–7. https://doi.org/10.1053/j.jfas.2016.03.006. Epub 2016 Apr 8
25. Miyamoto W, Takao M, Yasui Y, Miki S, Matsushita T. Endoscopic surgery for symptomatic unicameral bone cyst of the proximal femur. Arthrosc Tech. 2013;2(4):e467–71. https://doi.org/10.1016/j.eats.2013.07.001. eCollection 2013 Nov
26. Randelli P, Arrigoni P, Cabitza P, Denti M. Unicameral bone cyst of the humeral head: arthroscopic curettage and bone grafting. Orthopedics. 2009 Jan;32(1):54.
27. Choi Y, Kwak JM, Chung SH, Jung GH, Kim JD. Tumor treated by endoscopy. Clin Orthop Surg. 2014;6:72–9. https://doi.org/10.4055/cios.2014.6.1.72.
28. Dietz JF, Kachar SM, Nagle DJ. Endoscopically assisted excision of digital enchondroma. Arthroscopy. 2007;23:678.e1–4.
29. Teoh KH, Watts AC, Chee YH, Reid R, Porter DE. Predictive factors for recurrence of simple bone cyst of the proximal humerus. J Orthop Surg (Hong Kong). 2010;18:215–9.
30. Kaelin AJ, MacEwen GD. Unicameral bone cysts. Natural history and the risk of fracture. Int Orthop. 1989;13(4):275–82.
31. Spence KF, Sell KW, Brown RH. Solitary bone cyst: treatment with freeze-dried cancellous bone allograft. A study of one hundred seventy-seven cases. J Bone Joint Surg Am. 1969 Jan;51(1):87–96.
32. Capanna R, Dal Monte A, Gitelis S, Campanacci M. The natural history of unicameral bone cyst after steroid injection. Clin Orthop Relat Res. 1982;166:204–11.
33. Donaldson S, Chundamala J, Yandow S, Wright JG. Treatment for unicameral bone cysts in long bones: an evidence based review. Orthop Rev (Pavia). 2010;2(1):e13. https://doi.org/10.4081/or.2010.e13.
34. Ahn JI, Park JS. Pathological fractures secondary to unicameral bone cysts. Int Orthop. 1994 Feb;18(1):20–2.
35. Nakamura T, Takagi K, Kitagawa T, Harada M. Microdensity of solitary bone cyst after steroid injection. J Pediatr Orthop. 1988 Sep-Oct;8(5):566–8.
36. Mirels H. Metastatic disease in long bones. A proposed scoring system for diagnosing impending pathologic fractures. Clin Orthop Relat Res. 1989;249:256–64.

17

Coatings as the useful drug delivery system for the prevention of implant-related infections

Chenhao Pan[1], Zubin Zhou[1] and Xiaowei Yu[1,2]* (iD)

Abstract

Implant-related infections (IRIs) which led to a large amount of medical expenditure were caused by bacteria and fungi that involve the implants in the operation or in ward. Traditional treatments of IRIs were comprised of repeated radical debridement, replacement of internal fixators, and intravenous antibiotics. It needed a long time and numbers of surgeries to cure, which meant a catastrophe to patients. So how to prevent it was more important than to cure it. As an excellent local release system, coating is a good idea by its local drug infusion and barrier effect on resisting biofilms which were the main cause of IRIs. So in this review, materials used for coatings and evidences of prevention were elaborated.

Keywords: Implant-related infections, Coating, Osteomyelitis, Local drug delivery system, Biofilm

Background

Implant-related infections (IRIs) are the result of bacteria adhesion to an implant surface and subsequent biofilm formation at the implantation site [1]. The incidence of IRIs in orthopedic trauma patients was from 5 to 10% depending on the severity of the injury, condition of soft tissue, and the type of fracture [2]. It remains challenging and expensive to treat IRIs, despite advances in antibiotics and new operative techniques. The traditional management of IRIs includes irrigation and debridement, obliteration of dead space, intravenous antibiotics, and removal of the hardware [3]. Each year, 750,000–1,000,000 IRIs occur in the USA, and the government needs to spend more than $1.6 billion to cover the expense of the excess hospital charges [4]. Especially, with the widely use of orthopedic implants, the number of infected implants was continued to increase [5]. Even if the infected implants can be successfully removed by secondary surgery, the functionality of the limb and the fracture healing may be limited, which may eventually lead to fatal surgical operations such as amputation, joint arthroplasty, or arthrodesis.

So how to prevent the occurrence of fatal IRIs is more important than the treatment. IRIs are typically caused by microorganisms which grow in biofilms and adhere to the implant surface in a highly hydrated extracellular matrix. Avoiding biofilms forming can effectively prevent or treat IRIs [6–9]. As the elective surgery could not be performed under an absolutely sterile environment, bacteria may prefer to adhere to the surface of the bioinert titanium implants and form biofilms, especially when the host's immunological defense functions are compromised and/or the systemic antibiotic prophylaxis is not very effective [10, 11]. Bacteria which can resist immune responses in biofilms were much less susceptible to antibiotics [12]. Therefore, it is difficult to truly eliminate the biofilm infections and, typically, there are chronic recurring symptoms, even after antibiotic therapy. So the prevention of the growth of nosocomial pathogens is more important than the elimination of the biofilm in IRIs.

Because of the restrictions of traditional systemic drug treatment of bone infection, such as poor effect or hepatorenal toxicity, drugs for IRIs should be performed locally and specifically for implants sites at optimal concentrations over appropriate stages [13].

* Correspondence: yuxw@sjtu.edu.cn
Chenhao Pan and Zubin Zhou should be considered as equal first coauthors.
Chenhao Pan and Zubin Zhou contributed equally to this work.
[1]Department of Orthopaedic Surgery, Shanghai Jiao Tong University Affiliated Sixth People's Hospital, Shanghai 200233, China
[2]Department of Orthopaedic Surgery, Shanghai Sixth People's Hospital East Campus, Shanghai University of Medicine and Health Sciences, Shanghai 201306, China

Numerous strategies have been attempted to prevent and treat IRIs by either implant surface fabrication or incorporation of antibiotics into the implant devices. Recent developments in material science showed that implants with biodegradable polymer coatings can be used as controllable means to deliver antibiotics in a sustained fashion. Polymer coatings are capable of completely releasing all antibiotics in a sustained fashion thus minimizing any local or systemic toxicity associated with high fluctuating antibiotic concentrations. For example, Buchholz et al. [14] reported that implant with a synthetic polymers coating as a local drug delivery system significantly reduced the infections and representing a promising approach in the treatment of IRIs. One of the main advantages of implant surface coating-mediated local drug delivery is keeping other parts of the body out of affected so as to avoid serious systemic side effects [15]. A sustained and high antibiotic concentration over minimal inhibitory concentration (MIC) of pathogenic bacteria at the implant site is expected to inhibit bacterial adhesion, colonization, and biofilm formation [16].

The antibacterial implant coating can be divided into calcium or silicon bone cements, polymer hydrogels, and antibacterial ion coatings based on the materials selected by different manufacturing processes like spraying, smearing, and electroplating [17, 18]. In this review, we will focus on (1) implants coated with antimicrobial substances and (2) the usage of coating in prevention of IRIs.

Mechanism of the IRIs—biofilm

Biofilms are aggregates of microorganisms as a self-produced matrix of extracellular polymeric substances (EPS) where bacteria are frequently embedded. EPS adherent to the medically surface (skin, implants, wearing) are accounting for most of microbial infections in the internal fixation devices [16]. Bioinert surfaces attract the biofilm formation [18–20]. The ligand of bacterial fimbriae can be bound to electrovalent bond or hydrophobic bond on the surface of the material. The factors of a surface that determine initial bacterial attachment are its hydrophobicity and roughness [19–21].

In most previous studies on bacterial adhesion on titanium and ceramic surfaces, the quantity of bacterial adhesion showed a direct positive correlation with surface roughness [22–24]. From an atomic force microscopy (AFM) viewpoint, most surfaces are rough and all kinds of surfaces provide adequate conditions for bacterial adhesion [25]. According to the thermodynamic model of microbial adhesion, hydrophobic materials are preferentially colonized by hydrophobic bacteria [26–28]. Consequently, the adhesion properties of different bacteria are affected by the hydrophobicity of the bacterial cell surface [29, 30]. Both S. aureus and Methicillin-resistant Staphylococcus aureus (MRSA) which are common bacteria in IRIs are known to prefer hydrophobic surfaces

[31, 32]. Titanium implants are often bioinert, smooth (Ra = 280 nm) but enough for bacterial adhesion [33] and hydrophobicity to prevent blood clotting. Thus, biofilm formation occurs commonly [22–33].

Biofilms are complicated systems with high microorganisms' densities, ranging from 10^8 to 10^{11} bacteria g^{-1} wet weight [12]. Most of the biofilm biomass comprises hydrated EPS instead of bacteria. The intermolecular interactions among EPS components originating from self-organization of EPS matrix determine the mechanical characteristics and the biological activity of the matrix in the biofilm [12]. The biofilm architecture formation is a continuous process that creates a micro spatial organization where bacteria clusters present in the biofilm in micro colonies. As the ramparts of bacteria, biofilms have the feature of antibiotics tolerance.

Antibiotics tolerance of biofilms is due to the properties of the biofilm matrix and of the slow growth which occurs in biofilms. The components of EPS matrix can deactivate antimicrobial substances diffused through the biofilm as diffusion–reaction inhibition [34, 35]. Antimicrobial resistance may be promoted by diffusion–reaction inhibition form biofilms through decreasing the effective concentration of antimicrobials that bacteria are exposed to. On the other side, dormancy and slow growth rates have been considered to be ways of bacteria survival in biofilms being exposed to antimicrobials for a long time [36]. The formation and antibiotics resistance of biofilm is time-dependent. The initial bacterial attachment (within an hour) is crucial for the biofilm formation [37–39]. Cell wall-anchored (CWA) proteins of bacteria promote attachment to surfaces in the following 24 h bacteria adhesion stage. The scanning electron microscope (SEM) revealed implants surface was comprised of bacteria clusters always associated with fibrils, which was presumed as fibrin, and surrounded by diameter host cells [35, 37]. When the bacteria are anchored to the implants, biofilm formation begins to develop. There was a new structure which was called "lacunae" till day 7 [15, 35]. The lacunae is the shallow depressions consistent with the size of bacteria, which meant the matrix spaces left by dispersed bacteria. The accumulation of bacteria during biofilm formation is attributed only to the polysaccharide intercellular adhesin (PIA) [38–40]. Next, the biofilm proliferation and maturation remodeling by phenol-soluble modulins (PSMs) begin [41]. After 14–28 days, empty lacunae and a few bacteria were the main morphological characteristics of EPS matrix. This phenotype of EPS matrix remained the same till 6 months post-implantation and showed an unexpectedly outstanding stability of EPS mature biofilm in chronic implant-related infection [35]. In summary, typical biofilm formation is first shaping at day 7 and its growth diffusion peaks covering 30–40% of the implant is at 2 weeks.

Unlike the distinct biofilm formation phenotypes in vitro, the in vivo biofilm formation comprised of strains is hard to be indistinguishable [42]. The biofilm formation in vivo takes longer time than in vitro, which may be due to the "race to surface" between bacteria and host cells. Bacterial attachment and biofilm formation stage lasted 12–24 h, and the biofilm proliferation and maturation lasted 36–72 h for completion [43, 44]. The early infection may be defined up to 3–4 weeks during which debridement and antibiotic therapy with the retained stable implants were performed in the traditional management perspective [45, 46]. The residual biofilms on retained implants may cause the recurrence of IRIs in many clinical cases. Bioinert polymer coatings like polymethylmethacrylate (PMMA) [47] with antibacterial agents have been used to prevent early fibrin and bacteria adhesion through its barrier and antibacterial effect for IRIs [48, 49].

Over time, the complete biofilms are gradually formed, so is the antibiotic resistance. On the basis of time- and dose- dependent effect of antibiotic susceptibility [50–53], ideal cumulative prevention and cure antibiotics release kinetics of the coatings should have the releasing peak over the minimal bactericidal concentration (MBC) during 7–14 days that prevent biofilm formation followed by sustained release between the MIC and MBC over several weeks. By inhibiting the biofilm formation, cells are in a dominant position in the competition against bacteria for growth, so the ideal releasing should have the concentration above MIC over at least 28 days.

At least 1% bacteria in stationary phase in biofilms are tolerant to antibiotics [54]. As time goes on, more bacteria in the biofilm moved into the stationary phase. Hence, for some kinds of antibiotics like vancomycin, antibiotics tolerance of biofilms showed temporal correlation, which denoted that higher tolerance was shown in older biofilms for these antibiotics as well as metal nanoparticles like Ag [34]. Moreover, biofilms would always die from the outside-in instead of the inside-out [53]. According to the characteristics of biofilm, the treatment is more difficult than prevention. Depending on the type of fracture and contamination of the trauma, second operation for IRIs may be avoided by the use of coating with the ideal antibiotics release curve for prevention.

Main components of coating for IRIs
Bone cement coatings
Various forms of PMMA bone cements and the beads made of it with antibiotics have been used for more than 40 years in hip replacement or in acute and chronic osteomyelitis [45, 47, 55, 56]. There are several premixed cements that have been allowed the clinical use by American Food and Drug Administration (FDA): DePuy® (DePuy Orthpedics), Cobalt™ G-HV (Biomet), Cemex® Genta (Exactech), Palacos® G (Biomet), and Simplex® P (Stryker Orthpedics). However, these FDA approved antibiotics eluting PMMA bone cements are more appropriate being used as a preventative measure than for the treatment because of their lack of effect on active IRIs due to limited and burst release of embedded antibiotics [57, 58]. Antibiotics release from PMMA cements is mainly due to the diffusion through surface roughness, superficial pores, and surface erosion [46, 58, 59]. The release characteristic of PMMA was typically performed as a biphasic phase which included a burst head of initial release and a continued tail of ineffective release for weeks or months. The mechanical strength of PMMA is satisfactory, but the low efficiency of the local drug release is the main barriers for its clinical use in IRIs. Therefore, a variety of new biomaterials have been developed and manufactured as alternative antibiotic-eluting bone cements.

Calcium phosphate cements (CPC), beta-tricalciumphosphate (β-TCP) and hydroxyapatite (HA) are the calcium phosphate materials. The calcium phosphate materials are degradable and the end products are calcium and phosphate (Ca^{2+}, PO_4^{3-}) that are biocompatible, bioactive, and stimulate new bone growth [59–62]. The injectable CPCs are now commercial available that can be solidified after implantation. [60, 61]. There are commonly two phases before the CPCs solidified: the particles and the liquid for better performance. CPCs have the ability of self-set, self-molding, and no exothermic reaction which may be harmful for the bone and incorporated drug [59, 62]. The slow biodegradation in vivo and poor biomechanical strength have restricted the clinical application of CPCs [58]. In addition, the microstructures of CPCs are dense, lacking of macroporosity that are obviously not suitable for the adhesion, penetration, and colonization of cells and tissue regeneration [58].

Antibiotics, such as gentamicin [46, 63–66] and vancomycin [67, 68], can be mixed in the liquid phase of calcium phosphate cement, HA, or β-TCP [46] against S. aureus and MRSA. The apatite cements are made up of microcrystals that have a better biological performance in size and formation than HA particles [63], and show better antibacterial activity. HA nanoparticles can be propagated by wet chemical precipitation and show good bactericidal effect for implant-related pathogens through toxic effect of damaging bacterial membrane [69–71]. It was reported that a drug-chitosan compound was filled in the porous HA matrix and subsequently coated onto the implant smooth surface to obtain a Ti_6Al_4V implant with drug-chitosan-HA-coating [72–74]. The burst releasing peak continued in the first several hours, and the continued release were covered the post-operative time of perioperative period or 4–8 days. The rest releasing was lasting for more than 1 month. Though HA have better biomechanical properties, β-TCP seemed to be more suitable for drug release. Another coatings comprised of HA and TCP were defined as bi-phasic calcium phosphates (BCP). More ions dissolved in the BCP in the local releasing, which meant more carbonate hydroxyapatite on the surface [75]. A β-TCP coating contained doxycycline (BonyPid™) was described to form a steady, zero-order rate releasing up to 30 days to be capable of eliminating the contaminating bacteria [70]. Moreover, poly(lactic acid)(PLLA)/β-TCP coating presents a good result of infection as manifested by the microbiological, radiological, and histological analysis [67, 76]. At present, the releasing profiles of FDA-approved antibiotic eluting bone cements have the limitations of burst and limited release that are not sufficient to reach a desired constant and long-term sustained release effect to satisfy time- and dose-dependence of biofilms prevention.

Hydrogels coatings
Hydrogels are usually prepared from natural to synthetic polymers with high degree of hydration and represent promising biomaterials for tissue engineering and regenerative medicine. One class of natural polymers is polysaccharides (e.g., dextran, alginate, chitosan, fibrin, and proteins gelatin). Synthetic polymers include polyethylene oxide (PEO)/polyethylene glycol (PEG), poly (vinyl alcohol) (PVA), poly (acrylic acid) (PAA), and others [49]. Implant surface with PEG and/or PEO coating can endow the ability of anti-bacteria adhesion [77, 78]. There was a report that the inclusion of arginine-glycine-aspartic acid (RGD) array restored the function of local osteoblasts that were damaged by some synthetic polymer coatings [79]. A solubilizing surrounding was offered for the antimicrobials dissolution in local delivery system by the hydrophilic characteristic of hydrogels. Several antibiotics, like ciprofloxacin [80], amoxicillin [81], and gentamicin [82] can be embedded in the bioactive hydrogels. Hydrogels were recently designed by self-assembly formation of tripeptide (D)Leu--Phe-Phe with the incorporation of ciprofloxacin [49, 80]. During the self-assembly process, it showed that the antimicrobials played an active role in process to incorporate into the hydrogels formation directly. The non-covalent bond contributed to the antimicrobials integration in peptide structure [48, 49]. The final release was indicated to reach the effect of anti-infection.

The antibacterial properties of chitosan is due to the combination between positively charged amino groups of chitosan and negatively charged bacterial membranes, leading to bacteria membrane leakage [83]. However, because of the displayed weak positive charges on chitosan, coating with chitosan reveal only limited antibacterial effects [84]. Furthermore, the physical and chemical characteristics of chitosan are poorly for embrittlement at room temperature and in acid dissolution environment [85]. Another hydrogel similar to chitosan is a polysaccharide originated from natural chitin polymerization and has the antibacterial activity [86]. The bacterial adhesion and subsequent biofilm formation can be prevented by using chitosan alone. Several temperature-responsive structures of hydrogels (PLLA-PEG-PLLA, PDLA-CPC-PDLA, and PDLA-PEG-PDLA) were reported [87]. These hydrogels were performed to inhibit the growth of S. aureus and E. coli.

Titanium implants with different antibiotics (like gentamicin)-doped hydrogels coating significantly prevented the occurrence of infection. However, the methods of antibiotics hydrogel coating need to be optimized to reach suitable drug releasing profiles and optimal coating matrix degradation rate. Controlled delivery system loaded with drug on the titanium implants showed the double ability of antibacterial and osteogenesis forming by biodegradable sol-gel and polymers coating [88, 89]. The controlled releasing technology of nanostructured sol-gel provided a continuous and effective local delivery system for orthopedic instruments to prevent and cure IRIs [90].

Silver/silver ions coatings
Most of the metal ions coating is in the form of ionic or nanoparticles instead of bulk material [91]. Silver ion is bioactive by wrecking the cell membrane permeability and cellular metabolism [91, 92]. The sulfhydryl groups of metabolic enzymes and bacterial DNA are disrupted by Ag to the destruction of bacterial membranes, so the bacterial key metabolism and replication are inactivated [92]. Implants coated with silver can prevent bacteria adhesion and subsequent colonization (like S. aureus and S. epidermidis) in vitro [93, 94]. Titanium dioxide itself has been performed to be a kind of anti-infective biomaterials or cooperated with other factors [95, 96]. However, implant with low-dose silver coating (< 1 ppm) may be incapable of reducing the infection rates [97], while high-dose silver coating (> 1.5 ppm) may induce cytotoxicity [98]. However, cytotoxicity sensitivity is different among different cells [99–101]. Therefore, for the simple silver coating, the concentration of silver had better range from 1.8% to 6.5 wt% for inhibiting bacteria proliferation without decreasing osteoblast activity [99, 102]. No observable adverse effect level (NOAEL) of silver is up to 30 mg/kg [103]. The most serious adverse effect of silver is Argyria, which is not found at or below 1.7 g total silver in vivo. For a long time release, the minimum requirement for antibacterial effect was at the concentrations of at least 0.1 ppb [104, 105]. Another study reported that an optimal silver density on the implant surface was 1×10^{18} ions/cm^2, representing a balance

between corrosion resistance and antibacterial effect [106]. Unlike Ag^+ which is diffused to the surrounding tissue, a new antibacterial HA film was developed by immobilization of Ag in HA film through inositol hexaphosphate chelation. This antibacterial HA film coating demonstrated excellent antibacterial activity both in vitro and in vivo [107]. Data generated from a *S. aureus* induced in vivo osteomyelitis model demonstrated that no bacteria infection was detectable up to 21 days after implantation of implants with antibacterial HA film coating [107]. Ag-coated fracture external fixation pins were examined in human studies; however, these studies fail to demonstrate any advantages in reduction of pin site infections when silver-coated pins were used [108].

In summary, most studies have concentrated on these three kinds of materials coating. Other coating materials, such as iodine ions [109, 110], titanium oxide photocatalysis, nitric oxide, and graphene coating [111], have provided new ideas and alternative approaches for the prevention of IRIs.

Evidence of the anti-infective prophylactic therapy of coating

In vitro studies

Many studies using antimicrobial coatings have achieved on IRIs prevention in vitro. The therapeutic effects of antibacterial coating materials on the prevention of biofilm are usually evaluated by the in vitro zone inhibition of bacterial growth, such as *S.aureus* or MRSA [69, 112], antibiotic release profiles and bioactivities [70, 113, 114], cytotoxicity [67] of osteoblast, or other cell lines from the liver and kidney [104]. A characteristic time- and dose-dependent sustained antibiotics release is critical for the biofilm formation inhibition. David et al. tested a variety of antibiotics releasing efficacy and showed that all antibiotics used alone or in combination showed an initial burst release peak with dose-dependent antimicrobial effects and have no negative effects on osteoblast [112]. Local antibacterial spectrum and releasing curve for the biomaterial were needed to be considered when coating with antibiotics. The synthesized HA nanocrystals displayed antimicrobial effect against the IRIs by damaging bacteria membrane [69]. HA nanoparticles dispersed in the chitosan matrix lowered the burst releasing peak of the small molecule drug because of HA physisorption, which promoted persistent release kinetics up to 3 weeks [70]. The calcium phosphate coating can reduce burst release, which provided long-term release kinetics throughout 4 weeks [113]. Another team coated vancomycin onto PLLA/β-TCP composites to release antibiotics through dip coating. The PLLA/β-TCP coating was biocompatible on cell proliferation, adhesion, and mineralization [67]. While gentamicin-doped poly(D,L-lactic acid) (PDLLA) coatings had an initial

burst release and around 60% of incorporated drug was released within 1 min. Then, a subsequent slow and constant release of gentamycin was observed lasting 6 weeks from 40% down to 15% [114].

Implants with antibiotic-doped coating suffered from a problem that antibiotic therapeutic concentrations lasted for a limited period time. When the antibiotic was exhausted, the antibiotic concentration was down to the levels enabling bacteria to escape antibiotic and colonize the implants [115]. Alternative approaches have been developed to tethering antibiotics on the surface of metal implants through a bridge linker and forming an immobilized antibacterial coating. The immobilized antibacterial coating is expected to be functional throughout the whole life of implants. Various types of antibiotics and bacterial membrane destructing molecules are suitable candidates for the preparation of immobilized antibacterial coating [116]. Compared to antibiotics, antimicrobial peptide was highly specific and had minimal toxicity to cells without drug resistance [117]. However, antimicrobial peptides are preferred for the treatment of IRIs instead of prevention.

In vivo studies

For mouse and rat model, 10^5 colony-forming unit (CFU) bacterial suspension is often injected into the tibia bone marrow and fixed with different material steel pins [64, 118–120] Rat tibia implantation with bacterial infection[121] can be initiated by inoculation of a bacterial suspension at the site of implantation [122] or the use of a pre-colonized implant1. Mixed-models, involving the use of both a pre-colonized implant and a bacterial suspension [123], were reported to reproduce the clinical use of an infected implant and contaminated washing solutions at surgery, respectively. One limitation of the mixed models was the difficulty in distinguishing the biofilm formed on the implant from that of the inoculated bacterial suspension. Previous studies showed that inoculation of between 10^2 and 10^6 CFU of *S. aureus* showed similar histological changes [124, 125]. Results from in vivo were similar to in vitro demonstrating that biofilm was found on the implant surface on day 1 and then robustly proliferate on day 3, persisting until day 7. Biofilm formation was steady at 40% covering on day 14 [35]. Layer-by-layer (LBL) coatings were designed using the electrostatic multilayer assembly to get a programmable release [49], which was able to allow release antibiotics contained in upper layers in early stage that prevented the formation of biofilm followed by sustained antibiotics release in lower layers above MIC for 3–4 weeks [118]. These kinds of coatings provide two kinds of releasing curve to overcome drug deficiency during slow releasing. Beside antibiotics coatings, lysostaphin has been coated on the titanium implants and tested in a mouse model. Bacterial growth was almost totally inhibited, and a successful osseous healing was observed with lysostaphin-coated implants [119]. As mentioned earlier, ionic silver was immobilized on implant with hexaphosphate chelation by low heat immersion process. In mouse osteomyelitis model, there was no detectable bacterial presence 3 weeks after inoculation with *S. aureus* without burst releasing [107]. Gentamicin coating on titanium implants with gentamicin-sodiumdodecylsulfate (SDS) and tannic acid demonstrated a high preventive effect on IRIs, which showed successful rapid osseointegration [64]. The rapid osseointegration is necessary which meant repairing completed. Gentamicin palmitate coating also significantly reduced IRIs on the implants as well as systemic inflammation [120]. PLLA/β-TCP-coated implants loading with vancomycin presented favorable controlling IRIs and advancing bone osseointegration for 6 week [68].

Rabbit osteomyelitis model has been widely used for the evaluation of the antibacterial effect. Before fixed with different material steel pins, 10^6–10^8 CFU bacterial suspension is injected into the tibia bone marrow [126–128]. Polymer-Lipid Encapsulation MatriX (PLEX)-doxycycline-coated implants successfully avoided the occurrence of IRIs, even when rabbits were inoculation with a doxy-resistance strain [126]. The chitosan-calcium sulfate coating was reported to improve the therapeutic and preventive outcome of IRIs by prolonging the period of high releasing concentrations of antibiotic [127]. Ti$_6$Al$_4$V pin coated vancomycin–chitosan/HA [74] and phosphatidylcholine [128] reached the similar results for the prophylaxis and therapy of IRIs. Local antibiotics release system can be easily used in surgery for IRIs by inhibiting biofilm biofilms formation on the implant surface [74, 128]. The abovementioned coating strategies are based on the traditional user-friendly technology and have some limitations in the release curve. While LBL formation by the deposition of hydrolytically poly (b-amino ester), poly (acrylic acid), and gentamicin were constructed without pre-modification. Interestingly, a burst-release peak of drug was over several days and followed by stable continuous zero-order release for weeks by hydrolytic erosion [63].

There are relatively few studies reported in using large size (dogs, miniature pigs, goat) animal models. Tran et al. created a titanium oxide combined with siloxane polymer coating doped with silver on intramedullary nails by metal-organic methods and tested in a goat osteomyelitis model with fracture. The tibia shaft fractures were created followed by the injection of 2×10^4 CFU bacterial suspension in the osteotomy site. Then, a silver coated intramedullary nail was inserted for fixation. 5 weeks after fixation, the cured goat can walk by all four limbs without infection compared to the unwilling walking control, which suggested that the coated intramedullary implant as local antimicrobial releasing system for IRIs

was feasible and effective [102]. In this research, the injection of bacterial suspension is low. Salgado CJ et al. established a model of tibial osteomyelitis by the injection of 4×10^9 CFU bacterial suspension into osteotomy site [129]. However, there is lack of evidence to make sure the concentration of bacterial suspension for large size animal models.

Clinical studies

Until now, large randomized and multicenter clinical studies using antibacterial coating for the prevention of IRI were hard to be executed, because of the diversity of anti-infective coatings and the specificity of the manufacturing processes. Expert Tibia Nail (ETN) PROtect™ coated with a biodegradable gentamicin-laden polymer was used for IRIs. When it was used for the prophylaxis of osteomyelitis, no deep infections were observed after the placement of the gentamicin-coated nail and no side effects were reported that were linked to the implant coating [65, 130]. Conway et al. used antibiotic cement-coated (ACC) rods for the control of IRIs by providing both the mechanical stability and local delivery of antibiotics. In this research, 60% of the patients were cured after the first procedure using ACC for infected arthrodesis and infected non-union and gets better functional rehabilitation. At last follow-up, 5 patients need amputation, illustrating a limb salvage rate of 105/110 (95%) [131]. In the operating room Thonse et al. has used interlocking intramedullary nails coated with antibiotic cements before implantation. They found that the infection was well controlled in 95%(19/20) of treated patients, while the rest 1 patient had a union with infection and underwent an amputation unfortunately [132]. In a prospective, non-randomized case series, Fuchs et al. investigated the outcomes of 21 patients underwent surgical treatment with the gentamicin-loaded coating of an implant (UTN PROtect), and no implant-related infections occurred [133]. A 17-year-old man with grade IIIc tibial fractures was also treated by UTN-PROtect and has been successfully limb salvaged instead of prolonged external fixation or amputation which were the standard treatment [66]. Silver coated on the implant surface (Mutars® tumor endoprosthesis (Implantcast, Buxtehude, Germany)) reduced the infection rate from 17.6 to 5.9% in patients with bone sarcoma [134]. Knee arthrodesis nail based on Mutars® technology was successful in eradicating infection [135]. A case control study was conducted to examine the effect of silver-coated coatings, which showed the post-operative infection rate was 11.8% compared with 22.4% for the control group [136]. However, a report showed that local argyria occurred by Mutars® tumor endoprosthesis though the length of the implant did not influence the development of local argyria [137]. Implants coated with iodine can be effective for preventing and treating IRIs. Two case series indicated that the rate of preventing or treating IRIs was over 95% with cytotoxicity and adverse effects [109, 110]. A summary of above mentioned clinical studies was listed in Table 1. The evidence of the research was weak because of the number and design of cases although kinds of coatings showed excellent effective for preventing and treating IRIs.

Conclusion

Prevention is better and more important than treatment for IRIs. The characteristics of time- and dose-dependence of biofilm formation require a more constant and sustained antibiotics release from implant coatings. Surface coating as one of implant surface fabrication approaches has been extensively investigated for the purpose of preventing and treating IRIs by either local antibiotics eluting or forming an antibacterial surface to resist the biofilm formation. A desired antibacterial implant coating is expected to enhance the adhesion and growth of host cells, while inhibiting bacterial adhesion and biofilm formation, so that host cells can be the winner in the "race to surface." The formation of biofilm and antibiotic resistance are time- and dose-dependent, so that the antibacterial effect of coating should be sustained and constant at effective concentration at least for 4 weeks with a short-term releasing peak at 4–7 days. According to the characteristic of biofilms, layer by layer coating was more appropriate than monolayer coating for IRIs prevention.

S. aureus is one of the leading pathogens involved in IRIs [138]. As shown in Tande et al.'s [139] study that summarized the microbiological results of 2400 patients with IRIs, around 60% of IRIs was caused by S. aureus. Patients with S. aureus IRIs frequently have multiple medical comorbidities [140], such as diabetes (30 to 40%) [141] and rheumatoid arthritis (10 to 20%) [142]. Gentamicin and vancomycin are commonly used antibiotics for local drug eluting. For many years, antibiotic (gentamicin and vancomycin)-impregnated PMMA bone cement has been widely used to prevent IRIs [47]. Though PMMA cement is mechanically strong, the therapeutic efficacy of this treatment was questioned in recent studies. Major problems with antibiotic-loaded cements are their burst release and limited release of embedded antibiotics because of the diffusion through surface roughness, superficial pores, and surface erosion [46, 59]. It is estimated that over 90% of loaded antibiotics are retained within the PMMA cement [58]. Regarding the IRIs prevention, the polymers hydrogel coating significantly extended the antibiotics release. The hydrogels release the drug steadily through the crosslinking structure [78–81]. Drug release is closely related to gel degradation through chemical bonds or ionic bonds [82–85]. The silver or silver ion coating seems to be the best way of prevention because of its broad antibacterial spectrum, a stable time- and dose-releasing effect, stable structure. But it has certain side effects on the human body, even if it is partially sustained releasing.

There are great opportunities and challenges to construct an ideal local drug delivery system. It is necessary to further establish a polymer system that has appropriate mechanical

Table 1 Published clinical data of different coatings

Authors	Implant	Coating technology	Study type	Evidence level
Moghaddam et al. [65]	Tibia nail (ETN PROtect™)	Gentamicin PLLA with "dip coating process"	Case series	IV
Metsemakers et al. [130]	Tibia nail (ETN PROtect™)	Gentamicin PLLA with "dip coating process"	Case series	IV
Conway et al. [131]	Rods (antibiotic cement-coated)	Tobramycin and vancomycin cement (Biomet Cobalt) with metal molds or silicone tubing	Case series	IV
Thonse et al. [132]	Interlocking intramedullary (antibiotic cement-coated)	Antibiotic powder Interlocking intramedullary wrap-ped by cement (Zimmer, Warsaw, Indiana) with metal molds	Case series	IV
Fuchs et al. [133]	Tibia nail (UTN PROtect)	Gentamicin PLLA with dip coating process	Case series	IV
Raschke et al. [66]	Tibia nail (UTN PROtect)	Gentamicin PLLA with "dip coating process"	Case report	IV
Hardes et al. [134]	Endoprosthesis (Mutars)	Silver with galvanic deposition	Case control study	III
Wilding et al. [135]	Knee arthrodesis nail (Mutars)	Silver with galvanic deposition	Case series	IV
Wafa et al. [136]	Silver-enhanced custom-made endoprostheses	Silver with anodisation of the titanium alloy	Case control study	III
Glehr et al. [137]	Endoprosthesis (Mutars)	Silver with galvanic deposition	Case series	IV
Shirai et al. [109]	Kyocera Limb Salvage System KOBELCO K-MAX	Povidone-iodine electrolyte-based process	Case series	IV
Tsuchiya et al. [110]	Spinal instrumentation, plates, external fixator pins, prostheses, nails, cannulated screw	Povidone-iodine electrolyte-based process	Case series	IV

strength, matrix formation, desired drug-releasing profiles, and is biodegradable in clinical application. Through data generated from many in vivo and in vitro studies were promising, there was lack of clinical trials for further validation. Therefore, future research should be concentrated on the clinical evaluation of polymer systems such as their clinical efficiency and analysis of post-operative surface of coatings. As for functional groups, drugs and agents can be improved in embedding method to achieve an ideal releasing curve, active ingredient, and conventional drug in new use or effective factors loaded.

In short, for modified implants, translational medicine is important. Whether the antibacterial polymer coatings are effective for prevention of IRIs or not needs clinical validation.

Abbreviations

ACC: Antibiotic cement-coated; AFM: Atomic force microscopy; BCP: Biphasic calcium phosphates; CFU: Colony-forming units; CPC: Calcium phosphate cements; CWA: Cell wall-anchored; EPS: Extracellular polymeric substances; ETN: Expert Tibia Nail; FDA: American Food and Drug Administration; HA: Hydroxyapatite; IRIs: Implant related infections; LBL: Layer-by-layer; MBC: Minimal bactericidal concentration; MIC: Minimal inhibitory concentrations; MRSA: Methicillin resistant *Staphylococcus aureus*; NOAEL: No observable adverse effect level; PAA: Poly (acrylic acid); PDLLA: Poly(D,L-lactic acid); PEG: Polyethylene glycol; PEO: Polyethylene oxide; PIA: Polysaccharide intercellular adhesin; PLEX: Polymer-Lipid Encapsulation MatriX; PLLA: Poly(lactic acid); PMMA: Polymethylmethacrylate; PSMs: Phenol-soluble modulins; PVA: Poly (vinyl alcohol); RGD: Arginine-glycine-aspartic acid; SDS: Sodiumdodecylsulfate; SEM: Scanning electron microscope; β-TCP: Beta-tricalciumphosphate

Acknowledgements

We would like to express our sincere thanks to Prof. Changqing Zhang and Shanghai Jiao Tong University Affiliated Sixth People's Hospital who have lent us hands in the course of writing this paper. And thanks for the comments on the amendment of the grammar and the supplement of the content from Prof. Weiping Ren (Department of Biomedical Engineering, Wayne State University College of Engineering, Detroit, MI).

Funding

This project was supported by National Natural Science Foundation of China (81572155).

Authors' contributions

CP and ZZ contributed equally to this work and should be considered as equal first coauthors. CP and ZZ conceived, drafted, and finalized the paper. ZZ and XY contributed to writing and finalizing the manuscript. All authors read and approved the final manuscript.

Competing interests

The authors declare that they have no competing interests.

References

1. Mangram AJ, Horan TC, Pearson ML, Silver LC, Jarvis WR. Guideline for prevention of surgical site infection, 1999. Hospital infection control practices advisory committee. Infect Control Hosp Epidemiol. 1999;20(4):250–78. quiz 79-80
2. Richards JE, Kauffmann RM, Obremskey WT, May AK. Stress-induced hyperglycemia as a risk factor for surgical-site infection in nondiabetic orthopedic trauma patients admitted to the intensive care unit. J Orthop Trauma. 2013;27(1):16–21.
3. Cook GE, Markel DC, Ren W, et al. Infection in orthopaedics. J Orthop Trauma. 2015;29(Suppl 12):S19–23.
4. Edmiston CE, Spencer M, Lewis BD, et al. Reducing the risk of surgical site infections: did we really think SCIP was going to lead us to the promised land? Surg Infect. 2011;12(3):169–77.
5. Cataldo MA, Petrosillo N, Cipriani M, Cauda R, Tacconelli E. Prosthetic joint infection: recent developments in diagnosis and management. J Inf Secur. 2010;61(6):443–8.
6. Williams DL, Haymond BS, Beck JP, et al. In vivo efficacy of a silicone–cationic steroid antimicrobial coating to prevent implant-related infection. Biomaterials. 2012 Nov;33(33):8641–56.
7. Yilmaz C, Colak M, Yilmaz BC, et al. Bacteriophage therapy in implant-related infections: an experimental study. J Bone Joint Surg Am. 2013;95(2):117–25.
8. Drago L, De Vecchi E. Microbiological diagnosis of implant-related infections: scientific evidence and cost/benefit analysis of routine antibiofilm processing. Adv Exp Med Biol. 2017;971:51–67.
9. Lovati AB, Bottagisio M, de Vecchi E, Gallazzi E, Drago L. Animal models of implant-related low-grade infections. A twenty-year review. Adv Exp Med Biol. 2017;971:29–50.
10. Romanò CL, Scarponi S, Gallazzi E, et al. Antibacterial coating of implants in orthopaedics and trauma: a classification proposal in an evolving panorama. J Orthop Surg Res. 2015;10:157.
11. Esteban J, Molina-Manso D, Spiliopoulou I, et al. Biofilm development by clinical isolates of Staphylococcus spp. from retrieved orthopedic prostheses. Acta Orthop. 2010;81(6):674–9.
12. Flemming HC, Wingender J. The biofilm matrix. Nat Rev Microbiol. 2010;8(9): 623–33.
13. Drews J. Drug discovery: a historical perspective. Science. 2000;287(5460): 1960–4.
14. Buchholz HW, Elson RA, Engelbrecht E, et al. Management of deep infection of total hip replacement. J Bone Joint Surg Br. 1981;63-B(3):342–53.
15. Simchi A, Tamjid E, Pishbin F, Boccaccini AR. Recent progress in inorganic and composite coatings with bactericidal capability for orthopaedic applications. Nanomedicine. 2011;7(1):22–39.
16. Vert M, Doi Y, Hellwich KH, et al. Terminology for biorelated polymers and applications (IUPAC Recommendations 2012). Pure Appl Chem. 2014;63(11–12): 377–410.
17. Zhou K, Yu H, Li J, et al. No difference in implant survivorship and clinical outcomes between full-cementless and full-cemented fixation in primary total knee arthroplasty: a systematic review and meta-analysis. Int J Surg. 2018;53:312–9.
18. Qin S, Xu K, Nie B, Ji F, Zhang H. Approaches based on passive and active antibacterial coating on titanium to achieve antibacterial activity. J Biomed Mater Res A. 2018; https://doi.org/10.1002/jbm.a.36413.
19. Gkana EN, Doulgeraki AI, Chorianopoulos NG, Nychas GE. Anti-adhesion and anti-biofilm potential of organosilane nanoparticles against foodborne pathogens. Front Microbiol. 2017;11(8):1295.
20. Merghni A, Bekir K, Kadmi Y, et al. Adhesiveness of opportunistic Staphylococcus aureus to materials used in dental office: in vitro study. Microb Pathog. 2017;103: 129–34.
21. Berlanga M, Guerrero R. Living together in biofilms: the microbial cell factory and its biotechnological implications. Microb Cell Factories. 2016; 15(1):165.
22. Wassmann T, Kreis S, Behr M, Buergers R. The influence of surface texture and wettability on initial bacterial adhesion on titanium and zirconium oxide dental implants. Int J Implant Dent. 2017;3(1):32.
23. Liu P, Zhao Y, Yuan Z, et al. Construction of Zn-incorporated multilayer films to promote osteoblasts growth and reduce bacterial adhesion. Mater Sci Eng C Mater Biol Appl. 2017;75:998–1005.

24. Lorenzetti M, Dogša I, Stošicki T, et al. The influence of surface modification on bacterial adhesion to titanium-based substrates. ACS Appl Mater Interfaces. 2015;7(3):1644–51.

25. Poon CY, Bhushan B. Comparison of surface roughness measurements by stylus profiler, AFM and non-contact profiler. Wear. 1995;190:76–88.

26. Mabboux F, Ponsonnet L, Morrier JJ, Jaffrezic N, Barsotti O. Surface free energy and bacterial retention to saliva-coated dental implant materials—an in vitro study. Colloids Surf B Biointerfaces. 2004;25:199–205.

27. Weerkamp AH, van der Mei HC, Busscher HJ. The surface free energy of oral streptococci after being coated with saliva and its relation to adhesion in the mouth. J Dent Res. 1985;64:1204–10.

28. Verran J, Taylor RL, Lees GC. Bacterial adhesion to inert thermoplastic surfaces. J Mater Sci Mater Med. 1996;7:597.

29. Atefyekta S, Ercan B, Karlsson J, et al. Antimicrobial performance of mesoporous titania thin films: role of pore size, hydrophobicity, and antibiotic release. Int J Nanomedicine. 2016;11:977–90.

30. Grivet M, Morrier JJ, Benay G, Barsotti O. Effect of hydrophobicity on in vitro streptococcal adhesion to dental alloys. J Mater Sci Mater Med. 2000;11: 637–42.

31. Alam F, Balani K. Adhesion force of staphylococcus aureus on various biomaterial surfaces. J Mech Behav Biomed Mater. 2017;65:872–80.

32. Harris LG, Meredith DO, Eschbach L, Richards RG. Staphylococcus aureus adhesion to standard micro-rough and electropolished implant materials. J Mater Sci Mater Med. 2007;18(6):1151–6.

33. Albrektsson T, Wennerberg A. Oral implant surfaces: part 1—review focusing on topographic and chemical properties of different surfaces and in vivo responses to them. Int J Prosthodont. 2004;17:536–43.

34. Daddi Oubekka S, Briandet R, Fontaine-Aupart MP, Steenkeste K. Correlative time-resolved fluorescence microscopy to assess antibiotic diffusion-reaction in biofilms. Antimicrob Agents Chemother. 2012;56(6):3349–58.

35. Nishitani K, Sutipornpalangkul W, de Mesy Bentley KL, et al. Quantifying the natural history of biofilm formation in vivo during the establishment of chronic implant-associated Staphylococcus aureus osteomyelitis in mice to identify critical pathogen and host factors. J Orthop Res. 2015;33(9):1311–9.

36. Brown MR, Allison DG, Gilbert P. Resistance of bacterial biofilms to antibiotics: a growth-rate related effect? J Antimicrob Chemother. 1988; 22(6):777–80.

37. Foster TJ, Geoghegan JA, Ganesh VK, Höök M. Adhesion, invasion and evasion: the many functions of the surface proteins of Staphylococcus aureus. Nat Rev Microbiol. 2014;12(1):49–62.

38. Moormeier DE, Bayles KW. Staphylococcus aureus biofilm: a complex developmental organism. Mol Microbiol. 2017;104(3):365–76.

39. Heilmann C, Schweitzer O, Gerke C, et al. Molecular basis of intercellular adhesion in the biofilm-forming Staphylococcus epidermidis. Mol Microbiol. 1996;20(5):1083–91.

40. Arciola CR, Campoccia D, Ravaioli S, Montanaro L. Polysaccharide intercellular adhesin in biofilm: structural and regulatory aspects. Front Cell Infect Microbiol. 2015;5:7.

41. Le KY, Dastgheyb S, Ho TV, Otto M. Molecular determinants of staphylococcal biofilm dispersal and structuring. Front Cell Infect Microbiol. 2014;4:167.

42. Clarissa P, Waters EM, Rudkin JK, Schaeffer CR, Lohan AJ, Tong P, Loftus BJ, Pier GB, Fey PD, Massey RC. Methicillin resistance alters the biofilm phenotype and attenuates virulence inStaphylococcus aureus device-associated infections. PLoS Pathog. 2012;8(4):e1002626.

43. Sánchez MC, Llama-Palacios A, Fernández E, et al. An in vitro biofilm model associated to dental implants: structural and quantitative analysis of in vitro biofilm formation on different dental implant surfaces. Dent Mater. 2014; 30(10):1161–71.

44. Roehling S, Astasov-Frauenhoffer M, Hauser-Gerspach I, et al. In vitro biofilm formation on titanium and zirconia implant surfaces. J Periodontol. 2017; 88(3):298–307.

45. Jiranek WA, Hanssen AD, Greenwald AS. Antibiotic-loaded bone cement for infection prophylaxis in total joint replacement. J Bone Joint Surg Am. 2006; 88(11):2487–500.

46. Wu T, Zhang Q, Ren W, et al. Controlled release of gentamicin from gelatin/ genipin reinforced beta-tricalcium phosphate scaffold for the treatment of osteomyelitis. J Mater Chem B. 2013;1(26):3304–13.

47. Walenkamp GH, Kleijn LL, de Leeuw M. Osteomyelitis treated with gentamicin-PMMA beads: 100 patients followed for 1-12 years. Acta Orthop Scand. 1998;69(5):518–22.

48. Wei Q, Haag R. Universal polymer coatings and their representative biomedical applications. Mater Horiz. 2015;2(6):567–77.

49. Wei Q, Becherer T, Angioletti-Uberti S, et al. Protein interactions with polymer coatings and biomaterials. Angew Chem Int Ed Engl. 2014;53(31): 8004–31.

50. Boles BR, Thoendel M, Singh PK. Self-generated diversity produces "insurance effects" in biofilm communities. Proc Natl Acad Sci U S A. 2004; 101(47):16630–5.

51. Sanchez-Gomez S, Ferrer-Espada R, Stewart PS, et al. Antimicrobial activity of synthetic cationic peptides and lipopeptides derived from human lactoferricin against Pseudomonas aeruginosa planktonic cultures and biofilms. BMC Microbiol. 2015;15:137.

52. Davies JA, Harrison JJ, Marques LL, et al. The GacS sensor kinase controls phenotypic reversion of small colony variants isolated from biofilms of Pseudomonas aeruginosa PA14. FEMS Microbiol Ecol. 2007;59(1):32–46.

53. Harrison JJ, Ceri H, Turner RJ. Multimetal resistance and tolerance in microbial biofilms. Nat Rev Microbiol. 2007;5(12):928–38.

54. Maisonneuve E, Gerdes K. Molecular mechanisms underlying bacterial persisters. Cell. 2014;157(3):539–48.

55. Benoit MA, Mousset B, Delloye C, Bouillet R, Gillard J. Antibiotic-loaded plaster of Paris implants coated with poly lactide-co-glycolide as a controlled release delivery system for the treatment of bone infections. Int Orthop. 1997;21(6): 403–8.

56. Webb JC, Spencer RF. The role of polymethylmethacrylate bone cement in modern orthopaedic surgery. J Bone Joint Surg Br. 2007;89(7):851.

57. Zilberman M, Elsner JJ. Antibiotic-eluting medical devices for various applications. J Control Release. 2008;130(3):202–15.

58. Zhou Z, Seta J, Markel DC, et al. Release of vancomycin and tobramycin from polymethylmethacrylate cements impregnated with calcium polyphosphate hydrogel. J Biomed Mater Res B Appl Biomater. 2017; https://doi.org/10.1002/jbm.b.34063.

59. Wu TY, Zhou ZB, He ZW, et al. Reinforcement of a new calcium phosphate cement with RGD-chitosan-fiber. J Biomed Mater Res A. 2014;102(1):68–75.

60. Bohner M, Gbureck U, Barralet JE. Technological issues for the development of more efficient calcium phosphate bone cements: a critical assessment. Biomaterials. 2005;26(33):6423–9.

61. Wu T, Hua X, He Z, et al. The bactericidal and biocompatible characteristics of reinforced calcium phosphate cements. Biomed Mater. 2012;7(4):045003.

62. Chen WC, Lin JH, Ju CP. Transmission electron microscopic study on setting mechanism of tetracalcium phosphate/dicalcium phosphate anhydrous-based calcium phosphate cement. J Biomed Mater Res A. 2003;64(4):664–71.

63. Moskowitz JS, Blaisse MR, Samuel RE, et al. The effectiveness of the controlled release of gentamicin from polyelectrolyte multilayers in the treatment of Staphylococcus aureus infection in a rabbit bone model. Biomaterials. 2010;31(23):6019–30.

64. Diefenbeck M, Schrader C, Gras F, et al. Gentamicin coating of plasma chemical oxidized titanium alloy prevents implant-related osteomyelitis in rats. Biomaterials. 2016;101:156–64.

65. Moghaddam A, Graeser V, Westhauser F, et al. Patients' safety: is there a systemic release of gentamicin by gentamicin-coated tibia nails in clinical use? Ther Clin Risk Manag. 2016;12:1387–93.

66. Raschke M, Vordemvenne T, Fuchs T. Limb salvage or amputation? The use of a gentamicin coated nail in a severe, grade IIIc tibia fracture. Eur J Trauma Emerg Surg. 2010;36(6):605–8.

67. Kankilic B, Bayramli E, Kilic E, Dağdeviren S, Korkusuz F. Vancomycin containing PLLA/β-TCP controls MRSA in vitro. Clin Orthop Relat R. 2011;469(11):3222–8.

68. Kankilic B, Bilgic E, Korkusuz P, Korkusuz F. Vancomycin containing PLLA/ beta-TCP controls experimental osteomyelitis in vivo. J Orthop Surg Res. 2014;9:114.

69. Baskar K, Anusuya T, Devanand Venkatasubbu G. Mechanistic investigation on microbial toxicity of nano hydroxyapatite on implant associated pathogens. Mater Sci Eng C Mater Biol Appl. 2017;73:8–14.

70. Uskokovic V, Desai TA. In vitro analysis of nanoparticulate hydroxyapatite/chitosan composites as potential drug delivery platforms for the sustained release of antibiotics in the treatment of osteomyelitis. J Pharm Sci. 2014;103(2):567–79.

71. Xie XH, Yu XW, Zeng SX, et al. Enhanced osteointegration of orthopaedic implant gradient coating composed of bioactive glass and nanohydroxyapatite. J Mater Sci Mater Med. 2010;21(7):2165–73.

72. Xiu P, Jia Z, Lv J, et al. Hierarchical micropore/nanorod apatite hybrids in-situ grown from 3-D printed macroporous Ti6Al4V implants with improved bioactivity and osseointegration. J Mater Sci Technol. 2017;2:179–86.

73. Shah FA, Trobos M, Thomsen P, Palmquist A. Commercially pure titanium (cp-Ti) versus titanium alloy (Ti$_6$Al$_4$V) materials as bone anchored implants—is one truly better than the other? Mater Sci Eng C Mater Biol Appl. 2016;62:960–6.

74. Yang CC, Lin CC, Liao JW, Yen SK. Vancomycin–chitosan composite deposited on post porous hydroxyapatite coated Ti6Al4V implant for drug controlled release. Mater Sci Eng C Mater Biol Appl. 2013;33(4):2203–12.

75. Dorozhkin SV. Biphasic, triphasic and multiphasic calcium orthophosphates. Acta Biomater. 2012;8(3):963–77.

76. Polak SJ, Levengood SK, Wheeler MB, et al. Analysis of the roles of microporosity and BMP-2 on multiple measures of bone regeneration and healing in calcium phosphate scaffolds. Acta Biomater. 2011;7(4):1760–71.

77. Li X, Wei J, Aifantis KE, et al. Current investigations into magnetic nanoparticles for biomedical applications. J Biomed Mater Res A. 2016;104(5):1285–96.

78. Razavi M, Fathi M, Savabi O, Vashaee D, Tayebi L. In vivo study of nanostructured akermanite/PEO coating on biodegradable magnesium alloy for biomedical applications. J Biomed Mater Res A. 2015;103(5):1798–808.

79. Oh S, Moon KS, Lee SH. Effect of RGD peptide-coated TiO2 nanotubes on the attachment, proliferation, and functionality of bone-related cells. J Nanomater. 2013;2013(13):125–8.

80. Marchesan S, Qu Y, Waddington LJ, et al. Self-assembly of ciprofloxacin and a tripeptide into an antimicrobial nanostructured hydrogel. Biomaterials. 2013;34(14):3678–87.

81. Chang CH, Lin YH, Yeh CL, et al. Nanoparticles incorporated in pH-sensitive hydrogels as amoxicillin delivery for eradication of helicobacter pylori. Biomacromolecules. 2010;11(1):133.

82. Li H, Yang J, Hu X, et al. Superabsorbent polysaccharide hydrogels based on pullulan derivate as antibacterial release wound dressing. J Biomed Mater Res A. 2011;98(1):31.

83. Rabea EI, Badawy ET, Stevens CV, Smagghe G, Steurbaut W. Chitosan as antimicrobial agent: applications and mode of action. Biomacromolecules. 2015;4(6):1457.

84. Xiao B, Wan Y, Zhao M, Liu Y, Zhang S. Preparation and characterization of antimicrobial chitosan-N-arginine with different degrees of substitution. Carbohydr Polym. 2011;83(1):144–50.

85. Hashemi DA, Mirzadeh H, Imani M, Samadi N. Chitosan/polyethylene glycol fumarate blend film: physical and antibacterial properties. Carbohydr Polym. 2013;92(1):48–56.

86. Dai T, Tanaka M, Huang YY, Hamblin MR. Chitosan preparations for wounds and burns: antimicrobial and wound-healing effects. Expert Rev Anti-Infe. 2011;9(7):857.

87. Yan L, Kazuki F, Coady DJ, et al. Broad-spectrum antimicrobial and biofilm-disrupting hydrogels: stereocomplex-driven supramolecular assemblies. Angew Chem. 2013;52(2):674.

88. Guillaume O, Garric X, Lavigne JP, Van DBH, Coudane J. Multilayer, degradable coating as a carrier for the sustained release of antibiotics: preparation and antimicrobial efficacy in vitro. J Control Release. 2012;162(3):492–501.

89. Tang Y, Zhao Y, Wang H, et al. Layer-by-layer assembly of antibacterial coating on interbonded 3D fibrous scaffolds and its cytocompatibility assessment. J Biomed Mater Res A. 2012;100A(8):2071–8.

90. Qu H, Knabe C, Burke M, et al. Bactericidal micron-thin sol-gel films prevent pin tract and periprosthetic infection. Mil Med. 2014;179(8 Suppl):29–33.

91. Lemire JA, Harrison JJ, Turner RJ. Antimicrobial activity of metals: mechanisms, molecular targets and applications. Nat Rev Microbiol. 2013;11(6):371–84.

92. Feng QL, Wu J, Chen GQ, et al. A mechanistic study of the antibacterial effect of silver ions on Escherichia coli and Staphylococcus aureus. J Biomed Mater Res. 2015;52(4):662–8.

93. Chen W, Oh S, Ong AP, et al. Antibacterial and osteogenic properties of silver-containing hydroxyapatite coatings produced using a sol gel process. J Biomed Mater Res A. 2010;82A(4):899–906.

94. Zheng Z, Yin W, Zara JN, et al. The use of BMP-2 coupled - nanosilver-PLGA composite grafts to induce bone repair in grossly infected segmental defects. Biomaterials. 2010;31(35):9293–300.

95. Chernousova S, Epple M. Silver as antibacterial agent: ion, nanoparticle, and metal. Angew Chem Int Ed Engl. 2013;52(6):1636–53.

96. Mijnendonckx K, Leys N, Mahillon J, Silver S, Houdt RV. Antimicrobial silver: uses, toxicity and potential for resistance. Biometals. 2013;26(4):609.

97. Harrasser N, Gorkotte J, Obermeier A, et al. A new model of implant-related osteomyelitis in the metaphysis of rat tibiae. BMC Musculoskel Dis. 2016;17(1):1–11.

98. Agarwal A, Weis TL, Schurr MJ, et al. Surfaces modified with nanometer-thick silver-impregnated polymeric films that kill bacteria but support growth of mammalian cells. Biomaterials. 2010;31(4):680–90.

99. Bai X, Sandukas S, Appleford M, Ong JL, Rabiei A. Antibacterial effect and cytotoxicity of Ag-doped functionally graded hydroxyapatite coatings. J Biomed Mater Res B Appl Biomater. 2012;100(2):553–61.

100. Singh A, Dar MY, Joshi B, et al. Phytofabrication of silver nanoparticles: novel drug to overcome hepatocellular ailments. Toxicol Rep. 2018;5:333–42.

101. Dakal TC, Kumar A, Majumdar RS, Yadav V. Mechanistic basis of antimicrobial actions of silver nanoparticles. Front Microbiol. 2016;7:1831.

102. Tran N, Tran PA, Jarrell JD, et al. In vivo caprine model for osteomyelitis and evaluation of biofilm-resistant intramedullary nails. Biomed Res Int. 2013;2013:674378.

103. Kim YS, Song MY, Park JD. Subchronic oral toxicity of silver nanoparticles. Part Fibre Toxicol. 2010;7:20. https://doi.org/10.1186/1743-8977-7-20.

104. Nandi SK, Shivaram A, Bose S, Bandyopadhyay A. Silver nanoparticle deposited implants to treat osteomyelitis. J Biomed Mater Res B Appl Biomater. 2018;106(3):1073–83.

105. Kundu B, Nandi SK, Roy S, et al. Systematic approach to treat chronic osteomyelitis through ceftriaxone–sulbactam impregnated porous β-tri calcium phosphate localized delivery system. Ceram Int. 2012;38:1533–48.

106. Zhao J, Feng HJ, Tang HQ, Zheng JH. Bactericidal and corrosive properties of silver implanted TiN thin films coated on AISI317 stainless steel. Surf Coat Tech. 2007;201(9):5676–9.

107. Funao H, Nagai S, Sasaki A, et al. A novel hydroxyapatite film coated with ionic silver via inositol hexaphosphate chelation prevents implant-associated infection. Sci Rep. 2016;6:23238.

108. Coester LM, Nepola JV, Allen J, Marsh JL. The effects of silver coated external fixation pins. Iowa Orthop J. 2006;26:48–53.

109. Shirai T, Tsuchiya H, Nishida H, et al. Antimicrobial megaprostheses supported with iodine. J Biomater Appl. 2014;29(4):617–23.

110. Tsuchiya H, Shirai T, Nishida H, et al. Innovative antimicrobial coating of titanium implants with iodine. J Orthop Sci. 2012;17(5):595–604.

111. Zhou Z, Xu Z, Wang F, et al. New strategy to rescue the inhibition of osteogenesis of human bone marrow-derived mesenchymal stem cells under oxidative stress: combination of vitamin C and graphene foams. Oncotarget. 2016;7(44):71998–2010.

112. Back DA, Bormann N, Calafi A, et al. Testing of antibiotic releasing implant coatings to fight bacteria in combat-associated osteomyelitis - an in-vitro study. Int Orthop. 2016;40(5):1039–47.

113. Bastari K, Arshath M, Ng ZH, et al. A controlled release of antibiotics from calcium phosphate-coated poly(lactic-co-glycolic acid) particles and their in vitro efficacy against Staphylococcus aureus biofilm. J Mater Sci Mater Med. 2014;25(3):747–57.

114. Vester H, Wildemann B, Schmidmaier G, Stockle U, Lucke M. Gentamycin delivered from a PDLLA coating of metallic implants: in vivo and in vitro characterisation for local prophylaxis of implant-related osteomyelitis. Injury. 2010;41(10):1053–9.

115. Hickok NJ, Shapiro IM. Immobilized antibiotics to prevent orthopaedic implant infections ☆. Adv Drug Deliv Rev. 2012;64(12):1165–76.

116. Jr VA, Adams CS, Parvizi J, et al. The inhibition of Staphylococcus epidermidis biofilm formation by vancomycin-modified titanium alloy and implications for the treatment of periprosthetic infection. Biomaterials. 2008;29(35):4684–90.

117. Héquet A, Humblot V, Berjeaud JM, Pradier CM. Optimized grafting of antimicrobial peptides on stainless steel surface and biofilm resistance tests. Colloid Surfaces B. 2011;84(2):301–9.

118. Min J, Choi KY, Dreaden EC, et al. Designer dual therapy nanolayered implant coatings eradicate biofilms and accelerate bone tissue repair. ACS Nano. 2016;10(4):4441–50.

119. Windolf CD, Logters T, Scholz M, Windolf J, Flohe S. Lysostaphin-coated titan-implants preventing localized osteitis by Staphylococcus aureus in a mouse model. PLoS One. 2014;9(12):e115940.

120. Folsch C, Federmann M, Kuehn KD, et al. Coating with a novel gentamicinpalmitate formulation prevents implant-associated osteomyelitis induced by methicillin-susceptible Staphylococcus aureus in a rat model. Int Orthop. 2015;39(5):981–8.

121. Monzón M, García-Alvarez F, Laclériga A, et al. A simple infection model using pre-colonized implants to reproduce rat chronic Staphylococcus

aureus osteomyelitis and study antibiotic treatment. J Orthop Res. 2001; 19(5):820–6.

122. Power ME, Olson ME, Domingue PA, Costerton JW. A rat model of Staphylococcus aureus chronic osteomyelitis that provides a suitable system for studying the human infection. J Med Microbiol. 1990;33(3):189–98.

123. Gracia E, Laclériga A, Monzón M, et al. Application of a rat osteomyelitis model to compare in vivo and in vitro the antibiotic efficacy against bacteria with high capacity to form biofilms. J Surg Res. 1998;79(2):146–53.

124. Lucke M, Schmidmaier G, Sadoni S, et al. A new model of implant-related osteomyelitis in rats. J Biomed Mater Res B Appl Biomater. 2003;67(1):593–602.

125. Ren W, Muzik O, Jackson N, et al. Differentiation of septic and aseptic loosening by PET with both 11C-PK11195 and 18F-FDG in rat models. Nucl Med Commun. 2012;33(7):747–56.

126. Metsemakers WJ, Emanuel N, Cohen O, et al. A doxycycline-loaded polymer-lipid encapsulation matrix coating for the prevention of implant-related osteomyelitis due to doxycycline-resistant methicillin-resistant Staphylococcus aureus. J Control Release. 2015;209:47–56.

127. Beenken KE, Smith JK, Skinner RA, et al. Chitosan coating to enhance the therapeutic efficacy of calcium sulfate-based antibiotic therapy in the treatment of chronic osteomyelitis. J Biomater Appl. 2014;29(4): 514–23.

128. Jennings JA, Beenken KE, Skinner RA, et al. Antibiotic-loaded phosphatidylcholine inhibits staphylococcal bone infection. World J Orthop. 2016;7(8):467–74.

129. Salgado CJ, Jamali AA, Mardini S, Buchanan K, Veit B. A model for chronic osteomyelitis using Staphylococcus aureus in goats. Clin Orthop Relat Res. 2005;436:246–50.

130. Metsemakers WJ, Reul M, Nijs S. The use of gentamicin-coated nails in complex open tibia fracture and revision cases: a retrospective analysis of a single Centre case series and review of the literature. Injury. 2015;46(12): 2433–7.

131. Conway J, Mansour J, Kotze K, Specht S, Shabtai L. Antibiotic cement-coated rods: an effective treatment for infected long bones and prosthetic joint nonunions. Bone Joint J. 2014;96-b(10):1349–54.

132. Thonse R, Conway J. Antibiotic cement-coated interlocking nail for the treatment of infected nonunions and segmental bone defects. J Orthop Traum. 2007;21(4):258–68.

133. Fuchs T, Stange R, Schmidmaier G, Raschke MJ. The use of gentamicin-coated nails in the tibia: preliminary results of a prospective study. Arch Orthop Trauma Surg. 2011;131(10):1419–25.

134. Hardes J, von Eiff C, Streitbuerger A, et al. Reduction of periprosthetic infection with silver-coated megaprostheses in patients with bone sarcoma. J Surg Oncol. 2010;101(5):389–95.

135. Wilding CP, Cooper GA, Freeman AK, Parry MC, Jeys L. Can a silver-coated arthrodesis implant provide a viable alternative to above knee amputation in the unsalvageable, infected total knee arthroplasty? J Arthroplast. 2016; 31(11):2542–7.

136. Wafa H, Grimer RJ, Reddy K, Jeys L, Abudu A, Carter SR, Tillman RM. Retrospective evaluation of the incidence of early periprosthetic infection with silver-treated endoprostheses in high-risk patients: case-control study. Bone Joint J. 2015;97-B(2):252–7.

137. Glehr M, Leithner A, Friesenbichler J, et al. Argyria following the use of silver-coated megaprostheses: no association between the development of local argyria and elevated silver levels. Bone Joint J. 2013;95-B(7): 988–92.

138. Pulido L, Ghanem E, Joshi A, Purtill JJ, Parvizi J, et al. Periprosthetic joint infection: the incidence, timing, and predisposing factors. Clin Orthop Relat Res. 2008;466(7):1710–5.

139. Tande AJ, Patel R. Prosthetic joint infection. Clin Microbiol Rev. 2014;27(2): 302–45.

140. Sendi P, Banderet F, Graber P, Zimmerli W. Clinical comparison between exogenous and haematogenous periprosthetic joint infections caused by Staphylococcus aureus. Clin Microbiol Infect. 2011;17(7):1098–100.

141. Senneville E, Joulie D, Legout L, et al. Outcome and predictors of treatment failure in total hip/knee prosthetic joint infections due to Staphylococcus aureus. Clin Infect Dis. 2011;53(4):334–40.

142. Lora-Tamayo J, Murillo O, Iribarren JA, et al. A large multicenter study of methicillin-susceptible and methicillin-resistant Staphylococcus aureus prosthetic joint infections managed with implant retention. Clin Infect Dis. 2013;56(2):182–94.

18

Reliability and validity of the Spinal Appearance Questionnaire (SAQ) and the Trunk Appearance Perception Scale (TAPS)

Meinald T. Thielsch[1*] ⓘ, Mark Wetterkamp[2], Patrick Boertz[1], Georg Gosheger[3] and Tobias L. Schulte[2]

Abstract

Background: The Spinal Appearance Questionnaire (SAQ) and the Trunk Appearance Perception Scale (TAPS) are questionnaires that mostly rely on drawings to assess scoliosis patients' subjective viewpoints on their trunk deformity. Our aim was to perform an in-depth assessment of the psychometric quality of both measures, the SAQ (version 1.1) and TAPS, and compare them to provide practical recommendations.

Methods: Web-based survey study with 255 patients suffering from idiopathic scoliosis (age 30.0 ± 16.7 years, Cobb angle $43.5 \pm 20.9°$) and 189 matched healthy control individuals. Participants answered a broad set of validated questionnaires including SRS 22-r, PHQ-9, PANAS, FKS, WHO-5, BFI-S, and PTQ. We calculated reliability (Cronbach's a, test–retest correlations) as well as factorial, convergent, divergent, concurrent, and discriminant validity.

Results: Reliability was high (Cronbach's $a \geq .86$; test–retest $r \geq .80$), except for test–retest correlation of the SAQ Expectations scale ($r = 0.67$). Both the SAQ and TAPS measures showed clear factor solutions, indicating factorial validity. High correlations with theoretically related measures (e.g., SRS 22-r, overall stress, Cobb angle) indicated convergent validity. Moderate correlations occurred with concurrent criteria such as mood, depression, body dysmorphic disorder, and well-being. The matched-pair analysis revealed strong evidence for discriminant validity (Cohen's $d > 2$ for SAQ total score and TAPS). Subgroup analyses showed that patients with more severe Cobb angles ($\geq 40°$) and those ≥ 46 years of age had significantly worse SAQ and TAPS scores.

Conclusion: We recommend using the TAPS for future clinical workups and research, as it is much shorter and revealed slightly higher psychometric quality in comparison to the SAQ.

Keywords: Idiopathic scoliosis, Body image, Assessment, Psychometric properties, Validation

Background

In recent years, specific scales for the in-depth evaluation of scoliosis patients' subjective viewpoints on their trunk deformity have been developed [1–3]. Most of such scales use questions in the form of statements, yet two specific instruments encompass drawings: The Spinal Appearance Questionnaire (SAQ) and the Trunk Appearance Perception Scale (TAPS), both originating from the Walter Reed Visual Assessment Scale (WRVAS) [4–6].

The WRVAS focuses on patients' appearances, but it fails to ask about patients' satisfaction with their body image [6]. Also, as reported by Bago et al., some of the WRVAS drawings do not directly correlate with the equivalent radiological deformity, and adolescents can have difficulties in comprehending the questionnaire [5, 7]. Therefore, Sanders et al. created the SAQ, which was further modified by Carreon et al. to address these specific limitations [4, 8]. This current modified version of the SAQ, the SAQ v1.1, is the focus of the present study; for readability, we will refer to it only as SAQ (meaning SAQ v.1.1) in the following text. This questionnaire consists of 11 pictorial items and 22 questions regarding patients' expectations. Yet, based on data from 1802 patients, Carreon et al. found that only 14 of the items

* Correspondence: thielsch@uni-muenster.de
[1]Department of Psychology, University of Münster, Fliednerstr. 21, 48149 Münster, Germany
Full list of author information is available at the end of the article

loaded on two factors: The first ten drawings on the so-called Appearance factor and four questions (#12–15) on an Expectations factor. Thus, the authors recommended using only these 14 items. The authors also reported evidence for good reliability (Cronbach's $\alpha \geq 0.88$; test–retest correlation ≥ 0.81) and convergent validity of the SAQ in terms of correlations with the major curve magnitude ($0.324 \leq r \leq 0.361$, $P < 0.01$), and they argued for discriminant validity by showing significant differences between patients receiving different treatments [8]. Yet, they have not yet performed a comparison with healthy controls or a systematic analysis of further convergent criteria (especially psychological criteria and patients' well-being). Furthermore, Mulcahey et al. [7] found that a large percentage of younger patients (between 8 and 16 years old) had difficulties understanding items and illustrations in the child version of the SAQ. Finally, there is an imbalance between the SAQ Appearance and the SAQ Expectation scales, as the Appearance scale makes up about 70% of the total SAQ score. Thus, in psychometric analyses, both subscales should be examined in detail and separately.

The other questionnaire of interest in this study, the TAPS, was created by Bago et al. [5]. It consists of only three drawings illustrating the patient's trunk from three different angles: First, looking at the back of the patient in an upright position; second, looking at the front of the patient from their head towards the pelvis while the patient is bent over towards the observer; and third, looking at the front of the patient in an upright position (this third drawing has a version for females and a version for males) [9]. The authors tested 186 patients and found evidence for good to excellent reliability (Cronbach's $\alpha = 0.89$; test–retest correlation for $n = 35$ patients was 0.92). Furthermore, Bago et al. reported convergent validity in terms of high correlations with the SRS-22 and discriminant validity by finding high correlations between TAPS and the largest curve in terms of Cobb angle (CMAX) [5]. In additional studies, Misterka et al. reported high correlations between TAPS and the main Cobb angle ($r = -0.44$, $P < 0.05$, $n = 36$) [10]; Rigo et al. reported high correlations between TAPS and self-image and pain scales in the SRS-22 ($n = 71$) [11]. Nonetheless, currently, the TAPS has only been assessed with relatively small samples; it is still missing a factor analysis, a comparison to healthy controls, and further systematic analysis of additional convergent criteria.

Matamalas et al. was the first to directly compare the SAQ with the TAPS based on a sample of 80 patients (with Cobb angles $\geq 25°$, mean age 20.3 years). They found nearly identical reliability values (in terms of Cronbach's α) as the original studies, high correlation with the SRS-22 and with radiological magnitude of the curve, and a correlation of $r = -0.80$ between the SAQ

Appearance scale and TAPS. Matamalas et al. favored the TAPS over the SAQ because it is shorter [12]. Still, to validly compare the SAQ and the TAPS, there needs to be a broad prospective cohort study that (a) examines patients of different ages with a wide range of Cobb angles and (b) compares the SAQ (in its version 1.1) with the TAPS using a set of relevant convergent validity criteria, tests the factor structure, and investigates discriminative validity with a matched healthy control sample. Without such a study, it is impossible to further assess the psychometric quality of both instruments and their applicability in practice and research. As a consequence, the first aim of the present study is to assess the reliability and validity of SAQ and TAPS in detail, based on a large clinical sample and a matched healthy control group. The second aim is to compare both instruments in terms of their quality and provide recommendations for their use in research or by physicians.

Materials and methods

Patients were recruited from the Department of Orthopaedics at Münster University Hospital in Münster, Germany, and from the self-help group for scoliosis patients in Germany (*Bundesverband Skoliose-Selbsthilfe e.V.*). The online panel PsyWeb (http://psyweb.uni-muenster.de/) was used to establish a healthy control group. Participation in the study required a minimum age of 14 years and was completely voluntary, anonymous, and without any compensation. Informed consent was obtained from all individual participants included in the study. All participants were instructed at the beginning of the online survey about the purpose and responsible researcher (including contact opportunities), that all data will be used only for academic purposes, and that all participants will remain completely anonymous in this study. We asked for consent twice: (1) On the second and third page of the web survey information, consent forms were given. (2) Additionally, all participants were again asked for consent at the end of the study (thus, after they have seen all relevant questions). At this point, participants had the opportunity to withdraw their consent with a self-exclusion item. Data was acquired through self-reports, and data transfer was encrypted. The ethics committee of the Medical Faculty of the University of Münster approved the study (ref. no. 2014-660-f-S).

All study participants were surveyed about their age, gender, height, weight (body mass index was calculated), average level of back pain during the previous 6 months on the visual analogue scale (VAS), current degree of scoliosis (Cobb angle of the most severe curve), history of scoliosis treatment, and current treatment. Afterwards, participants answered several scoliosis-related questionnaires including the SAQ and TAPS. In the SAQ, the first 11 items consist of standardized drawings showing the varying severity of several components of spinal deformity [8]. There are five response options (1–5) with a higher score indicating a more severe deformity. The questionnaire goes on with 22 questions concerning patients' impressions regarding their appearance with the following answer options (patients choose one): Not true (1), A little true (2), Somewhat true (3), Fairly true (4), and Very true (5). A higher score indicated a worse deformity [8]. The answers to drawings 1 to 10 result in the SAQ Appearance score and questions 12 to 15 in the SAQ Expectations score [8]. Answers to questions/drawings 1 to 10 and 12 to 15 give the SAQ total score (see scoring sheet in Additional file 1: Appendix 1). Sum scores and, for better comparability of the scales, additional mean scores were calculated (Table 1). The TAPS consists of three drawings scored from 1 (greatest deformity) to 5 (smallest deformity), and a mean score is obtained by adding the scores for the three drawings and dividing by 3 (see Additional file 1: Appendix 2). The SAQ Appearance scale and the TAPS are non-verbal. The four verbal items of the SAQ Expectations scale (as well as additional, not analyzed SAQ items and instructions) were systematically translated by a professional medical translator into German and retranslated by a different medical translator into English. Both English versions were compared, and no relevant discrepancies were found. The final German version of the SAQ is attached in Additional file 1: Appendix 1.

Furthermore, all participants answered several validated questionnaires including the Scoliosis Research Society 22-r (SRS 22-r) [1], Patient Health Questionnaire (PHQ-9) [13], Positive and Negative Affect Schedule (PANAS; only the negative scale was applied in this study) [14], Questionnaire on Body Dysmorphic Symptoms (*Fragebogen körperdysmorpher Symptome*, FKS) [15], neuroticism subscale from GSOEP Big Five Inventory (BFI-S) [16], and Perseverative Thinking Questionnaire (PTQ) [17]. The study contained three additional questions created by the authors: (1) Do you think your back's shape will lead to less success in your professional career (job-related worries)? (2) Do you think your back's shape will lead to less satisfaction in your private life (social life-related worries)? (Answer scale for these two questions is Definitely not (1), Rather not (2), Maybe (3), Probably yes (4), and Definitely yes (5)). 3. All in all, how stressed are you by the look of your back (overall stress)? (Answer scale for this question is Not at all (1), A little bit (2), Moderately (3), Very (4), and Extremely (5)). Due to time restrictions, the WHO-5 Well-Being Index (WHO-5) [18] was only added during a retest measure. At the end of each data collection, participants were thanked, had the opportunity to give additional comments, and could exclude their data from subsequent analysis.

The survey was available online between March 2015 and March 2016. Data were partly used in the validation of the German Body Image Disturbance Questionnaire-Scoliosis (G-BIDQ-S) [19] and the German Quality of Life Profile for Spinal Disorders (G-QLPSD) [20] but were never previously analyzed with respect to the SAQ or TAPS. Further, G-BIDQ-S [19] and the G-QLPSD [20] have a different focus (patients' specific worries, life quality), following a completely different measurement approach by using verbal items (instead of drawings in SAQ and TAPS), and the main focus of prior publications was an investigation with respect to the success of a German translation; the present paper focuses on psychometric qualities of SAQ and TAPS in general and a recommendation for future application.

Statistical analyses were performed using SPSS, version 23.

Results

A total number of 677 patients started the questionnaire, yet $n = 149$ dropped out before completing it. Further, we excluded $n = 181$ who reported a spinal deformity other than idiopathic scoliosis, $n = 87$ who reported a Cobb angle below 10°, and $n = 5$ who did not give consent for analyzing their data. Thus, questionnaires of 255 patients (37.67%) were included. An additional 626 individuals were surveyed as healthy controls without scoliosis (of them, $n = 347$ dropped out before completing the questionnaire). This led to a subsample of 189 perfectly matched pairs according to age (full years) and gender (i.e., 74.12% of analyzed patients could be matched).

As the last item of the TAPS showed different drawings for men and women [5], we checked for gender differences in answering behavior before conducting further analysis. In the present study, no significant difference occurred ($M_{men} = 3.03 \pm 1.10$ $M_{women} = 3.14 \pm 0.93$; $T = - 0.67$, df = 253, $P = 0.51$); thus, item 3 was jointly analyzed for both genders. Basic data, demographics, and the results of the SAQ, TAPS, and the other questionnaires are presented in Table 1.

Reliability

Reliability was tested in terms of internal consistency (i.e., Cronbach's α) and test–retest reliability (stability over time, see Table 2). Cronbach's α was 0.93 for the SAQ Appearance scale, 0.86 for SAQ Expectations, and 0.91 for SAQ total score; the TAPS had an internal consistency of 0.86. Thus, both measures are highly consistent.

The retest was conducted about 8 weeks after the primary test (on average 55.44 ± 26.32 days). Participants received SAQ and TAPS again, and at both measurement points, some additional measures not pertinent to the current study. There were no significant differences in the means of the SAQ Expectations scale and SAQ total scores. Yet, the SAQ Appearance scale score was a little lower in

Table 1 Basic data, demographics, and results of questionnaires in the scoliosis group and control group

Parameter	Scoliosis group (n = 255)	Scoliosis subgroup for matched-pair analysis (n = 189)	Controls for matched-pair analysis (n = 189)
Age (years)	30.0 ± 16.7	33.6 ± 17.0	33.6 ± 17.0
Gender			
Male	38	17	17
Female	217	172	172
Weight (kg)	63.1 ± 11.6	64.1 ± 11.9	67.7 ± 14.4[b]
Height (cm)	169.6 ± 9.5	168.7 ± 9.0	169.1 ± 7.1[c]
BMI (kg/m^2)	22.0 ± 4.0	22.6 ± 4.2	23.6 ± 4.7[d]
Cobb angle (°)	43.5 ± 20.9	47.8 ± 20.3	–
Academic level			
Secondary school	13	11	2
Junior high	65	47	18
Technical college entry qualification	25	21	10
High school	83	54	67
University degree	69	56	92
Scoliosis treatment[a]			
Physiotherapy	222	160	0
Brace	182	127	0
Surgery	84	73	0
SAQ total score (range 14, i.e., best, to 70, i.e., worst), sum score (mean, range 1, i.e., best, to 5, i.e., worst)	37.29 ± 10.72 (2.87 ± 0.85)	38.58 ± 11.15 (2.94 ± 0.88)	19.19 ± 5.06 (1.45 ± 0.50)[e]
SAQ Appearance (range 10, i.e., best, to 50, i.e., worst), sum score (mean, range 1, i.e., best, to 5, i.e., worst)	23.93 ± 7.59 (2.39 ± 0.76)	25.15 ± 7.83 (2.52 ± 0.78)	12.66 ± 2.49 (1.27 ± 0.25)[e]
SAQ Expectations (range 4, i.e., best, to 20, i.e., worst), sum score (mean, range 1, i.e., best, to 5, i.e., worst)	13.36 ± 4.86 (3.34 ± 1.21)	13.43 ± 4.87 (3.36 ± 1.22)	6.53 ± 3.43 (1.63 ± 0.86)[e]
TAPS (range 5, i.e., best, to 1, i.e., worst)	3.21 ± 0.89	3.07 ± 0.91	4.81 ± 0.31[e]
SRS 22-r score (range 5, i.e., best, to 1, i.e., worst)			
Overall mean	3.76 ± 0.61		
Function	3.89 ± 0.65		
Pain	3.90 ± 0.90		
Self-image	3.46 ± 0.75		
Mental health	3.77 ± 0.78		
Satisfaction	3.77 ± 0.98		
Job-related worries (range 1, i.e., best, to 5, i.e., worst)	2.42 ± 1.24		
Social life-related worries (range 1, i.e., best, to 5, i.e., worst)	2.75 ± 1.29		
Overall stress (range 1, i.e., best, to 5, i.e., worst)	2.37 ± 1.12		
VAS (pain) (range 0, i.e., best, to 10, i.e., worst)	4.20 ± 2.61		
PANAS (mood) (range 10, i.e., best, to 50, i.e., worst)	13.94 ± 5.41		
PHQ-9 (range 0, i.e., best, to 27, i.e., worst)	4.95 ± 4.63		
FKS (body dysmorphic disorder) (range 0, i.e., best, to 64, i.e., worst)	12.17 ± 9.57		
BFI-S (neuroticism) (range 1, i.e., best, to 7, i.e., worst)	3.71 ± 1.52		
PTQ (negative thinking) (range 0, i.e., best, to 48, i.e., worst)	18.99 ± 12.43		
WHO-5 (well-being) (range 25, i.e., best, to 0, i.e., worst)	13.50 ± 5.75 (n = 133)[f]		

BMI body mass index, *SAQ* Spinal Appearance Questionnaire, *TAPS* Trunk Appearance Perception Scale, *SRS* Scoliosis Research Society, *VAS* visual analogue scale, *PANAS* Positive and Negative Affect Schedule, *PHQ-9* Patient Health Questionnaire, *BFI-S* neuroticism subscale of the Big Five Inventory—short, *FKS Fragebogen körperdysmorpher Symptome*, Questionnaire on Body Dysmorphic Symptoms, *PTQ* Perseverative Thinking Questionnaire, *WHO-5* The WHO-5 Well-Being Index

[a]Binomials included

[b]Difference in weight is significant ($T = -2.63$, df = 376, $P < 0.01$); effect size is rather small ($d = -0.27$)

[c]Difference in height is not significant ($T = -0.50$, df = 374, $P = 0.62$)

[d]Difference in BMI is significant ($T = -2.24$, df = 374, $P = 0.03$); effect size is rather small ($d = -0.23$)

[e]Differences between scoliosis subgroup and controls are significant with $P < .01$, see the "Discriminate validity" section

[f]Only given during at the second time of measurement (retest)

Table 2 Reliability of the SAQ and TAPS

	SAQ Appearance	SAQ Expectations	SAQ total score	TAPS	n
Cronbach's α	0.93	0.86	0.91	0.86	255
Test–retest reliability	0.84**	0.67**	0.80**	0.84**	133

All patients were invited to the retest, $n = 133$ took part; **$P < 0.01$

the retest (T1 25.48 ± 7.87, T2 24.65 ± 8.61; $T = 2.04$, df = 132, $P = 0.04$), and the TAPS score was slightly elevated in the retest (TAPS: T1 3.05 ± 0.93, T2 3.22 ± 0.94; $T = -3.82$, df = 132, $P < 0.01$). The retest reliability was good ($r \geq 0.80$, $P < 0.01$) for both measures, except for the SAQ Expectations scale ($r = 0.67$, $P < 0.01$).

Validity
Factorial validity
An exploratory factor analysis (EFA) was used to investigate the structure of both measures. In the analysis of the SAQ, items 1 to 10 and 12 to 15 were included as proposed by Carreon et al. [8]. A value of 0.91 in the Kaiser–Meyer–Olkin (KMO) test indicated high suitability of the data for factor analysis [21]. Screeplot and factor solution reflected exactly the proposed structure of the SAQ with two factors, explaining 58.13% of variance. Factor loadings were between 0.47 and 0.89 for SAQ Appearance items and between 0.70 and 0.81 for SAQ Expectation items (see Additional file 1: Appendix 3). Both scales were correlated ($r = 0.46$, $P < 0.01$, see Additional file 1: Appendix 4).

In the factor analysis of the TAPS, a value of 0.73 in the Kaiser–Meyer–Olkin (KMO) test indicated a middling suitability of the data for factor analysis [21]. The screeplot clearly indicated one single factor, explaining 67.02% of variance. Factor loadings were between 0.77 and 0.85.

In sum, both measures showed clear factor solutions, which indicate high factorial validity.

Convergent validity
Convergent validity is the extent of agreement among theoretically highly related measures [22]. The SAQ and its two subscales showed significant correlations with each domain in the SRS 22-r, especially with the SRS self-image scale (see Table 3). Thus, a higher (poorer) SAQ score is associated with a lower (poorer) SRS 22-r score. The same pattern occurred for the TAPS (due to coding, correlations were positive).

Furthermore, high correlations were found for both measures with overall stress. In addition, worsening SAQ Appearance and TAPS scores were associated with higher Cobb angles, which was further investigated in a subgroup analysis (see below).

Divergent validity
Divergent validity refers to the degree of disagreement between theoretically unrelated (or less related) constructs

[22]. We expected the SAQ and the TAPS to correlate with the BMI at a low level. Surprisingly, we found relatively high correlations between the BMI and the SAQ Appearance scale ($r = 0.41$), the SAQ total score ($r = 0.34$), and the TAPS ($r = -0.35$; see Table 3).

Concurrent validity
Concurrent validity refers to the ability of a measure to predict a concurrently assessed criterion [22]. The concurrently evaluated criteria (PANAS, PHQ-9, FKS, WHO-5, PTQ, and BFI-S) showed mostly moderate correlations with the SAQ Appearance, Expectations, and total score as well as the TAPS (see Table 3).

Discriminant validity
In the context of the present research, discriminant validity refers to the ability of a measure to distinguish between patients with scoliosis and individuals in a healthy control group. In a matched-pair analysis, the scoliosis group and the control group showed very clear differences in both measures: The average SAQ total score was twice as high in patients (see Table 1; $F = 474.62$, df = 1, 376, $P < 0.01$, $d = 2.24$), and the same applied to the SAQ Appearance scale ($F = 436.72$, df = 1, 376, $P < 0.01$, $d = 2.15$) and the SAQ Expectations scale ($F = 253.69$, df = 1, 376, $P < 0.01$, $d = 1.64$). Likewise, the TAPS score was quite lower (i.e., worse) in patients (see Table 1, $T = -24.78$, df = 231.52, $P < 0.01$, $d = -2.56$). The effect sizes $(d)^1$ were very large for all tested differences between patients and controls. Thus, both instruments are highly capable of distinguishing between scoliosis patients and healthy persons.

Subgroup analysis: Cobb angle and age
A subgroup analysis of patients with Cobb angles of less than 40° and those with $\geq 40°$ revealed significant differences for SAQ and TAPS, but not for the SAQ Expectations scale (see Table 4). Patients were divided into three age groups (14–17 years, $n = 59$; 18–45 years, $n = 130$; and 46 years and older, $n = 66$). The underage patients group as well as the young adults group showed lower (better) SAQ scores; however, the older patients group showed significantly higher (worse) SAQ scores. Answers given on the TAPS revealed a similar pattern.

Discussion
In line with prior research, both instruments showed very good results with respect to reliability in terms of

Table 3 Correlations for convergent, divergent, and concurrent validity

	SAQ Appearance	SAQ Expectations	SAQ total score	TAPS	N
SRS 22-r					
- Overall mean	− 0.49**	− 0.40**	− 0.53**	0.48**	255
- Function	− 0.40**	− 0.20**	− 0.37**	0.40**	255
- Pain	− 0.37**	− 0.24**	− 0.37**	0.36**	255
- Self-image	− 0.53**	− 0.49**	− 0.60**	0.50**	255
- Mental health	− 0.28**	− 0.31**	− 0.34**	0.27**	255
- Satisfaction	− 0.25**	− 0.28**	− 0.31**	0.26**	255
Job-related worries	0.33**	0.31**	0.38**	− 0.33**	255
Social life-related worries	0.26**	0.38**	0.36**	− 0.27**	255
Overall stress	0.51**	0.52**	0.60**	− 0.51**	255
VAS (pain)	0.36**	0.27**	0.38**	− 0.33**	255
Cobb angle	0.55**	0.10	0.44**	− 0.51**	255
BMI	0.41**	0.11	0.34**	− 0.35**	253
PANAS (mood)	0.27**	0.24**	0.30**	− 0.26**	255
PHQ-9 (depression)	0.31**	0.30**	0.35**	− 0.26**	255
FKS (body dysmorphic disorder)	0.26**	0.32**	0.33**	− 0.24**	255
WHO-5 (well-being)	− 0.38**	− 0.24**	− 0.38**	0.33**	133
PTQ (negative thinking)	0.08	0.21**	0.16*	− 0.10	255
BFI-S (neuroticism)	0.16**	0.20**	0.21**	− 0.12*	255

Convergent validation = SRS-22r, job-related worries, social life-related worries, overall stress, VAS, Cobb angle
Divergent validation = BMI
Concurrent validation = PANAS, PHQ-9, FKS, WHO-5, PTQ, BFI-S
*$P < 0.05$, **$P < 0.01$

Cronbach's α [5, 8, 12]. The TAPS showed good test–retest reliability with a correlation of 0.84. The retest was good for the SAQ Appearance scale (0.84) and the SAQ total score (0.80) but was lower for the SAQ Expectation scale (0.67). Similar values were also reached by Carreon et al. (0.81 for the SAQ Appearance scale and 0.89 for the SAQ total score), but better scores were achieved for the SAQ Expectations scale (0.91) [8]. This difference might be explained by the shorter time period of only

2 weeks between both investigations, in comparison to about 8 weeks after the first interrogation in our study. In light of these results, the long-term stability of the SAQ Expectation scale is at least in doubt and below the requirement ($r = 0.7$) for use in practice [23].

Regarding the convergent validity, the drawings in both questionnaires highly correlate with the Cobb angle (SAQ Appearance: $r = 0.55$, TAPS: $r = -0.51$), which was also reported in earlier studies and is a lot higher than

Table 4 Subgroup and age analysis

	SAQ Appearance	SAQ Expectations	SAQ total score	TAPS
Cobb angle 10 to 39° ($n = 133$)	20.62 ± 4.83	12.89 ± 4.75	33.51 ± 8.22	3.57 ± 0.62
Cobb angle ≥ 40° ($n = 122$)	27.54 ± 8.38	13.88 ± 4.94	41.42 ± 11.61	2.81 ± 0.97
Significance of differences in Cobb angle groups	$F = 30.26$, df = 1, 252, $P < 0.01$	$F = 1.11$, df = 1, 252, $P = 0.29$	$F = 8.68$, df = 1, 252, $P < 0.01$	$F = 23.11$, df = 1, 252, $P < 0.01$
Correlations with age	0.58**	0.18**	0.49**	− 0.59**
Age 14 to < 18 years ($n = 59$)	21.20 ± 5.78	13.92 ± 4.68	35.12 ± 8.55	3.57 ± 0.64
Age 18 to 45 years ($n = 130$)	21.35 ± 5.49	12.18 ± 4.81	33.54 ± 8.93	3.48 ± 0.69
Age ≥ 46 years ($n = 66$)	31.44 ± 7.64	15.20 ± 4.50	46.64 ± 10.24	2.35 ± 0.89
Significance of differences in age groups	$F = 40.41$, df = 1, 252, $P < 0.01$	$F = 1.16$, df = 1, 252, $P = 0.28$	$F = 10.89$, df = 1, 252, $P < 0.01$	$F = 44.44$, df = 1, 252, $P < 0.01$

Means and standard deviations of SAQ sum scores and TAPS mean score are presented; for displayed correlations: **$P < 0.01$; F values result from a MANCOVA with Cobb angle as independent variable, age as covariate, and SAQ and TAPS as dependent variables

values found for verbal questionnaires such as the G-BIDQ-S ($r = 0.30$) or G-QLPSD ($r = 0.28$) [12, 19, 20]. The correlation between Cobb angle and both the SAQ Appearance scale and TAPS was even higher than in Carreon et al. (SAQ, $r = 0.36$) and Misterska et al. (TAPS, $r = -0.44$) [8, 10]. Thus, the use of such drawings might reflect the scoliosis perception of patients much better than verbal questions.

There were also high correlations between the SRS 22-r total score and both questionnaires (SAQ total score $r = -0.63$ vs. TAPS $r = 0.48$). The highest correlations were reported between the self-image domain of the SRS and the SAQ Appearance scale ($r = -0.53$) as well as the TAPS ($r = 0.50$). These results match the findings of Carreon et al. (SAQ $r = -0.39$) and Bago et al. (TAPS $r = 0.54$) [5, 8] and could be explained by the fact that both measures are focused on patients' body image. Moreover, the overall stress item showed high correlations with both instruments (SAQ, $r = 0.60$ vs. TAPS, $r = -0.51$), indicating a psychological burden on the patients. The study also revealed evidence for very high discriminant validity: Patients with scoliosis had a significantly higher (worse) SAQ score on both scales as well as for the total score. Similarly, the TAPS score is lower (worse) in patients. This corresponds with earlier findings that patients with scoliosis have a worse body image than healthy controls [19]. Taking everything into account, the SAQ and TAPS showed similar results with regard to various correlations in validation.

The two subgroups of patients with higher and lower Cobb angles (cut-off = 40° according to the international literature, which recommends different treatments for patients below and above 40°) showed similar results on the SAQ Expectations scale. However, patients with more severe deformities had worse scores in the SAQ Appearance scale and the TAPS, which reflects earlier findings in similar studies [10, 12, 19]. Regarding patient age, there seemed to be no relevant difference between underage patients and adults up to the age of 45. However, older scoliosis patients reported worse SAQ and TAPS scores. To date, no studies had been performed concerning this issue; therefore, further research is needed.

With a total number of 255 patients with idiopathic scoliosis, this is the largest collective that has ever answered both the SAQ and the TAPS for the purpose of comparison. Such a sample provides a sound basis for stable estimates of correlations [24]. With regard to factor analysis, most sample size requirements for producing a reliable factor solution were met, although a definitive identification of a multifactorial model might require larger sample sizes [25, 26]. Two further limitations might be considered when interpreting the present study: First, data were acquired via a web-based study relying on self-reports, and no radiographic data for patients were taken into account—as it was most feasible, we only used the main Cobb angle. Second, there might be additional constructs relevant for scoliosis patients' body image and well-being not covered in the present validation of SAQ and TAPS.

Finally, we aimed to answer the question of which instrument—the SAQ or TAPS—should be recommended for clinical or scientific use. For scientific projects, both could be of value. In clinical everyday situations, the number of questionnaires should be limited due to time restrictions and practicability. Based on the present findings, to investigate patients' subjective body image, we clearly recommend using the TAPS. Thus, here, we confirm and extend the results of the comparison study performed by Matamalas et al. [12]. The reasons for our recommendation are that, first, the SAQ Appearance scale and TAPS are highly correlated ($r = 0.85$, $P < 0.01$), but the TAPS only consists of three items vs. the ten items on the SAQ's Appearance scale. Thus, less time is needed to fill out the questionnaire while there is no loss in psychometric quality. Second, as Carreon et al. recommend using only four out of the 22 remaining items of the SAQ [8], using other measures instead of the SAQ Expectations scale seems more efficient and promising. Patient expectations and worries could be better assessed with scales such as the BIDQ-S [2, 19], and scoliosis patients' quality of life could be better assessed with a measure such as the QLPSD [3, 20].

In general, for treating patients in research, combining different measures is useful in an extensive anamnesis. In doing so, patient questionnaires are of high value for refining a medical diagnosis, understanding a patient's needs, and assessing the potential need to offer psychotherapeutic support. For clinical use, a compilation of questionnaires is recommended depending on the goals of the caregiver. As a general recommendation, we suggest applying a combination of the TAPS, BIDQ-S, and SRS-22 or alternatively QLPSD as screening instruments for scoliosis patients about twice a year.

Conclusions

In respect to our first aim, we can state that both instruments show high psychometric qualities; only the stability of the SAQ Expectations scale seems to be impaired. For our second aim, comparing the instruments, we clearly recommend using the TAPS for future clinical workups and research.

Endnotes

[1]According to the guidelines provided by Cohen, standardized mean differences of 0.2, 0.5, and 0.8 and more are considered to represent small, medium, and large effects, respectively [27].

Abbreviations
BFI-S: GSOEP Big Five Inventory; BMI: Body mass index; FKS: Fragebogen körperdysmorpher Symptome [Questionnaire on Body Dysmorphic Symptoms]; G-BIDQ-S: German Body Image Disturbance Questionnaire-Scoliosis; G-QLPSD: German Quality of Life Profile for Spinal Disorders; PANAS: Positive and Negative Affect Schedule; PHQ-9: Patient Health Questionnaire; PTQ: Perseverative Thinking Questionnaire; SAQ: Spinal Appearance Questionnaire; SRS 22-r: Scoliosis Research Society 22-r; TAPS: Trunk Appearance Perception Scale; VAS: Visual analogue scale; WRVAS: Walter Reed Visual Assessment Scale

Acknowledgements
We would like to thank Jan Henrik Terheyden for his support in acquiring patients and Friederike Jansen for her support in sampling and data preparation for analyses. We would also like to thank Dr. Celeste Brennecka for proofreading the manuscript as well as Dr. Michael Robertson and Petra Hölzle for professionally translating the Spinal Appearance Questionnaire from English to German and vice versa.

Funding
We acknowledge support from the Open Access Publication Fund of the University of Muenster.

Authors' contributions
MT conceived, designed and performed the study, contributed materials/analysis tools, analyzed the data, prepared the tables, drafted the work, and revised it critically for important content. MW conceived, designed and performed the study, contributed materials/analysis tools, drafted the work, and revised it critically for important content. PB conceived, designed and performed the study, and contributed materials/analysis tools. GG contributed materials/analysis tools. TS conceived and designed the study, contributed materials/analysis tools, drafted the work, and revised it critically for important content. All authors read and approved the final manuscript.

Consent for publication
The study was performed in a web-based format. Thus, all participants were instructed via the online survey website about the purpose and responsible researcher (including contact opportunities), that all data will be used only for academic purposes, and that all participants will remain completely anonymous in this study. We asked for consent twice: (1) On the second and third page of the web survey information, consent forms were given. Consent forms were draw up in consultation with the ethics committee of the Medical Faculty of the University of Münster and approved for the study by the ethics committee (ref. no. 2014-660-f-S). Forms were stored electronically, as the study was performed in a web-based manner. If needed, English translations of German forms can be provided via the corresponding author. (2) Additionally, all participants were again asked for consent at the end of the study (thus, after they have seen all relevant questions). Participants had the opportunity to withdraw their consent (and consequently delete all of their data) with a self-exclusion item at the end of the study (see the "Materials and methods" section of our manuscript). This question was given automatically and individually.
In line with the standards provided by the German Council for Market and Social Research (see http://rat-marktforschung.de/fileadmin/user_upload/pdf/R05_RDMS.pdf) and according to the German law effective at the time of the study, parental consent was not obtained for participants aged between 14 und 17.

Competing interests
The authors declare that they have no competing interests.

Author details
[1]Department of Psychology, University of Münster, Fliednerstr. 21, 48149 Münster, Germany. [2]St. Josef-Hospital, Ruhr University Bochum, Bochum, Germany. [3]Universitätsklinikum Münster, Münster, Germany.

References
1. Niemeyer T, Schubert C, Halm HF, Herberts T, Leichtle C, Gesicki M. Validity and reliability of an adapted German version of scoliosis research society-22 questionnaire. Spine. 2009;34:818–21.
2. Auerbach JD, Lonner BS, Crerand CE, Shah SA, Flynn JM, Bastrom T, Penn P, Ahn J, Toombs C, Bharucha N, et al. Body image in patients with adolescent idiopathic scoliosis: validation of the body image disturbance questionnaire--scoliosis version. J Bone Joint Surg Am. 2014;96:e61-1–8.
3. Climent JM, Reig A, Sanchez J, Roda C. Construction and validation of a specific quality of life instrument for adolescents with spine deformities. Spine. 1995;20:2006–11.
4. Sanders JO, Harrast JJ, Kuklo TR, Polly DW, Bridwell KH, Diab M, Dormans JP, Drummond DS, Emans JB, Johnston CE, et al. The Spinal Appearance Questionnaire: results of reliability, validity, and responsiveness testing in patients with idiopathic scoliosis. Spine. 2007;32:2719–22.
5. Bago J, Sanchez-Raya J, Perez-Grueso FJS, Climent JM. The Trunk Appearance Perception Scale (TAPS): a new tool to evaluate subjective impression of trunk deformity in patients with idiopathic scoliosis. Scoliosis. 2010;5:6.
6. Sanders JO, Polly DW Jr, Cats-Baril W, Jones J, Lenke LG, O'Brien MF, Stephens Richards B, Sucato DJ. Analysis of patient and parent assessment of deformity in idiopathic scoliosis using the Walter Reed Visual Assessment Scale. Spine. 2003;28:2158–63.
7. Mulcahey MJ, Chafetz RS, Santangelo AM, Costello K, Merenda LA, Calhoun C, Samdani AF, Betz RR. Cognitive testing of the spinal appearance questionnaire with typically developing youth and youth with idiopathic scoliosis. J Pediatr Orthop. 2011;31:661–7.
8. Carreon LY, Sanders JO, Polly DW, Sucato DJ, Parent S, Roy-Beaudry M, Hopkins J, McClung A, Bratcher KR, Diamond BE. Spinal appearance questionnaire: factor analysis, scoring, reliability, and validity testing. Spine. 2011;36:4.
9. Bagó J, Climent JM, Pérez-Grueso FJS, Pellisé F. Outcome instruments to assess scoliosis surgery. Eur Spine J. 22(Suppl 2):195–202.
10. Misterska E, Glowacki M, Latuszewska J, Adamczyk K. Perception of stress level, trunk appearance, body function and mental health in females with adolescent idiopathic scoliosis treated conservatively: a longitudinal analysis. Qual Life Res. 2013;22:1633–45.
11. Rigo M, D'agata E, Jelacic M. Trunk Appearance Perception Scale (TAPS) discrepancy between scoliosis children and their parents influence the SRS-22 secore. Scoliosis. 2012;7:O3.
12. Matamalas A, Bago J, D'Agata E, Pellise F. Body image in idiopathic scoliosis: a comparison study of psychometric properties between four patient-reported outcome instruments. Health Qual Life Outcomes. 2014;12:81.
13. Kroenke K, Spitzer RL, Williams JBW. The PHQ-9: validity of a brief depression severity measure. J Gen Intern Med. 2001;16(9):606–13.
14. Watson D, Clark LA, Tellegen A. Development and validation of brief measures of positive and negative affect. The PANAS scales. J Pers Soc Psychol. 1988;54:1063–70.
15. Buhlmann U, Wilhelm S, Glaesmer H, Brähler E, Rief W. Fragebogen körperdysmorpher Symptome (FKS). Ein Screening-Instrument Verhaltenstherapie. 2009;19:237–42.
16. Schupp J, Gerlitz JY. Big Five Inventory-SOEP (BFI-S). Zusammenstellung sozialwissenschaftlicher Items und Skalen. 2014. https://doi.org/10.6102/zis54.
17. Ehring T, Zetsche U, Weidacker K, Wahl K, Schonfeld S, Ehlers A. The Perseverative Thinking Questionnaire (PTQ): validation of a content-independent measure of repetitive negative thinking. J Behav Ther Exp Psychiatry. 2011;42:225–32.
18. Topp CW, Østergaard SD, Søndergaard S, Bech P. The WHO-5 Well-Being Index: a systematic review of the literature. Psychother Psychosom. 2015;84: 167–76.
19. Wetterkamp M, Thielsch MT, Gosheger G, Boertz P, Terheyden, JH, Schulte TL. German Validation of the BIDQ-S questionnaire on body image disturbance in idiopathic scoliosis. Eur Spine J. 2017;26(2):309–15.

20. Schulte TL, Thielsch MT, Gosheger G, Boertz P, Terheyden JH, Wetterkamp M. German Validation of the Quality of Life Profile for Spinal Disorders (QLPSD). Eur Spine J. 2018;27(1):83–92.

21. Dziuban CD, Shirkey EC. When is a correlation matrix appropriate for factor analysis? Some decision rules. Psychol Bull. 1974;81:358–61.

22. Nunnally JC, Bernstein IH. Psychometric theory. 3rd ed. New York: McGraw-Hill; 1994.

23. Cook DA, Beckman TJ. Current concepts in validity and reliability for psychometric instruments: theory and application. Am J Med. 2006;119:166.e7–166.e16.

24. Schönbrodt FD, Perugini M. At what sample size do correlations stabilize? J Res Pers. 2013;47:609–12.

25. Hirschfeld G, von Brachel R, Thielsch MT. Selecting items for Big Five questionnaires. At what sample size do factor loadings stabilize? J Res Pers. 2014;53:54–63.

26. Beavers AS, Lounsbury JW, Richards JK, Huck SW, Skolits GJ, Esquivel SL. Practical Considerations for Using Exploratory Factor Analysis in Educational Research. Pract Assess Res Eval. 2013;18(6). Available at: https://www.pareonline.net/getvn.asp?v=18&n=6.

27. Cohen J. Statistical power analysis for the behavioral sciences. 2nd ed. Hillsdale: Erlbaum; 1988.

19

Effect of lycopene on titanium implant osseointegration in ovariectomized rats

Xiaojie Li[*] , Wenli Xue, Yong Cao, Yanming Long and Mengsheng Xie

Abstract

Background: Lycopene prevents bone loss in osteopenic models. However, the role of lycopene in the success rate of dental implants under osteopenic conditions remains unknown. The aim of this study was to evaluate whether lycopene prevents delayed implant osseointegration in an ovariectomized (OVX) rat model.

Methods: Thirty female Sprague-Dawley rats were randomly divided into the following groups: OVX with vehicle (OVX group), OVX with lycopene (OVX + lycopene group) and sham-operated with vehicle (sham group). Twelve weeks after ovariectomy or sham operation, titanium implants were placed into the distal metaphysis of the bilateral femurs of each rat. These rats were subsequently gavaged with lycopene (50 mg/kg/day) or vehicle. After 12 weeks of gavage, all rats were sacrificed, and specimens were harvested. Sample osseointegration was evaluated by biomechanical testing, 3D micro-computed tomography (micro-CT) analysis and histomorphometric analysis.

Results: Compared with the OVX group, the OVX + lycopene group showed a 69.3% increase in the maximum push-out force ($p < 0.01$). Micro-CT data for the femurs in the OVX + lycopene group showed significantly higher bone volume, trabecular thickness and less trabecular space than did those in the OVX group. The bone area (BA) around the implant and bone contact (BC) with the implant were increased by 72.3% ($p < 0.01$) and 51.4% ($p < 0.01$) in the OVX + lycopene group, respectively, compared with those in the OVX group. There was no significant difference in the mechanical test, micro-CT scanning and histomorphometric data between the OVX + lycopene and sham groups ($p > 0.05$).

Conclusions: Lycopene improved implant osseointegration, fixation and bone formation under osteopenic conditions, suggesting that lycopene is a promising therapeutic agent to prevent delayed implant osseointegration and bone loss under osteopenic conditions.

Keywords: Osteoporosis, Osseointegration, Implant fixation, Lycopene, Ovariectomized, Biomechanical test

Background

Implant-based treatment has been widely used in the fields of orthopaedics and dentistry. Regarding patient characteristics, aside from smoking and periodontitis as negative risk factors [1], the successful fixation and stability of dental implants depend on the implant site (mandible vs. maxillary) [2, 3] and bone quality and quantity around the implant [4]. Osteoporosis is a systemic skeletal metabolic disease characterized by low bone mass and micro-architectural bone deterioration, with a high risk of fragility fracture [5]. Although osteoporosis is not considered as a risk factor for dental

implant failure [6, 7], initial implant stability can be influenced by both local and skeletal bone densities, and osteoporotic patients need more healing time [8, 9]. Proper implant osseointegration, i.e. direct contact between the implant and surrounding bone, is desired for mechanical fixation of the implant [10]. In a rat model, the quantity and quality of osseointegration remained significantly impaired under osteopenic conditions 12 weeks after implantation, leading to decreased implant fixation [11]. Various therapeutic agents have been investigated and verified to be effective in promoting implant osseointegration in osteopenic bone [12]. Although adverse events are rare among approved osteoporosis treatment agents, in some cases, bisphosphonates and denosumab could cause osteonecrosis of

* Correspondence: d52xiao@126.com
Department of Prosthodontics, College and Hospital of Stomatology, Guangxi Medical University, 10th Shuangyong Road, Nanning 530021, China

the jaw, raloxifene may increase the risks of thrombus and stroke and teriparatide may cause nausea and other side effects [13]. Thus, new safe, cost-effective drugs that can accelerate implant osseointegration under osteoporotic conditions are still in demand.

The bone remodelling process is similar between osseointegration and fracture healing [10]. Some researchers have proposed that oxidative stress and antioxidants might play a role in fracture healing [14, 15]. Immediately after fracture, oxidative stress significantly increases due to severe bone loss and ischaemia [14]. Reactive oxygen species (ROS) can cause cell DNA damage, accumulate in the injury site and have detrimental effects on bone healing [15]. During normal healing, the antioxidants in the body increase correspondingly to scavenge excessive ROS [14]. However, in cases when the antioxidant system is compromised, elevated ROS activity leads to oxidative stress, which inhibits osteogenesis and can reduce bone regenerative capacity [15]. Thus, an imbalance between excessive ROS generation and an insufficient antioxidant defence mechanism makes these fractures difficult to heal. Bednarek-Tupikowksa et al. demonstrated higher oxidative biomarkers and reduce d antioxidative potency in postmenopausal women than in premenopausal women [16]; these findings are associated with compromised bone healing capacity due to osteoporosis. However, antioxidant treatment promoted bone healing in rats with severe bone loss [17]. Furthermore, an antioxidant-based diet prevented bone loss in menopausal women [18], and a case-control study showed that the antioxidant intake score was inversely associated with hip fracture risk in ever-smokers but not in never-smokers [19]. Therefore, antioxidant therapy might be useful in promoting osseointegration under osteoporotic conditions.

Lycopene, a carotenoid found in red fruits and vegetables, is one of the most potent natural antioxidants and has the highest scavenging capacity for singlet oxygen molecules among all carotenoids [20]. Lycopene has been used for decades to prevent chronic diseases [21]. Lycopene exerts its antioxidant effect mainly through activating the antioxidant response element/electrophile response element (ARE) transcription system by disrupting the cytosolic interactions between the major ARE-activating transcription factor, nuclear factor erythroid 2-related factor 2 (Nrf2) and its inhibitor, Kelch-like ECH-associated protein 1 (Keap1) [22]. Recently, Mackinnon et al. showed that a lycopene-restricted diet significantly decreased circulating lycopene and decreased biomarkers of oxidative stress and bone resorption in healthy postmenopausal women [23]. In addition, in a pilot study using a small group of healthy postmenopausal women, the same group showed that lycopene supplementation significantly decreased the detection of oxidative stress markers and a bone resorption marker [24].

These findings suggest that lycopene has a positive effect on bone metabolism by reducing the rate of bone resorption. Interestingly, a prospective cohort study of 946 men and women reported that lycopene intake is inversely associated with the risk of osteoporotic hip fracture [25]. Moreover, lycopene supplementation prevents bone loss and maintains bone strength in ovariectomized (OVX) rats [26]. However, the role of lycopene in implant osseointegration under osteopenic conditions remains unknown.

OVX rats have been widely used as a model of postmenopausal osteoporosis in humans [27]. OVX rats have also been used in many studies on implant osseointegration under osteopenic conditions [12]. Implant osseointegration could be achieved in OVX rats, but according to histomorphometric and functional analysis, less osseointegration occurred in OVX rats than in sham rats within 2–12 weeks [11, 28, 29]. These results indicated that a longer healing time was needed due to compromised healing capacity under osteopenic conditions, which is similar to the implant healing process of humans.

We hypothesized that lycopene prevents delayed implant osseointegration under osteopenic conditions. In our study, we used OVX rats as an osteopenic model and analysed the effect of lycopene on titanium-based implant osseointegration.

Methods

Implant preparation

Sixty titanium cylindrical implants (2.5 mm in diameter and 4 mm in length) were custom-made of TA3 pure titanium (Fox Ti Tech, Shanghai, China). The surfaces of the implants were blasted with aluminium oxide to obtain a rough appearance without any coating. Next, the implants were washed three times with distilled water, sonicated for 10 min in high concentrations of trichloroethylene and ethanol, autoclaved at 134 °C and under 0.205 MPa for 8 min and stored in a drying cabinet.

Animals

Thirty female Sprague-Dawley rats (Animal Centre of Guangxi Medical University), aged 12 weeks old with a weight of 245 ± 7.46 g, were used in this study. Animals were given a standard laboratory diet and tap water and were maintained under climate-controlled conditions (25 °C; 55% relative humidity; 12 h light and 12 h darkness). All procedures followed were in accordance with the ethical standards of Animal Care and Use of Guangxi Medical University. The study protocol was approved by the Animal Experimental Ethical Committee of Guangxi Medical University (ID Number: 201601007).

Ovariectomy and implantation procedures

After 1 week of acclimatisation, 30 rats were randomly divided into the following groups: OVX with vehicle

(OVX group, $n = 10$), OVX with lycopene (OVX + lycopene group, $n = 10$) and sham-operated with vehicle (sham group, $n = 10$). Rats in the OVX group and OVX + lycopene group underwent bilateral ovariectomy following a previously described procedure [30], and ten rats underwent sham surgery (sham group). After surgery, the rats were fed with standard rat chow for 12 weeks.

Twelve weeks after ovariectomy, titanium implants were inserted bilaterally into the distal femur using a previously described procedure [30]. Briefly, the rats were anaesthetized by intraperitoneal injection of 10% chloral hydrate (3.0 ml/kg; Kelon Biosciences, Chengdu, China) and were incised above the knee of the hind limb to expose the knee (Fig. 1a). A channel was drilled from the intercondylar notch to the medullary canal in a longitudinal direction parallel to the long axis of the femur using a straight fissure bur (2.0 mm in diameter) with a speed of 800 rotations per minute (RPM). Cold (4 °C) saline irrigation was applied during the entire drilling procedure. Titanium implants were inserted into the channels with a titanium mallet to a position at which the distal implant surface was approximately 1 mm below the cartilage surface (Fig. 1b, c). The incision was then closed with sutures. For pain control, subcutaneous injection of 5% carprofen (0.3 ml/kg; Vland Biotech, Qingdao, China) was administered for 2 days following the procedure.

Drug intervention

Ardawi et al. [26] reported that lycopene prevented bone loss in OVX rats in a dose-dependent manner. In their study, the highest dosage of the OVX + lycopene group, which was 45 mg/kg/day, showed the best effect on bone mass in OVX rats. Therefore, for easy calculations, a dosage of 50 mg/kg/day, which is closest to the highest dosage used in their study, was chose0n. After implantation surgery, rats in the OVX + lycopene group were gavaged with lycopene (50 mg/kg/day, Hezhong Biosciences,

Wuhan, China) dissolved in corn oil (10 mg lycopene/ml) for 12 weeks, while rats in the OVX and sham groups were gavaged with corn oil (5 ml/kg/day). During the 12-week gavage period, three rats died (one in each group), possibly due to oesophageal damage. Twelve weeks after implantation, the rats were sacrificed, and both femurs were harvested. For each rat, the left femur was used for histological analysis, and the right femur was used for biomechanical testing and micro-computed tomography (micro-CT) analysis. For each group, nine specimens were used for histological analysis, and nine specimens were used for mechanical testing and micro-CT analysis.

Biomechanical testing

Immediately after sacrifice, the femurs were trimmed to expose both ends of the implant (Fig. 2a) with a high-speed dental handpiece and a diamond bur (SF-12C, Mani, Japan) without damaging the implants. By placing the distal end of the specimen on a flat surface to check whether the sample was evenly placed, the excess bone tissue was trimmed, and a flat specimen surface level to the distal end of the implant was obtained to increase the stability during the mechanical test. Samples were wrapped in gauze soaked with saline and were then stored at − 20 °C. Three days later, after all of the samples were prepared, they were thawed at 4 °C overnight and then delivered on ice for biomechanical testing. The biomechanical properties of bone-implant interfaces were tested by the push-out test method [30] using a universal mechanical testing machine (AGS-X; Shimadzu, Kyoto, Japan). The specimen was evenly placed on a jig hole 0.5 mm larger than the implant diameter (Fig. 2b), with the proximal end facing upwards. The push-out rod was moved as close to the specimen as possible without touching it. Next, a vertical force (parallel to the longitudinal axis of the implant) with a displacement speed of 0.5 mm/min was applied

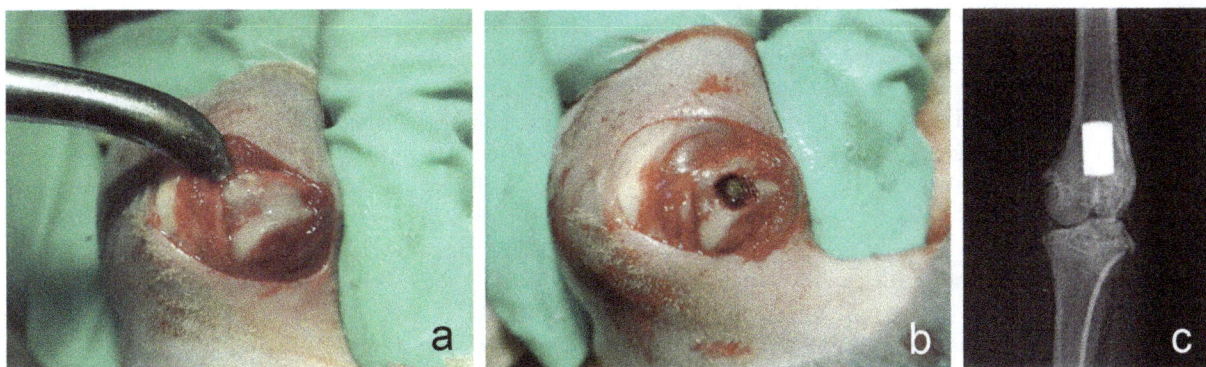

Fig. 1 The operative location of the implant. **a** The exposed knee joint. **b** An implant was inserted into the channel. **c** Radiograph of the implant in the distal metaphysis of femur after surgery

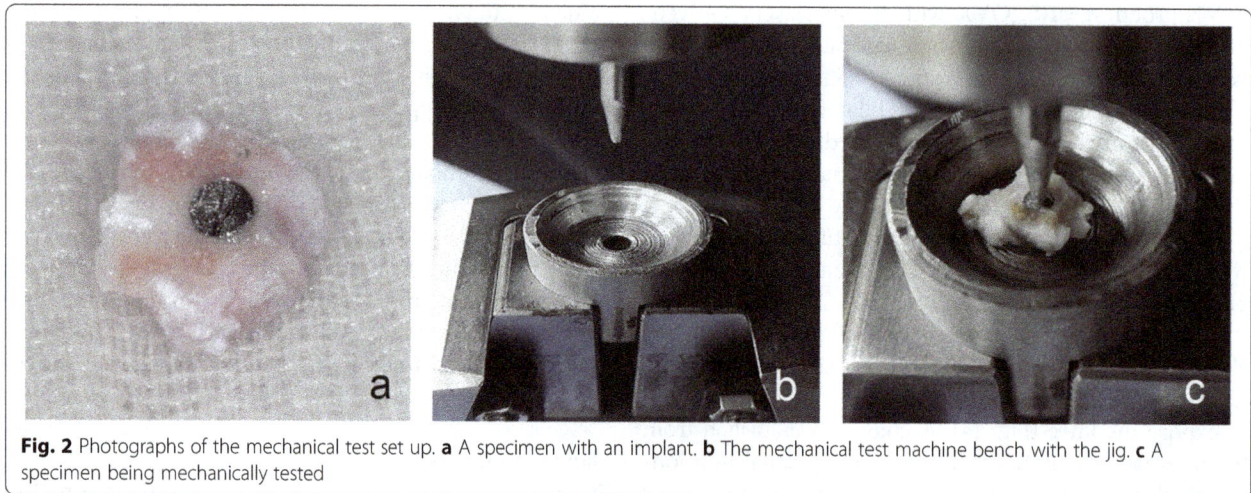

Fig. 2 Photographs of the mechanical test set up. **a** A specimen with an implant. **b** The mechanical test machine bench with the jig. **c** A specimen being mechanically tested

to the implant (Fig. 2c). The test was stopped when the implant was completely free from the bone. The peak force was then recorded in Newtons (N).

Micro-CT evaluation

In our pilot test, we scanned the sample with the implant before the push-out test and found that there were many metal artefacts that appeared as streaks or shadows, which compromised the readability of the image around the implant. To avoid metal artefacts, we gently removed the implants after mechanical testing and stored the bone tissue in 70% ethanol for micro-CT detection. The specimens were scanned using a micro-CT scanner (60 kV, 667 μA; ZKKS-MCT-Sharp; Kaisheng Technology, Guangzhou, China) at a high resolution and an isotropic voxel size of 20 μm. The scanning axis was along the axis of the femur. ZKKS-Micro-CT.3.0 software was used for 3D reconstruction and for 3D and quantitative evaluation. For the analysis of peri-implant bone tissue, the volume of interest (VOI) included the trabecular compartment extending 250 μm from the surface of the implant, assuming that the implant had not been removed. An equally long VOI was chosen for all samples, including 100 slices (2000 μm) beneath the lowest part of the growth plate, but the cortical bone was excluded semi-automatically if it was within the VOI. The bone volume/total bone (BV/TV) ratio, bone mineral density (BMD), trabecular thickness (Tb.Th), trabecular separation (Tb.Sp) and trabecular number (Tb.N) were calculated.

Histological evaluation

Samples were trimmed with a high-speed handpiece and a diamond bur (SF-12C, Mani) to expose both ends of the implants. Then, the femurs with implants were fixed in 10% neutral formalin for 48 h and decalcified with 10% neutral ethylene-diamine-tetraacetic acid for 30 days. Next, the whole samples were placed on the mechanical

test jig with the proximal end facing upwards, and the implants were gently pushed out along the axis of the implant with the push-out rod by hand. Specimens without implants were then dehydrated in graded ethanol and embedded in paraffin. Transverse 5-μm-thick sections were cut with a paraffin ultra-thin slicer (RM2235; Lecia, Heidelberger, Germany). The section at the growth plate level was selected as the section of interest and was stained with haematoxylin-eosin (HE). Histomorphometry was performed to semi-quantify the percentages of the bone area (BA) and bone contact (BC) with the implant for each sample using a semi-automated digital image analysis system, consisting of an optical microscope (BX61VS; OLYMPUS, Tokyo, Japan), OLYMPUS VS-ASW image collecting software and Image-Pro Plus 6.0 software (Media Cybernetics, Rockville, USA). Assuming that the implant had not been removed, BA was defined as the percentage area of the bone tissue found within an annulus of 0.25 mm around the implant to the total area of the annulus [31], while BC was defined as the percentage length of the direct bone-implant interface to the total implant surface [32].

Statistical analysis

Data are expressed as the mean ± standard deviation (SD). Statistical analyses were performed with the SPSS 17.0 statistics package, using one-way analysis of variance (ANOVA) to compare three groups and the Student-Newman-Keuls test to perform multiple comparisons between two groups. A p value below 0.05 was set as the significance level.

Results
Biomechanical test

Biomechanical testing data indicated that implant fixation decreased in the OVX group, while lycopene treatment almost prevented this effect. Compared with the sham group, the OVX group showed a 50.8% ($p < 0.01$) decrease in the maximum push-out force, while compared with the OVX group, the OVX + lycopene group showed a 69.3% ($p < 0.01$) decrease. There was no significant difference in the push-out force between the OVX + lycopene and sham groups ($p > 0.05$) (Fig. 3).

Micro-CT analysis

In 2D and 3D transverse micro-CT images, the peri-implant bone volume was lower in the OVX group than in the sham group, while the volume was higher in the OVX + lycopene group than in the OVX group (Fig. 4). In the quantitative analysis of the peri-implant bone volume and trabecular micro-architecture within VOI, compared with the sham group, the OVX group showed a 33.1% decrease in the BV/TV ratio ($p < 0.01$), 26.9% in Tb.Th ($p < 0.01$), 20.0% in BMD ($p < 0.01$) and 5.1% in Tb.N ($p < 0.05$) (Fig. 5). Interestingly, compared with the OVX group, the OVX + lycopene group showed a 45.8% increase in the BV/TV ratio ($p < 0.01$), 31.5% in Tb.Th ($p < 0.01$), 20.0% in BMD ($p < 0.01$) and 3.4% in Tb.N ($p > 0.05$). Tb.Sp was 16.7% ($p < 0.01$) higher in the OVX group than in the sham group and was 7.7% ($p < 0.05$) lower in the OVX + lycopene group than in the OVX group. There was no significant difference between the OVX + lycopene and sham groups in BV/TV, BMD, Tb.N, Tb.Th and Tb.Sp ($p > 0.05$) (Fig. 5).

Histological analysis

The decalcified sections showed the destructive effects of OVX surgery on implant osseointegration and peri-implant bone mass, while those values were increased in the OVX + lycopene group (Fig. 6). In quantitative analysis within a region of interest (ROI), compared with BA and BC in the sham group, BA and BC in the OVX group decreased by 45.6% ($p < 0.01$) and 37.0% ($p < 0.01$),

respectively. However, BA and BC were 72.3% ($p < 0.01$) and 51.4% ($p < 0.01$) higher in the OVX + lycopene group than in the OVX group, respectively. There was no significant difference in BA and BC between the OVX + lycopene and sham groups ($p > 0.05$) (Fig. 7).

Discussion

Osteoporosis, a common disease in elderly people, is characterized by low BMD and loss of structural and biomechanical properties [33]. The compromised bone healing capacity under osteopenic conditions shows adverse effects on implant fixation and osseointegration 2–12 weeks after implantation [11, 28, 29] and affects the initial stability and healing time of the implant in osteoporotic patients [8, 9]. Implant fixation can be mostly explained by the degree of osseointegration [34]. In this study, we histomorphometrically and functionally investigated the effects of lycopene on implant osseointegration in osteopenic rats. As expected, the sham group had more mechanical implant fixation, BC and bone mass than did the OVX group, indicating the destructive effect of osteopenia on implant osseointegration. Furthermore, as expected, lycopene maintained mechanical implant fixation, BC and bone mass around the implant in the OVX + lycopene group to almost the same level as that in the sham group. These results indicate that lycopene could prevent bone loss and maintain osseointegration in OVX rats 12 weeks after implantation. These findings suggest that lycopene might be a new therapeutic agent for preventing delayed osseointegration under osteopenic conditions.

The OVX rat model is most commonly used to simulate postmenopausal osteoporosis [35]. In our study, compared with sham rats, OVX rats showed significantly decreased BMD and compromised bone tissue micro-structure surrounding the implant. These results indicate that OVX can induce osteopenia in rats, in accordance with published data on the effects of OVX on bone mass [11]. In addition, osseointegration, implant fixation and micro-structure of the bone surrounding the implant were significantly lower in OVX rats than in sham rats. These results were in accordance with those of other studies [11, 32, 36, 37], indicating the adverse impact of OVX on osseointegration in rats.

Lycopene is a natural potent antioxidant that is considered a human nutritional supplement by the United States Food and Drug Administration (US FDA) [38]. The recommended dosages for humans are 5–7 mg/day to prevent chronic diseases and 35–75 mg/day to treat cancer and cardiovascular diseases [21]. The largest dosage reported for rats was 3000 mg/kg/day for 13 weeks without any adverse effects observed [39]. The only side effects in cases of excessive intake of lycopene were alterations in the skin and liver colouration, which

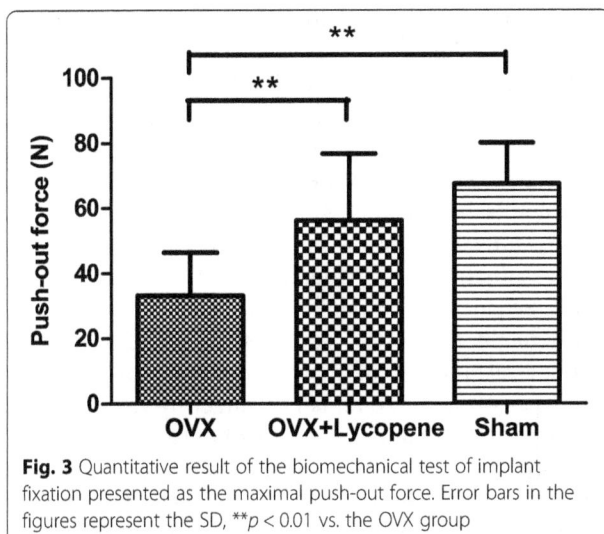

Fig. 3 Quantitative result of the biomechanical test of implant fixation presented as the maximal push-out force. Error bars in the figures represent the SD, **$p < 0.01$ vs. the OVX group

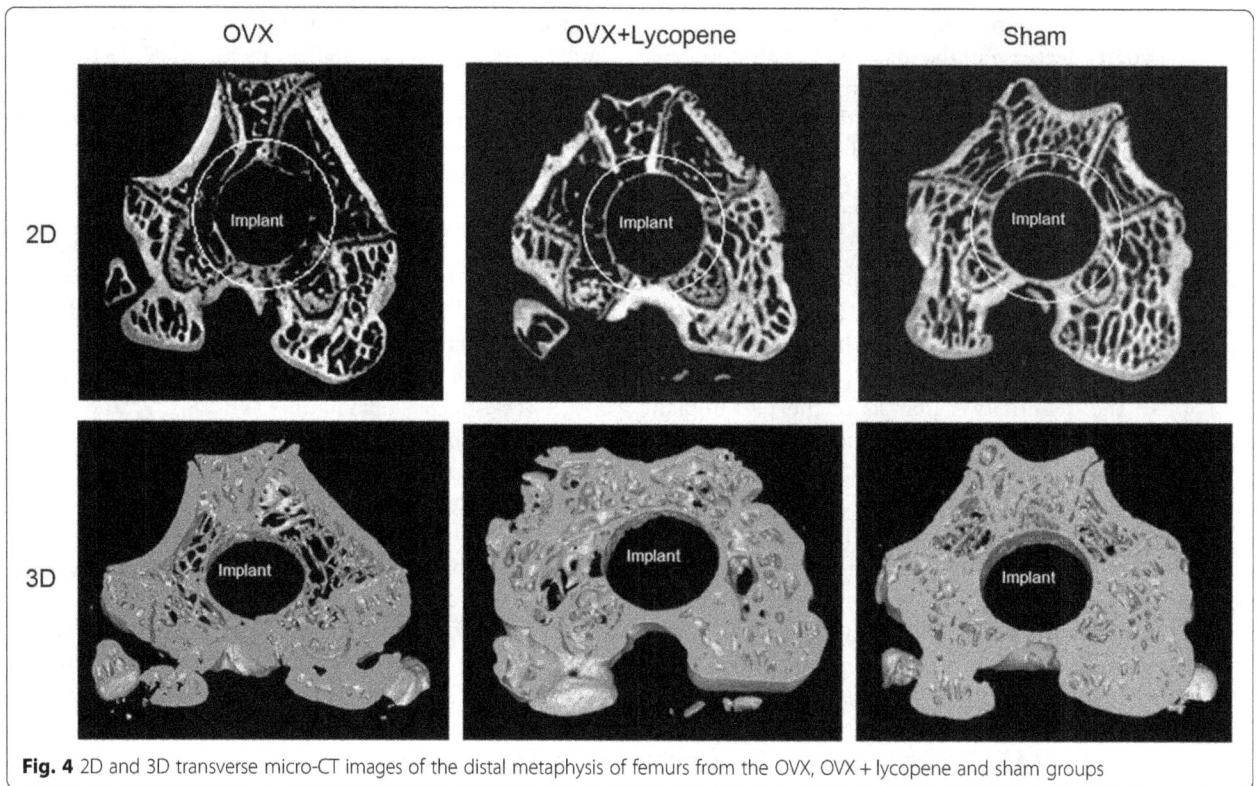

Fig. 4 2D and 3D transverse micro-CT images of the distal metaphysis of femurs from the OVX, OVX + lycopene and sham groups

were non-toxic and reversible [40]. Ardawi et al. [26] demonstrated the dose-dependent effect of lycopene on bone loss prevention in OVX rats. In their study, the highest dosage of the OVX + lycopene group, which was 45 mg/kg/day, showed the best effect on bone mass in OVX rats. In our study, 50 mg/kg/day lycopene was given to OVX rats by gavage for 12 weeks, and no adverse effects were observed. Therefore, lycopene is a relatively safe medication.

A number of studies have demonstrated the beneficial effects of lycopene on bone metabolism [23, 24, 26, 41–43]. In vitro studies have shown that lycopene promotes proliferation and differentiation of osteoblasts [26, 44] and suppresses osteoclastogenesis and differentiation of osteoclasts in normal and OVX rats [26, 45]. Lycopene treatment can increase the expression of bone formation biomarkers in rats [42] and can decrease the expression of bone resorption biomarkers in osteoporotic patients [24, 41]. Taken together, these findings indicate that lycopene has both anabolic and anti-catabolic effects on bone metabolism. In our study, histomorphometric and micro-CT analyses showed significantly increased BA, BMD and the micro-structure of the bone surrounding the implants in OVX rats, demonstrating the treatment effects of lycopene on local osteopenic bone. Our findings were consistent with the results of Ardawi et al. [26] and Iimura et al. [43], which both reported that

lycopene prevented bone loss in OVX rats. Therefore, lycopene could be an effective therapeutic agent for osteoporosis.

Several drugs reportedly promote osseointegration and implant fixation by improving the micro-structure of the bone surrounding the implants in rats [36, 37, 46]. At the tissue level, osseointegration could be affected by the quantity and quality of the bone around the implant. Li et al. [11] reported impaired implant osseointegration and fixation in OVX rats with compromised peri-implant bone micro-structure. In our study, lycopene increased BA, BV/TV, BMD and Tb.Th and decreased Tb.Sp of peri-implant bone in OVX rats. Consistent with the results of the aforementioned studies, these results revealed that the role of lycopene in osseointegration might be mediated by altering the peri-implant bone mass and trabecular micro-architecture.

Our study has several limitations. First, the experimental situation is not representative of clinical situations. Second, measuring the decalcification of bone tissue might not be the best method for performing a histological analysis of the osseointegration rate. The interfaces of the bone remained intact by visual inspection after the implants were pushed out from the femur, as they did after embedding and sectioning. One possible reason why the interface between the implant and adjacent tissues was not apparently damaged is that

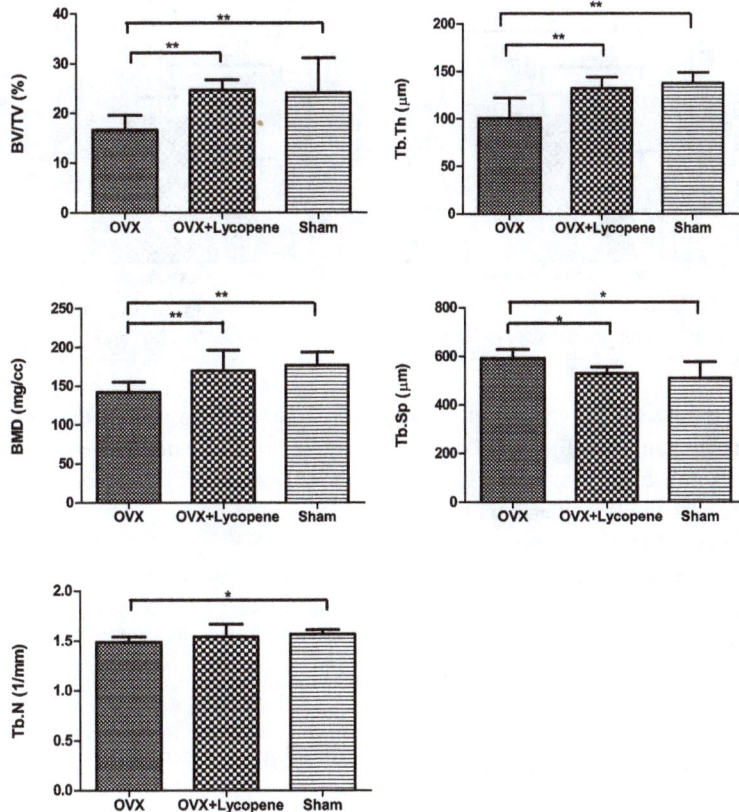

Fig. 5 Quantitative results of peri-implant bone volume and trabecular micro-architecture by micro-CT analysis. BV/TV, percent bone volume; Tb.Th, mean trabecular thickness; BMD, bone mineral density; Tb.Sp, mean trabecular separation; Tb.N, mean trabecular number. Error bars in the figures represent the SD, *$p < 0.05$ and **$p < 0.01$ vs. the OVX group

the surface of the implant had no threads and was basically smooth. Another reason is that damage might occur only at small interfacial points and did not affect the calculation of BA and BC. However, the bone tissue on the slides was deformed to different degrees during the process of staining, possibly because the decalcified bone tissue was prone to exfoliation from the slides, making the inner boundary of the bone irregular and complicating the calculation of BA and BC. Based on this study, applying non-decalcified bone to the slide to maintain the original shape of the bone for better analysis of the osseointegration rate might be more

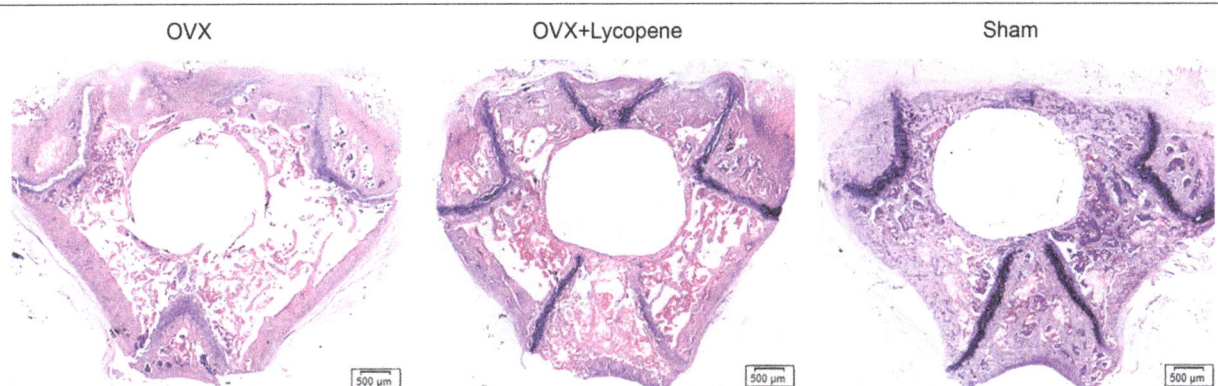

Fig. 6 Light microscope images of transverse histological sections at the epiphyseal plate level of the distal metaphysis of femurs from the OVX, OVX + lycopene and sham groups. HE staining

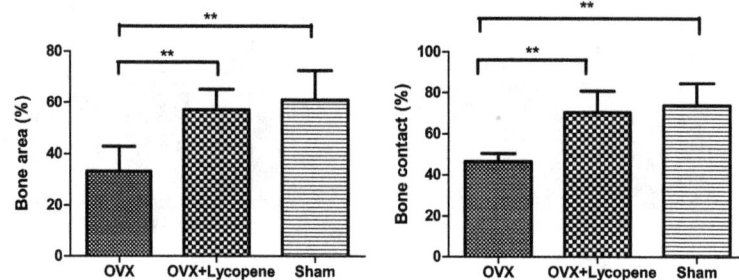

Fig. 7 Quantitative results of histomorphometric analysis presented as bone area (BA) around the implant and bone contact (BC) with implant, assuming that the implant had not been removed. Error bars in the figures represent the SD, *$p < 0.05$ and **$p < 0.01$ vs. the OVX group

appropriate. Third, we did not examine the condition of the bone at the time of implant placement. Lycopene-treated rats had better osseointegration than did OVX + vehicle rats at 12 weeks post-implant placement. This difference may have occurred due to the prevention of further bone loss between 12 and 24 weeks post-OVX or through a positive effect of lycopene on the healing process. Because we did not examine the condition of the bone at the time of implant placement, we cannot know whether lycopene improved or maintained osseointegration in the lycopene-treated group. Fourth, we did not record the uterine weights or examine oestrogen production levels before and after lycopene treatment (lower body weight was observed in lycopene-treated rats than in OVX + vehicle rats after 12 weeks of gavage, but the difference was non-significant; data not shown). Several authors have found that oestrogen production is stimulated by treatment with lycopene and other carotenoid derivatives [42, 47]. This stimulation is reflected in uterine hypertrophy [26] and could be responsible for the positive bone effects of lycopene treatment, making the effects of lycopene indirect. Due to a lack of recording of the variation in uterine weights and oestrogen production levels before and after the treatment, we cannot determine whether lycopene performed its role through oestrogen production. If lycopene's mode of action is through oestrogen, then it will not have similar effects on male rats or non-OVX-induced osteopenic rats. Therefore, the specific mechanism of how lycopene promotes osseointegration under osteopenic conditions needs further study.

Conclusions

We evaluated the influence of systematically administered lycopene on implant osseointegration in an OVX rat model. The results indicated that lycopene significantly increased implant osseointegration, fixation and bone mass in OVX rats to the level of those in sham rats. Within the limitations of the study, lycopene may be an effective medication for preventing delayed osseointegration under osteopenic conditions. Further

research is warranted to determine the specific mechanism of how lycopene prevents delayed osseointegration under osteopenic conditions.

Abbreviations
ARE: Antioxidant response element/electrophile response element; BA: Bone area; BC: Bone contact; BMD: Bone mineral density; BV/TV: Bone volume/total bone; HE: Haematoxylin-eosin; Keap1: Kelch-like ECH-associated protein 1; micro-CT: Micro-computed tomography; OVX: Ovariectomized; ROS: Reactive oxygen species; Tb.N: Trabecular number; Tb.Sp: Trabecular separation; Tb.Th: Trabecular thickness; VOI: Volume of interest

Funding
This study was funded by the Nature Science Foundation of Guangxi Province (grant number: 2013GXNSFBA019162), Basic Skills Improving Program of Young Teachers in Guangxi Colleges and Universities (grant number: 2017KY0092) and Guangxi Medical University Youth Science Fund (grant number: GXMUYSF201634).

Authors' contributions
XL designed the whole study and was a major contributor in writing the manuscript. WX acquired, analysed and interpreted all the data in the manuscript. YC performed the OVX and implant surgery on the rats. YL prepared the specimens for biomechanical testing and micro-CT analysis. MX performed the histological examination of the samples. All authors read and approved the final manuscript.

Competing interests
The authors declare that they have no competing interests.

References

1. Liddelow G, Klineberg I. Patient-related risk factors for implant therapy. A critique of pertinent literature. Aust Dent J. 2011;56(4):417–26; quiz 441. https://doi.org/10.1111/j.1834-7819.2011.01367.x.
2. French D, Larjava H, Ofec R. Retrospective cohort study of 4591 Straumann implants in private practice setting, with up to 10-year follow-up. Part 1: multivariate survival analysis. Clin Oral Implants Res. 2015;26(11):1345–54. https://doi.org/10.1111/clr.12463.
3. French D, Larjava H, Tallarico M. Retrospective study of 1087 anodized implants placed in private practice: risk indicators associated with implant failure and relationship between bone levels and soft tissue health. Implant Dent. 2018. https://doi.org/10.1097/id.0000000000000743.
4. Goiato MC, dos Santos DM, Santiago JF Jr, Moreno A, Pellizzer EP. Longevity of dental implants in type IV bone: a systematic review. Int J Oral Maxillofac Surg. 2014;43(9):1108–16. https://doi.org/10.1016/j.ijom.2014.02.016.
5. Phetfong J, Sanvoranart T, Nartprayut K, Nimsanor N, Seenprachawong K, Prachayasittikul V, Supokawej A. Osteoporosis: the current status of mesenchymal stem cell-based therapy. Cell Mol Biol Lett. 2016;21:12. https://doi.org/10.1186/s11658-016-0013-1.
6. Giro G, Chambrone L, Goldstein A, Rodrigues JA, Zenobio E, Feres M, Figueiredo LC, Cassoni A, Shibli JA. Impact of osteoporosis in dental implants: a systematic review. World J Orthop. 2015;6(2):311–5. https://doi.org/10.5312/wjo.v6.i2.311.
7. de Medeiros F, Kudo GAH, Leme BG, Saraiva PP, Verri FR, Honorio HM, Pellizzer EP, Santiago Junior JF. Dental implants in patients with osteoporosis: a systematic review with meta-analysis. Int J Oral Maxillofac Surg. 2018;47(4):480–91. https://doi.org/10.1016/j.ijom.2017.05.021.
8. Merheb J, Temmerman A, Rasmusson L, Kubler A, Thor A, Quirynen M. Influence of skeletal and local bone density on dental implant stability in patients with osteoporosis. Clin Implant Dent Relat Res. 2016;18(2):253–60. https://doi.org/10.1111/cid.12290.
9. Aro HT, Alm JJ, Moritz N, Makinen TJ, Lankinen P. Low BMD affects initial stability and delays stem osseointegration in cementless total hip arthroplasty in women: a 2-year RSA study of 39 patients. Acta Orthop. 2012;83(2):107–14. https://doi.org/10.3109/17453674.2012.678798.
10. Mavrogenis AF, Dimitriou R, Parvizi J, Babis GC. Biology of implant osseointegration. J Musculoskelet Neuronal Interact. 2009;9(2):61–71.
11. Li Y, He S, Hua Y, Hu J. Effect of osteoporosis on fixation of osseointegrated implants in rats. J Biomed Mater Res B Appl Biomater. 2017;105(8):2426–32. https://doi.org/10.1002/jbm.b.33787.
12. Ross RD, Hamilton JL, Wilson BM, Sumner DR, Virdi AS. Pharmacologic augmentation of implant fixation in osteopenic bone. Curr Osteoporos Rep. 2014;12(1):55–64. https://doi.org/10.1007/s11914-013-0182-z.
13. Khan M, Cheung AM, Khan AA. Drug-related adverse events of osteoporosis therapy. Endocrinol Metab Clin N Am. 2017;46(1):181–92. https://doi.org/10.1016/j.ecl.2016.09.009.
14. Prasad G, Dhillon MS, Khullar M, Nagi ON. Evaluation of oxidative stress after fractures. A preliminary study. Acta Orthop Belg. 2003;69(6):546–51.
15. Sheweita SA, Khoshhal KI. Calcium metabolism and oxidative stress in bone fractures: role of antioxidants. Curr Drug Metab. 2007;8(5):519–25.
16. Bednarek-Tupikowska G, Tworowska U, Jedrychowska I, Radomska B, Tupikowski K, Bidzinska-Speichert B, Milewicz A. Effects of oestradiol and oestroprogestin on erythrocyte antioxidative enzyme system activity in postmenopausal women. Clin Endocrinol. 2006;64(4):463–8. https://doi.org/10.1111/j.1365-2265.2006.02494.x.
17. Ilyas A, Odatsu T, Shah A, Monte F, Kim HK, Kramer P, Aswath PB, Varanasi VG. Amorphous silica: a new antioxidant role for rapid critical-sized bone defect healing. Adv Healthc Mater. 2016;5(17):2199–213. https://doi.org/10.1002/adhm.201600203.
18. De Franca NA, Camargo MB, Lazaretti-Castro M, Martini LA. Antioxidant intake and bone status in a cross-sectional study of Brazilian women with osteoporosis. Nutr Health. 2013;22(2):133–42. https://doi.org/10.1177/0260106014563445.
19. Zhang J, Munger RG, West NA, Cutler DR, Wengreen HJ, Corcoran CD. Antioxidant intake and risk of osteoporotic hip fracture in Utah: an effect modified by smoking status. Am J Epidemiol. 2006;163(1):9–17. https://doi.org/10.1093/aje/kwj005.
20. Wang XD. Lycopene metabolism and its biological significance. Am J Clin Nutr. 2012;96(5):1214S–22S. https://doi.org/10.3945/ajcn.111.032359.
21. Rao AV, Rao LG. Carotenoids and human health. Pharmacol Res. 2007;55(3):207–16. https://doi.org/10.1016/j.phrs.2007.01.012.
22. Kelkel M, Schumacher M, Dicato M, Diederich M. Antioxidant and anti-proliferative properties of lycopene. Free Radic Res. 2011;45(8):925–40. https://doi.org/10.3109/10715762.2011.564168.
23. Mackinnon ES, Rao AV, Rao LG. Dietary restriction of lycopene for a period of one month resulted in significantly increased biomarkers of oxidative stress and bone resorption in postmenopausal women. J Nutr Health Aging. 2011;15(2):133–8.
24. Mackinnon ES, Rao AV, Josse RG, Rao LG. Supplementation with the antioxidant lycopene significantly decreases oxidative stress parameters and the bone resorption marker N-telopeptide of type I collagen in postmenopausal women. Osteoporos Int. 2011;22(4):1091–101. https://doi.org/10.1007/s00198-010-1308-0.
25. Sahni S, Hannan MT, Blumberg J, Cupples LA, Kiel DP, Tucker KL. Protective effect of total carotenoid and lycopene intake on the risk of hip fracture: a 17-year follow-up from the Framingham Osteoporosis Study. J Bone Miner Res. 2009;24(6):1086–94. https://doi.org/10.1359/jbmr.090102.
26. Ardawi MS, Badawoud MH, Hassan SM, Rouzi AA, Ardawi JM, AlNosani NM, Qari MH, Mousa SA. Lycopene treatment against loss of bone mass, microarchitecture and strength in relation to regulatory mechanisms in a postmenopausal osteoporosis model. Bone. 2016;83:127–40. https://doi.org/10.1016/j.bone.2015.10.017.
27. Yamazaki I, Yamaguchi H. Characteristics of an ovariectomized osteopenic rat model. J Bone Miner Res. 1989;4(1):13–22. https://doi.org/10.1002/jbmr.5650040104.
28. Ozawa S, Ogawa T, Iida K, Sukotjo C, Hasegawa H, Nishimura RD, Nishimura I. Ovariectomy hinders the early stage of bone-implant integration: histomorphometric, biomechanical, and molecular analyses. Bone. 2002;30(1):137–43.
29. Duarte PM, Cesar Neto JB, Goncalves PF, Sallum EA, Nociti J F. Estrogen deficiency affects bone healing around titanium implants: a histometric study in rats. Implant Dent. 2003;12(4):340–6.
30. Alghamdi HS, van den Beucken JJ, Jansen JA. Osteoporotic rat models for evaluation of osseointegration of bone implants. Tissue Eng Part C Methods. 2014;20(6):493–505. https://doi.org/10.1089/ten.TEC.2013.0327.
31. Alghamdi HS, Cuijpers VM, Wolke JG, van den Beucken JJ, Jansen JA. Calcium-phosphate-coated oral implants promote osseointegration in osteoporosis. J Dent Res. 2013;92(11):982–8. https://doi.org/10.1177/0022034513505769.
32. Ying G, Bo L, Yanjun J, Lina W, Binquan W. Effect of a local, one time, low-dose injection of zoledronic acid on titanium implant osseointegration in ovariectomized rats. Arc Med Sci. 2016;12(5):941–9. https://doi.org/10.5114/aoms.2016.61908.
33. Edwards MH, Dennison EM, Aihie Sayer A, Fielding R, Cooper C. Osteoporosis and sarcopenia in older age. Bone. 2015;80:126–30. https://doi.org/10.1016/j.bone.2015.04.016.
34. Virdi AS, Irish J, Sena K, Liu M, Ke HZ, McNulty MA, Sumner DR. Sclerostin antibody treatment improves implant fixation in a model of severe osteoporosis. J Bone Joint Surg Am. 2015;97(2):133–40. https://doi.org/10.2106/JBJS.N.00654.
35. Johnston BD, Ward WE. The ovariectomized rat as a model for studying alveolar bone loss in postmenopausal women. Biomed Res Int. 2015;2015:635023. https://doi.org/10.1155/2015/635023.
36. Gao Y, Luo E, Hu J, Xue J, Zhu S, Li J. Effect of combined local treatment with zoledronic acid and basic fibroblast growth factor on implant fixation in ovariectomized rats. Bone. 2009;44(2):225–32. https://doi.org/10.1016/j.bone.2008.10.054.
37. Dikicier E, Karacayli U, Dikicier S, Gunaydin Y. Effect of systemic administered zoledronic acid on osseointegration of a titanium implant in ovariectomized rats. J Craniomaxillofac Surg. 2014;42(7):1106–11. https://doi.org/10.1016/j.jcms.2014.01.039.
38. Rao AV, Ray MR, Rao LG. Lycopene. Adv Food Nutr Res. 2006;51:99–164. https://doi.org/10.1016/s1043-4526(06)51002-2.
39. Mellert W, Deckardt K, Gembardt C, Schulte S, Van Ravenzwaay B, Slesinski R. Thirteen-week oral toxicity study of synthetic lycopene products in rats. Food Chem Toxicol. 2002;40(11):1581–8.
40. Michael McClain R, Bausch J. Summary of safety studies conducted with synthetic lycopene. Regul Toxicol Pharmacol. 2003;37(2):274–85.

41. Rao LG, Mackinnon ES, Josse RG, Murray TM, Strauss A, Rao AV. Lycopene consumption decreases oxidative stress and bone resorption markers in postmenopausal women. Osteoporos Int. 2007;18(1):109–15. https://doi.org/10.1007/s00198-006-0205-z.

42. Liang H, Yu F, Tong Z, Zeng W. Lycopene effects on serum mineral elements and bone strength in rats. Molecules. 2012;17(6):7093–102. https://doi.org/10.3390/molecules17067093.

43. Iimura Y, Agata U, Takeda S, Kobayashi Y, Yoshida S, Ezawa I, Omi N. The protective effect of lycopene intake on bone loss in ovariectomized rats. J Bone Miner Metab. 2015;33(3):270–8. https://doi.org/10.1007/s00774-014-0596-4.

44. Kim L, Rao AV, Rao LG. Lycopene II--effect on osteoblasts: the carotenoid lycopene stimulates cell proliferation and alkaline phosphatase activity of SaOS-2 cells. J Med Food. 2003;6(2):79–86. https://doi.org/10.1089/109662003322233468.

45. Rao LG, Krishnadev N, Banasikowska K, Rao AV. Lycopene I--effect on osteoclasts: lycopene inhibits basal and parathyroid hormone-stimulated osteoclast formation and mineral resorption mediated by reactive oxygen species in rat bone marrow cultures. J Med Food. 2003;6(2):69–78. https://doi.org/10.1089/109662003322233459.

46. Liu Y, Hu J, Liu B, Jiang X, Li Y. The effect of osteoprotegerin on implant osseointegration in ovariectomized rats. Arch Med Sci. 2017;13(2):489–95. https://doi.org/10.5114/aoms.2017.65468.

47. Veprik A, Khanin M, Linnewiel-Hermoni K, Danilenko M, Levy J, Sharoni Y. Polyphenols, isothiocyanates, and carotenoid derivatives enhance estrogenic activity in bone cells but inhibit it in breast cancer cells. Am J Phys Endocrinol Metab. 2012;303(7):E815–24. https://doi.org/10.1152/ajpendo.00142.2011.

20

Chemokine analysis as a novel diagnostic modality in the early prediction of the outcome of non-union therapy: a matched pair analysis

Patrick Haubruck[1,2]* , Anja Solte[1], Raban Heller[1], Volker Daniel[3], Michael Tanner[1], Arash Moghaddam[1,4], Gerhard Schmidmaier[1] and Christian Fischer[1]

Abstract

Background: Despite the regenerative capability of skeletal tissue fracture, non-union is common. Treatment of non-unions remains challenging, and early determination of the outcome is impossible. Chemokines play an important role in promoting the formation of new bone and remodeling existing bone. Despite their importance regarding the regulation of bone biology, the potential of chemokines as biological markers reflecting osseous regeneration is unknown.

The purpose of this study was to determine (1) if serum chemokine expression levels correlate with the outcome of non-union surgery and (2) if chemokine expression analysis can be used to identify patients at risk for treatment failure.

Methods: Non-union patients receiving surgical therapy in our institution between March 2012 and March 2014 were prospectively enrolled in a clinical observer study. Regular clinical and radiological follow-up was conducted for 12 months including collection of blood during the first 12 weeks. Based on the outcome, patients were declared as responders or non-responders to the therapy. To minimize biases, patients were matched (age, sex, body mass index (BMI)) and two groups of patients could be formed: responders (R, $n = 10$) and non-responders (NR, $n = 10$). Serum chemokine expression (CCL-2, CCL-3, CCL-4, CXCL-10, CCL-11, and interferon gamma (IFN-γ)) was analyzed using Luminex assays. Data was compared and correlated to the outcome.

Results: CCL-3 expression in NR was significantly higher during the course of the study compared to R ($p = 0.002$), and the expression pattern of CCL-4 correlated with CCL-3 in both groups (NR: $p < 0.001$ and $r = 0.63$). IFN-γ expression in NR was continuously higher than in R ($p < 0.001$), and utilization of CCL-3 and IFN-γ serum expression levels 2 weeks after the treatment resulted in a predictive model that had an AUC of 0.92 (CI 0.74–1.00).

Conclusion: Serum chemokine expression analysis over time is a valid and promising diagnostic tool. The chemokine expression pattern correlates with the outcome of the Masquelet therapy of lower limb non-unions. Utilization of the serum analysis of CCL-3 and IFN-γ 2 weeks after the treatment resulted in an early predictive value regarding the differentiation between patients that are likely to heal and those that are prone to high risk of treatment failure.

Keywords: Bone regeneration, Non-union, Chemokine, Cytokine, Diagnostics, Prediction

* Correspondence: patrick.haubruck@med.uni-heidelberg.de
[1]HTRG—Heidelberg Trauma Research Group, Center for Orthopedics, Trauma Surgery and Spinal Cord Injury, Trauma and Reconstructive Surgery, Heidelberg University Hospital, Schlierbacher Landstrasse 200a, 69118 Heidelberg, Germany
[2]Raymond Purves Bone and Joint Research Laboratories, Kolling Institute of Medical Research, Institute of Bone and Joint Research, University of Sydney, St Leonards, New South Wales 2065, Australia
Full list of author information is available at the end of the article

Background

Bone is one of the few tissues that can heal without a fibrous scar, thereby osseous healing is considered as a form of tissue regeneration [1]. The osseous healing cascade is a complex physiological process involving multiple parameters both on a molecular and cellular level [1, 2] that need to act concertedly. Aberrations in this biological process can result in delayed healing or in the development of a non-union [1]. Despite the regenerative capability of skeletal tissue, fracture non-union is a common (up to 30% of fractures fail to heal) and persistent complication [3, 4]. Treatment of non-unions remains a challenge in orthopedics and trauma surgery [4] while multiple treatment modalities have been introduced lately. The Masquelet therapy was established as a safe and clinically effective treatment modality in the treatment of large non-unions [5]. Despite studies showing satisfying clinical results subsequent to the Masquelet therapy [6, 7], early determination of the outcome remains impossible. At present, the outcome is usually assessed as early as 6 months after surgery based on radiologic findings that require ionizing radiation (computed tomography and X-rays) [8]. In addition, no valid marker exists identifying patients that are prone to high risk of treatment failure. Early identification of those patients at risk would assist treating physicians in the postoperative management and provide a rationale for adjunct non-union treatment or timely revision surgery.

Chemokines are a family of signaling proteins secreted by cells that are specific to vertebrates [9]. They can be assigned to two major subfamilies: CXC (C–X–C motif) and CC (C–C motif) chemokine [10]. Members of these subfamilies play an important role in bone biology [9] and promote bone formation developmentally and in response to mechanical stimuli [11]. In particular, they modulate the formation of new bone and remodeling of existing bone by coordinating cellular homing, osteoblastogenesis, and osteoclastogenesis [10]. Due to their important role regarding the regulation of bone biology, recent research focus has shifted towards several chemokines and their mechanisms of action associated with bone remodeling [10]. Thus, exploration of chemokines as biological markers reflecting osseous regeneration seems natural.

In previous studies [11, 12], the serum cytokine analysis was established as a valid method investigating into biological processes occurring during bone regeneration subsequent to non-union therapy. Hence, this study was aimed to determine primarily if serum cytokine expression levels of distinct chemokines correlate with the outcome of non-union surgery. Secondly, the possibility to determine a prognostic model regarding the outcome of non-union therapy based on the expression levels of chemokines was investigated. Due to their importance in bone healing, CCL-2, CCL-3, CCL-4, CXCL-10, CCL-11, and interferon gamma (IFN-γ) [9, 10, 13, 14] were included and analyzed. The hypothesis of the study was that the expression patterns of distinct cytokines correlate with bone regeneration occurring during non-union therapy and can be used to identify patients at risk at an early stage.

Methods

Study design

To answer the research questions, a prospective clinical observer study was performed. The study was conducted at the Department of Orthopedics and Traumatology at the Heidelberg University Hospital (a level 1 trauma center). A total of 207 patients suffering from long-bone non-union and receiving surgery between March 2012 and March 2014 in our department were enrolled in the study. Due to the highly sensitive chemokine measurement, strict inclusion and exclusion criteria were applied and ultimately patients were matched in order to reduce confounders and influences onto the results of this study. Inclusion of patients started after approval of the local institutional ethics committee (S-636/2011). In addition, the study was conducted in accordance with the latest version of the Declaration of Helsinki.

Inclusion and exclusion criteria

Patients suffering from failed bone healing after diaphyseal fractures of the tibia or femur that were between 18 and 80 years old and gave a written declaration of consent were included in the study. Initially, patients that were unable or unwilling to give a written consent, suffering from chronic inflammatory diseases or malignancies, needed to take immunosuppressive medication, or suffered from renal or hepatic failure were excluded from the study. In addition, patients that required additional surgical interventions or re-revisions were excluded during the course of the study.

Rationale for group assignment

Patients that failed to show consolidation within 12 months after the second step of the Masquelet therapy were determined as non-responders, whereas patients that showed proper consolidation were determined as responders. Based on the outcome, patients were matched based on three established criteria (age, sex, and BMI) [11] and two groups were formed:

1. Responders to the therapy (group: R/N = 10)
2. Non-responders to the therapy (group NR/N = 10)

If more than one match was found for a patient, then the patient with the most similar type of non-union was chosen (Table 1).

Table 1 Patient characteristics

Patients	All	Responders	Non-responders	Significance
Sex				
Male	12	6	6	$p = 1.000$
Female	8	4	4	
Age	50.75 ± 11.49	50.8 ± 13.05	50.7 ± 10.40	$p = 0.4277$
BMI	30.08 ± 6.57	27.92 ± 6.45	32.235 ± 6.25	$p = 0.3946$
Smoking				
S	8	3	5	$p = 0.2865$
NS	10	5	5	
FS	2	2	0	
Diabetes				
Yes	3	1	2	$p = 1.0000$
No	17	9	8	
Localization				
Tibia	10	7	3	$p = 0.1797$
Femur	10	3	7	
Fixation				
Nail	8	3	5	$p = 0.6481$
Plate	12	7	5	
Previous surgeries	3.15 ± 2.03	2.5 ± 1.08	3.8 ± 2.57	$p = 0.7715$

S active smoker, NS nonsmoker, FS former smoker; age is presented in years

Intervention

According to the "diamond concept" [15], there are several core factors necessary to achieve fracture consolidation and bone regeneration [15] (vascularity, growth factors, mechanical stability, osteogenic cells, and osteoconductive scaffolds). The Masquelet therapy, also called induced membrane technique, was specifically designed to treat challenging non-unions [5] by enhancing local bone biology and inducing osseous regeneration via two steps [5, 16]. In the initial surgical treatment (step I), the non-union tissue, surrounding avital bone and avital surrounding soft tissue, is debrided leaving a defect site. In the same surgery, this defect is filled with polymethyl methacrylate (PMMA) that is impregnated with antibiotics. The emerging foreign body reaction induces the vascularized Masquelet membrane [17]. Harvesting of tissue samples occurs during the first step that is subsequently microbiologically examined. The first step is repeated until asepsis is achieved and guaranteed by negative microbiological results, and afterwards, the spacer is left in situ for 6 weeks to enable a fully grown Masquelet membrane [18]. In a second step, the spacer is removed while leaving the membrane intact and the defect site is filled with a combination of autologous bone graft and additional growth factors (3.3 mg of bone morphogenetic protein 7) [5, 18–20]. De novo osteosynthesis

is performed during the first or second step based on the anatomical localization and morphology of non-union. Thereby, the Masquelet therapy provides all factors necessary for bone healing according to the "diamond concept."

Postoperative care and determination of outcome

According to previously published protocols [6, 11, 12], clinical and radiologic examination was performed as part of a dedicated follow-up program. In addition, patient data was thoroughly assessed preoperatively and during each follow-up visit. Examination occurred prior and 2 days as well as 1 week subsequent to each step. In addition, examination was performed 2, 4, and 6 weeks, as well as 3, 6, and 12 months, after the second step. Blood samples were collected until 3 months after the second step of the treatment (Additional file 1: Figure S1). Patients included in the study were completing most of all follow-up examination. However, due to unavailability, occasionally, single isolated blood samples were not obtained. Outcome was evaluated 12 months after the final surgical treatment and based on radiologic signs of consolidation (bridging in three out of four cortices in conventional X-rays) and mechanical stability and full weight-bearing [21–23].

Sample acquisition and measurement

Venous blood samples were taken (S Monovette 7.5 ml, Sarstedt AG, Germany) from all patients following a highly standardized previously published protocol [12]. Analysis of C-reactive protein (CRP) and leukocytes was conducted directly after the blood was drawn. The quantitative analysis was performed with Luminex Performance Human High Sensitivity Assays (Quantikine®, RD Systems, Minneapolis, MN, USA) strictly according to the manufacturer's instructions. The lab technician performing the Luminex assays was blinded to both patient data and clinical outcome.

Determination of sample size

Prior to commencement of the study, sample size determination was performed based on previously published data [24]. In particular, the sample size calculation for this study was performed in R [3.2.3] using the package "pwr." Assuming an alpha level of .05 and a power of .80 as well as an equal number of subjects in the experimental and control groups, 9.41 patients per group were estimated to be required. Thus, a total of 10 patients per group were included.

Patients demographics

Forty-nine patients were eligible for the current study (Fig. 1). According to our established matched-pair analysis, a total of 20 non-union patients were included into the current study (8 females and 12 males). Included

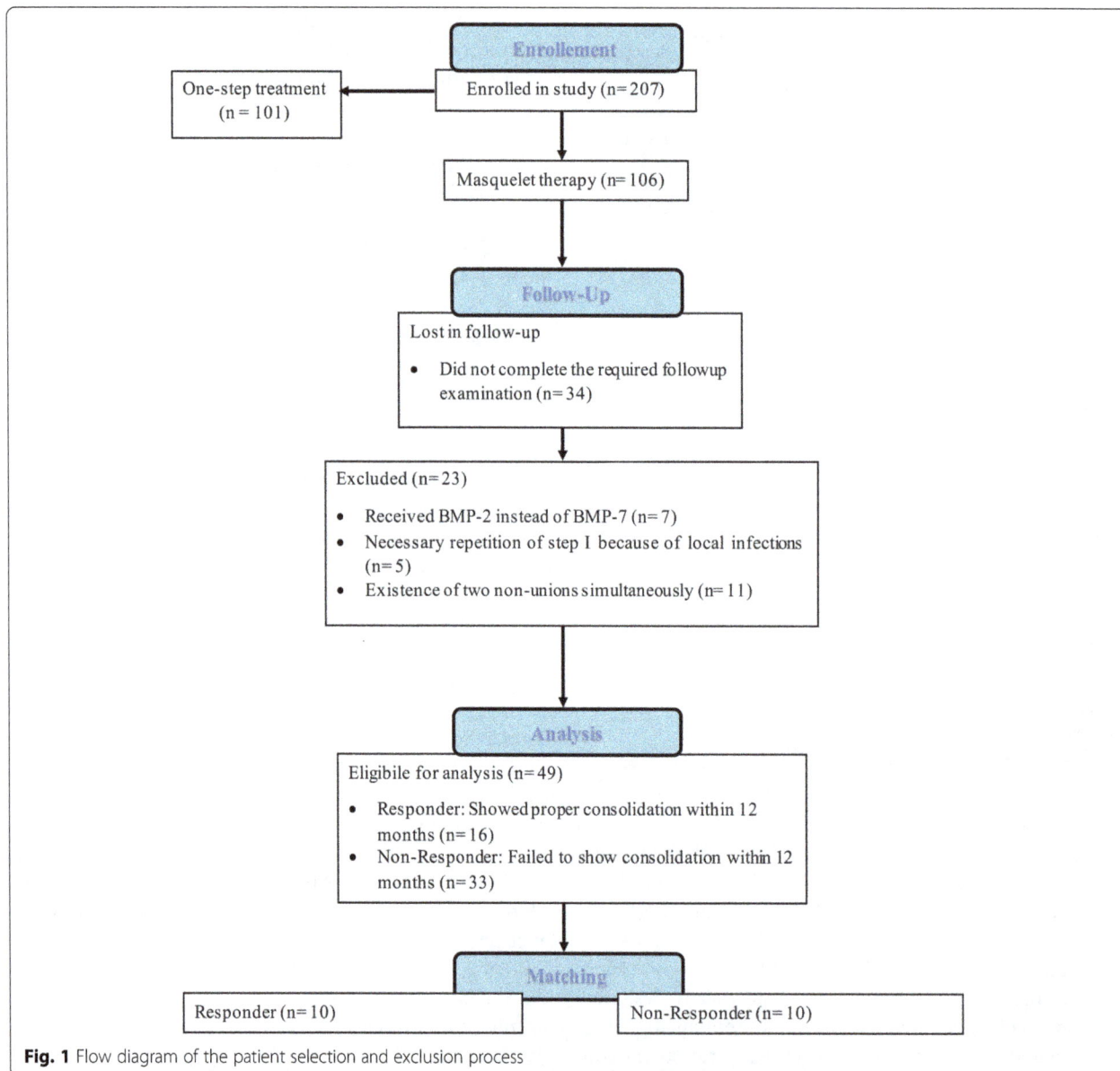

Fig. 1 Flow diagram of the patient selection and exclusion process

patients were an average of 50.8 ± 11.5 years old. Statistically, patients of both groups had resembling characteristics regarding gender, age, BMI, smoking habits, diabetes, localization of the non-union, nail or plate fixation, and count of previous surgeries. Further details regarding patient characteristics in each group can be found in Table 1.

Statistics

Explorative correlation analyses were conducted between all cytokine variables. Nonparametric test methods were assessed to investigate location shifts between groups (Mann–Whitney U test). Categorical variables were evaluated using the chi-square test. In order to assess if analysis of the expression pattern of the measured chemokines was able to predict the outcome of the therapy, multiple

binary logistic regression models were utilized. Patients with incomplete data points were excluded from this analysis. Variables included were standardized. All initially available clinical variables (e.g., sex, age) as well as any serum parameters were included in the process to ensure valid assessment of the additional predictive power of the remaining potential covariates. Model selection was performed via AIC (Akaike information criterion) comparison. Predictive performance was assessed by estimation of the AUC (area under the curve) of the ROC (receiver operating characteristic) curve and the corresponding confidence interval. All p values quoted are to be interpreted in a descriptive way as they were not adjusted for multiple testing as this is an exploratory post hoc analysis. All statistical calculations were performed with R version 3.2.3

[25]. Figures were created by using the package "ggplot2" [26]. Serum levels are expressed as absolute mean concentrations ± SEM (standard error of mean), and statistical significance was determined as $p < 0.05$.

Results

Evaluation of inflammatory response
Independent inflammatory markers (CRP and leukocytes) revealed a physiological expression pattern without significant differences between groups. Both CRP and leukocyte count returned to normal 4 weeks after surgery (Table 2).

Evaluation of CCL-3 and CCL-4 serum expression
Following baseline expression, serum levels of CCL-3 in R slightly decreased until reaching a minimum prior to step II (18.51 ± 4.46 pg/ml); afterwards, expression in R was continuously lower than in NR reaching its peek 4 weeks after the treatment (27.54 ± 6.01 pg/ml). Starting 2 days after the initial surgery, expression of CCL-3 in NR was higher than in R throughout the study period. Analysis showed that expression of CCL-3 6 weeks after the treatment was significantly higher in NR compared to R ($p = 0.036$). Additionally, combined expression of CCL-3 in NR was significantly higher during the course of the study compared to R ($p = 0.002$ (Fig. 2a)). The expression pattern of CCL-4 was similar to the expression pattern of CCL-3 in both groups. Differences of CCL-4 between groups were at a nonsignificant extent (Fig. 2b). Expression pattern of CCL-3 and CCL-4 correlated significantly in NR to the therapy at 1 week after the first step ($p = 0.001$), prior to the second step ($p = 0.047$), and two days ($p = 0.013$) and one week after the second step ($p = 0.040$).

Analysis of CCL-2 and CCL-11 serum expression
In R, the CCL-2 values were the highest prior to the surgical treatment (preoperatively, 566.21 ± 56.35 pg/ml) and the lowest two weeks after the second step (467.85 ± 32.90 pg/ml). In contrast, mean CCL-2 values in NR showed a minimum immediately after the first step (409.29 ± 39.82 pg/ml) and peak serum levels were reached 6 weeks following step II (608.23 ± 97.41 pg/ml). Statistical analysis revealed that differences between groups were at a nonsignificant extent during the course of the study. Interestingly, similar to CCL-3 and CCL-4, baseline expression of CCL-2 in R was higher compared to NR (Fig. 3a). Four weeks after step II, serum values of CCL-11 were significantly higher in responders to the therapy (R, 402.45 ± 51.24 pg/ml vs. NR, 261.06 ± 12.65 pg/ml; $p = 0.047$). Interestingly, peak values of CCL-11 in R were reached 3 months after the treatment (406.54 ± 83.07 pg/ml), whereas peak values in NR occurred 6 weeks after the treatment (351.51 ± 58.93 pg/ml) (Fig. 3b).

Analysis of CXCL-10 and IFN-γ serum expression
CXCL-10 expression was slightly lower in R compared to NR and differences being significant 1 week after the initial treatment ($p = 0.043$). Expression was lowest in both groups immediately after step I (R, 58.45 ± 10.33 pg/ml vs. NR, 62.81 ± 9.31 pg/ml). Interestingly, expression in R showed a minimum immediately after each surgical treatment, whereas expression in NR only showed that minimum after the first step. Expression in NR peaked 4 weeks after step II (127.65 ± 18.49 pg/ml) and in R 2 weeks after the second step (108.94 ± 15.59 pg/ml) (Fig. 4a). Peak expression of IFN-γ in NR was higher (2 weeks after the treatment: 10.21 ± 3.91 pg/ml) compared to the peak reached in R (4 weeks after the treatment: 4.07 ± 1.56 pg/ml). Afterwards, values decreased until the end of the study. Combined expression of IFN-γ in NR was significantly higher than in R ($p < 0.001$) (Fig. 4b).

Binary logistic modeling regarding the predictive power
Statistical analysis revealed that the best performing model was the one including only CCL-3 and IFN-γ serum expression levels 2 weeks after the second step of the Masquelet therapy. Regarding its predictive capabilities, the utilized model had an AUC of 0.92 (CI 0.74–1.00) and the resulting ROC is depicted in Fig. 5.

Table 2 Analysis of independent infectious parameters

Group	Measurement	Time point							
		Pre-op step I	2 days	1 week	Pre-op step II	2 days	1 week	2 weeks	4 weeks
Responders	L (mean ± SEM in 1000/µL)	7.434 ± 0.56	8.376 ± 0.83	7.331 ± 0.91	7.17 ± 0.71	8.156 ± 1.11	7.54 ± 0.89	7.285 ± 1.66	7.005 ± 1.01
	CRP (mean ± SEM in mg/L)	8.74 ± 2.85	100.4 ± 12.82	32.35 ± 9.96	14.32 ± 4.99	97.3 ± 14.89	47.29 ± 10.56	38.25 ± 12.70	8.05 ± 6.05
Non-responders	L (mean ± SEM in 1000/µL)	7.126 ± 0.52	7.391 ± 0.70	6.232 ± 0.47	6.559 ± 0.65	7.223 ± 0.70	6.952 ± 0.83	7.877 ± 1.50	5.53 ± 1.08
	CRP (mean ± SEM in mg/L)	9.06 ± 3.01	91.06 ± 12.44	35.33 ± 8.81	15.178 ± 9.06	105.275 ± 18.46	48.1 ± 8.72	15.033 ± 6.07	19.15 ± 13.95

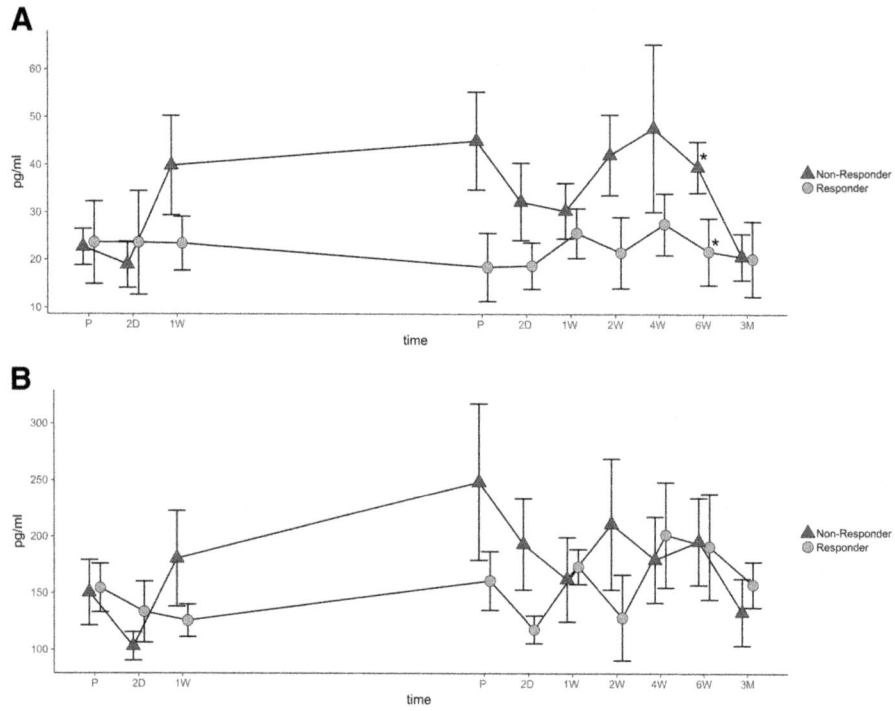

Fig. 2 Analysis of CCL-3 and CCL-4. The average concentration and SEM (pg/ml) of CCL-3 (**a**) and CCL-4 (**b**) are shown during both steps of treatment and follow-up. Dark triangles display non-responders, and gray points indicate responders. Significant differences are indicated by a star ($p < 0.05$). Abbreviations: preoperatively (P), postoperative days (D), and weeks (W)

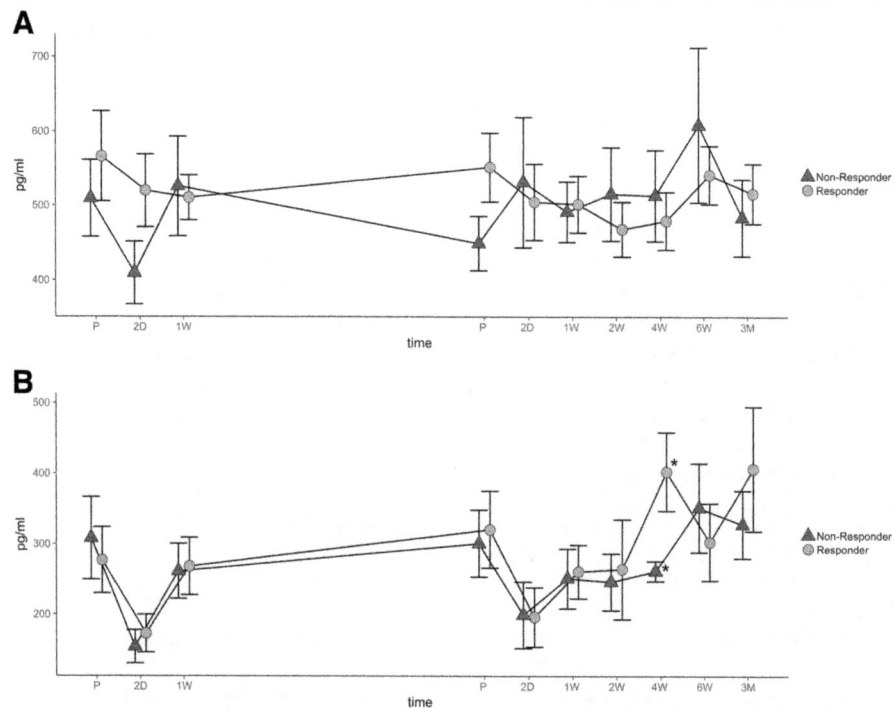

Fig. 3 Analysis of CCL-2 and CCL-11. The average concentration and SEM (pg/ml) of CCL-2 (**a**) and CCL-11 (**b**) are shown during both steps of treatment and follow-up. Dark triangles display non-responders, and gray points indicate responders. Significant differences are indicated by a star ($p < 0.05$). Abbreviations: preoperatively (P), postoperative days (D), and weeks (W)

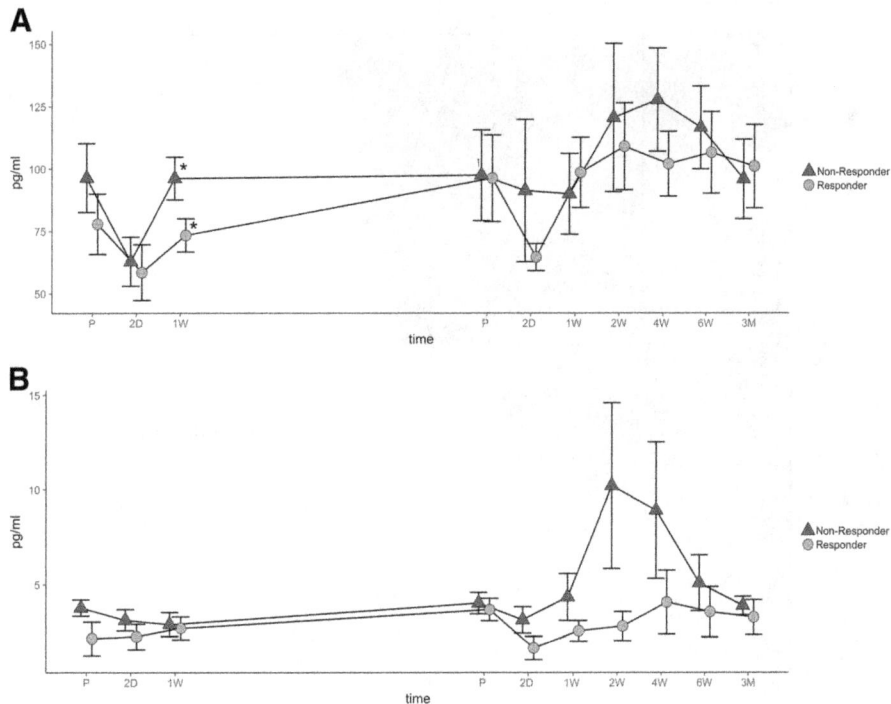

Fig. 4 Analysis of CXCL-10 and IFN-γ. The average concentration and SEM (pg/ml) of CXCL-10 (**a**) and IFN-γ (**b**) are shown during both steps of treatment and follow-up. Dark triangles display non-responders, and gray points indicate responders. Significant differences are indicated by a star ($p < 0.05$). Abbreviations: preoperatively (P), postoperative days (D), and weeks (W)

Discussion

The findings of the current study provide important information regarding both research questions. Serum chemokine expression analysis over time of treatment is a valid and promising novel tool in the analysis of the expression pattern of distinct chemokines in context with non-union therapy. This data indicates that the chemokine expression pattern correlates with the outcome of the Masquelet therapy of lower limb non-unions. Ultimately, the analysis of CCL-3 and IFN-γ 2 weeks after the second step was able to identify patients that are at high risk for failure of the treatment.

The initial phase of fracture healing and bone regeneration is characterized by its inflammatory character [1]. CCL-2, also called monocyte chemotactic protein-1 (MCP-1), and its receptor CCR2 have been shown to induce the early inflammatory phase of tissue healing [27] and therefore play an important role during the early phase of fracture healing [27, 28]. Deletion of CCR2 only in the early phase of fracture healing has caused delayed fracture healing indicating the importance of increased CCL-2 expression for normal fracture healing [27]. In the current study, NR showed a minimum subsequent to the initial surgical treatment, whereas values in R only slightly decreased. The first step of the Masquelet therapy is intended to induce a vascularized membrane via a foreign body reaction [18, 29]. Interestingly, the foreign

body reaction is initiated by an inflammatory response to the biomaterial similar to the response in early fracture healing [30]. Lower levels of CCL-2 after the first step in NR might correlate with an abnormal initial inflammatory response during the enfolding foreign body reaction that influences the outcome of the following bone regeneration.

Macrophage inflammatory protein 1 (MIP1) is a chemokine subfamily consisting of four members [31]. Relevant roles of CCL-3 expression, also called macrophage inflammatory protein 1 α (MIP1α), have been described for a variety of diseases [31]. However, no evidence exists regarding the role of CCL-3 during bone regeneration. In this study, beginning 1 week after the initial treatment, CCL-3 levels were constantly higher in NR. This elevated expression of CCL-3 might correlate with an increased osteoclastogenesis and active bone degradation resulting in an unfavorable microenvironment regarding the integration of the bone graft. This postulation is supported by findings from the literature. Expression of CCL-3 has been described in context with osteoclastogenesis and osteolysis [32]. Additionally, elevated expression of CCL-3 can be found in aseptic implant loosening and osteomyelitis [32] providing evidence of CCL-3 inducing differentiation of monocytes to bone-resorbing osteoclasts [32]. In particular, strong evidence exists regarding CCL-3 expression correlating with bone degeneration in patients with

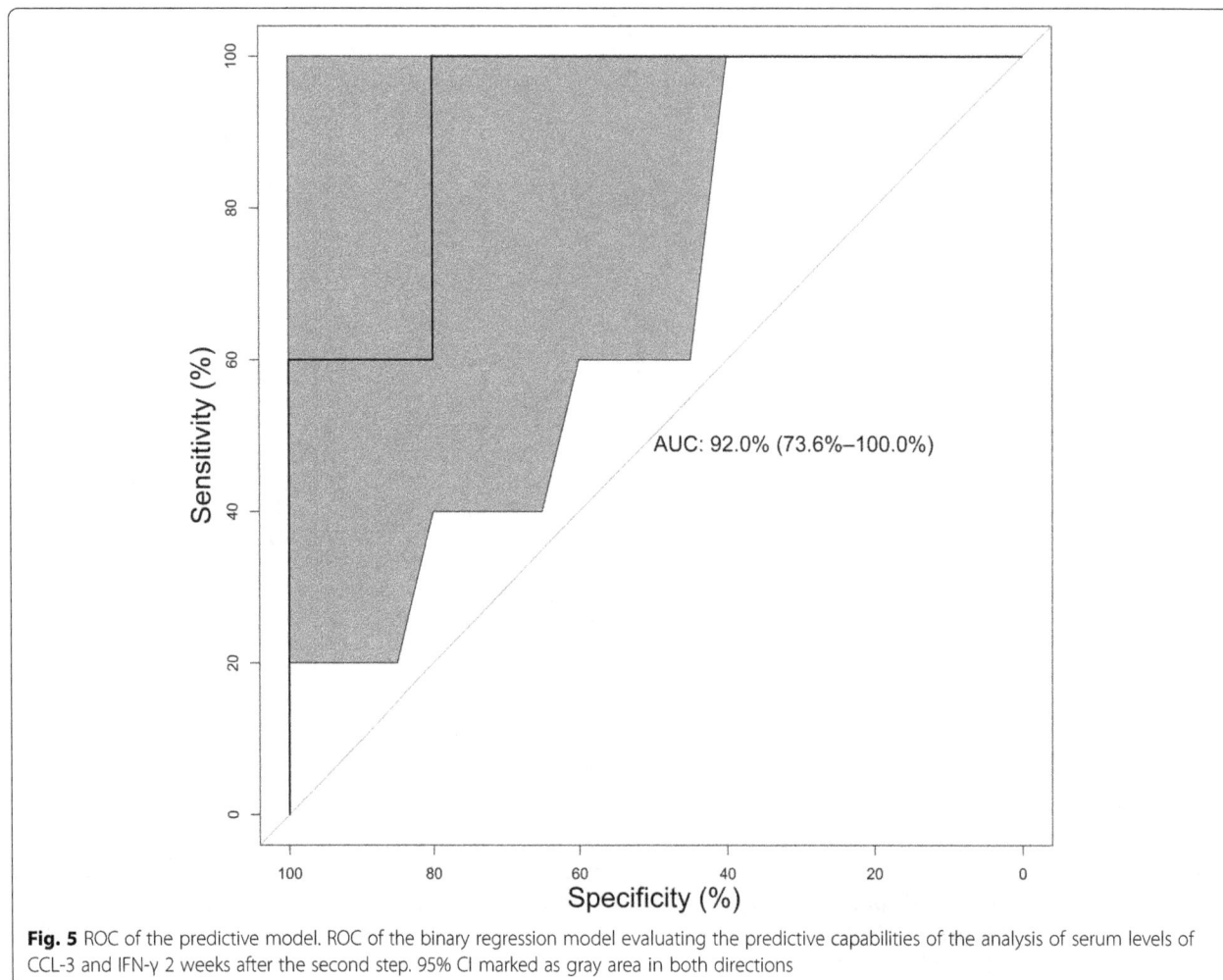

Fig. 5 ROC of the predictive model. ROC of the binary regression model evaluating the predictive capabilities of the analysis of serum levels of CCL-3 and IFN-γ 2 weeks after the second step. 95% CI marked as gray area in both directions

multiple myeloma providing proof regarding a link between CCL-3 activation and bone degradation [32–34]. Biological function of CCL-4, also called MIP1β, is closely connected to CCL-3 [35]. Studies have shown that CCL-3 and CCL-4 are predominant factors responsible for the enhancement of bone resorption in multiple myeloma [36] and play a causal role in the development of lytic bone lesions in vivo. In the current study, serum expression of CCL-4 correlated significantly with the expression pattern of CCL-3. Thus, expression of CCL-4 was higher in NR during most time of the study. This correlation supports previous findings by indicating that both CCL-3 and CCL-4 act in concert.

CCL-11, also called eotaxin-1, is a chemokine that is produced by a variety of cells including endothelial cells and chondrocytes [37]. In mice suffering from an inflammatory bone resorption, CCL-11 expression was higher compared to healthy controls [37], whereas in patients with chronic nonbacterial osteomyelitis, CCL-11 expression was lower compared to healthy controls [38]. Interestingly, the authors stated that expression of CCL-11

varied between different groups [38]. In bone regeneration subsequent to the Masquelet therapy, expression of CCL-11 was similar during the initial 10 weeks of the treatment. Hereafter, serum expression of CCL-11 was significantly higher in patients that responded to the therapy. Previous studies reported a chemokine-dependent amplification loop in bone metabolism [38, 39]. In particular, in aseptic conditions, CCL-11 was expressed by normal osteoblasts, while in inflammatory conditions, elevated CCL-11 levels stimulated migration of osteoclast precursors in addition to bone resorption [38]. Despite being initiated by an inflammatory response, bone regeneration in the current study occurred in aseptic conditions. Therefore, higher levels of CCL-11 in responders during bone integration might correlate with bone remodeling necessary to integrate the graft. However, the exact nature of this mechanism remains a speculation and is beyond the scope of this report.

The chemokine CXCL-10 is induced by IFN-γ resulting in its alternative name interferon-gamma-inducible protein 10 (IP-10) [40]. A relevant role for CXCL-10 was shown for chronic Th1 inflammatory diseases [40]. In particular, serum levels of CXCL-10 were elevated in patients suffering from a rheumatoid arthritis [40] and expression of CXCL-10 caused the recruitment of inflammatory cells and is involved in bone erosion in inflamed joints [41]. Interestingly, a recent study has shown increased CXCL-10 levels in the acute graft-versus-host disease (aGvHD) subsequent to bone marrow transplantation [42]. Thereby, measurement of CXCL-10 was postulated as possible biomarker in context with aGvHD [42]. In the current study, patients received autologous bone grafts and usually no graft-versus-host response is expected. However, a syndrome similar to GvHD has been reported to occur spontaneously in 8% of patients receiving autologous bone [43]. Interestingly, expression of CXCL-10 was elevated in non-responders in the initial 10 weeks of the treatment and peak levels were reached subsequent to the implantation of autologous bone graft. This elevated CXCL-10 might correlate with an abnormal response of the body to the transplanted autologous bone graft resulting in failure of the treatment. This altered host response regarding autologous bone might pose as an interesting approach in understanding factors influencing the outcome of bone regeneration and warrants further investigation.

IFN-γ is the only type II interferon and was originally associated with the host defense regarding a viral infection [44]. However, substantial evidence exists regarding the influence of IFN-γ onto bone healing. In particular, IFN-γ decreased the bone healing capability of mesenchymal stem cells (MSC) and MSC treated with IFN-γ underwent apoptosis [44]. Thereby, an anti-osteogenic function was associated with IFN- [44]. Another study showed that IFN-γ and tumor necrosis factor alpha synergistically induced MSC deficiency resulting in osteoporosis [44]. Autologous bone graft induces bone healing due to its osteoinductivity based on high concentrations of MSC [15]. In this study, initial expression of IFN-γ was similar during the first step of the treatment and only after the transplantation of autologous bone values were higher in non-responders to the therapy. These high levels of IFN-γ might inhibit the function of MSCs in the implanted graft causing an impaired osseous induction ultimately resulting in failure of the treatment.

Up to date, no valid biomarker exists capable of identifying patients that are at risk for an unsuccessful non-union treatment. Evaluation of the outcome relies on radiological diagnostics that require radiation exposure [8], and earliest determination is achievable 6–12 months postoperatively. Recalcitrant non-unions are associated with a low quality of life, long period of recovery, and strenuous surgical treatments that eventually fail. As traditional X-ray or CT scans are not able to determine the outcome at an early stage, the resulting uncertainty represents a considerable psychological burden for concerned patients. Thus,

an early prediction of the outcome might contribute towards both an improved patient satisfaction and stratification of the postoperative management regarding the individual risk. In addition, early identification might provide rationale for additional postoperative non-union therapies, such as low-intensity pulsed ultrasound [45]. Results from this study introduced the measurement of CCL-3 and IFN-γ 2 weeks subsequent to the second step of the Masquelet therapy as promising novel diagnostic modality. In particular, evaluation based on these biological markers had a high sensitivity and good specificity in detecting patients at risk for poor outcome. Due to the commercial availability of the used Luminex assays, the low direct costs, and the short time necessary to perform the analysis, this method is easy to both implement and perform in all centers having a clinical laboratory. The promising results of the current study are intended to encourage surgeons to evaluate this diagnostic modality in their own setting. Ultimately, the findings of this study might contribute towards an improved patient safety in context with non-union therapy.

Despite relevant findings, our study has limitations. Non-unions are a severe and clinically relevant complication, whereas absolute numbers remain relatively small. In addition, serum cytokine and chemokine analysis are highly sensitive and can be influenced by various factors; therefore, a close matching of patients next to our strict inclusion and exclusion criteria was used to reduce the differences between groups. This explains the small patient collective of this study. In the context of current literature and recent studies [12, 46], the patient collective size is still sufficient to provide reliable results. Results of this study may be influenced by a systemic inflammation; therefore, the CRP and leukocyte serum patterns were assessed in the initial 4 weeks subsequent to the procedure. The data showed comparable CRP values during the course of the study in both groups; in addition, leukocytes remained in a physiological range during the whole time, thereby indicating that no systemic inflammation was present. The current study provided first evidence regarding the predictive capabilities of chemokine expression analysis in context with non-union therapy. However, further studies are needed that involve a larger non-matched patient collective in order to assess the influence of individual patient characteristics and establish a threshold for the introduced CCL-3 and IFN-γ test.

Conclusions
The results of the current study introduce the serum analysis of the expression pattern of distinct chemokines as a novel diagnostic modality in context with bone regeneration occurring during non-union therapy. As bone regeneration occurs in the Masquelet therapy and the treatment is both highly standardized and regularly

monitored, this treatment has become valuable in studying biological processes occurring during bone regeneration. The expression pattern of chemokines (CCL-2, CCL-3, CCL-4, CCL-11, CXCL-10, and IFN-γ) correlates with the outcome of the Masquelet therapy of lower limb non-unions. Furthermore, the analysis of CCL-3 and IFN-γ serum levels 2 weeks after step II of the therapy predicts the likelihood of successful induction of bone regeneration during the Masquelet therapy and provides an additional predictive value regarding the early identification of patients that are at high risk for failure of the treatment. Based on these results, the current study introduces an early predictive value regarding the differentiation between patients that are likely to heal and those that are at high risk for a poor outcome.

Abbreviations
AIC: Akaike information criterion; AUC: Area under the curve; BMI: Body mass index; CCL: CC (C–C motif) chemokine; CI: Confidence interval; CRP: C-reactive protein; CXCL: CXC (C–X–C motif) chemokine; INF-y: Interferon-gamma; L: Leucocytes; NR: Non-responders; PMMA: Polymethyl methacrylate; R: Responders; ROC: Receiver operating characteristic; SEM: Standard error of mean

Acknowledgements
We would like to thank Martina Kutsche-Bauer for performing the Luminex assays. We acknowledge the financial support by Deutsche Forschungsgemeinschaft within the funding program Open Access Publishing, by the Baden-Württemberg Ministry of Science, Research and Arts, and by the Ruprechts-Karls-Universität Heidelberg.

Authors' contributions
PH, AS, MT, AM, GS, and CF carried out the conceptualization. PH, RH, and CF contributed to the data curation. PH and CF did the funding acquisition. PH, AS, RH, VD, AM, GS, and CF contributed to the investigation. PH, MT, GS, and CF administered the project. VD, AM, and CF obtained the resources. VD, MT, GS, and CF supervised the study. PH did the validation. AS and RH contributed to the visualization. PH, AS, RH, and CF wrote the original draft. PH, AS, VD, MT, AM, GS, and CF wrote the review and contributed to the editing. All authors read and approved the final version of this manuscript. Authorship eligibility guidelines according to the ICMJE were followed. The use of professional writers is not intended.

Competing interests
The authors declare that they have no competing interests.

Author details
[1]HTRG—Heidelberg Trauma Research Group, Center for Orthopedics, Trauma Surgery and Spinal Cord Injury, Trauma and Reconstructive Surgery, Heidelberg University Hospital, Schlierbacher Landstrasse 200a, 69118 Heidelberg, Germany. [2]Raymond Purves Bone and Joint Research Laboratories, Kolling Institute of Medical Research, Institute of Bone and Joint Research, University of Sydney, St Leonards, New South Wales 2065, Australia. [3]Department of Transplantation Immunology, Institute of Immunology, University of Heidelberg, Im Neuenheimer Feld 305, 69120 Heidelberg, Germany. [4]ATORG—Aschaffenburg Trauma and Orthopedic Research Group, Center for Trauma Surgery, Orthopedics and Sports Medicine, Am Hasenkopf 1, 63739 Aschaffenburg, Germany.

References
1. Marsell R, Einhorn TA. The biology of fracture healing. Injury. 2011. https://doi.org/10.1016/j.injury.2011.03.031.
2. Phillips AM. Overview of the fracture healing cascade. Injury. 2005. https://doi.org/10.1016/j.injury.2005.07.027.
3. Audige L, Griffin D, Bhandari M, Kellam J, Ruedi TP. Path analysis of factors for delayed healing and nonunion in 416 operatively treated tibial shaft fractures. Clin Orthop Relat Res. 2005. https://doi.org/10.1097/01.blo.0000163836.66906.74.
4. Schmidmaier G, Moghaddam A. Long bone nonunion. Z Orthop Unfall. 2015. https://doi.org/10.1055/s-0035-1558259.
5. Masquelet AC, Begue T. The concept of induced membrane for reconstruction of long bone defects. Orthop Clin North Am. 2010. https://doi.org/10.1016/j.ocl.2009.07.011.
6. Moghaddam A, Thaler B, Bruckner T, Tanner M, Schmidmaier G. Treatment of atrophic femoral non-unions according to the diamond concept: results of one- and two-step surgical procedure. J Orthop. 2017. https://doi.org/10.1016/j.jor.2016.10.003.
7. Moghaddam A, Zietzschmann S, Bruckner T, Schmidmaier G. Treatment of atrophic tibia non-unions according to 'diamond concept': results of one- and two-step treatment. Injury. 2015. https://doi.org/10.1016/s0020-1383(15)30017-6.
8. Fischer C, Preuss EM, Tanner M, Bruckner T, Krix M, Amarteifio E, et al. Dynamic contrast-enhanced sonography and dynamic contrast-enhanced magnetic resonance imaging for preoperative diagnosis of infected nonunions. J Ultrasound Med. 2016. https://doi.org/10.7863/ultra.15.06107.
9. Gilchrist A, Stern PH. Chemokines and bone. Clin Rev Bone Miner Metab. 2015. https://doi.org/10.1007/s12018-015-9184-y.
10. Smith JT, Schneider AD, Katchko KM, Yun C, Hsu EL. Environmental factors impacting bone-relevant chemokines. Front Endocrinol (Lausanne). 2017. https://doi.org/10.3389/fendo.2017.00022.
11. Haubruck P, Kammerer A, Korff S, Apitz P, Xiao K, Buchler A, et al. The treatment of nonunions with application of BMP-7 increases the expression pattern for angiogenic and inflammable cytokines: a matched pair analysis. J Inflamm Res. 2016. https://doi.org/10.2147/JIR.S110621.
12. Moghaddam A, Muller U, Roth HJ, Wentzensen A, Grutzner PA, Zimmermann G. TRACP 5b and CTX as osteological markers of delayed fracture healing. Injury. 2011. https://doi.org/10.1016/j.injury.2010.11.017.
13. Einhorn TA. The cell and molecular biology of fracture healing. Clin Orthop Relat Res. 1998;355(Suppl 1):7–21.
14. Sun T, Wang X, Liu Z, Chen X, Zhang J. Plasma concentrations of pro- and anti-inflammatory cytokines and outcome prediction in elderly hip fracture patients. Injury. 2011. https://doi.org/10.1016/j.injury.2011.01.010.
15. Giannoudis PV, Einhorn TA, Marsh D. Fracture healing: the diamond concept. Injury. 2007. https://doi.org/10.1016/S0020-1383(08)70003-2.
16. Moghaddam A, Child C, Bruckner T, Gerner HJ, Daniel V, Biglari B. Posttraumatic inflammation as a key to neuroregeneration after traumatic spinal cord injury. Int J Mol Sci. 2015. https://doi.org/10.3390/ijms16047900.
17. Bosemark P, Perdikouri C, Pelkonen M, Isaksson H, Tagil M. The masquelet induced membrane technique with BMP and a synthetic scaffold can heal a rat femoral critical size defect. J Orthop Res. 2015. https://doi.org/10.1002/jor.22815.
18. Pelissier P, Masquelet AC, Bareille R, Pelissier SM, Amedee J. Induced membranes secrete growth factors including vascular and osteoinductive factors and could stimulate bone regeneration. J Orthop Res. 2004. https://doi.org/10.1016/S0736-0266(03)00165-7.
19. Moghaddam-Alvandi A, Zimmermann G, Buchler A, Elleser C, Biglari B, Grutzner PA, et al. Results of nonunion treatment with bone morphogenetic protein 7 (BMP-7). Unfallchirurg. 2012. https://doi.org/10.1007/s00113-011-2100-0.
20. Karger C, Kishi T, Schneider L, Fitoussi F, Masquelet AC. Treatment of posttraumatic bone defects by the induced membrane technique. Orthop Traumatol Surg Res. 2012. https://doi.org/10.1016/j.otsr.2011.11.001.
21. Kuhlman JE, Fishman EK, Magid D, Scott WW Jr, Brooker AF, Siegelman SS. Fracture nonunion: CT assessment with multiplanar reconstruction. Radiology. 1988. https://doi.org/10.1148/radiology.167.2.3357959.
22. Savolaine ER, Ebraheim N. Assessment of femoral neck nonunion with multiplanar computed tomography reconstruction. Orthopedics. 2000. https://doi.org/10.3928/0147-7447-20000701-19.

23. Slade JF 3rd, Gillon T. Retrospective review of 234 scaphoid fractures and nonunions treated with arthroscopy for union and complications. Scand J Surg. 2008. https://doi.org/10.1177/145749690809700402.

24. Haubruck P, Heller R, Apitz P, Kammerer A, Alamouti A, Daniel V, et al. Evaluation of matrix metalloproteases as early biomarkers for bone regeneration during the applied Masquelet therapy for non-unions. Injury. 2018. https://doi.org/10.1016/j.injury.2018.07.015.

25. R Development Core Team. R: a language and environment for statistical computing. Vienna: R Foundation for Statistical Computing; 2015.

26. Wickham H. ggplot2: elegant graphics for data analysis. New York: Springer-Verlag; 2009.

27. Ishikawa M, Ito H, Kitaori T, Murata K, Shibuya H, Furu M, et al. MCP/CCR2 signaling is essential for recruitment of mesenchymal progenitor cells during the early phase of fracture healing. PLoS One. 2014. https://doi.org/10.1371/journal.pone.0104954.

28. Xing Z, Lu C, Hu D, Yu YY, Wang X, Colnot C, et al. Multiple roles for CCR2 during fracture healing. Dis Model Mech. 2010. https://doi.org/10.1242/dmm.003186.

29. Giannoudis PV, Faour O, Goff T, Kanakaris N, Dimitriou R. Masquelet technique for the treatment of bone defects: tips-tricks and future directions. Injury. 2011;42(6):591-8. https://doi.org/10.1016/j.injury.2011.03.036. Epub 2011 May 4.

30. Anderson JM, Rodriguez A, Chang DT. Foreign body reaction to biomaterials. Semin Immunol. 2008. https://doi.org/10.1016/j.smim.2007.11.004.

31. Maurer M, von Stebut E. Macrophage inflammatory protein-1. Int J Biochem Cell Biol. 2004. https://doi.org/10.1016/j.biocel.2003.10.019.

32. Dapunt U, Maurer S, Giese T, Gaida MM, Hansch GM. The macrophage inflammatory proteins MIP1alpha (CCL3) and MIP2alpha (CXCL2) in implant-associated osteomyelitis: linking inflammation to bone degradation. Mediat Inflamm. 2014. https://doi.org/10.1155/2014/728619.

33. Abe M, Hiura K, Wilde J, Moriyama K, Hashimoto T, Ozaki S, et al. Role for macrophage inflammatory protein (MIP)-1alpha and MIP-1beta in the development of osteolytic lesions in multiple myeloma. Blood. 2002;100: 2195–202.

34. Watanabe T, Kukita T, Kukita A, Wada N, Toh K, Nagata K, et al. Direct stimulation of osteoclastogenesis by MIP-1alpha: evidence obtained from studies using RAW264 cell clone highly responsive to RANKL. J Endocrinol. 2004. https://doi.org/10.1677/joe.0.1800193.

35. Guan E, Wang J, Norcross MA. Identification of human macrophage inflammatory proteins 1alpha and 1beta as a native secreted heterodimer. J Biol Chem. 2001. https://doi.org/10.1074/jbc.M006327200.

36. Abe M, Hiura K, Ozaki S, Kido S, Matsumoto T. Vicious cycle between myeloma cell binding to bone marrow stromal cells via VLA-4-VCAM-1 adhesion and macrophage inflammatory protein-1alpha and MIP-1beta production. J Bone Miner Metab. 2009. https://doi.org/10.1007/s00774-008-0012-z.

37. Kindstedt E, Holm CK, Sulniute R, Martinez-Carrasco I, Lundmark R, Lundberg P. CCL11, a novel mediator of inflammatory bone resorption. Sci Rep. 2017. https://doi.org/10.1038/s41598-017-05654-w.

38. Hofmann SR, Bottger F, Range U, Luck C, Morbach H, Girschick HJ, et al. Serum interleukin-6 and CCL11/eotaxin may be suitable biomarkers for the diagnosis of chronic nonbacterial osteomyelitis. Front Pediatr. 2017. https://doi.org/10.3389/fped.2017.00256.

39. Hoshino A, Iimura T, Ueha S, Hanada S, Maruoka Y, Mayahara M, et al. Deficiency of chemokine receptor CCR1 causes osteopenia due to impaired functions of osteoclasts and osteoblasts. J Biol Chem. 2010. https://doi.org/10.1074/jbc.M109.099424.

40. Lee JH, Kim B, Jin WJ, Kim HH, Ha H, Lee ZH. Pathogenic roles of CXCL10 signaling through CXCR3 and TLR4 in macrophages and T cells: relevance for arthritis. Arthritis Res Ther. 2017. https://doi.org/10.1186/s13075-017-1353-6.

41. Kwak HB, Ha H, Kim HN, Lee JH, Kim HS, Lee S, et al. Reciprocal cross-talk between RANKL and interferon-gamma-inducible protein 10 is responsible for bone-erosive experimental arthritis. Arthritis Rheum. 2008. https://doi.org/10.1002/art.23372.

42. Ahmed SS, Wang XN, Norden J, Pearce K, El-Gezawy E, Atarod S, et al. Identification and validation of biomarkers associated with acute and chronic graft versus host disease. Bone Marrow Transplant. 2015. https://doi.org/10.1038/bmt.2015.191.

43. Jones RJ, Vogelsang GB, Hess AD, Farmer ER, Mann RB, Geller RB, et al. Induction of graft-versus-host disease after autologous bone marrow transplantation. Lancet. 1989. https://doi.org/10.1016/S0140-6736(89)90826-X.

44. Liu J, Chen B, Yan F, Yang W. The influence of inflammatory cytokines on the proliferation and osteoblastic differentiation of MSCs. Curr Stem Cell Res Ther. 2017. https://doi.org/10.2174/1574888X12666170509102222.

45. Mishima H, Sugaya H, Yoshioka T, Wada H, Aoto K, Hyodo K, et al. 2. The effect of combined therapy, percutaneous autologous concentrated bone marrow grafting and low-intensity pulsed ultrasound (LIPUS), on the treatment of non-unions. J Orthop Trauma. 2016. https://doi.org/10.1097/01.bot.0000489987.43355.1d.

46. Westhauser F, Zimmermann G, Moghaddam S, Bruckner T, Schmidmaier G, Biglari B, et al. Reaming in treatment of non-unions in long bones: cytokine expression course as a tool for evaluation of non-union therapy. Arch Orthop Trauma Surg. 2015. https://doi.org/10.1007/s00402-015-2253-3.

Cross-cultural adaptation and validation of the Simplified Chinese version of Copenhagen Hip and Groin Outcome Score (HAGOS) for total hip arthroplasty

Shiqi Cao[1,2*†] ⓘ, Jia Cao[2†], Sirui Li[3†], Wei Wang[4*], Qirong Qian[2*] and Yu Ding[1]

Abstract

Background: To translate and cross-culturally adapt the Copenhagen Hip and Groin Outcome Score (HAGOS) into a Simplified Chinese version (HAGOS-C) and evaluate the reliability, validity, and responsiveness of the HAGOS-C in total hip arthroplasty (THA) patients.

Methods: The cross-cultural adaptation was performed according to the internationally recognized guidelines of the American Academy of Orthopaedic Surgeons Outcome Committee. A total of 192 participants were recruited in this study. The intra-class correlation coefficient (ICC) was used to determine reliability. Construct validity was analyzed by evaluating the correlations between HAGOS-C and EuroQoL 5-dimension (EQ-5D), as well as the short form (36) health survey (SF-36). Responsiveness of HAGOS-C was evaluated according to standard response means (SRM) and standard effect size (ES) between the first test and the third test (6 months after primary THA).

Results: The original version of the HAGOS was well cross-culturally adapted and translated into Simplified Chinese. HAGOS-C was indicated to have excellent reliability (ICC = 0.748–0.936, Cronbach's alpha = 0.787–0.886). Moderate to substantial correlations between subscales of HAGOS-C and EQ-5D ($r = 0.544$–0.751, $p < 0.001$), as well as physical function ($r = 0.567$–0.640, $p < 0.001$), role physical ($r = 0.570$–0.613, $p < 0.001$), bodily pain ($r = 0.467$–0.604, $p < 0.001$), and general health ($r = 0.387$–0.432, $p < 0.001$) subscales of SF-36, were observed. The ES of 0.805–1.100 and SRM of 1.408–2.067 revealed high responsiveness of HAGOS-C.

Conclusions: HAGOS-C was demonstrated to have excellent acceptability, reliability, validity, and responsiveness in THA, which could be recommended for patients in mainland China.

Keywords: HAGOS, Total hip arthroplasty, Reliability, Validity, Responsiveness, Quality of life

Background

Total hip arthroplasty (THA) has demonstrated among the most successful operations in medicine [1, 2] and proven effective in patients with hip diseases [3, 4], which has a profound impact on health-related quality of life (HRQoL) [5]. For a better understanding of patient disorder severity and more appropriate therapeutic approach [6], a large body of patient-based HRQoL questionnaires have been developed [7], such as Copenhagen Hip and Groin Outcome Score (HAGOS) [8]. This need has become more essential with the growing number of multicenter studies among different countries and cultures [7], which provide more statistical power of evidence-based trials [9]. When one reliable, valid questionnaire is used in populations with different cultures, it is necessary to test the psychometric properties of the questionnaire rather than simply translating the content to avoid bias due to cultural variety [10, 11].

---

* Correspondence: sq_cao@126.com; 345880492@qq.com; qianqr@163.com
†Shiqi Cao, Jia Cao and Sirui Li contributed equally to this work.
[1]Department of Rehabilitation, Minimally Invasive Spine Center, Navy General Hospital, No. 6, Fucheng Road, Haidian District, Beijing 100048, People's Republic of China
[4]Department of Orthopaedics, Chengdu Military General Hospital, No. 270, Tianhui Road, Jinniu District, Chengdu 610083, People's Republic of China
[2]Joint Surgery and Sports Medicine Department, Changzheng Hospital, Navy Medical University, No. 415, Fengyang Road, Huangpu District, Shanghai 200003, People's Republic of China
Full list of author information is available at the end of the article

The HAGOS, published in 2012, consists of 37 items in six subscales: symptoms (7 items), pain (10 items), function in daily living (5 items), function in sport and recreation (8 items), participation in physical activities (2 items), and hip- and/or groin-related quality of life (5 items) [8]. A Danish, English, Swedish, and Dutch version of HAGOS was distinguished in good reliability and validity [8, 12, 13] and has been widely used in assessing patients with hip disorders. Chinese is the language spoken by the largest population in the world, and China has one of the largest population of patients performed with total joint arthroplasty and arthroscopy. However, there is no HAGOS in Chinese version for this population so far. Besides, as a scale evaluating hip problems, no study has been performed to validate HAGOS in arthroplasty patients.

Considering the cultural gap and social environment between China and western countries, the purpose of this study was to translate, adapt the original version of HAGOS into a Simplified Chinese version (HAGOS-C) cross-culturally, and evaluate the reliability, validity, and responsiveness of HAGOS-C in native Chinese-speaking patients who underwent THA.

Methods

Translation and cross-cultural adaptation

The steps of translation and trans-cultural adaptation were followed by previous guidelines in five steps [7, 14]. Forward translation—two bilingual translators translated the scale from English to simplified Chinese independently. One of the translators was an orthopedic surgeon in the author's hospital; the other one was a professional translator without medical background. Synthesis of the translation—two translators and other researchers unified contradictions regarding language expression and cultural difference after a consensus meeting and obtained the first HAGOS-C. Backward translation—two native English speakers with fluent English and blind to the previous original English version of HAGOS independently translated the first HAGOS-C back into English version. Summarization of prefinal HAGOS-C—a consensus meeting with all researchers including four forward and backward translators was held to resolve all discrepancies, ambiguities, or any other verbal issues to reach a prefinal HAGOS-C. Determination of final HAGOS-C—researchers invited 20 patients to preliminarily test the prefinal version and collect feedback from them.

Eventually, all researchers involved in this study discussed issues in translation and developed the final HAGOS-C.

Patients and data collection

From August 2015 to September 2017, 192 participants were recruited from patients suffering from developmental dysplasia of hip joint, osteonecrosis of the femoral head, or hip osteoarthritis for total hip arthroplasty in two hospitals of authors. The inclusion criteria were as follows: age > 18 years of age, literate native Chinese speakers, and patients diagnosed with diseases above that required THA. Participants were excluded for similar symptoms at contralateral limb; inflammatory joint diseases, such as ankylosing spondylitis and rheumatoid arthritis; hip operation history; history of spine surgery or any surgery in the recent 1 month; other diseases that limited patient sport or movement ability; other uncontrolled systematic disorders, such as diabetes mellitus, malignant tumor, or hepatitis. Participants who met the inclusion criteria and presented no item in the exclusion criteria were recruited in this study. The number of patients also needed to meet the standard proposed by Terwee et al. [15] that the study should include at least 50 patients for floor or ceiling effects, reliability, and validity analysis. All included participants were required to sign informed consent, and the study was approved by the clinical research Ethics Committees of hospitals of authors.

Patients should provide demographic data regarding gender, year of age, side of affected joint, and diagnosis at the first day approving to participate the study and then finished the HAGOS-C, EuroQoL 5-dimension (EQ-5D), and the short form (36) health survey (SF-36). All participants filled in the HAGOS-C for the second time 7–14 days later before surgery to assess its test-retest reliability and were contacted 6 months postoperatively to complete HAGOS-C to assess its responsiveness.

Instruments

The Hip and Groin Outcome Score (HAGOS) is a disease-specific questionnaire for people suffering from hip and/or groin complaints [8]. It consists of 37 items in six subscales, symptoms (7 items), pain (10 items), function in daily living (ADL, 5 items), function in sport and recreation (sport/rec, 8 items), participation in physical activities (PA, 2 items), and hip- and/or groin-related quality of life (QoL, 5 items). In this questionnaire, all questions are answered from extreme symptoms to no symptoms, corresponding to 0 to 4 scores. Total points for each subscale are calculated according to the average score of all answered questions (eliminating missing value) and then multiplied by 25 into the centesimal system (0–100 scores). Higher scores refer to better outcome.

The EQ-5D is a self-reported questionnaire which consists of two pages, EQ-5D descriptive system, and EQ visual analog scale (EQ-VAS). EQ-5D descriptive system records the level of problems in five dimensions including mobility, self-care, usual activities, pain/discomfort, and anxiety/depression, and EQ-VAS records the respondent's self-rated health on a visual analog scale where the endpoints are labeled "best imaginable health state" and "worst imaginable health state" [16]. SF-36 is a questionnaire assessing the general quality of life. It is composed of 36 items in eight subscales to evaluate the patient's general condition. Scores for each subscale range from 0 (poor) to 100 (good) [17]. Both of the scales above have been translated into Chinese and proven good reliability and validity [18–20].

Psychometric assessments and statistical analysis

To assess the acceptability of HAGOS-C, patients were asked for the difficulties encountered. Statistical analysis for score distribution was performed. Floor and ceiling effects were defined as being present if more than 15% of patients reported lowest (0) or highest (100) possible scores [8, 21].

Reliability was examined in terms of test-retest reliability and internal consistency. The test-retest reliability was tested by comparing outcomes when the same patient without changes in health answered HAGOS-C at two separated situations with proper duration interval. It was evaluated by the intra-class correlation coefficient (ICC), which derived from a two-way analysis of variance in a random effect model. ICC > 0.8 and > 0.9 were considered as good and excellent reliability [22]. Bland-Altman plots were carried out to estimate systematic bias between the two measures [23]. Meanwhile, Cronbach's alpha was used to assess the internal consistency of the questionnaire, and > 0.7, 0.8, and 0.9 was considered as acceptable, good, and excellent internal consistency, respectively [15].

Validity tests for HAGOS-C included content validity and construct validity. To assess content validity, one rehabilitation therapist and three orthopedists were invited to analyze the correlation between content in each item and state of disease. Good construct validity meant that the questionnaire correlated well with measures of the same construct (convergent validity) and correlated poorly with measures of different constructs (divergent or discriminant validity) [24]. On account of this theory, we assumed that the score of HAGOS-C should be in accordance with EQ-VAS and disease-related subscales of EQ-5D and SF-36, but not with other subscales of EQ-5D and SF-36. Under such hypothesis, we calculated Pearson correlation coefficient * between HAGOS-C and EQ-VAS and subscales of EQ-5D and SF-36. Then, the construct validity for HAGOS-C was evaluated by comparing how data conformed to the calculated correlations, judged as poor ($r = 0$–0.2), fair ($r = 0.2$–0.4), moderate ($r = 0.4$–0.6), substantial ($r = 0.6$–0.8), or almost perfect ($r = 0.8$–1.0) [24].

The responsiveness of HAGOS-C was evaluated according to standard response means (SRM) and standard effect size (ES) between the first test and the third test (6 months after primary THA). SRM represented the mean change score divided by the SD of the change score. The ES was calculated as the mean change in score divided by the SD of the baseline score [25]. SRM

was considered large if larger than 0.80, moderate if between 0.50 and 0.79, and small if between 0.2 and 0.49. For ES, a value of 0.80 or higher was considered as high responsiveness.

Statistical Package for the Social Sciences, version 20.0 (SPSS, Chicago, IL) was used to analyze data. p values of 0.05 or less were considered significant.

Results

Participants

From August 2015 to September 2017, 238 patients were invited to participate in our study, and 192 of them (80.7%) agreed to participate in the study. All patients completed two rounds of instruments without withdrawn cases, in which 158 (82.3% of patients included) finished the third round of instrument assessing responsiveness. Detailed demographic and clinical characteristics of participants were listed in Table 1.

Translation and cross-cultural adaptation process

There were no major problems in the forward and back translations of HAGOS. However, "vacuuming" in the item A5 listed in the original English version of HAGOS were less popular among Chinese and were adapted cross-culturally into "sweeping floors." After the adaptation, no special issue was raised by the participants in the prefinal test. In consequence, the final version of HAGOS-C could be used to evaluate the patients' condition in further research.

Acceptability and score distribution

In formal investigation, no participants complained that any content was too difficult to understand at the first time of completing HAGOS-C. The answer rate was 100%.

Neither ceiling effect nor floor effect was significant in all subscales of HAGOS-C, except floor effect for the subscale PA (20.3%) (Table 2).

Table 1 Demographic and clinical characteristics of participants

Characteristics	Number or mean ± SD
Age (years)	64.1 ± 12.7
Range	28–88
Gender	Total ($N = 192$)
Female	112 (58.3%)
Male	80 (41.7%)
Side	
Right	85 (44.3%)
Left	107 (55.7%)
Diagnosis	
Developmental dysplasia of hip joint	87 (45.3%)
Osteonecrosis of the femoral head	73 (38.0%)
Hip osteoarthritis	32 (16.7%)

Table 2 Score distribution and floor-ceiling effects of the subscales of HAGOS-C

Subscale	Mean ± SD	Observed range	Theoretical range	Floor effect (%)*	Ceiling effect (%)*
Symptoms	44.9 ± 16.9	3.6–82.1	0–100	0	0
Pain	39.2 ± 15.8	0–87.5	0–100	2.1	0
ADL	49.3 ± 23.9	0–100	0–100	0.5	1.6
Sport/rec	36.5 ± 19.3	0–90.6	0–100	3.1	0
PAsss	26.3 ± 24.0	0–100	0–100	20.3	1.0
QoL	34.1 ± 21.2	0–95	0–100	6.3	0

*Percentage of patients with the worst (floor effect) and the best (ceiling effect) condition
HAGOS-C Chinese version of the Copenhagen Hip and Groin Outcome Score, ADL physical function in daily living, sport/rec physical function in sport and recreation, PA participation in physical activities, QoL hip and or/groin-related quality of life

Reliability

Mean scores of each subscale in the retest was comparable with the first test (Table 3). ICCs ranged from 0.748 to 0.936, demonstrating good or excellent test-retest reliability of HAGOS-C. Bland-Altman plots for the two measures revealed no systematic error (Fig. 1), which suggested good test-retest accordance and reproducibility of HAGOS-C [23]. Cronbach's alpha coefficient was calculated for each subscale ranging from 0.787 to 0.886, indicating a high internal consistency.

Validity

According to the evaluation of rehabilitation expert and orthopedic experts, the content validity was good in HAGOS-C and the information derived from all items was adequate to assess the function of included patients.

Table 4 lists the data of construct validity of HAGOS-C. All subscales of the HAGOS-C showed significant correlations with the EQ-5D-S total score and the EQ-5D-S VAS score (Table 4). When comparing HAGOS-C with SF-36, correlation coefficients for subscales of physical function ($r = 0.567$–0.640, $p < 0.001$), role physical ($r = 0.570$–0.613, $p < 0.001$), bodily pain ($r = 0.467$–0.604, $p < 0.001$), and general health ($r = 0.387$–0.432, $p < 0.001$) were moderate to substantial; meanwhile, this correlation was just weak to fair for vitality ($r = 0.195$–0.256, $p = 0.001$–0.007), social function ($r = 0.240$–0.313, $p < 0.001$), role emotional

($r = 0.141$–0.247, $p = 0.001$–0.051), and mental health ($r = 0.168$–0.276, $p = 0.001$–0.020), which consistently matches our hypothesis.

Responsiveness

To assess responsiveness, 158 participants completed the third round of instrument approximately 6 months after primary THA. ES ranged from 0.805 to 1.100, and SRM ranged from 1.408 to 2.067 (Table 3). Both ES and SRM were greater than 0.80, indicating high responsiveness for all subscales.

Discussion

In this study, the English version of HAGOS was successfully translated and cross-culturally adapted into Simplified Chinese. The HAGOS-C had good reliability, validity, and responsiveness in evaluating patients who underwent THA in mainland China.

HRQoL questionnaires are very important and valuable in the quantification of patients' function and data analysis among studies. Nowadays, with the invigorating strategy through science, technology and education, and greater science and technology input in China, the number of papers annually published in China is the second largest all over the world [24, 26, 27]. Therefore, valid questionnaires are urgently needed to support this huge amount of clinical research.

Table 3 Reliability and responsiveness of the HAGOS-C

Subscale	1st test (mean ± SD)	2nd test (mean ± SD)	3rd test (mean ± SD)	ICC (CI range)	ES	SRM	Cronbach's alpha
Symptoms	45.3 ± 16.9	45.1 ± 19.5	64.3 ± 16.2	0.824 (0.773–0.865)	1.100	1.868	0.812
Pain	38.8 ± 15.8	39.9 ± 18.5	56.2 ± 13.7	0.806 (0.750–0.850)	1.096	1.949	0.787
ADL	47.6 ± 23.9	49.0 ± 25.8	69.6 ± 20.2	0.902 (0.872–0.926)	0.849	2.067	0.886
Sport/rec	36.5 ± 19.3	35.6 ± 20.4	57.2 ± 18.6	0.913 (0.886–0.934)	1.057	1.797	0.858
PA	27.5 ± 24.0	32.7 ± 25.7	48.4 ± 24.2	0.793 (0.734–0.840)	0.805	1.408	0.866
QoL	33.8 ± 21.2	35.8 ± 22.2	54.5 ± 21.0	0.946 (0.929–0.959)	0.944	1.644	0.873

*The 1st test was conducted at the beginning of this research (192 patients), the 2nd test was conducted 1 week later to calculate the test-retest reliability (ICC) of the HAGOS-C (192 patients), and the 3rd test was conducted 6 months later to calculate the responsiveness (ES, SRM) of the HAGOS-C (158 patients)
ICC intra-class correlation coefficient, ES effect size, SRM standardized response mean, CI 95% confidence interval, HAGOS-C Chinese version of the Copenhagen Hip and Groin Outcome Score

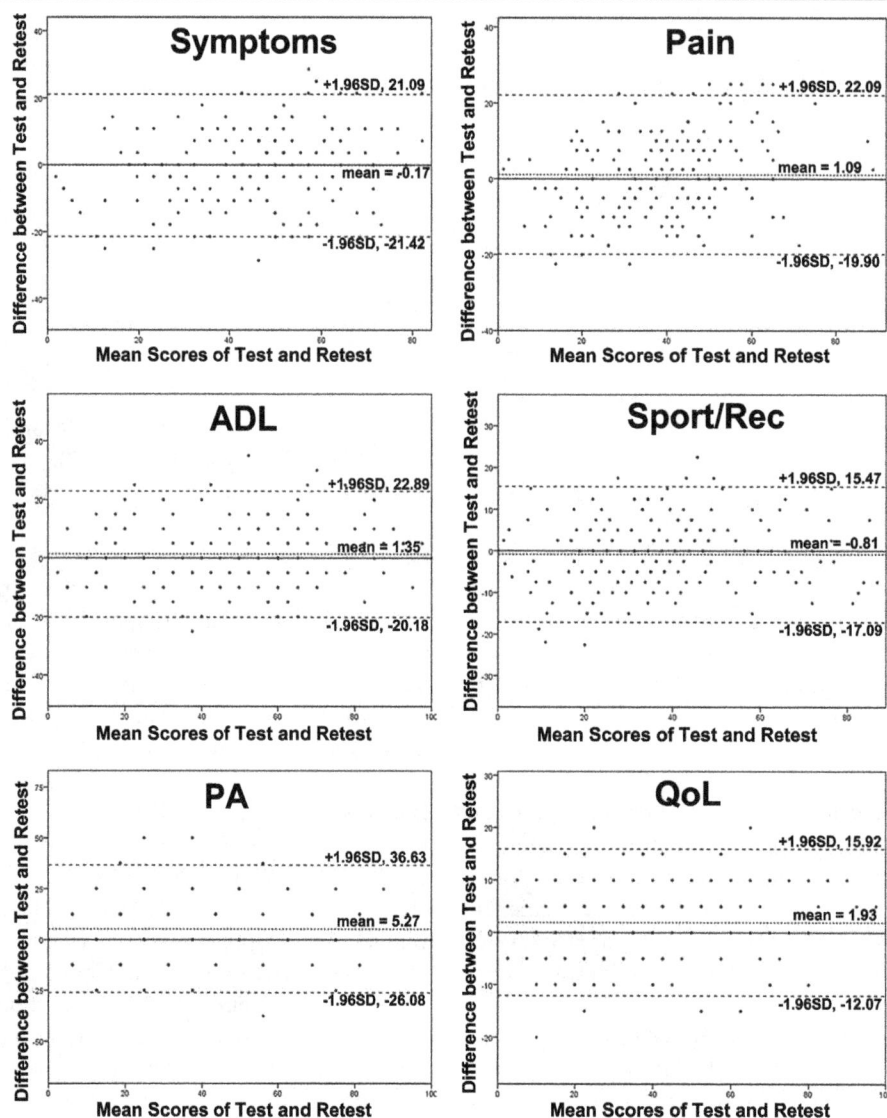

Fig. 1 The Bland-Altman plot for test-retest agreement of HAGOS. The differences between scores for HAGOS from first two test sessions were plotted against the mean of the test and retest. The line indicates mean difference value of the two sessions and the 95% (mean ± 1.96 standard deviation) limits of agreement

In the process of translation and adaptation, authors strictly followed the standardized procedure listed in the literature. In item A5, "vacuuming" written in the original English version of HAGOS were less popular among Chinese and were adapted cross-culturally into "sweeping floors". Interestingly, with the popularity of price-friendly "sweeping and mopping robot" in China, better examples listed in A5 in HAGOS-C might be explored to substitute "scrubbing and sweeping floors".

A floor effect of 20.8% was observed in the subscale of PA in HAGOS-C, which was also detected in literature before [8, 12, 13]. This relative high floor effect might be due to the following reasons. Firstly, there are only two

items listed in this subscale, which makes it easy to choose both of the items with the lowest score. Besides, some of the patients who underwent THA suffered from end-stage hip diseases, which restricted patients from participation in physical activities naturally.

In our study, all subscales of HAGOS-C showed very good internal consistency (Cronbach's alpha = 0.787–0.886) and test-retest reliability (ICC = 0.793–0.946). The results above were basically in agreement with the data reported by Thorborg et al. (Danish HAGOS), Thomeé et al. (Swedish HAGOS), and Brans et al. (Dutch HAGOS) [8, 12, 13]. The ICC for the QoL subscale (ICC = 0.946) is the highest among all subscales, which might due to the fact that

Table 4 Construct validity of the HAGOS-C

Correlation coefficient r_s (p value)*	HAGOS-C subscales					
	Symptoms	Pain	ADL	Sport/rec	PA	QoL
EQ-5D						
Total score	0.751 (< 0.001)	0.637 (< 0.001)	0.605 (< 0.001)	0.637 (< 0.001)	0.544 (< 0.001)	0.625 (< 0.001)
Health status (VAS)	0.671 (< 0.001)	0.534 (< 0.001)	0.495 (< 0.001)	0.523 (< 0.001)	0.513 (< 0.001)	0.523 (< 0.001)
SF-36 subscales						
Physical function	0.601 (< 0.001)	0.568 (< 0.001)	0.640 (< 0.001)	0.602 (< 0.001)	0.567 (< 0.001)	0.593 (< 0.001)
Role-physical	0.589 (< 0.001)	0.598 (< 0.001)	0.579 (< 0.001)	0.613 (< 0.001)	0.573 (< 0.001)	0.570 (< 0.001)
Bodily pain	0.567 (< 0.001)	0.604 (< 0.001)	0.490 (< 0.001)	0.557 (< 0.001)	0.467 (< 0.001)	0.541 (< 0.001)
General health	0.432 (< 0.001)	0.391 (< 0.001)	0.407 (< 0.001)	0.406 (< 0.001)	0.406 (< 0.001)	0.387 (< 0.001)
Vitality	0.195 (0.007)	0.243 (0.001)	0.218 (0.002)	0.232 (0.001)	0.256 (< 0.001)	0.221 (0.002)
Social function	0.282 (< 0.001)	0.278 (< 0.001)	0.240 (0.001)	0.286 (< 0.001)	0.313 (< 0.001)	0.282 (< 0.001)
Role-emotional	0.168 (0.020)	0.141 (0.051)	0.169 (0.019)	0.178 (0.014)	0.247 (0.001)	0.180 (0.012)
Mental health	0.177 (0.014)	0.203 (0.005)	0.168 (0.020)	0.195 (0.007)	0.276 (< 0.001)	0.198 (0.006)

*Calculated by the Pearson correlation coefficient of the HAGOS-C with EQ-5D and SF-36

HAGOS-C Chinese version of the Copenhagen Hip and Groin Outcome Score, *EQ-5D* EuroQol-5 dimensions, *SF-36* short form 36, *ADL* physical function in daily living, *sport/rec* physical function in sport and recreation, *PA* participation in physical activities, *QoL* hip and or/groin-related quality of life

quality of life for patients changed with least possibility in the duration interval of 1 to 2 weeks among the perspectives assessed in HAGOS-C.

The correlation between the subscales of HAGOS-C and EQ-5D total score, EQ-VAS, as well as SF-36 subscales, was in accordance with our hypothesis. Almost all correlations between HAGOS-C subscales and EQ-5D total score, EQ-VAS, as well as SF-36 subscales, were significant, except the correlation between pain subscale of HAGOS-C and role-emotional subscale of SF-36. However, the r value for these correlations varied a lot. In our study, HAGOS-C subscales correlated better with the EQ-5D total score, EQ-VAS, and physical function, role physical, and bodily pain subscales of SF-36, whereas these correlations were weaker between HAGOS-C subscales and vitality, social function, role-emotional, and mental health subscales of SF-36. One possible reason might be that HAGOS-C was designed for the evaluation of function and symptoms in the hip and groin region, and vitality, social function, role-emotional, and mental health subscales of SF-36 indicated psychological or social state of patients, which could be affected by many factors other than physical situation and symptoms comparing with other scales of high correlation with HAGOS-C. Interestingly, the correlation between symptoms, pain, and sport/rec subscales of HAGOS-C and EQ-5D and physical function, role-physical, bodily pain, and general health subscales of SF-36 were the slightly higher other subscales of HAGOS-C. Likewise, this might contribute to the fact that symptoms, pain, and sport/rec subscales of HAGOS-C indicated direct symptoms of patients, which were affected more by the disease itself with less interference of other matters. All of these suggested

satisfied divergent or discriminant validity for HAGOS-C in THA patients.

The responsiveness was tested to detect changes between the preoperative and 6-month postoperative conditions. As our hypothesis, SRM and ES were defined as large after 6 months of postoperative rehabilitation. This outcome is similar to some part of other versions of the HAGOS. The ESs for the change in the score on the Danish version of HAGOS were – 1.29 to – 0.60, 0.01 to 0.19, and 0.77 to 1.78, in "much worse" and "worse" group, "somewhat worse" and "not changed" and "somewhat better," and "much better" and "better" group, respectively[8]. Analogously, ESs on the Swedish version were – 0.44 to – 0.19, 0.23 to 0.54, and 1.07 to 1.87 in 20 points lower, ± 20 points, and 20 points higher of global perceived effect group, respectively [13]. The ESs in our study was much larger than the first two groups in both of the studies above, but comparable with the third group in these two studies. In the original Danish study, authors included patients seeking medical care presenting with hip and/or groin who had received treatment for the symptom, and in the cross-cultural study on Swedish, patients requiring hip arthroscopy for femoroacetabular impingement were investigated. Meanwhile, only patients who underwent THA were included in our study. Under the circumstances, the patients' symptom severity in both of the studies above was milder than our study. As we know, THA has demonstrated among the most successful operations in medicine [1, 2], which has been proven effective in patients with hip diseases [3, 4]; so, it is reasonable that larger ESs were shown among patients who underwent THA.

There are several limitations to our study. First, the sample was limited in size and may not fully represent the Chinese population. Second, although Simplified Chinese is the official language in China, China is a country with multiple nationalities, most of which have their own language. Thus, the problem of national cultural differences should be noted. Finally, patients with symptoms in the hip and/or groin region who were not performed with THA were not evaluated, which could be carried out in future studies.

Conclusion
The HAGOS was successfully translated and cross-culturally adapted into Simplified Chinese. The HAGOS-C had good reliability, validity, and responsiveness in evaluating patients who underwent THA in mainland China.

Abbreviations
ADL: Function in daily living; EQ-5D: EuroQoL 5-dimension; EQ-VAS: EQ visual analog scale; ES: Effect size; HAGOS: Copenhagen Hip and Groin Outcome Score; HAGOS-C: Simplified Chinese version of Copenhagen Hip and Groin Outcome Score; HRQoL: Health-related quality of life; ICC: Intra-class correlation coefficient; PA: Participation in physical activities; QoL: Groin-related quality of life; SF-36: Short form (36) health survey; Sport/rec: Function in sport and recreation; SRM: Standard response means; THA: Total hip arthroplasty

Acknowledgements
This study was funded by the National Natural Science Foundation of China (grant number: 81171727).
We sincerely thank Rong Zhou and Shu Chen for their work in the translation and cross-cultural adaptation.

Funding
This project was funded by the National Natural Science Foundation of China (grant number: 81171727).

Authors' contributions
SQC, WW, and QRQ contributed to the study design. SQC and SRL contributed to the data analysis. JC, SRL, and YD contributed to the collection of data. SQC and WW contributed to the writing of the manuscript. SQC, JC, and SRL contributed to the modification of the manuscript. All authors read and approved the final manuscript.

Competing interests
The authors declare that they have no competing interests.

Author details
[1]Department of Rehabilitation, Minimally Invasive Spine Center, Navy General Hospital, No. 6, Fucheng Road, Haidian District, Beijing 100048, People's Republic of China. [2]Joint Surgery and Sports Medicine Department, Changzheng Hospital, Navy Medical University, No. 415, Fengyang Road, Huangpu District, Shanghai 200003, People's Republic of China. [3]College of Basic Medicine, Army Medical University, Chongqing 400038, People's Republic of China. [4]Department of Orthopaedics, Chengdu Military General Hospital, No. 270, Tianhui Road, Jinniu District, Chengdu 610083, People's Republic of China.

References
1. Balck F, Kirschner S, Jeszenszky C, Lippmann M, Gunther KP. Validity and reliability of the German version of the HSS Expectation Questionnaire on Hip Joint Replacement. Z Orthop Unfall. 2016;154:606.
2. Brown JM, Mistry JB, Cherian JJ, Elmallah RK, Chughtai M, Harwin SF, Mont MA. Femoral component revision of total hip arthroplasty. Orthopedics. 2016;39:e1129.
3. Wang D, Li LL, Wang HY, Pei FX, Zhou ZK. Long-term results of cementless total hip arthroplasty with subtrochanteric shortening osteotomy in Crowe type IV developmental dysplasia. J Arthroplast. 2016;32(4).
4. Bause L. Short stem total hip arthroplasty in patients with rheumatoid arthritis. Orthopedics. 2015;38:S46.
5. Veenhof C, Huisman PA, Barten JA, Takken T, Pisters MF. Factors associated with physical activity in patients with osteoarthritis of the hip or knee: a systematic review. Osteoarthr Cartil. 2012;20:6.
6. Guyatt GH, Feeny DH, Patrick DL. Measuring health-related quality of life. Ann Intern Med. 1993;118:622.
7. Guillemin F, Bombardier C, Beaton D. Cross-cultural adaptation of health-related quality of life measures: literature review and proposed guidelines. J Clin Epidemiol. 1993;46:1417.
8. Thorborg K, Holmich P, Christensen R, Petersen J, Roos EM. The Copenhagen Hip and Groin Outcome Score (HAGOS): development and validation according to the COSMIN checklist. Br J Sports Med. 2011;45:478.
9. Freedman KB, Back S, Bernstein J. Sample size and statistical power of randomised, controlled trials in orthopaedics. J Bone Joint Surg Br. 2001;83:397.
10. Pynsent PB. Choosing an outcome measure. J Bone Joint Surg Br. 2001;83:792.
11. Zheng W, Li J, Zhao J, Liu D, Xu W. Development of a valid simplified Chinese version of the Oxford hip score in patients with hip osteoarthritis. Clin Orthop Relat Res. 2014;472:1545.
12. Brans E, de Graaf JS, Munzebrock AV, Bessem B, Reininga IH. Cross-cultural adaptation and validation of the Dutch version of the Hip and Groin Outcome Score (HAGOS-NL). PLoS One. 2016;11:e0148119.
13. Thomee R, Jonasson P, Thorborg K, Sansone M, Ahlden M, Thomee C, Karlsson J, Baranto A. Cross-cultural adaptation to Swedish and validation of the Copenhagen Hip and Groin Outcome Score (HAGOS) for pain, symptoms and physical function in patients with hip and groin disability due to femoro-acetabular impingement. Knee Surg Sports Traumatol Arthrosc. 2014;22:835.
14. Beaton DE, Bombardier C, Guillemin F, Ferraz MB. Guidelines for the process of cross-cultural adaptation of self-report measures. Spine (Phila Pa 1976). 2000;25:3186.
15. Terwee CB, Bot SD, de Boer MR, van der Windt DA, Knol DL, Dekker J, Bouter LM, de Vet HC. Quality criteria were proposed for measurement properties of health status questionnaires. J Clin Epidemiol. 2007;60:34.
16. Rabin R, de Charro F. EQ-5D: a measure of health status from the EuroQol Group. Ann Med. 2001;33:337.
17. Brazier JE, Harper R, Jones NM, O'Cathain A, Thomas KJ, Usherwood T, Westlake L. Validating the SF-36 health survey questionnaire: new outcome measure for primary care. BMJ. 1992;305:160.
18. Gao F, Ng GY, Cheung YB, Thumboo J, Pang G, Koo WH, Sethi VK, Wee J, Goh C. The Singaporean English and Chinese versions of the EQ-5D achieved measurement equivalence in cancer patients. J Clin Epidemiol. 2009;62:206.
19. Wang HM, Patrick DL, Edwards TC, Skalicky AM, Zeng HY, Gu WW. Validation of the EQ-5D in a general population sample in urban China. Qual Life Res. 2012;21:155.

Cross-cultural adaptation and validation of the Simplified Chinese version of Copenhagen Hip and Groin...

191

20. Li L, Wang HM, Shen Y. Chinese SF-36 Health Survey: translation, cultural adaptation, validation, and normalisation. J Epidemiol Community Health. 2003;57:259.

21. McHorney CA, Tarlov AR. Individual-patient monitoring in clinical practice: are available health status surveys adequate? Qual Life Res. 1995;4:293.

22. Landis JR, Koch GG. The measurement of observer agreement for categorical data. Biometrics. 1977;33:159.

23. Bland JM, Altman DG. Measuring agreement in method comparison studies. Stat Methods Med Res. 1999;8:135.

24. Wei X, Wang Z, Yang C, Wu B, Liu X, Yi H, Chen Z, Wang F, Bai Y, Li J, Zhu X, Li M. Development of a simplified Chinese version of the Hip Disability and Osteoarthritis Outcome Score (HOOS): cross-cultural adaptation and psychometric evaluation. Osteoarthr Cartil. 2012;20:1563.

25. Husted JA, Cook RJ, Farewell VT, Gladman DD. Methods for assessing responsiveness: a critical review and recommendations. J Clin Epidemiol. 2000;53:459.

26. Cao S, Liu N, Han W, Zi Y, Peng F, Li L, Fu Q, Chen Y, Zheng W, Qian Q. Simplified Chinese version of the forgotten joint score (FJS) for patients who underwent joint arthroplasty: cross-cultural adaptation and validation. J Orthop Surg Res. 2017;12:6.

27. Cao S, Liu N, Li L, Lv H, Chen Y, Qian Q. Simplified Chinese version of University of California at Los Angeles Activity Score for Arthroplasty and Arthroscopy: cross-cultural adaptation and validation. J Arthroplast. 2017;32:2706.

Association between SMAD3 gene polymorphisms and osteoarthritis risk: a systematic review and meta-analysis

Jian-qiao Hong[†], Yang-xin Wang[†], Si-hao Li, Guang-yao Jiang, Bin Hu, Yu-te Yang, Jia-hong Meng and Shi-gui Yan[*] ⓘ

Abstract

Objective: Several studies have been performed to investigate the association between SMAD3 gene polymorphism and osteoarthritis (OA), but the results were inconclusive. This study aims to determine whether SMAD3 polymorphism is associated with risk of OA.

Method: A comprehensive literature search in PubMed, Embase, and ISI Web of Science for relevant studies was performed. After extracting data from eligible studies, we chose the fixed or random effect model according to the heterogeneity test. Estimation of publication bias and sensitivity analysis were conducted to confirm the stability of this meta-analysis.

Results: In total, 10 studies from 6 articles with 5093 OA patients and 5699 controls were enrolled in this meta-analysis. The combined results revealed significant association between SMAD3 rs12901499 polymorphism and the risk of OA (allele model: OR 1.21, 95% CI 1.07–1.38). Subgroup analysis revealed that G allele increased the risk of OA in Caucasians, but not in Asians (allele model: Caucasians: OR 1.31, 95% CI 1.18–1.44; Asians: OR 1.24, 95% CI 0.95–1.61). And the pooled results revealed significant association between SMAD3 rs12901499 polymorphism and both knee and hip OA (knee OA: OR 1.18, 95% CI 1.04–1.34; hip OA: OR 1.31, 95% CI 1.18–1.44).

Conclusion: The current meta-analysis revealed that the G variant of SMAD3 rs12901499 polymorphism increased the risk of OA in Caucasians. Further well-designed studies with larger sample size in different ethnic populations are required to confirm these results.

Keywords: SMAD3, Polymorphism, Osteoarthritis, Meta-analysis

Background

Osteoarthritis (OA), a late-onset musculoskeletal disease in the elder, is featured by the gradual degradation of articular cartilage with further lesion to the synovium, subchondral bone, or the other joint tissues. The osteoarthritis could cause chronic joint pain with swelling and restricted range of motion through the pathologic process including narrowing of joint space and osteophyte formation [1–3]. It was estimated that over 15% of the population suffered from OA, and the number tends to be doubled by 2020 due to the increasing elder population [4, 5]. Though the mechanism of osteoarthritis still has not been fully clarified,

a large number of risk factors have been reported, including age, sex, obesity, trauma in the joint, environmental factors, and genetic factors [3, 6, 7].

The SMAD3 (SMAD family member 3) gene, located on chromosome 15q22.33, acts a critical role in the joint homeostasis [8, 9]. It is known as a downstream mediator in the TGF-B (transforming growth factor-b) signaling pathway which plays a key role in anabolism of chondrocytes [9]. The genetic variations of TGF-B signaling have been reported significant relationship to the OA [10]. In TGF-β signaling pathway, SMAD3 translocates into the nucleus and regulates target gene transcription and produces the phenotype in cartilage by interaction with DNA and transcription factors [11]. Several studies have been performed to investigate the association between SMAD3 polymorphisms and OA susceptibility, but the results

---

* Correspondence: zrjwsj@zju.edu.cn

[†]Jian-qiao Hong and Yang-xin Wang contributed equally to this work.
Department of Orthopaedic Surgery, The Second Affiliated Hospital, Zhejiang University School of Medicine, No.88 Jiefang Road, Hangzhou 310009, People's Republic of China

remained unclear. Valdes [12] revealed that the SMAD3 gene rs12901499 polymorphism was associated with hip and knee OA in European populations. However, the results reported by other subsequent studies remain inconsistent and inconclusive [13–17]. In this study, we therefore performed a meta-analysis to evaluate whether the SMAD3 gene polymorphisms are associated with the risk of OA.

Materials and methods

Literature search strategy

We conducted a comprehensive literature search using the electronic databases PubMed, Embase, and ISI Web of Science for relevant studies published in English (last search was updated on April 10, 2018). The search strategy was based on the following keywords: ("SMAD3" OR "SMAD family member 3") AND ("polymorphism" OR "variant" OR "SNP") AND ("osteoarthritis" OR "OA"). References of clinical trials and review articles were also searched manually for additional articles. All the literature search was performed according to the Preferred Reporting Items for Systematic Reviews and Meta-Analyses (PRISMA) guidelines (Additional file 1: Table S1) [18].

Inclusion criteria

Two researchers screened the relevant investigations and further determined the eligible studies which met the following inclusion criteria: (1) case-control or cohort design; (2) evaluating the association between SMAD3 polymorphisms and knee/hip OA susceptibility; (3) patients with OA were diagnosed based on clinical manifestation and radiographic findings, or received total joint arthroplasty because of primary OA; and (4) enough data on genotype or allele frequency for calculation of odds ratio (OR) and corresponding 95% confidence interval (CI). The animal model research, review, case reports, or the studies without sufficient data were excluded. If several articles reported findings for repeated study populations, we only selected the most recent study or the one with the largest sample size.

Data extraction

For each eligible study, two independent investigators extracted the following data: first author's name, publication year, country and ethnicity of study population, study design, OA sites, sample size, demographics of enrolled subjects, genotyping method, studied polymorphisms, and genotype distributions.

Quality assessment

According to the Newcastle-Ottawa Quality Assessment Scale (NOS) [19], the quality score of each study was based on three categories: selection (4 items, 1 point each), comparability (1 item, up to 2 points), and exposure/outcome (3 items, 1 point each). Each

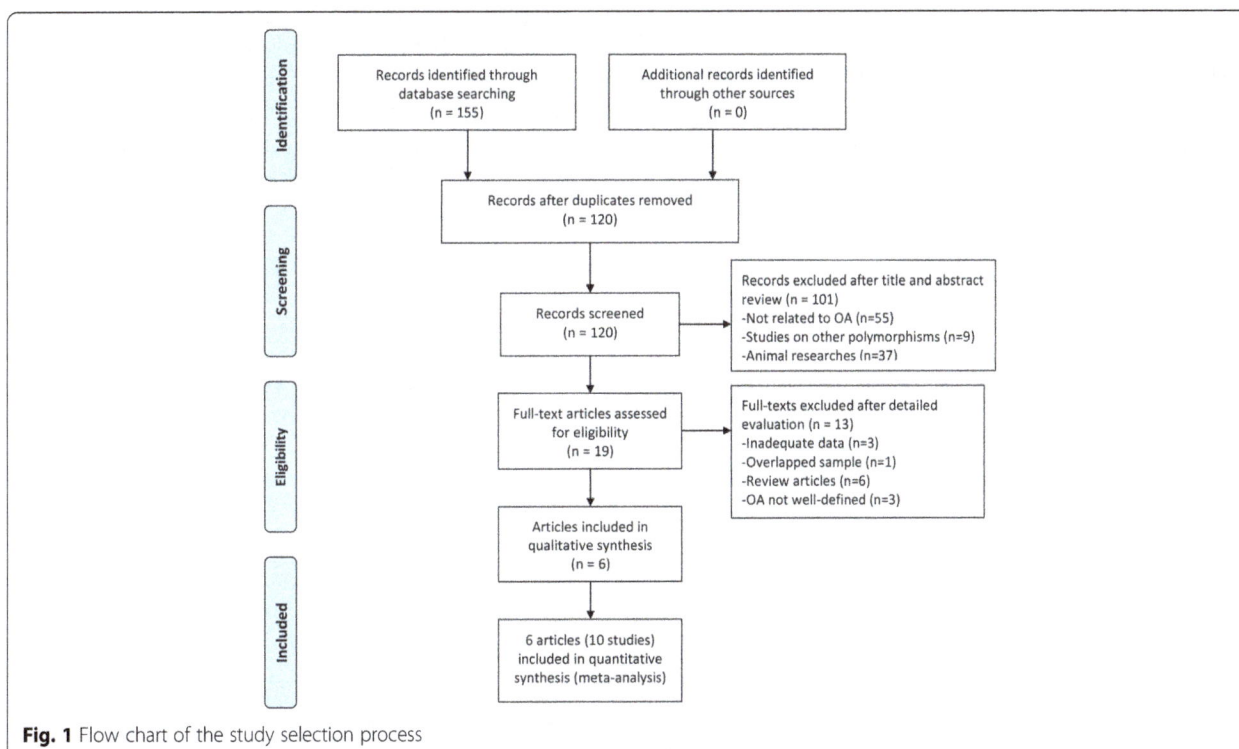

Fig. 1 Flow chart of the study selection process

Table 1 Characteristics of included studies

Study	Year	Country	Ethnicity	Design	OA site	Genotyping method	Sample size (F/M)		HWE	NOS
							OA	Control		
Valdes-Discovery set	2010	UK	Caucasian	CC	Knee, hip	Allele-specific PCR	477 (NA)	520 (NA)	Y	7
Valdes-Nottingham	2010	UK	Caucasian	CC	Knee, hip	Allele-specific PCR	2014 (NA)	733 (NA)	Y	7
Valdes-Chingford	2010	UK	Caucasian	Cohort	Knee, hip	Allele-specific PCR	317 (317/0)	488 (488/0)	Y	9
Valdes-Hertfordshire	2010	UK	Caucasian	Cohort	Knee	Allele-specific PCR	167 (NA)	867 (NA)	Y	8
Valdes-Estonia	2010	Estonia	Caucasian	Cohort	Knee	Allele-specific PCR	68 (NA)	449 (NA)	Y	8
Jiang	2013	China	Asian	CC	Knee	PCR-RFLP	232 (159/73)	236 (91/145)	Y	7
Su	2015	China	Asian	CC	Knee	PCR-RFLP	518 (328/190)	468 (261/207)	Y	7
Sharma	2017	India	Asian	CC	Knee	Allele-specific PCR	450 (230/220)	458 (234/224)	Y	8
Zhang	2018	China	Asian	CC	Knee	Allele-specific PCR	350 (99/251)	400 (110/210)	Y	8
Zhong	2018	China	Asian	CC	Hip	Allele-specific PCR	500 (260/240)	1080 (580/500)	Y	8

CC case-control, *F* female, *M* male, *NA* number of each gender not available, *HWE* Hardy-Weinberg equilibrium, *NOS* Newcastle-Ottawa Quality Assessment Scale

study scored from 0 point (worst) to 9 points (best), and scored 6 or less were classified as low quality, whereas studies scoring 7 or higher were defined as high quality.

Statistical analysis

All statistical analyses were conducted with STATA version 12.0 (STATA Corporation, College Station, TX, USA), and *p* value < 0.05 was considered significant except for the I^2 statistic. To assess the correlation between SMAD3 polymorphisms and OA susceptibility, we calculated pooled ORs with 95% CI and analyzed five genetic models: allele model, dominant model, recessive model, homozygous model, and heterozygous model.

Heterogeneity between studies was measured using *Q* and I^2 statistics [20]. If $I^2 > 50\%$ and *p* value of *Q* statistic < 0.10, the DerSimonian-Laird random effect model was applied to calculate pooled ORs and 95% CIs [21].

Otherwise, a fixed effect model was used as the pooling method [22].

Subgroup analysis was conducted by ethnicity, OA site. Sensitivity analysis was also performed by removing individual study sequentially in order to evaluate the stability of pooled results. We evaluated the publication bias by funnel plot and Egger's regression test.

Results
Study selection

Figure 1 presented the selection process and reasons for exclusion. One hundred fifty-five articles were retrieved totally from a systematic literature search, 35 articles were removed because of duplications, and 101 articles were excluded after review of title and abstract; only 19 full-text articles remained for further evaluation. Subsequently, 4 articles were excluded because of inadequate data, 1 article was excluded due to overlapped

Table 2 Genotype and allele distributions of SMAD3 rs12901499 polymorphism in the included studies

Study	Genotype distribution						Allele distribution				Association findings
	OA			Control			OA		Control		
	AA	AG	GG	AA	AG	GG	A	G	A	G	
Valdes-Discovery set	NA	NA	NA	NA	NA	NA	419	635	489	551	G allele↑
Valdes-Nottingham	NA	NA	NA	NA	NA	NA	1788	2336	698	768	G allele↑
Valdes-Chingford	NA	NA	NA	NA	NA	NA	316	388	477	499	NS
Valdes-Hertfordshire	NA	NA	NA	NA	NA	NA	134	200	779	955	NS
Valdes-Estonia	NA	NA	NA	NA	NA	NA	67	79	481	417	NS
Jiang	47	141	25	114	83	23	235	191	311	129	G allele↑, GG genotype↑
Su	142	247	129	116	228	124	531	505	460	476	NS
Sharma	85	70	75	90	92	52	240	220	272	196	G allele↑, GG genotype↑
Zhang	82	173	91	81	202	111	337	355	364	424	GG genotype↓
Zhong	10	200	290	20	610	450	220	780	650	1510	G allele↑, GG genotype↑

NA data not available, ↑/↓ increase/decrease the risk of OA, *NS* not significant

Table 3 Pooled results on the association between SMAD3 rs12901499 polymorphism and OA risk

Genetic model	Sub-group	No. of studies	Test of association		Statistical model	Test of heterogeneity	
			OR (95% CI)	p		I^2 (%)	p
Allele model (G vs. A)	Overall	10	1.21 (1.07–1.38)	0.003	Random	75.4	0.000
	Ethnicity						
	Asian	5	1.24 (0.95–1.61)	0.115	Random	88.7	0.000
	Caucasian	5	1.20 (1.11–1.31)	0.000	Fixed	0.0	0.891
	OA site						
	Knee OA	9	1.18 (1.04–1.34)	0.011	Random	67.1	0.002
	Hip OA	4	1.31 (1.18–1.44)	0.000	Fixed	39.9	0.172

samples, and 8 review articles were removed; 3 articles studied generalized OA, temporomandibular joint OA, and spinal OA, respectively, and were not included because the OA patients included by those studies were not well defined.

Finally, 6 articles met our inclusion criteria [12–17]. One article provided by Valdes included 5 different study populations; these 5 studies were analyzed independently. Therefore, 10 independent studies from 6 articles were included in our meta-analysis.

Characteristics of included studies

Table 1 shows the main characteristics of included studies, and Table 2 presents the genotype and allele distributions of the SMAD3 rs12901499 polymorphism. A total of 5093 OA patients and 5699 controls were included in this study, which involved 5 Caucasian and 5

Asian populations. Patients diagnosed with OA were recruited according to clinical and radiographic results or ascertained by total joint arthroplasty. The genotype distribution of the control group showed conformation to Hardy-Weinberg equilibrium in all the included studies. As for the sites of OA, 9 studies examined knee OA, and 4 studies examined hip OA. Regarding the NOS scale, the quality of all the included studies was fairly high (Additional file 2: Table S2). Eventually, all the 10 studies from the articles as stated above were included in the meta-analysis for further research.

Association between SMAD3 rs12901499 polymorphism and OA susceptibility

Table 3 and Fig. 2 summarize the meta-analysis results on the association between *SMAD3 rs12901499* polymorphism and risk of OA. Because genotype distribution data

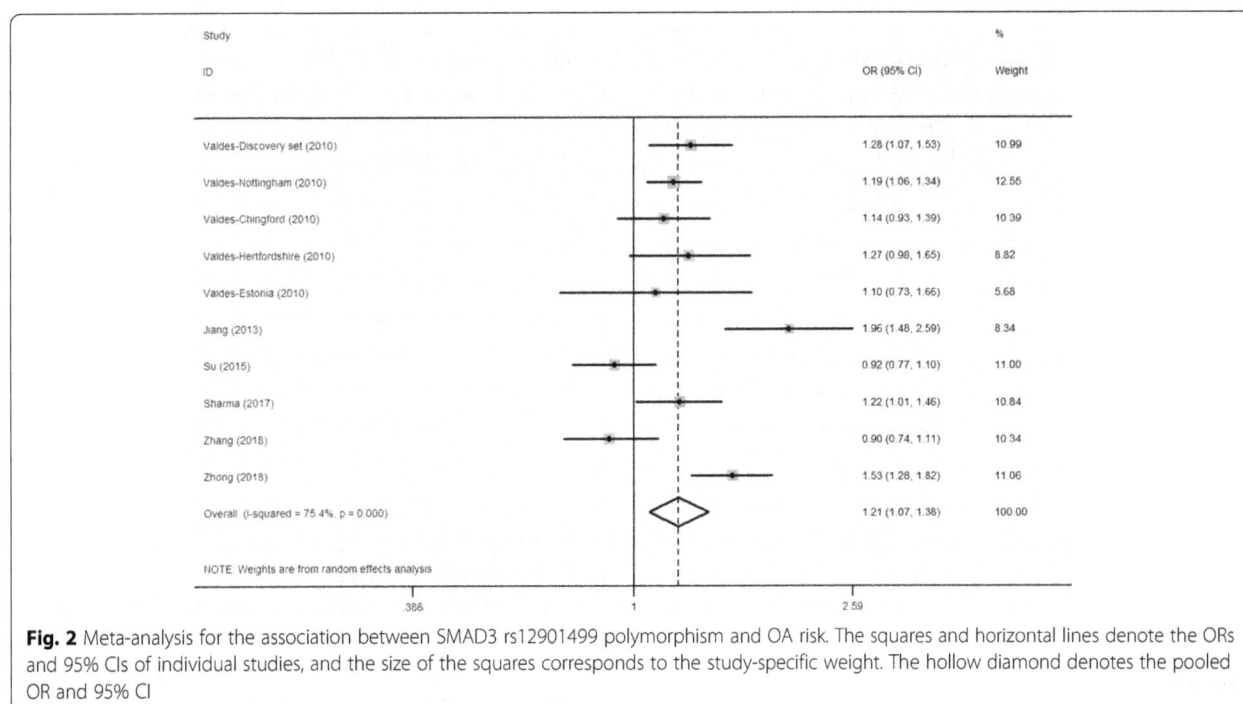

Fig. 2 Meta-analysis for the association between SMAD3 rs12901499 polymorphism and OA risk. The squares and horizontal lines denote the ORs and 95% CIs of individual studies, and the size of the squares corresponds to the study-specific weight. The hollow diamond denotes the pooled OR and 95% CI

Table 4 Pooled results on the association between SMAD3 rs12901499 polymorphism and OA risk in Asians

Genetic model	No. of studies	Test of association		Statistical model	Test of heterogeneity	
		OR (95% CI)	p		I^2 (%)	p
Allele model (G vs. A)	5	1.28 (0.87–1.88)	0.203	Random	90.1	0.000
Dominant model (GG+AG vs. AA)	5	1.18 (0.70–2.00)	0.529	Random	90.2	0.000
Recessive model (GG vs. AG+AA)	5	1.29 (0.90–1.86)	0.166	Random	85.3	0.000
Homozygote model (GG vs. AA)	5	1.21 (0.83–1.77)	0.324	Random	70.6	0.009
Heterozygote model (AG vs. AA)	5	1.06 (0.56–1.99)	0.857	Random	92.3	0.000

was not reported by Valdes, only allele model was analyzed in the overall population and European population. Overall, the combined results revealed a significant association between SMAD3 rs12901499 polymorphism and the risk of OA (allele model: OR 1.21, 95% CI 1.07–1.38); (Table 3; Fig. 2).

When we divided the participants according to ethnicity, G allele was associated with increased risk of OA in Caucasian rather than in Asians (allele model: Caucasian: OR 1.31, 95% CI 1.18–1.44; Asian: OR 1.24, 95% CI 0.95–1.61) (Table 3). What is more, stratification by OA site showed that SMAD3 rs12901499 polymorphism was significantly associated with the risk of both knee OA and hip OA (knee OA: OR 1.18, 95% CI 1.04–1.34; hip OA: OR 1.31, 95% CI 1.18–1.44) (Table 3).

For Asian subgroup, other genetic models were also analyzed (allele model: OR 1.28, 95% CI 0.87–1.88; dominant model: OR 1.18, 95% CI 0.70–2.00; recessive model: OR 1.29, 95% CI 0.90–1.86; homozygote model: OR 1.21, 95% CI 0.83–1.77; heterozygote model: OR 1.06, 95% CI 0.56–1.99) (Table 4).

Sensitivity and publication bias analysis

With the aid of funnel plots and Egger's test (Table 3; p egger = 0.692), we find no significant publication bias (Fig. 3). Furthermore, by using sensitivity analysis (Fig. 4), the combined results remained stable after

removing individual studies. The robustness of summarized estimate was shown by the data above.

Discussion

OA, known as a degenerative disease in the aging population, is the most universal cause of joint disease which could finally result in physical disability [23]. Although OA is considered as a multifactorial disease, genetic factors are reported as vital determinants in the pathogenesis of this disorder [6, 7]. Enormous attention has been paid to the association between gene SNPs and risk of osteoarthritis, and SMAD3 SNP rs12901499 was studied by several researchers. In different studies, the results ranged from no association to the strong linkage between the SNPs and the disorder [12, 14, 16, 17]. The inconsistent findings on the associations between OA and SMAD3 rs12901499 polymorphism in Asians from relatively underpowered studies above may be attributed to factors like small sample size and different population. So we conducted this systematic review and meta-analysis to draw a more definitive conclusion.

To obtain compelling evidence of the linkage between SMAD3 rs12901499 polymorphism and risk of OA, we enrolled a total of 5093 OA patients and 5699 controls from 10 studies in this meta-analysis. The pooled results showed there is an association between OA and rs12901499 polymorphism in the overall population. And subgroup analysis stratified by ethnicity demonstrated that G allele increased the risk of OA in Caucasian. While in Asians, no association was found between SMAD3 rs12901499 polymorphism and OA risk. The results seem intriguing that there is association in the overall population but without positive result in Asian. It could be probably statistically insufficient when the majority of cases of the study were originated from Caucasian (6100/10792). And one other possibility may relate to the different expression patterns of Smad3 in non-homogeneous ethnic populations.

Sensitivity analysis and bias estimation warrant the stability of our meta-analysis.

Based on the present analysis, we propose that patients harboring the G allele of SMAD rs12901499 polymorphism experience an increased susceptibility to OA in Caucasian, though the mechanism underlying the association between

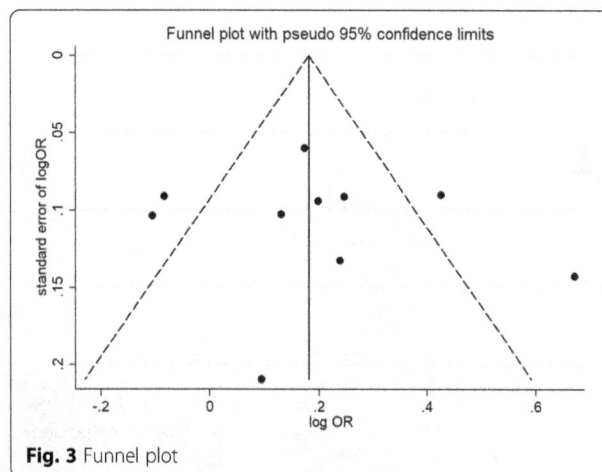

Fig. 3 Funnel plot

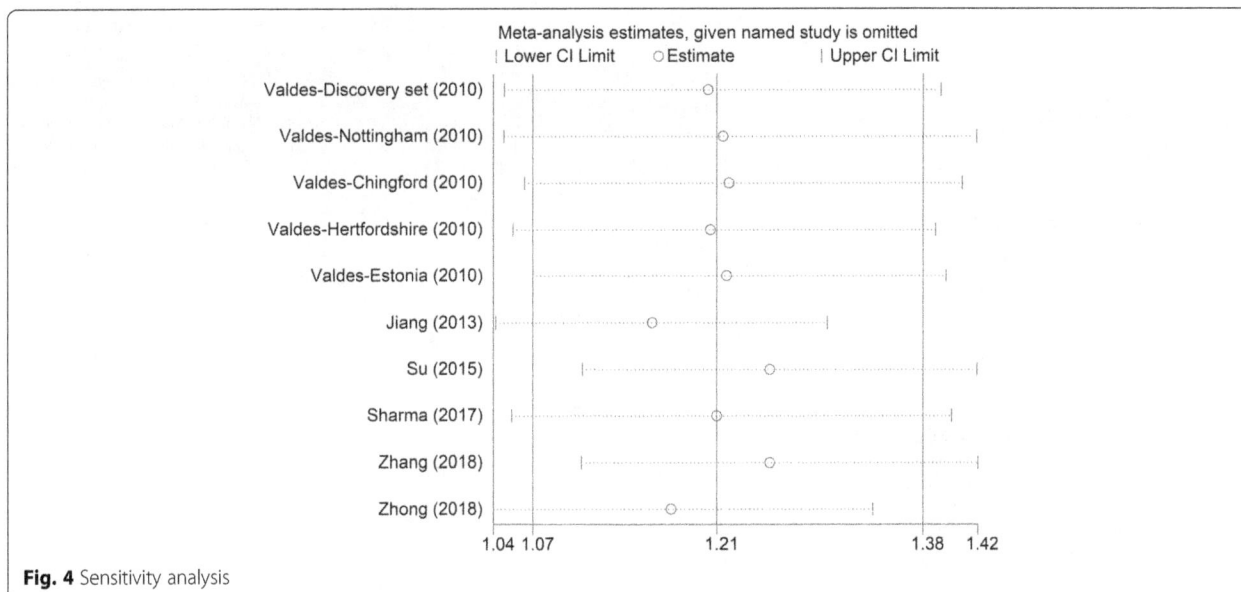

Fig. 4 Sensitivity analysis

SMAD3 rs12901499 polymorphism and osteoarthritis is temporarily unknown. It was reported that SMAD2/3 molecules, known as a part of the TGF-B signaling, have been linked to the chondrocyte anabolism. Previous study showed mutation of SMAD3 could lead to lower expression of type II collagen [17]. Through an in vivo study, Wu et al. found that loss of Smad3 could enhance the BMP signaling to induce articular chondrocytes hypertrophy and lose its normal phenotype [24]. Further functional studies are required to identify the role of SNP rs12901499 in OA susceptibility.

The meta-analysis presented does have some limitations. Firstly, the genotype distribution data was not available in Valdes' study and only allele model among overall population was analyzed to assess the association. Secondly, OA was considered as a multifactorial disease; however, the interactions between the gene and environment were not fully addressed in this meta-analysis, which may magnify the role of Smad3 polymorphism in osteoarthritis. Thirdly, heterogeneity, which comes from different designation about interventions, participants, or outcomes in amount of studies, was inevitably existed though partially addressed by subgroup analysis stratified by ethnic groups and OA sites. Fourthly, since the data is not completely available, the subgroup analysis stratified by every potential confounders in including BMI, age, and gender could not be performed, which may lead to relatively inaccurate pooled results. Last, though there was no obvious publication bias revealed by funnel plot and Egger's test, the selection bias could not be completely removed because only studies published in English were included.

Conclusion

In conclusion, the present meta-analysis demonstrated that the G variant of SMAD3 rs12901499 polymorphism increased the risk of OA in Caucasians. By contrast, SMAD3 rs12901499 polymorphism was not associated with OA risk in Asians. Due to the limitations of our study, further well-designed studies with larger sample size in different ethnic populations should be performed to confirm these results.

Abbreviations
OA: Osteoarthritis; OR: Odds ratio; SMAD3: SMAD family member 3; SNP: Single nucleotide polymorphisms; TGF: Transforming growth factor

Acknowledgements
This study was supported by grants from Zhejiang Province Natural Science Foundation (NO.LQ18H060001), Zhejiang Province medical and health project (NO.2018269731), and Zhejiang Province Chinese medicine project (NO. 2015ZB028).

Authors' contributions
JQH and YXW contributed to the design of the study and retrieval of the literatures, extracted and analyzed the data, and wrote the manuscript. SHL contributed to the retrieval of the literatures and extracted and analyzed data. GYJ contributed to the search strategies and extracted the data. BH participated in the statistical analysis. YTY and JHM helped to screen the manuscript and to review the result of statistical analysis. SGY participated in its design and coordination and helped to review the manuscript. All authors read and approved the final manuscript.

Competing interests

The authors declare that they have no competing interests.

References

1. Brandt KD, Dieppe P, Radin EL. Etiopathogenesis of osteoarthritis. Rheum Dis Clin N Am. 2008;34(3):531–59.
2. Brown KA, Pietenpol JA, Moses HL. A tale of two proteins: differential roles and regulation of Smad2 and Smad3 in TGF-beta signaling. J Cell Biochem. 2007;101(1):9–33.
3. Neogi T, Zhang Y. Epidemiology of osteoarthritis. Rheum Dis Clin N Am. 2013;39(1):1–19.
4. Lawrence RC, et al. Estimates of the prevalence of arthritis and other rheumatic conditions in the United States. Part II. Arthritis Rheum. 2008; 58(1):26–35.
5. Guccione AA, et al. The effects of specific medical conditions on the functional limitations of elders in the Framingham Study. Am J Public Health. 1994;84(3):351–8.
6. Cooper C, et al. Risk factors for the incidence and progression of radiographic knee osteoarthritis. Arthritis Rheum. 2000;43(5):995–1000.
7. Vaughan MW, et al. Perceived community environmental factors and risk of five-year participation restriction among older adults with or at risk of knee osteoarthritis. Arthritis Care Res (Hoboken). 2017;69(7):952–8.
8. Li Y, et al. SMAD3 regulates follicle-stimulating hormone synthesis by pituitary gonadotrope cells in vivo. J Biol Chem. 2017;292(6):2301–14.
9. van der Kraan PM, et al. TGF-beta signaling in chondrocyte terminal differentiation and osteoarthritis: modulation and integration of signaling pathways through receptor-Smads. Osteoarthr Cartil. 2009;17(12):1539–45.
10. Finnson KW, et al. TGF-b signaling in cartilage homeostasis and osteoarthritis. Front Biosci (Schol Ed). 2012;4:251–68.
11. Finnson KW, et al. Endoglin differentially regulates TGF-beta-induced Smad2/3 and Smad1/5 signalling and its expression correlates with extracellular matrix production and cellular differentiation state in human chondrocytes. Osteoarthr Cartil. 2010;18(11):1518–27.
12. Valdes AM, et al. Genetic variation in the SMAD3 gene is associated with hip and knee osteoarthritis. Arthritis Rheum. 2010;62(8):2347–52.
13. Liying J, et al. A SMAD3 gene polymorphism is related with osteoarthritis in a Northeast Chinese population. Rheumatol Int. 2013;33(7):1763–8.
14. Su SL, et al. Gene-gene interactions between TGF-beta/Smad3 signalling pathway polymorphisms affect susceptibility to knee osteoarthritis. BMJ Open. 2015;5(6):e007931.
15. Sharma AC, et al. Association between single nucleotide polymorphisms of SMAD3 and BMP5 with the risk of knee osteoarthritis. J Clin Diagn Res. 2017;11(6):Gc01–gc04.
16. Zhang L, et al. Association between SMAD3 gene rs12901499 polymorphism and knee osteoarthritis in a Chinese population. J Clin Lab Anal. 2018;32:e22383.
17. Zhong F, et al. Genetic variation of SMAD3 is associated with hip osteoarthritis in a Chinese Han population. J Int Med Res. 2018;46:1178–86.
18. Moher D, et al. Preferred reporting items for systematic reviews and meta-analyses: the PRISMA statement. BMJ. 2009;339:b2535.
19. Stang A. Critical evaluation of the Newcastle-Ottawa scale for the assessment of the quality of nonrandomized studies in meta-analyses. Eur J Epidemiol. 2010;25(9):603–5.
20. Bowden J, et al. Quantifying, displaying and accounting for heterogeneity in the meta-analysis of RCTs using standard and generalised Q statistics. BMC Med Res Methodol. 2011;11:41.
21. DerSimonian R, Laird N. Meta-analysis in clinical trials. Control Clin Trials. 1986;7(3):177–88.
22. Mantel N, Haenszel W. Statistical aspects of the analysis of data from retrospective studies of disease. J Natl Cancer Inst. 1959;22(4):719–48.
23. Arden N, Nevitt MC. Osteoarthritis: epidemiology. Best Pract Res Clin Rheumatol. 2006;20(1):3–25.
24. Wu Q, et al. Induction of an osteoarthritis-like phenotype and degradation of phosphorylated Smad3 by Smurf2 in transgenic mice. Arthritis Rheum. 2008;58(10):3132–44.

Outcomes and factors of elbow arthroscopy upon returning to sports for throwing athletes with osteoarthritis

Shun-Wun Jhan[1], Wen-Yi Chou[1]* (iD), Kuan-Ting Wu[1], Ching-Jen Wang[1,2], Ya-Ju Yang[1] and Jih-Yang Ko[1,2]

Abstract

Background: Elbow arthroscopy had good functional outcome for throwing athletes. Returning to sports is a major concern for all athletes, but only a few reports have investigated the clinical factors related to the duration of returning to sports. The present study evaluates the efficacy of elbow arthroscopic surgery on throwing elbows with osteoarthritis and defines the clinical factors related to the duration of the returning to sports.

Methods: This was a retrospective study with fifteen active baseball throwing athletes with elbow osteoarthritis who were treated with elbow arthroscopy. Perioperative clinical factors were analyzed for functional outcomes. A multiple linear regression analysis was used to analyze the clinical factors associated with the duration of returning to training and sports.

Results: The 15 patients' mean age was 27 years. The mean follow-up time was 2.6 years. The mean procedural complexity was 3.1 ± 1.6 (range 1–6). The elbow total range of motion (ROM) improved significantly from $100.7 \pm 28.7°$ to $125.7 \pm 18.5°$ ($p = 0.001$). The terminal flexion range of the elbow increased significantly from $116.0 \pm 22.6°$ to $130.0 \pm 13.2°$ ($p = 0.001$), and the terminal extension range improved from $15.3 \pm 11.1°$ to $4.3 \pm 5.9°$ ($p = 0.001$). Before the operation, the average subjective patient outcome for return to sports (SPORTS) score was 3.4 ± 1.5, which increased significantly to 9.67 ± 0.45 ($p = 0.003$) at the last follow-up. The multiple linear regression analysis revealed that higher procedural complexity hinders the athletes from returning to competition.

Conclusions: Elbow arthroscopy offered highly satisfactory results in the throwing elbows of elite athletes and significantly improved the range of motion and SPORTS score. The procedural complexity was significantly related to the duration of returning to competition. Early and aggressive arthroscopic intervention is recommended for elite throwing athletes with elbow osteoarthritis who fail to respond to conservative treatment.

Keywords: Elbow arthroscope, Athletes, Returning to sports, Osteoarthritis

Background

Common causes of elbow arthritis include primary osteoarthritis, septic arthritis, post-traumatic arthritis, rheumatoid arthritis, crystalline arthropathy, and hemophilia [1]. Throwing athletes sustain consistent valgus extension overload stress on the elbow, which often leads to early traumatic arthritis due to the high demands in their daily activities. Chronic overuse with repetitive micro-trauma often results in subsequent scarring, contracture, and osteoarthritic changes [2, 3].

Valgus extension overload syndrome (VEOS) is a condition characterized by pathology in lateral radiocapitellum compression, medial collateral ligament tension, and posterior extension overload. Despite the increasing ulnar collateral ligament tears, osteoarthritis of the elbow is more common in throwing athletes [4, 5]. The clinical manifestation includes pain, catching or locking sensations, limited range of motion (ROM), and sensory paresthesia. The pathological changes within the elbow articulation include cartilage fragmentation, osteophyte formation, loose bodies within the joint, and capsular contracture.

* Correspondence: murraychou@yahoo.com.tw
[1]Department of Orthopedic Surgery, Kaohsiung Chang Gung Memorial Hospital and Chang Gung University College of Medicine, 123 Ta Pei Road, Niao Sung Dist, Kaohsiung, Taiwan
Full list of author information is available at the end of the article

The treatment options for osteoarthritis of the throwing elbow include anti-inflammatory medicine, activity modification with active rest, physical therapy, flexor-pronator strengthening, platelet-rich plasma injection, and arthroscopic debridement [6]. Due to the earlier recovery and its less invasive nature, elbow arthroscopic surgery has become a mainstay among surgical interventions when conservative treatments for the throwing elbow have failed. Compared to the shoulder arthroscopy in common throwing shoulder diseases, such as superior labral anterior-posterior lesion or rotator cuff tear, the result of elbow arthroscopy is superior in return to sports rate [7–9]. The indications for elbow arthroscopy include debridement for osteoarthritis, removal of loose bodies, synovectomy for inflammatory arthritis, contracture release, and osteochondral defect treatment [10, 11]. Complications related to elbow arthroscopy include superficial wound infection, wound complication, transient sensory paresthesia, deep intra-articular infection, persistent drainage, heterotrophic ossification, vascular injuries, and peripheral nerve injuries [12–14].

Previous reports have shown that elbow arthroscopy improves pain relief and the range of motion. It also has good functional outcomes and rates of returning to sports, which is a major concern for all athletes [15–17]. However, few reports have investigated the clinical factors related to the duration of returning to sports, which can be divided into returning to training and returning to competition. Therefore, the purpose of the present study is to evaluate the efficacy of elbow arthroscopic surgery in throwing elbows with osteoarthritis and to define the clinical factors related to the duration of returning to sports.

Materials and methods

Since 2014, elbow arthroscopic debridement was used to treat athletes with elbow pain due to osteoarthritis who failed to respond to rest, oral medication, and physiotherapy for more than 3 months. The patients recruited were active overhead athletes who participated in a professional ball club or national team for at least 1 year. Osteoarthritis of the elbow was identified and classified radiologically using the Hasting and Rettig elbow osteoarthritis classification system. This system is a useful tool for predicting the surgical outcome of arthroscopic debridement for primary elbow osteoarthritis [18]. The system also shows substantial intraobserver and interobserver reliability for primary elbow osteoarthritis [19].

The diagnosis was initially made according to the clinical presentation and plain radiographs. Ultrasound or magnetic resonance imaging (MRI) was used to confirm the diagnosis and to exclude the possibility of ulnar collateral ligament tears or other conditions, including tears of the common extensor tendon or common flexor tendon. Contraindications for elbow arthroscopic included prior trauma, surgical

scarring, and previous ulnar nerve transposition. All surgeries were performed by one orthopedic surgeon (W.Y.C.) who had subspecialty training in shoulder and elbow arthroscopy.

General demographic data were recorded, including age, gender, sport, affected elbow, and stage of elbow osteoarthritis. The preoperative factors recorded for the analysis were the duration of symptoms, preoperative terminal flexion, extension and ROM, and scores on the "subjective patient outcome for return to sports" (SPORTS) scale. The SPORTS score is a scoring system that is specifically designed to assess the return to sports, the level of performance, and the degree of residual impairment associated with doing sports [9]. It ranks the level of performance using five scales. Players receive a score of 10 if they can perform the same sports at the same level of effort and performance as before the onset of impairment and with no pain. Players who sustain mild pain receive a score of 9. Players who can perform the same sports at the same level of effort but reduced performance level compared to before onset of impairment receive a score of 6. Players who perform the same sports but at reduced levels of effort and performance compared to before the onset of impairment receive a score of 3. Players who are unable to return to the same sport receive a score of 0. A previous report shows that the SPORTS score is a valid and reliable scoring system for assessing the functional outcome and quantifying the return to sports [20].

The intraoperative factors examined were the olecranon process/fossa spurs, loose bodies, capitellum chondromalacia, and procedural complexity. The procedural complexity scale was adopted as one of the prognostic factors. This scale, which was first developed by Nelson et al. in 2014, ranges from 1 to 9, and its contributing factors include procedural specifics (scored as 1–5 points), tourniquet time (scored as 0–2 points), and the number of portals used (scored as 0–2 points). The procedural specifics included limited debridement, extensive debridement, capsular release, and osteocapsular arthroplasty, ranging from 1 point to 4 points, and release of posterior band of medial collateral ligament or medial epicondylectomy had an additional 1 point. The tourniquet time less than or equal to 60 min got 0 point and more than 90 min got 2 points. The portal number less than or equal to 2 got 0 point and more than 4 got 2 points [21]. Total complexity scores less than 4 are considered low, and scores greater than 5 are high. The postoperative factors include postoperative terminal flexion, extension and total ROM, and SPORTS scores.

All of these factors were utilized for the outcome assessment and to match the relationship of duration of returning to training and duration of returning to competition. The definition of duration of returning to training is the interval that athletes return to training without disruption by the symptoms after the surgery. Returning to competition was defined as the duration that athletes returned to the game according to the official game record after the surgery.

Arthroscopic approach and rehabilitation

The patients were placed in a lateral decubitus position under general anesthesia. The operative arm was supported with an arm scaffold to allow complete arthroscopic examination of the elbow joint without antecubital fossa impingement. A tourniquet was applied to all patients to control bleeding. Standard 30° 4.5-mm arthroscope equipment was used.

Before the beginning of the operation, we mapped the course of the ulnar nerve and marked bony landmarks including the medial epicondyle, lateral epicondyle, radiocapitellar joint, and olecranon. Before portal placement, 20 ml of normal saline was injected to inflate the joint through an 18-gauge needle. Usually, a midlateral portal was created first to evaluate the radiocapitellum joint and olecranon fossa. An anterior lateral portal or posterior portal was created to facilitate the debridement, capsular lysis, removal of loose bodies, and the excision of osteophytes. The capsular release was also carried out based on the intraoperative findings and usually started from the posterior compartment to medial/lateral, sometimes anterior capsule if necessary. The presented cases revealed common intraoperative findings, including loose bodies and olecranon fossa spurs (Fig. 1a, b).

The patients were encouraged to perform passive or active-assisted motion on the next day after the surgery if the pain and swelling were tolerable. Aggressive active motions of the elbow were carried out in the third week post-operation, including pronation/supination and flexion/extension. Partial resistance training with an elastic rope or tubing started in the fourth to sixth weeks post-operation. The return to interval throwing usually started in the seventh week post-operation.

Statistical analysis

All statistical analyses were performed using the SPSS software package (version 22.0; SPSS, Chicago, IL). A normality test of each variable was performed using the Shapiro-Wilk test, and comparisons of these variables were made with nonparametric tests ($P < 0.05$). The Wilcoxon signed-rank test was used to compare pre-operative and post-operative functional scores. Multiple linear regression analysis was used to determine the relative significance of each clinical factor associated with the duration of returning to training and sports.

Results

From January 2014 to December 2016, we used elbow arthroscopic debridement and release to treat athletes with sustained elbow pain due to osteoarthritis who

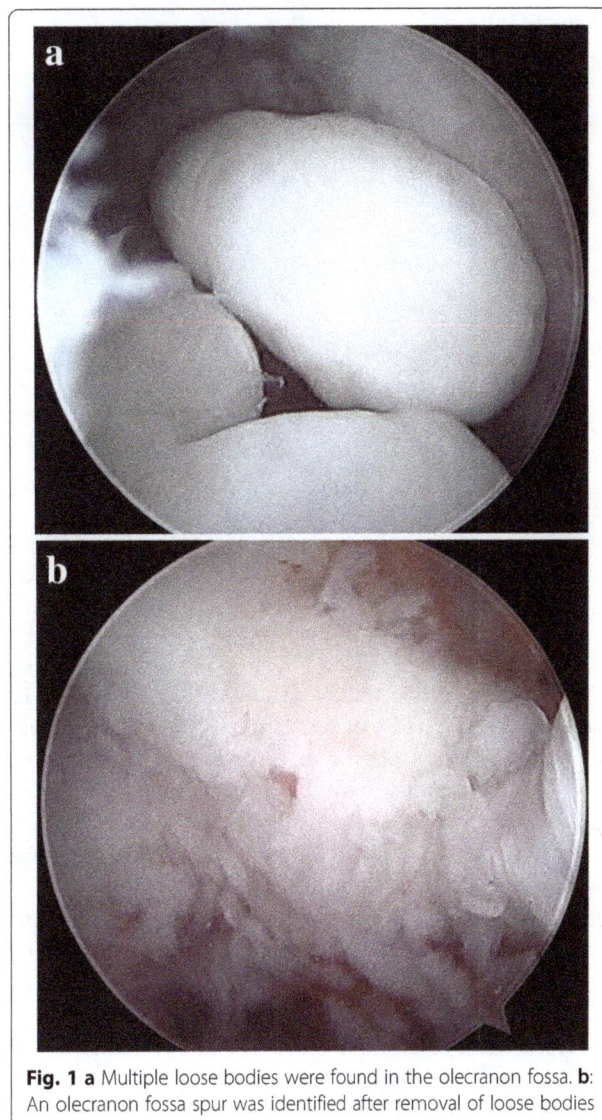

Fig. 1 a Multiple loose bodies were found in the olecranon fossa. **b**: An olecranon fossa spur was identified after removal of loose bodies

failed to respond to oral medication, physiotherapy, and other conservative treatments for more than 3 months. After the exclusion of two athletes who were lost to follow-up within 6 months, a total of 15 throwing elbows were recruited in the analysis. There were 12 professional baseball players and 3 amateurs with 12 right elbows and 3 left elbows involved. The mean age was 27 years (range 19–34 years). The mean follow-up time was 2.6 years (range 1.5–3.5 years) (Table 1).

The mean procedural complexity was 3.1 ± 1.6 (range 1–6). Before the operation, the duration of symptoms that kept the athletes from participating in routine training or competition was 7.9 ± 3.1 months (range 4–12 months) (Table 2). Regarding the stages of elbow osteoarthritis, three patients sustained grade II osteoarthritis, and the rest of the 12 elbows had grade I osteoarthritis. The preoperative ROM was $100.7 \pm 28.7°$ (range 45–140°).

Table 1 Demographic characteristics

Case	Age	Gender	Involved elbow	Sport	Level	Stages of osteoarthritis	Procedural complexity	Follow-up (years)
1	30	M	R	Baseball	Professional	II	1	3.5
2	33	M	L	Baseball	Professional	I	3	3.5
3	31	M	R	Baseball	Professional	I	4	3.1
4	19	M	L	Baseball	Semi-professional	I	3	3.1
5	24	M	R	Baseball	Professional	I	3	3
6	21	M	L	Baseball	Semi-professional	I	4	2.9
7	27	M	R	Baseball	Professional	I	5	2.8
8	27	M	R	Baseball	Professional	II	4	2.8
9	30	M	R	Baseball	Professional	I	5	2.7
10	28	M	R	Baseball	Professional	I	2	2.5
11	34	M	R	Baseball	Professional	I	2	2.4
12	27	M	R	Baseball	Professional	I	2	2.1
13	26	M	R	Baseball	Professional	II	6	1.5
14	20	M	R	Baseball	Semi-professional	I	1	1.5
15	26	M	R	Baseball	Professional	I	1	1.5

The intraoperative findings showed that 14 out of 15 patients (93.3%) had olecranon process spurs, and 5 patients (33.3%) had olecranon fossa impingement spurs. There were 10 patients (66.7%) who had loose bodies in the olecranon fossa and 4 patients (26.7%) with capitellum chondromalacia. The elbow terminal flexion range significantly increased from $116.0 \pm 22.6°$ to $130.0 \pm 13.2°$ ($p = 0.001$), and the terminal extension range also improved from $15.3 \pm 11.1°$ to $4.3 \pm 5.9°$ ($p = 0.001$). The total elbow ROM improved significantly from a mean of $100.7 \pm 28.7°$ to $125.7 \pm 18.5°$ ($p = 0.001$).

Before the operation, the average SPORTS score was 3.4 ± 1.5, which increased significantly to 9.67 ± 0.45 ($p = 0.003$) at the last follow up. In this analysis, all patients had SPORTS score less than 6 before the operation and had returned to the same level of competition after elbow arthroscopy as of the last follow-up. The mean follow-up interval was 2.59 years (range 1.5–3.5 years). The mean interval of returning to training was 2.0 ± 1.5 months (range 0.25–5 months) postoperatively, and the mean interval of returning to competition was 4.5 ± 1.5 months (range 2–6 months). There were no perioperative complications in this series, and no further surgical intervention was required at the last follow-up (Table 2).

In the multiple linear regression analysis, all the preoperative, intraoperative, and postoperative factors did not show significance regarding the duration of returning to training (Table 3). However, the procedural complexity demonstrated an influence on returning to competition (Table 4). The results implied that the complexity of elbow osteoarthritis is significantly related to the duration of returning to competition.

Discussion

In this series, we found consistent satisfactory results of arthroscopic debridement and release regarding osteoarthritis of the throwing elbow, as in previous reports. All the athletes could return to sports without complications in the mean follow-up period of 2.6 years. The mean durations of returning to training and competition were 2.0 ± 1.5 and 4.5 ± 1.5 months, respectively, which could be a reference for athletes and coaches to estimate the duration of returning to play (Table 2). Another principle finding is that the procedural complexity was significantly related to the duration of returning to competition, which indicated that the complexity of elbow osteoarthritis hindered the interval of returning to competition. Early and aggressive intervention for throwing elbows with osteoarthritis should be considered in patients who fail to respond to conservative treatments for more than 3 months.

According to Morrey et al., the elbow motion necessary for most daily activities in a functional arc of motion, which ranges from 30 to 130° [22]. Conservative treatments such as medication, splinting, and rehabilitation should be considered in patients with early osteoarthritis of the elbow or minor elbow contracture. However, the functional arc of motion might not be applicable to patients with highly demanding circumstances, such as throwing athletes. In this subpopulation, arthroscopic debridement and capsular release offer a minimally invasive modality to relieve symptoms and allow an earlier return to sports compared to traditional open procedures.

Tucker et al. concluded that elbow arthroscopy performed by an experienced doctor can produce better results than open release [17]. Previous studies show that

Table 2 Functional outcome assessment

Case	Terminal flexion		Terminal extension		Total ROM		SPORTS		Duration of symptoms (months)	Duration of returning to training (months)	Duration of returning to sports (months)
	Pre-op	Post-op	Pre-op	Post-op	Pre-op	Post-op	Pre-op	Post-op			
1	125	135	0	0	125	135	3	10	6	0.5	4
2	90	135	10	0	80	135	3	10	12	1	5
3	125	135	10	0	115	135	3	10	6	2	6
4	125	135	10	0	115	135	6	10	5	2	3
5	70	130	25	10	45	120	3	10	8	1	2
6	130	135	40	10	90	125	3	9	12	4	6
7	90	130	25	10	65	120	0	10	7	3	6
8	100	100	30	15	70	85	6	9	12	0.25	6
9	135	140	10	0	125	140	3	10	6	5	6
10	140	140	10	5	130	135	3	9	6	3	4
11	140	140	20	0	120	140	6	10	12	2	3
12	130	135	10	0	120	135	3	10	12	3	5
13	90	100	20	15	70	85	3	9	5	0.75	6
14	140	140	0	0	140	140	3	10	4	2	3
15	110	120	10	0	100	120	3	10	6	0.25	3
Mean	116.0 ± 22.6° (70–140°)	130.0 ± 13.2° (100–140°)	15.3 ± 11.1° (0–40°)	4.3 ± 5.9° (0–15°)	100.7 ± 28.7° (45–140°)	125.7 ± 18.5° (85–140°)	3.4 ± 1.5 (0–6)	9.67 ± 0.45 (9–10)	7.9 ± 3.1 (4–12)	2.0 ± 1.5 (0.25–5)	4.5 ± 1.5 (2–6)
P value	0.001[a]		0.001[a]		0.001[a]		0.003[a]				

ROM range of motion, SPORTS subjective patient outcome for return to sports, Pre-op preoperative, Post-op postoperative

[a]A p value of < 0.05 was considered to be statistically significant

Table 3 Multiple linear regression analysis of factors associated with duration of return to training

Variable	Coefficients	S.E.	p value
Preoperative factors			
Duration of symptoms	0.050	0.179	0.808
Preoperative terminal Flexion	0.016	0.039	0.729
Preoperative terminal extension	0.037	0.064	0.621
Preoperative ROM	0.017	0.013	0.204
Preoperative SPORTS	0.009	0.348	0.981
Intraoperative factors			
Procedural complexity	0.324	0.468	0.560
Olecranon fossa spur	0.947	1.258	0.530
Olecranon process spur	2.150	2.740	0.515
Loose bodies	− 0.497	1.141	0.706
Capitellum chondromalacia	1.686	1.846	0.457
Postoperative factors			
Postoperative terminal flexion	0.092	0.065	0.293
Postoperative terminal extension	− 0.080	0.222	0.753
Postoperative ROM	0.037	0.019	0.074
Postoperative SPORTS	− 1.248	2.108	0.614

S.E standard error of coefficient, Pre-op pre-operative, Post-op post-operative, ROM range of motion
SPORTS subjective patient outcome for return to sports

Table 4 Multiple linear regression analysis of factors associated with duration of return to competition

Variable	Coefficients	S.E	p value
Preoperative factors			
Duration of symptoms	0.149	0.071	0.171
Preoperative terminal flexion	0.014	0.016	0.463
Preoperative terminal extension	− 0.024	0.026	0.452
Preoperative ROM	− 0.009	0.014	0.542
Preoperative SPORTS	− 0.355	0.139	0.125
Intraoperative factors			
Procedural complexity	1.406	0.186	0.017[a]
Olecranon fossa spur	1.198	0.502	0.140
Olecranon process spur	− 3.590	1.092	0.081
Loose bodies	0.104	0.455	0.840
Capitellum chondromalacia	− 1.446	0.736	0.188
Postoperative factors			
Postoperative terminal flexion	− 0.017	0.026	0.581
Postoperative terminal extension	− 0.164	0.088	0.205
Postoperative ROM	− 0.029	0.021	0.195
Postoperative SPORTS	− 1.567	0.841	0.203

S.E. standard error of coefficient, Pre-op pre-operative, Post-op post-operative, ROM range of motion
SPORTS: subjective patient outcome for return to sports
[a]A p value of < 0.05 was considered to be statistically significant

elbow arthroscopic debridement and arthrolysis contribute significantly to the improvement of the elbow's ROM. Somanchi et al. reported improvements in elbow flexion and extension of 6° and 12.5° after elbow arthroscopic lysis, respectively [23]. Nguyen et al. retrospectively reviewed 22 patients who underwent elbow arthroscopy with an improvement of 19° terminal flexion and 19° terminal extension after 1 year of follow-up [16]. Meluzinová et al. and Cefo et al. both reported significant improvements in the average elbow ROM after arthroscopic treatment for the post-traumatic stiff elbow joint [24, 25]. Adams et al. reviewed 41 patients with 42 cases of primary osteoarthritis of the elbow who received arthroscopy for more than 2 years. The mean flexion, extension, and supination had significant improvements of 14.3°, 13.0°, and 7.9°, respectively [26]. In the present analysis, the improvement of ROM, terminal flexion, and extension correspond to the previous reports, but the follow-up was longer (mean 2.6 years).

Risks of elbow arthroscopy are believed to be related to the complications of the procedure. Kelly et al. reported that the minor complication rate after arthroscopic procedures was about 11%, and the complications would resolve spontaneously. Major complications such as deep joint infection were rare (0.8%) [12]. Nelson et al. reported that the complication rate of elbow arthroscopy was about 14% of cases. The major complication rate was about 5%, and repeated surgeries were needed in these cases [21]. Some investigators showed one superficial portal site infection in 14 patients after a 1-year follow-up [15]. Blonna et al. reported three cases of delayed-onset ulnar neuropathy in 26 patients who received arthroscopic treatment for terminal extension restoration. Two of them required further ulnar nerve transposition surgery [9]. It is reported that the elbow arthroscopy is limited in treating posterolateral rotatory instability and septic arthritis [11]. In addition, ulnar nerve compromise also should be highlighted for the athletes with the history of ulnar nerve transposition. In the present series, all of the elbows were sports-related osteoarthritis in which the results of arthroscopy are encouraging and our results were in line with the previous reports. Although the anterior bundle of ulnar collateral ligament contributes the majority of medial elbow stability, Terzini et al. also reported that the posterior bundle provides the stability in higher flexion angle [27]. The osteoarthritic elbow with collateral ligament injury-related instability was excluded from the present study since the ligamentous reconstruction, such as ulnar collateral ligament reconstruction, were done with extra-articular open procedure nowadays. There were no complications in the present study, which may due to the limited number of cases, the exclusion of elderly patients and patients with post-traumatic osteoarthritis, and the relatively low procedural complexity.

Ward et al. retrospectively reviewed 36 athletes who received elbow arthroscopy and reported that the most commonly treated lesions were loose bodies and impingement spurs, which were compatible with the present analysis. There was also a significant improvement in the subjective functional outcome score [28]. Somanchi reported an 87% satisfaction rate in 26 elbow arthroscopic patients in a 2-year follow-up study [23]. Blonna et al. revealed that 25 out of 26 athletes were restored to normal or near-normal function. Most importantly, 90% of patients returned to the same performance level as before the onset of impairment [9]. Even in advanced elbow capitellar osteochondritis dissecans, surgical intervention with autologous osteochondral mosaicplasty also had a high return to pre-injury competitive level rate (91%) [29]. In our study, all 15 athletes could return to the same competition level after the operation without recurrence in the mean follow-up of 2.6 years. The mean postoperative SPORTS score was 9.67, which is significantly improved from the score of 3.4, which indicated a high subjective patient outcome regarding the return to sports.

The multiple linear regression analysis excluded postulated clinical factors that might hinder the durations of returning to training and competition, including the duration of symptoms, terminal flexion and extension, total ROM, olecranon spurs, loose bodies, capitellum chondromalacia, and SPORTS score. But the procedural complexity scale was significantly related to the return to competition. This points out the complexities of elbow osteoarthritis, such as the involvement of more than two compartments or extensive capsular release that requires longer surgical time. These are factors that hindered the athletes from returning to competition due to the highly intensive demands during games rather than training. In terms of procedure complexity scale, early arthroscopic intervention for the athletes with osteoarthritis of the elbow is recommended for the arthritis retardation and the early return to competition.

The present study had some limitations. First, the retrospective analysis had selection bias. Second, there was no control group, such as athletes without surgical intervention, which restricted the performance of a comprehensive comparison. Third, the limited case numbers weakened the statistical analysis. Fourth, the procedural complexity scale had subjective components. For example,the tourniquet time and portal number might be influenced by the operation room equipment condition and the surgeon's experience since elbow arthroscopy is an operator-dependent procedure. However, there was a range between each point, which might reduce the subjective effect. In spite of the limitations, however, the present study offers the consistent results of arthroscopic treatment for throwing elbows. We also determined that the procedural complexity is a factor that hinders the return to competition.

Conclusions

In conclusion, elbow arthroscopy offered consistent and highly satisfactory results in throwing elbows with osteoarthritis, as shown in the improvement of ROM, SPORTS scores, and the 100% return to sports in a mean follow-up period of 2.6 years. The mean durations of returning to training and competition were 2 and 4.5 months, respectively, which could be a reference for practitioners to estimate the duration of returning to play. The procedural complexity was significantly related to the duration of returning to competition. Early and aggressive intervention for throwing elbows with osteoarthritis should be considered in athletes who have failed to respond to conservative treatments for more than 3 months.

Abbreviations
MRI: Magnetic resonance imaging; ROM: Range of motion; SPORTS: Subjective patient outcome for return to sports; VEOS: Valgus extension overload syndrome

Acknowledgements
Not applicable.

Funding
The authors received no financial support for the research, authorship, and/or publication of this article.

Authors' contributions
WYC, CJW, and JYK participated in the study design and coordination. SWJ and KTW collected the data. YJY contributed to the analysis and interpretation of data. SWJ drafted the manuscript, and WYC revised it. All authors read and approved the final manuscript.

Competing interests
The authors declare that they have competing interests.

Author details
[1]Department of Orthopedic Surgery, Kaohsiung Chang Gung Memorial Hospital and Chang Gung University College of Medicine, 123 Ta Pei Road, Niao Sung Dist, Kaohsiung, Taiwan. [2]Center for Shockwave Medicine and Tissue Engineering, Department of Medical Research, Kaohsiung Chang Gung Memorial Hospital and Chang Gung University College of Medicine, Kaohsiung, Taiwan.

References

1. Kokkalis ZT, Schmidt CC, Sotereanos DG. Elbow arthritis: current concepts. J Hand Surg. 2009;34:761–8.
2. Cain EL Jr, Dugas JR, Wolf RS, Andrews JR. Elbow injuries in throwing athletes: a current concepts review. Am J Sports Med. 2003;31:621–35.
3. Gregory B, Nyland J. Medial elbow injury in young throwing athletes. Muscles Ligaments Tendons J. 2013;3:91–100.
4. Ahmad CS, ElAttrache NS. Valgus extension overload syndrome and stress injury of the olecranon. Clin Sports Med. 2004;23:665–76 x.
5. Paulino FE, Villacis DC, Ahmad CS. Valgus extension overload in baseball players. Am J Orthop (Belle Mead NJ). 2016;45:144–51.
6. Cheung EV, Adams R, Morrey BF. Primary osteoarthritis of the elbow: current treatment options. J Am Acad Orthop Surg. 2008;16:77–87.
7. Gilliam BD, Douglas L, Fleisig GS, Aune KT, Mason KA, Dugas JR, Cain EL Jr, Ostrander RV, Andrews JR. Return to play and outcomes in baseball players after superior labral anterior-posterior repairs. Am J Sports Med. 2018;46: 109–15.
8. Weiss LJ, Wang D, Hendel M, Buzzerio P, Rodeo SA. Management of rotator cuff injuries in the elite athlete. Curr Rev Musculoskelet Med. 2018;11:102–12.
9. Blonna D, Lee GC, O'Driscoll SW. Arthroscopic restoration of terminal elbow extension in high-level athletes. Am J Sports Med. 2010;38:2509–15.
10. Adams JE, King GJ, Steinmann SP, Cohen MS. Elbow arthroscopy: indications, techniques, outcomes, and complications. J Am Acad Orthop Surg. 2014;22:810–8.
11. Yeoh KM, King GJ, Faber KJ, Glazebrook MA, Athwal GS. Evidence-based indications for elbow arthroscopy. Arthroscopy. 2012;28:272–82.
12. Kelly EW, Morrey BF, O'Driscoll SW. Complications of elbow arthroscopy. J Bone Joint Surg Am. 2001;83-a:25–34.
13. Gofton WT, King GJ. Heterotopic ossification following elbow arthroscopy. Arthroscopy. 2001;17:E2.
14. Ruch DS, Poehling GG. Anterior interosseus nerve injury following elbow arthroscopy. Arthroscopy. 1997;13:756–8.
15. Ball CM, Meunier M, Galatz LM, Calfee R, Yamaguchi K. Arthroscopic treatment of post-traumatic elbow contracture. J Shoulder Elb Surg. 2002;11:624–9.
16. Nguyen D, Proper SI, MacDermid JC, King GJ, Faber KJ. Functional outcomes of arthroscopic capsular release of the elbow. Arthroscopy. 2006;22:842–9.
17. Tucker SA, Savoie FH 3rd, O'Brien MJ. Arthroscopic management of the post-traumatic stiff elbow. J Shoulder Elb Surg. 2011;20:S83–9.
18. Rettig LA, Hastings H 2nd, Feinberg JR. Primary osteoarthritis of the elbow: lack of radiographic evidence for morphologic predisposition, results of operative debridement at intermediate follow-up, and basis for a new radiographic classification system. J Shoulder Elb Surg. 2008;17:97–105.
19. Amini MH, Sykes JB, Olson ST, Smith RA, Mauck BM, Azar FM, Throckmorton TW. Reliability testing of two classification systems for osteoarthritis and post-traumatic arthritis of the elbow. J Shoulder Elb Surg. 2015;24:353–7.
20. Blonna D, Castoldi F, Delicio D, Bruzzone M, Dettoni F, Bonasia DE, Rossi R. Validity and reliability of the SPORTS score. Knee Surg Sports Traumatol Arthrosc. 2012;20:356–60.
21. Nelson GN, Wu T, Galatz LM, Yamaguchi K, Keener JD. Elbow arthroscopy: early complications and associated risk factors. J Shoulder Elb Surg. 2014;23:273–8.
22. Morrey BF, Askew LJ, Chao EY. A biomechanical study of normal functional elbow motion. J Bone Joint Surg Am. 1981;63:872–7.
23. Somanchi BV, Funk L. Evaluation of functional outcome and patient satisfaction after arthroscopic elbow arthrolysis. Acta Orthop Belg. 2008;74:17–23.
24. Meluzinova P, Kopp L, Edelmann K, Obruba P, Avenarius J. Elbow arthroscopy in the surgical treatment of post-traumatic changes of the elbow joint. Acta Chir Orthop Traumatol Cechoslov. 2014;81:399–406.
25. Cefo I, Eygendaal D. Arthroscopic arthrolysis for posttraumatic elbow stiffness. J Shoulder Elb Surg. 2011;20:434–9.
26. Adams JE, Wolff LH 3rd, Merten SM, Steinmann SP. Osteoarthritis of the elbow: results of arthroscopic osteophyte resection and capsulectomy. J Shoulder Elb Surg. 2008;17:126–31.
27. Terzini M, Zanetti EM, Audenino AL, Putame G, Gastaldi L, Pastorelli S, Panero E, Sard A, Bignardi C. Multibody modelling of ligamentous and bony stabilizers in the human elbow. Muscles Ligaments Tendons J. 2017;7:493–502.
28. Ward WG, Anderson TE. Elbow arthroscopy in a mostly athletic population. J Hand Surg Am. 1993;18:220–4.
29. Funakoshi T, Momma D, Matsui Y, Kamishima T, Kawamura D, Nagano Y, Iwasaki N. Autologous osteochondral mosaicplasty for centrally and laterally located, advanced capitellar osteochondritis dissecans in teenage athletes: clinical outcomes, radiography, and magnetic resonance imaging findings. Am J Sports Med. 2018;46:1943–51.

24

Pressure distributions inside intervertebral discs under unilateral pedicle screw fixation in a porcine spine model

Zhao Meng[1*], Chen Wang[1], Li-Jun Tian[2], Xue-Jun Zhang[3], Dong Guo[3] and Yan Zou[1]

Abstract

Background: Little data are available regarding the effects of pedicle screws on the intervertebral disc stress for different spinal segments. The aim of this study was to analyze the intervertebral disc stress in response to the placement of pedicle screws.

Methods: T3–4, T11–12, T15–L1, L3–4, and L4–5 intervertebral disc segments from six porcine spine specimens were harvested. A compressive load of 200 N was applied both before and after the pedicle screw was implanted on the left side of each target segment; the resulting pressure was measured during vertical, 5° anterior flexion, 5° posterior extension, and 5° lateral bending.

Results: The posterior intradiscal pressures of the intervertebral disc were significantly lower in the fixed group than in the unfixed group for all segments during vertical, 5° anterior flexion, and 5° posterior extension. The left pressures of the intervertebral disc were significantly lower in the fixation group for all segments. During 5° lateral bending, the left intervertebral disc pressures were significantly lower in the fixation group. Lower mean pressures were observed in the fixed group.

Conclusions: Unilateral pedicle screws can effectively reduce the pressure of the fixed lateral intervertebral disc. Moreover, it can change the pressure distribution of the intervertebral disc and reduce the pressure of the entire intervertebral disc, especially the posterior side of the intervertebral disc.

Keywords: Intervertebral disc, Pressure, Pedicle screw fixation, Porcine, Spine, Unilateral

Background

Scoliosis, one of the complex three-dimensional deformities of the spine, refers to a lateral curvature of the spine in the coronal plane of more than 10°. It has a high prevalence of about 1/1000 and is usually complicated with the spine rotation and change of numbers of the sagittal dorsal or anterior processes, as well as uneven rib levels, the pelvic rotation and tilt, and paraspinal ligament and muscle abnormalities [1, 2]. Scoliosis is often used generically to refer to all spinal deformities in children. It can be categorized into three major types, congenital, syndromic, and idiopathic [3, 4]. Progressive scoliosis will seriously affect the children's skeletal growth and the development of various organs, and severe idiopathic scoliosis and most of congenital scoliosis require surgery.

Growing rods have been the mainstay surgical treatment of scoliosis. As early as 1963, Harrington first advocated the use of non-fusion method of internal fixation surgery for scoliosis [5]. Similarly, in 2001, Blakemore et al. reported a new generation of non-fusion internal fixation; although only a preliminary report, a significant improvement of the Cobb angle was observed post-operation [6]. Recently, pedicle screw-rod constructs have become increasingly popular in the treatment of spinal deformities, as they have excellent biomechanical properties and are suitable for the transfer and subsequent maintenance of large correction forces in all planes [7].

However, most biomechanical studies of scoliosis focus on pathology and morphology, and regarding the scoliosis internal fixation system, most studies focus on the

* Correspondence: mengzhao88@yeah.net
[1]Department of Orthopaedics, Children's Hospital of Hebei Province, No.133, Jianhua Street, Yuhua District, Shijiazhuang 050031, China
Full list of author information is available at the end of the article

clinical efficacy. To our knowledge, there are little available data regarding the effects of pedicle screws on the intervertebral disc stress for different spinal segments. At present, the clinical application of unilateral pedicle screw fixation for the treatment of scoliosis in children has been established; thus, the purpose of this study was to explore the feasibility of unilateral pedicle screw fixation for scoliosis based on bilateral pedicle screw fixation, with less interference and fewer implants to achieve the same control and orthopedic purposes. However, there is a lack of biomechanical basis and little data are available regarding the effects of unilateral pedicle screws on the intervertebral disc stress for different spinal segments. Most of the studies used sensors and probes in order to evaluate the pressure data of the intervertebral disc, and a shortcoming is that the results are only from certain points and also not intuitive. Pressure-sensitive film can intuitively display the pressure characteristics of each segment in the upper thoracic and lumbar spine [8] and thus is more appropriate in investigating the pressure distribution of the intervertebral disc. In this study, this approach was used to observe the pressure conditions of the intervertebral disc. Immature pigs are usually used as animal models to test the spinal internal fixation system for scoliosis modeling, because they have a similar anatomical structure to humans and their growth cycle is suitable for disease progress research. Therefore, we chose the porcine spine as the experimental subjects [9–11]. Accordingly, our study was established to analyze the intervertebral disc stress in response to the placement of unilateral pedicle screws. The data might be helpful for the clinical management of scoliosis.

Methods
Segmentation of specimens
Six spine specimens of 6-week-old female pigs were obtained from the Kangning Co., Ltd., Zhuozhou City, China. Spines were examined by CT scan; all six porcine spines showed no deformity, tumor, fracture, and other lesions. The characteristic spinal segments were taken as follows: T3–4, T11–12, T15–L1, L3–4, L4–5 segments and their adjacent superior and inferior vertebral bodies. The study was approved by the ethics committee of the local hospital.

Biomechanics experiment
All specimens were sealed with polyethylene films and stored at − 20 °C. The specimens were equilibrated for about 12 h at 3 °C and wrapped in polyethylene films to maintain the humidity [12]. Then, the sections of the up- and down-ends of specimens were embedded properly with self-condensing dental base acrylic resin powder with a thickness of 1 cm. The experimental environment was

maintained at a temperature of 20 °C and a humidity of 44%. After being placed onto the biomechanics experimental machine (Model CSS-44020, Changchun Research Institute for Testing Machines, China), an axial vertical compressive load of 300 N was applied for each segment to reduce the impact of the over-hydration effect of the intervertebral disc [12].The target segment intervertebral disc was carefully cut, without destroying the anterior and posterior longitudinal ligament and articular process. Then, the shape-adjusted and pressure-sensitive film was placed in the intervertebral disc and sealed with plastic membrane. The prepared spinal segments were again fixed in the biomechanical experimental machine, and a vertical compressive load of 200 N was applied; before the loading, three times of the pre-loading were applied in order to eliminate the viscoelasticity. The 2-min method was used for the pressure-sensitive film detection, that is, after development for 5 s, the film was maintained for 2 min to get a more stable and uniform image. A consecutive pressure loading was applied for the same spinal segment, and each pressure was loaded after the replacement of pressure-sensitive film. When the results of the three experiments are similar, the last pressure-sensitive film was analyzed. In order to simulate 5° anterior flexion, posterior extension, and lateral bending, a 5° wedge-shaped bevel was prepared by self-condensing dental base acrylic resin powder (type II, Shanghai Medical Devices Co., Ltd., China) and placed between the experimental machine and the model before loading the compressive force [13]. Thereafter, the posterior cervical fixation pedicle screw system (Shandong Weigao Orthopedic Device Co., Ltd., China) was implanted on one side (left side) of each target segment (Fig. 1); after the placement was confirmed by X-ray examination, the loading procedure was repeated. The appropriate pressure-sensitive film was retained for both the unfixed and fixed groups (for representative images, see Fig. 2).

Groups and data analysis
For both of the unfixed and fixed groups, the following pressure data were recorded and analyzed: the left, right, posterior, and mean pressure under vertical loading; the left, right, posterior, and mean pressure under 5° anterior flexion or posterior extension; and the left pressure under 5° lateral bending. Data were extracted from the double-sided pressure-sensitive paper (super low-pressure type: LLW) using pressure prescale spectrophotometer (Fujitsu, Japan); the same data was recorded by the same researcher in 1 mm successively, and then, an appropriate range was selected to calculate the mean pressure. The range of the posterior intervertebral disc is the posterior one third of the vertebral body and the intervertebral disc. The range of the front annulus is the anterior two thirds of the vertebral body and the intervertebral disc. The mean pressure

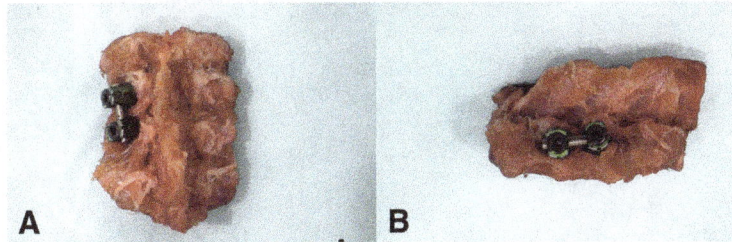

Fig. 1 Representative images of the posterior cervical fixation pedicle screw system. **a** Back view of the T11–12 segment. **b** Side view of the T11–12 segment

was calculated as the average value of the entire intervertebral disc; the range of the 5° anterior flexion, posterior extension, or lateral bending is separated by the middle line.

Statistical analysis

The experimental data were expressed as mean ± standard deviation. The data were analyzed by SPSS13.0 statistical software (SPSS Inc., IL, USA). The data of each group were analyzed by Shapiro-Wilk normality test and paired Student's t test. A value of $P < 0.05$ was considered statistically significant.

Results

The posterior intradiscal pressures under different loading conditions

When comparing the posterior intradiscal pressures of intervertebral disc (Table 1), in the unfixed group, generally, there was no significant difference among different loading conditions; however, the posterior intradiscal pressure under 5° posterior extension for the T3–4 segment was significantly lower than those under vertical or 5° anterior flexion conditions ($P < 0.05$). And for the comparison between the fixed and unfixed groups, under vertical loading condition, the posterior intradiscal

pressures in the fixed group were significantly lower than those in the unfixed group for all spinal segments (except the T3–4 segment) ($P < 0.05$). Under 5° anterior flexion loading condition, the posterior intradiscal pressures in the fixed group were significantly lower than those in the unfixed group for all spinal segments (except the L4–5 segment) ($P < 0.05$). Under 5° posterior extension condition, the posterior intradiscal pressures in the fixed group were significantly lower than in those the unfixed group for all spinal segments (except the T3–4 segment) ($P < 0.05$).

Left and right disc pressures under different loading conditions

The left and right pressures under different loading conditions in the unfixed and fixed groups were shown in Table 2. As for the unfixed group, there were no significant difference regarding the intervertebral disc pressures between the left and right sides for all spinal segments under the loading condition of vertical, 5° anterior flexion, and 5°posterior extension. As for the fixed group, left intervertebral disc had significantly lower pressures for all spinal segments under vertical loading condition ($P < 0.05$), lower pressures for all spinal segments (except the T3–4 segment) under 5°

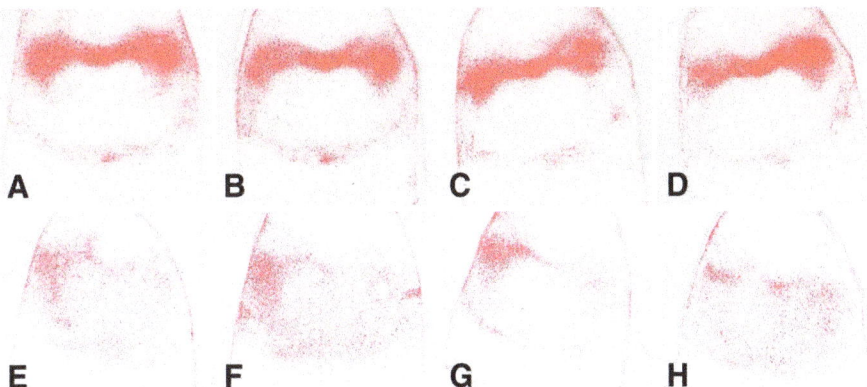

Fig. 2 Representative images (T11–L2) of pressure-sensitive film in the unfixed and fixed groups under different loading conditions. **a–d** Vertical, 5° anterior flexion, 5° posterior extension, and 5° lateral bending in the unfixed group. **e–h** Vertical, 5° anterior flexion, 5° posterior extension, and 5° lateral bending in the fixed group

Table 1 The posterior intradiscal pressures under different loading conditions in the unfixed and fixed groups (MPa)

Segment	Vertical		5° anterior flexion		5° posterior extension	
	Unfixed	Fixed	Unfixed	Fixed	Unfixed	Fixed
T3–4	1.83 ± 0.23	1.48 ± 0.25	1.95 ± 0.22	1.31 ± 0.16[†]	1.15 ± 0.12*	1.90 ± 0.27
T11–12	2.88 ± 0.27	1.02 ± 0.17[†]	2.66 ± 0.44	0.98 ± 0.18[†]	3.07 ± 0.39	1.11 ± 0.20[†]
T15–L1	2.51 ± 0.47	0.70 ± 0.14[†]	2.39 ± 0.279	0.67 ± 0.15[†]	2.31 ± 0.30	0.87 ± 0.10[†]
L3–4	1.94 ± 0.30	0.88 ± 0.20[†]	1.69 ± 0.33	0.86 ± 0.14[†]	1.87 ± 0.16	1.27 ± 0.23[†]
L4–5	1.87 ± 0.51	1.09 ± 0.20[†]	1.67 ± 0.33	1.15 ± 0.20	1.91 ± 0.36	1.10 ± 0.22[†]

*$P < 0.05$ versus the corresponding values of the unfixed group under vertical or 5° anterior flexion loading condition
[†]$P < 0.05$ versus the corresponding values of the unfixed group under different loading conditions

anterior flexion ($P < 0.05$), and lower pressures for all spinal segments (except the T3–4 and T15–L1 segments) under 5° posterior extension ($P < 0.05$), when compared to those of the right side.

In the unfixed group, the left intervertebral disc pressures for all spinal segments under 5° left lateral bending were significantly higher than those under vertical loading condition ($P < 0.05$). The fixed group had significantly lower left intervertebral disc pressures for all spinal segments (except the T3–4 segment) under vertical loading condition ($P < 0.05$), lower values for all spinal segments under 5° anterior flexion ($P < 0.05$), lower values for all spinal segments (except the T3–4 segment) under 5°posterior extension ($P < 0.05$), and lower values for all spinal segments under 5° left lateral

bending ($P < 0.05$), when compared to those in the unfixed group.

Disc pressures of the entire intervertebral disc under different loading conditions

The mean pressures of intervertebral disc were analyzed (Table 3). The fixed group had lower mean pressures in all segments (except the T3–4 segment) under vertical loading condition ($P < 0.05$), lower mean pressures in all segments (except the T3–4 and L4–5 segments) under 5° anterior flexion loading condition ($P < 0.05$), and lower mean pressures in all segments (except the T3–4 and L3–4 segments) under 5° posterior extension loading condition ($P < 0.05$), when compared to the unfixed group.

Table 2 The left and right pressures under different loading conditions in the unfixed and fixed groups (MPa)

Segment	T3–4	T11–12	T15–L1	L3–4	L4–5
Vertical					
Unfixed (L)	1.22 ± 0.25	1.39 ± 0.23	1.44 ± 0.24	1.23 ± 0.18	1.30 ± 0.17
Unfixed (R)	1.30 ± 0.28	1.46 ± 0.18	1.52 ± 0.25	1.32 ± 0.20	1.27 ± 0.21
Fixed (L)	1.05 ± 0.13[a]	0.59 ± 0.10[a,b]	0.45 ± 0.08[a,b]	0.75 ± 0.18[a,b]	0.76 ± 0.13[a,b]
Fixed (R)	1.46 ± 0.35	1.14 ± 0.12	0.81 ± 0.11	1.16 ± 0.16	1.53 ± 0.28
5° anterior flexion					
Unfixed (L)	1.43 ± 0.24	1.68 ± 0.23	1.48 ± 0.30	1.47 ± 0.12	1.12 ± 0.25
Unfixed (R)	1.49 ± 0.32	1.41 ± 0.31	1.53 ± 0.22	1.56 ± 0.32	1.00 ± 0.15
Fixed (L)	1.04 ± 0.14[b]	0.63 ± 0.11[a,b]	0.51 ± 0.07[a,b]	0.60 ± 0.08[a,b]	0.73 ± 0.06[a,b]
Fixed (R)	1.22 ± 0.14	1.31 ± 0.29	0.72 ± 0.07	0.86 ± 0.07	1.36 ± 0.29
5° posterior extension					
Unfixed (L)	0.93 ± 0.03	1.70 ± 0.29	1.41 ± 0.30	0.91 ± 0.13	1.48 ± 0.28
Unfixed (R)	1.01 ± 0.16	1.86 ± 0.22	1.65 ± 0.25	1.02 ± 0.18	1.34 ± 0.24
Fixed (L)	1.26 ± 0.23[b]	0.44 ± 0.07[a, b]	0.65 ± 0.12[b]	0.67 ± 0.14[a,b]	0.68 ± 0.11[a,b]
Fixed (R)	1.39 ± 0.27	1.35 ± 0.20	0.82 ± 0.11	1.32 ± 0.20	1.36 ± 0.23
5° left lateral bending					
Unfixed (L)	1.70 ± 0.18[c,d]	1.79 ± 0.14[c,d]	1.84 ± 0.22[c,d]	1.74 ± 0.28[c,d]	1.60 ± 0.23[c,d]
Fixed (L)	0.83 ± 0.12	0.93 ± 0.12	0.50 ± 0.05	0.60 ± 0.10	0.55 ± 0.08

[a]$P < 0.05$ versus the corresponding right pressures of the fixed group under different loading conditions
[b]$P < 0.05$ versus the corresponding left pressures of the unfixed group under different loading conditions
[c]$P < 0.05$ versus the left pressures of the unfixed group under vertical loading condition
[d]$P < 0.05$ versus the corresponding left pressures of the fixed group under 5° left lateral bending loading condition

Table 3 The mean pressure under different loading conditions in the unfixed and fixed groups (MPa)

Segments	Vertical			5° anterior flexion			5° posterior extension		
	Unfixed	Fixed	Unfixed/fixed (%)	Unfixed	Fixed	Unfixed/fixed (%)	Unfixed	Fixed	Unfixed/fixed (%)
T3–4	1.29 ± 0.22	1.16 ± 0.24	89.64	1.52 ± 0.19	1.17 ± 0.18	77.03	1.06 ± 0.11	1.23 ± 0.25	115.86
T11–12	1.69 ± 0.34	0.93 ± 0.17*	54.95	1.86 ± 0.33	0.91 ± 0.16*	48.95	1.93 ± 0.20	0.90 ± 0.16*	46.60
T15–L1	1.53 ± 0.32	0.67 ± 0.04*	43.80	1.73 ± 0.28	0.58 ± 0.11*	33.66	1.39 ± 0.25	0.75 ± 0.14*	53.82
L3–4	1.30 ± 0.18	0.93 ± 0.14*	71.24	0.97 ± 0.19	0.86 ± 0.12*	88.57	1.22 ± 0.20	1.09 ± 0.22	89.10
L4–5	1.48 ± 0.26	1.11 ± 0.18*	74.71	1.11 ± 0.21	1.05 ± 0.22	95.21	1.47 ± 0.27	1.06 ± 0.18*	72.10

*$P < 0.05$ versus the corresponding value of the unfixed group

The percentage of the mean pressure of the fixed group to that of unfixed group was calculated. Higher percentage indicated less effects of the fixation between specific intervertebral discs. The highest percentage was found in the T3–4 segment, and the lowest value was found in the T15–L1 segment under vertical loading condition. The highest percentage was found in the L4–5 segment, and the lowest in the T15–L1 segment under 5° anterior flexion loading condition. The highest percentage was found in the T3–4 segment, and the lowest in the T11–12 segment under 5° posterior extension loading condition.

Discussion

Previously, scoliosis-related studies mainly focused on the histomorphology, microscopic examination, and radiographic analysis [14–19]. However, limited information is available regarding the specific pressure data of intervertebral disc when an asymmetry stress was present, and most of the studies used sensors and probes in order to evaluate the pressure, and a shortcoming is that the results are only from certain points and also not intuitive [13, 20]. In contrast, the pressure-sensitive film method is more appropriate in investigating the pressure distribution of the intervertebral disc [8]. In the present study, pressure characteristics for different spinal segments under compression were recorded and analyzed using the pressure-sensitive film method. Previously, pigs are widely used for experimental purposes in spinal research and implant testing, mainly because of the anatomical similarities to humans [9–11]; therefore, we chose the porcine spine as the experimental subjects.

At present, there are many methods for the treatment of congenital scoliosis clinically, such as anterior and posterior convex epiphysiodesis, hemivertebra resection, and vertical expandable prosthetic titanium rib [21]. Some of these technologies have good effects, while some have not achieved the desired results; the unsatisfactory curative effect may partially be due to the lack of experimental research on spine biomechanics details or depth. Our study may lay foundation for further research on the biomechanics of the spinal column and provide ideas for the improvement and optimization of clinical therapy techniques. Our study proved that short-segment pedicle screw fixation is a minimally invasive and effective treatment method, which can significantly reduce the pressure on the fixed side of the spine and improve the unbalanced force distribution. This technique can be used for the surgical intervention of short-segment malformations in patients with congenital scoliosis, as well as severe long-spine-affected scoliosis, thereby achieving spinal deformity control with less vertebral body interference and implants, as well as minimizing the impact on children's spine development.

Regarding the non-fixed status, darker color in the back side of the film, which indicated higher pressure, was observed under vertical, 5° flexion, and 5°posterior extension loading conditions for all the spinal segments. In previous studies, the frontside pressure increased under the flexion, whereas the backside pressure decreased, and vice versa under the posterior extension [13, 22–24]. Notably, in this study, the backside pressure of the T3–4 segment was significantly reduced under posterior extension as compared with under vertical or 5° anterior flexion loading condition, and there was no significant difference in the backside pressure values among the other groups under different loading conditions for the same segment, although an increasing tendency was observed for the T11–12, L4–5 segments when under 5° posterior extension. The special physiological structure of the T3–4 segment may contribute to the effect observed in the present study, as the upper thoracic discs were relatively smaller, with more vertebral posterior column structures, the pressure was partially taken by articular process and therefore the intervertebral disc may take less pressure as expected under posterior extension [12, 25].

The left and right side pressures were basically the same under different loading conditions for all the spinal segments without significant differences. When under the 5° left lateral bending, as expected, the balance of pressure receiving between the two sides was broken; higher pressure was recorded on the concave side compared to the convex side, which is also consistent with a previous report [26].

For the fixed group, asymmetric pressures were observed between the left and right side under vertical, 5° flexion, and 5° posterior extension conditions, and this phenomenon has been reported previously [24]. As expected, the fixed side pressure was less than those of the unfixed side; significant differences were found for most of the spinal segments.

In this study, we obtained the specific pressure value of different spinal segments under asymmetric stress, which is valuable to test the effects of the pedicle screw fixation system on correcting of asymmetric stress. When under 5° left lateral bending condition, the left side pressures were significantly reduced as compared with the unfixed group for segments. It is generally believed that the wedge deformation of the vertebral body and intervertebral disc is essential to the development of scoliosis [26–31], which follows the Hueter-Volkmann principle [32]; growth is retarded by increased mechanical compression and accelerated by reduced loading. The morphological changes of the scoliosis are highly correlated with the asymmetric stress of intervertebral discs. Collectively, our data showed evidence that unilateral pedicle screw fixation can effectively reduce the pressure of the fixed side of the intervertebral disc and therefore be able to correct unbalanced stress.

When considering the average pressure, in the fixed group, the value of each segment was decreased compared to that in the unfixed group, suggesting that unilateral pedicle screw fixation can alleviate the overall stress of the intervertebral disc. We further calculated the percentage of the mean pressure of the fixed group to that of the unfixed group; results showed that the most contributable segments of the pedicle screw fixation system include the lower thoracic and thoracolumbar vertebrae.

Our study has several limitations. Firstly, porcine animal model with important differences to human beings (intradiscal pressure and anatomy) was used, because the availability of human cadaver material is very limited, particularly from the younger population. Therefore, the applicability of our strategy to human beings requires further study. Secondly, to compare the stress differences between the fixed side and the unfixed side, this study only focused on the unilateral pedicle screw fixation and the force of the spine was not fully revealed. Lastly, only some of the representative spinal segments were studied in this study, and the biomechanical data of the whole spine could not be fully reflected. Thus, further study regarding the biomechanical data of the whole spine and the difference between bilateral and unilateral pedicle screw fixation based on human beings is required in future.

Conclusion

Unilateral pedicle screws can effectively reduce the pressure of the fixed lateral intervertebral disc. In addition, it can change the pressure distribution of the intervertebral disc and reduce the press. The pressure characteristics obtained from the present study may be helpful in understanding the effects of the pedicle screw fixation system on the treatment of scoliosis.

Acknowledgements
We thank the Institute of Orthopaedics Affiliated to the Third Hospital of Hebei Medical University for providing the biomechanics experimental machine.

Funding
The study was approved by the Key Project of Medical Scientific Research of Hebei Province (no. 04096) and Key Research and Development Plan of Hebei Province (no. 18277745D). The funders had no role in the study design, data collection and analysis, decision to publish, or preparation of the manuscript.

Authors' contributions
ZM conceived the design and drafted the manuscript. CW carried out biomechanical analysis and participated in coordination. LT carried out the model validation. XZ and DG provided the critical revision of the manuscript. YZ performed the data assembly and analysis. All authors read and approved the final manuscript.

Competing interests
The authors declare that they have no competing interests.

Author details
[1]Department of Orthopaedics, Children's Hospital of Hebei Province, No.133, Jianhua Street, Yuhua District, Shijiazhuang 050031, China. [2]Department of Orthopaedics, the Third Hospital of Shijiazhuang, No. 15 South of Tiyu Street, Shijiazhuang 050011, Hebei, China. [3]Department of Orthopaedics, Beijing Children's Hospital, Capital Medical University, No. 56 Nan-li-shi Road, Beijing 100045, China.

References
1. Hedequist D, Emans J. Congenital scoliosis: a review and update. J Pediatr Orthop. 2007;27(1):106–16. https://doi.org/10.1097/BPO.0b013e31802b4993.
2. Shakil H, Iqbal ZA, Al-Ghadir AH. Scoliosis: review of types of curves, etiological theories and conservative treatment. J Back Musculoskelet Rehabil. 2014;27(2):111–5. https://doi.org/10.3233/BMR-130438.
3. El-Hawary R, Chukwunyerenwa C. Update on evaluation and treatment of scoliosis. Pediatr Clin N Am. 2014;61(6):1223–41. https://doi.org/10.1016/j.pcl.2014.08.007.
4. MacEwen GD, Shands AR Jr. Scoliosis—a deforming childhood problem. Clin Pediatr (Phila). 1967;6(4):210–6. https://doi.org/10.1177/000992286700600406.

5. Harrington PR. Scoliosis in the growing spine. Pediatr Clin N Am. 1963;10:225–45.

6. Blakemore LC, Scoles PV, Poe-Kochert C, Thompson GH. Submuscular Isola rod with or without limited apical fusion in the management of severe spinal deformities in young children: preliminary report. Spine (Phila Pa 1976). 2001;26(18):2044–8.

7. Rose PS, Lenke LG, Bridwell KH, Mulconrey DS, Cronen GA, Buchowski JM, et al. Pedicle screw instrumentation for adult idiopathic scoliosis: an improvement over hook/hybrid fixation. Spine (Phila Pa 1976). 2009;34(8): 852–7; discussion 8. https://doi.org/10.1097/BRS.0b013e31818e5962.

8. Xin-wei L, Shuo-gui X, Chun-cai Z, Qing-ge F, Pan-feng W. Biomechanical study of posterior wall acetabular fracture fixation using acetabular tridimensional memory alloy-fixation system. Clin Biomech (Bristol, Avon). 2010;25(4):312–7. https://doi.org/10.1016/j.clinbiomech.2010.01.008.

9. Zhou CS, Xu YF, Zhang Y, Chen Z, Lv H. Biomechanical testing of a unique built-in expandable anterior spinal internal fixation system. BMC Musculoskelet Disord. 2014;15:424. https://doi.org/10.1186/1471-2474-15-424.

10. Le Cann S, Cachon T, Viguier E, Miladi L, Odent T, Rossi JM, et al. Pedicle screw fixation study in immature porcine spines to improve pullout resistance during animal testing. PLoS One. 2015;10(10):e0127463. https:// doi.org/10.1371/journal.pone.0127463.

11. Shi YM, Zhu FZ, Wei X, Chen BY. Study of transpedicular screw fixation on spine development in a piglet model. J Orthopaedic Surg Res. 2016;11:8. https://doi.org/10.1186/s13018-015-0302-9.

12. Adams MA, McNally DS, Dolan P. 'Stress' distributions inside intervertebral discs. The effects of age and degeneration. J Bone Joint Surg Br. 1996;78(6):965–72.

13. Edwards WT, Ordway NR, Zheng Y, McCullen G, Han Z, Yuan HA. Peak stresses observed in the posterior lateral anulus. Spine (Phila Pa 1976). 2001; 26(16):1753–9.

14. Caballero A, Barrios C, Burgos J, Hevia E, Correa C. Vertebral growth modulation by hemicircumferential electrocoagulation: an experimental study in pigs. Eur Spine J. 2011;20(Suppl 3):367–75. https://doi.org/10.1007/ s00586-011-1909-0.

15. Fekete TF, Kleinstuck FS, Mannion AF, Kendik ZS, Jeszenszky DJ. Prospective study of the effect of pedicle screw placement on development of the immature vertebra in an in vivo porcine model. Eur Spine J. 2011;20(11): 1892–8. https://doi.org/10.1007/s00586-011-1889-0.

16. Odent T, Cachon T, Peultier B, Gournay J, Jolivet E, Elie C, et al. Porcine model of early onset scoliosis based on animal growth created with posterior mini-invasive spinal offset tethering: a preliminary report. Eur Spine J. 2011;20(11):1869–76. https://doi.org/10.1007/s00586-011-1830-6.

17. Patel A, Schwab F, Lafage R, Lafage V, Farcy JP. Does removing the spinal tether in a porcine scoliosis model result in persistent deformity? A pilot study. Clin Orthop Relat Res. 2011;469(5):1368–74. https://doi.org/10.1007/ s11999-010-1750-5.

18. Shea KG, Ford T, Bloebaum RD, D'Astous J, King H. A comparison of the microarchitectural bone adaptations of the concave and convex thoracic spinal facets in idiopathic scoliosis. J Bone Joint Surg Am. 2004;86-A(5):1000–6.

19. Zhu F, Qiu Y, Yeung HY, Lee KM, Cheng JC. Histomorphometric study of the spinal growth plates in idiopathic scoliosis and congenital scoliosis. Pediatr Int. 2006;48(6):591–8. https://doi.org/10.1111/j.1442-200X.2006.02277.x.

20. McMillan DW, McNally DS, Garbutt G, Adams MA. Stress distributions inside intervertebral discs: the validity of experimental "stress profilometry". Proc Inst Mech Eng H. 1996;210(2):81–7.

21. Kaspiris A, Grivas TB, Weiss HR, Turnbull D. Surgical and conservative treatment of patients with congenital scoliosis: alpha search for long-term results. Scoliosis. 2011;6:12. https://doi.org/10.1186/1748-7161-6-12.

22. Cil A, Yazici M, Daglioglu K, Aydingoz U, Alanay A, Acaroglu RE, et al. The effect of pedicle screw placement with or without application of compression across the neurocentral cartilage on the morphology of the spinal canal and pedicle in immature pigs. Spine (Phila Pa 1976). 2005;30(11):1287–93.

23. Steffen T, Baramki HG, Rubin R, Antoniou J, Aebi M. Lumbar intradiscal pressure measured in the anterior and posterolateral annular regions during asymmetrical loading. Clin Biomech (Bristol, Avon). 1998;13(7):495–505.

24. Zhang H, Sucato DJ. Unilateral pedicle screw epiphysiodesis of the neurocentral synchondrosis. Production of idiopathic-like scoliosis in an immature animal model. J Bone Joint Surg (American Volume). 2008;90(11): 2460–9. https://doi.org/10.2106/JBJS.G.01493.

25. McAfee PC, Yuan HA, Fredrickson BE, Lubicky JP. The value of computed tomography in thoracolumbar fractures. An analysis of one hundred consecutive cases and a new classification. J Bone Joint Surg (Am Vol). 1983;65(4):461–73.

26. Stokes IA, Iatridis JC. Mechanical conditions that accelerate intervertebral disc degeneration: overload versus immobilization. Spine (Phila Pa 1976). 2004;29(23):2724–32.

27. Mente PL, Aronsson DD, Stokes IA, Iatridis JC. Mechanical modulation of growth for the correction of vertebral wedge deformities. J Orthop Res. 1999;17(4):518–24. https://doi.org/10.1002/jor.1100170409.

28. Mente PL, Stokes IA, Spence H, Aronsson DD. Progression of vertebral wedging in an asymmetrically loaded rat tail model. Spine (Phila Pa 1976). 1997;22(12):1292–6.

29. Perdriolle R, Becchetti S, Vidal J, Lopez P. Mechanical process and growth cartilages. Essential factors in the progression of scoliosis. Spine (Phila Pa 1976). 1993;18(3):343–9.

30. Stokes IA, Aronsson DD. Disc and vertebral wedging in patients with progressive scoliosis. J Spinal Disord. 2001;14(4):317–22.

31. Stokes IA, Spence H, Aronsson DD, Kilmer N. Mechanical modulation of vertebral body growth. Implications for scoliosis progression. Spine (Phila Pa 1976). 1996;21(10):1162–7.

32. Mehlman CT, Araghi A, Roy DR. Hyphenated history: the Hueter-Volkmann law. Am J Orthop (Belle Mead NJ). 1997;26(11):798–800.

25

A comparative study to evaluate the feasibility of preoperative percutaneous catheter drainage for the treatment of lumbar spinal tuberculosis with psoas abscess

Zhen Lai, Shiyuan Shi*, Jun Fei, Guihe Han and Shengping Hu

Abstract

Background: Spinal tuberculosis is a frequent cause of psoas abscess (PA), and PA largely negates the efficacy of antituberculosis therapy. This study aimed to investigate the clinical outcome of preoperative percutaneous catheter drainage (PCD) in patients with lumbar spinal tuberculosis and PA.

Methods: Between January 2015 and January 2017, 72 patients with lumbar spinal tuberculosis with PA were assigned to group A (preoperative PCD) and group B ($n = 36$ per group). All patients received posterior pedicle screw fixation and anterior focal debridement and fusion. Data on intraoperative blood loss, the duration of the surgery, and the length of the anterior incision were recorded, as well as the postoperative anal exhaust time, visual analogue scale (VAS), Cobb angle, lumbar vertebra function, erythrocyte sedimentation rate (ESR), C-reactive protein (CRP) level, and sinus tract formation.

Results: Sixty-eight patients were followed up for an average time of 13 months (range 6–21 months). Until the final follow-up, no mixed infections, recurrence of tuberculosis, pedicle screw loosening, or screw pullout had occurred. There were significant between-group differences in blood loss, surgery duration, anterior incisional length, postoperative anal exhaust time, and sinus tract formation. As compared with group B, the ESR and CRP levels of the patients in group A were markedly improved following 3 weeks of antituberculosis therapy and 1 week postsurgery.

Conclusion: Preoperative PCD helps to increase the efficacy of antituberculosis therapy prior to surgery, reduce surgical trauma, and avoid postoperative complications, making it a safe and feasible treatment option for lumbar spinal tuberculosis with PA.

Keywords: Lumbar vertebra, Tuberculosis, Spine, Psoas abscess, Catheter drainage

* Correspondence: shiyuansss563@sina.com
Department of Orthopedics, Hospital of Integrated Traditional Chinese and Western medicine in Zhejiang Province, 208 Huancheng E.Rd, Hangzhou 310003, Zhejiang Province, People's Republic of China

Introduction

Psoas abscess (PA) is a result of myositis, which is caused by many types of bacteria, fungi, parasites, and viruses [1]. PA affects adjacent tissues and has serious public health implications. Spinal tuberculosis is considered a frequent cause of PA in developed countries [2]. According to a recent study, approximately 75–83% of patients with spinal tuberculosis may suffer from a paraspinal abscess or PA [3]. The latter arises when spinal tuberculosis advances through the periosteum, thereby causing inflammation and abscesses.

Chemotherapy plays a significant role in treating spinal tuberculosis. There is evidence that some patients with tuberculous PA may respond to medical therapy, such as antituberculosis treatment, with antituberculosis drugs reaching inhibitory concentrations in lesions [4]. However, a large number of patients fail to respond to medical therapy, necessitating surgical treatment. In recent years, studies have reported good clinical outcomes with posterior pedicle screw fixation combined with anterior focal debridement and fusion in treating lumbar spinal tuberculosis with PA [5, 6]. For instance, after debridement for spinal tuberculosis with a bilateral paraspinal abscess or PA, Li et al. treated the tuberculous lesions with gelatin sponges containing 5 g of streptomycin. They reported that streptomycin was released gradually and that local concentrations of the drug were maintained in the lesions [7]. However, following necrosis, with liquefaction of the PA region and thickening of pus walls, preoperative antituberculosis drugs have difficulty in penetrating the wall of a pyogenic abscess, which often leads to an unsatisfactory outcome. Therefore, in cases of PA, it is best to remove the abscess before surgery to improve the outcome of preoperative antituberculosis therapy.

During the past 10 years, accumulating evidence has strongly suggested that percutaneous catheter drainage (PCD) prior to surgery may be a new practical approach in the management of lumbar spinal tuberculosis with PA [8–10]. As documented previously, PCD is easy to perform, results in less post-surgical pain, and avoids complications associated with anterior surgery. Ye et al. reported that in comparison with anterior PCD, posterior PCD minimized the duration of surgery, reduced surgical trauma, and facilitated the recovery of patients with tuberculous PA [11]. The risk of complications with posterior PCD was also lower than with anterior PCD in these patients. The clinical outcome of preoperative PCD in treating lumbar spinal tuberculosis with PA has been seldom paid attention. The present prospective controlled study investigated short-term outcomes of preoperative PCD in the treatment of lumbar spinal tuberculosis with PA.

Materials and methods

Diagnostic criteria for lumbar spine tuberculosis

Lumbar spinal tuberculosis was diagnosed based on a comprehensive medical history, clinical manifestations, imageological diagnosis, as well as staining of pus and microscopy. All the enrolled patients had a history of lumbago, restricted lumbar vertebral function, partial pressing pain, and percussion pain. X-rays and computed tomography (CT) revealed osteoclasia and sequestra, and magnetic resonance imaging (MRI) showed an abscess near the pathological vertebrae and PA. Tuberculosis was confirmed by a staining and microscopic examination of pus drained from the abscess, followed by rapid liquid culture using the BACTEC MGIT 960 system (BD Biosciences, USA) and GeneXpert assay (MTB/RIF, BD, USA).

Inclusion and exclusion criteria

The inclusion criteria were (1) patients who fulfilled the diagnostic standard for lumbar spinal tuberculosis with PA with an abscess diameter ≥ 3 cm, (2) patients who had indications for spinal tuberculosis surgery (i.e., the presence of spinal compression, a sequestrum, overt bony destruction, and vertebral instability), (3) patients who underwent posterior pedicle screw fixation, anterior debridement, and bone graft fusion, and (4) patients who cooperated with the clinical research and provided signed informed consent.

Patients with one or more of the following were excluded: (1) patients with surgical contraindications, including those with other organ diseases who could not tolerate a long surgery and anesthesia and those with active pulmonary tuberculosis; (2) patients whose surgery had to be postponed because their ESR and CRP levels did not decrease after receiving antituberculosis treatment for 3 weeks; (3) patients with mental illness who could not cooperate with the surgical treatment; (4) patients whose antituberculosis schedules had to be changed during the 3 weeks of treatment; (5) patients who received anterior debridement and bone graft fusion in more than one segment; and (6) patients with a follow-up period less than 6 months.

General data

In this prospective study, 72 consecutive patients with lumbar spine tuberculosis companied with PA who presented to the Hospital of Integrated Traditional Chinese and Western Medicine in Zhejiang Province (Hangzhou, China) from January 2015 to January 2017 were included. Informed consent was obtained from all the patients and this study was approved by the ethics committee of the Hospital of Integrated Traditional Chinese and Western Medicine in Zhejiang Province. All the patients received a standard antituberculosis regimen containing rifampicin (0.45–0.6 g/d), ethambutol (0.75 g/d), isoniazid (0.3 g/d), and pyrazinamide (1.5 g/d).

The participants were randomly divided into two groups: group A ($n = 36$) and group B ($n = 36$). Briefly, the randomization was performed using opaque sequentially numbered envelopes labeled with the name of the treatment group (group A and B). Briefly, the randomization was performed using opaque sequentially numbered envelopes labeled with the name of the treatment group (group A and B). These envelopes were sealed, shuffled, and then numbered in sequential order. For each new patient entering the study, an envelope was opened. Thus, this procedure avoided the chance of having more patients in one group than another. All the patients in group A underwent preoperative PCD immediately after hospital admission. Four patients in group B were excluded in accordance with the exclusion criterion (4) after 3 weeks of antituberculosis treatment. There were 20 males and 16 females in group A (age range 24–73 years; mean age 42.5 ± 10.2 years) and 18 males and 14 females in group B (age range 23–75 years; mean age 42.3 ± 9.8 years). There were no statistically significances in the sex, age, ESR, CRP levels, or involved segments of the patients (Table 1).

Operative techniques

All patients in group A underwent ultrasound-guided PCD before surgery. Briefly, the location of the maximum diameter of the PA cavity was confirmed by ultrasound guidance after standard skin disinfection procedures and local anesthesia. Puncture needles were then inserted into the abscess cavities. The needle cores were removed when the ultrasound examination confirmed the correct position of the puncture needle. Drainage catheters were inserted into deep abscess to extract pus, followed by a smear test under a microscope to detect acid-fast bacillus. The specimens were detected using the Mycobacterial Growth Indicator Tube 960 (MGIT 960, BD Biosciences, USA) rapid liquid culture method and GeneXpert MTB/RIF assay (Cepheid Inc., USA). Finally, drainage tubes were fixed and connected with drainage bags (Fig. 1). Patients with bilateral PA also underwent bilateral puncture catheter drainage.

All patients in both groups were treated with antituberculosis drugs for 3 weeks, followed by posterior pedicle screw fixation and anterior debridement and fusion, which were performed by the same physicians (Figs. 1 and 2). The drainage bags were replaced each day during the 3-week treatment period. In all patients, anterior fusion was achieved using an autogenous bone graft from the iliac crest. Under general anesthesia, a straight incision was made in the middle of the spinous processes, with the patient in a prone position. After pedicle screw fixation, the length of the posterior incision was determined by the fixed segment. The pedicle screws were inserted into the cephalic and caudal adjacent lumbar spinal vertebral segments. The patients were then moved to a lateral position, and an anterior incision was made according to the site of segmental lesions and the size of PA, followed by blunt dissection of the obliquus externus abdominis, obliquus internus abdominis, transverses abdominis along the direction of the fibers. After exposing the peritoneum, the posterior peritoneum and the intestinal canal were pushed away to expose the psoas, reproductive nerves, and ureter. After exposure of the pathological vertebrae using a longitudinal dissociation of the psoas, a pathological examination was performed. Anterior debridement and fusion were conducted, and streptomycin (2 g) and isoniazid (0.6 g) were then administered.

Observation indexes

The intraoperative blood loss, duration of the surgery, and anterior incision length, as well as the postoperative anal exhaust time, visual analogue scale (VAS) (1 month postsurgery), Cobb angle (1 month postsurgery), ESR and CRP levels (1 week, 1 month and 6 months postsurgery), sinus tract formation and spinal cord injury were evaluated.

The amount of anterior blood loss was considered the blood loss mediated by vacuum aspiration and the blood volume absorbed by the gauze packing. Blood mediated by vacuum aspiration was calculated using the following formula: the amount of liquid in aspirator − (the flushing fluid volume + the amount of pus). The blood volume absorbed by the gauze packing was calculated as follows: the amount of absorbed blood in the gauze packing = the

Table 1 Comparison of baseline data in the two groups

Groups	Cases (n)	Sex		Age (years)	ESR (mm/h)	CRP (mg/L)	The involved segments single biarticulate triarticular		
		Male	Female				single	biarticulate	triarticular
A	36	20	16	42.5 ± 10.2	74.5 ± 8.2	83.4 ± 7.0	23	10	3
B	32	18	14	42.3 ± 9.8	73.3 ± 9.8	82.8 ± 6.1	21	9	2
Statistic		$\chi^2 = 0.002$		$t = 0.928$	$t = 0.126$	$t = 0.268$	$\chi^2 = 0.328$		
P value		0.964		0.360	0.901	0.790	0.848		

ESR erythrocyte sedimentation rate, *CRP* C-reactive protein

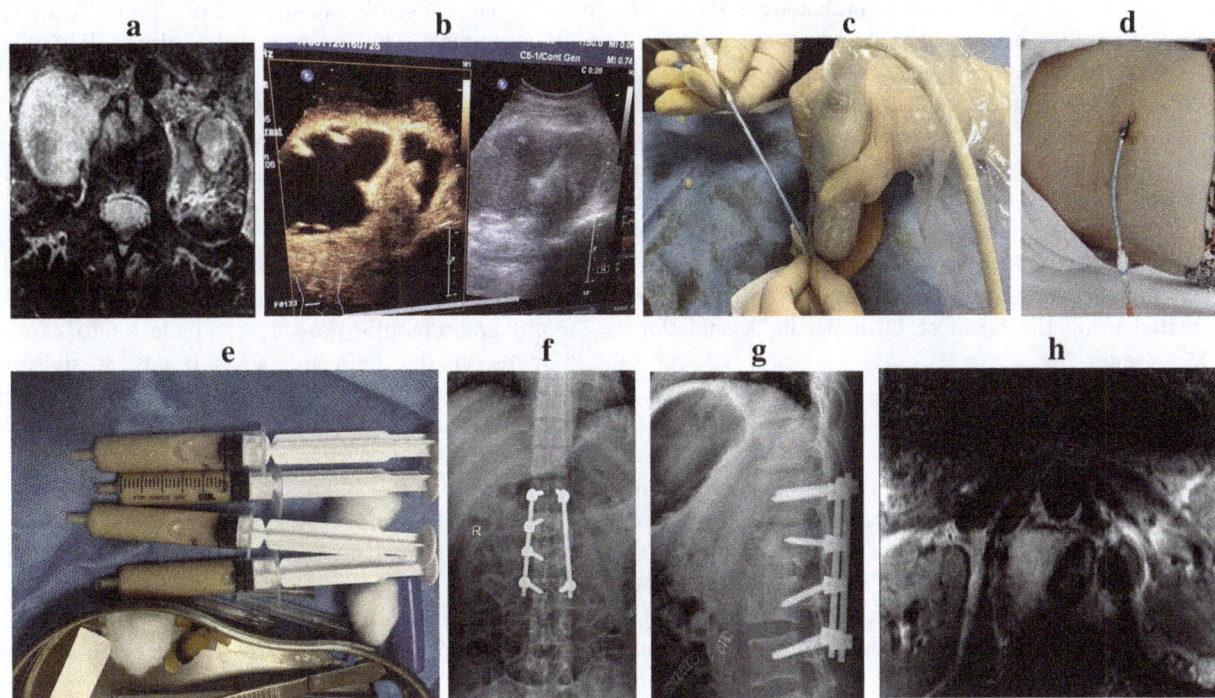

Fig. 1 A 46-year-old female patient with tuberculosis of the L1/2 lumbar vertebrae and PA underwent preoperative PCD under ultrasound guidance, antituberculosis therapy for 3 weeks, posterior pedicle screw fixation, and anterior debridement and bone graft fusion. **a.** Preoperative magnetic resonance imaging (MRI) showing lumbar spinal tuberculosis, with abscess formation. **b–e.** PCD was performed under ultrasound guidance. **f, g.** The X-ray image 3 days after surgery showed good internal fixation and bone grafting. **h.** Postoperative MRI performed at the 3-month follow-up showed complete debridement and no obvious abscess

total weight of wet gauze – (the weight of a single gauze pad × the total number of gauze pads).

The duration of surgery was determined as the time of starting cutting the skin until suture of the incision.

Due to the use of preoperative PCD in group A, the severity of PA may have differed in group A and group B. Thus, the length of the anterior incision may have been different. After suturing the anterior incision, the anterior incision length was measured.

The pain index was analyzed using the VAS to evaluate the clinical status of the patients before surgery and one month following surgery. Pains scores of 0, 1–3, 4–6, and 7–10 were judged as no pain, mild pain, moderate pain, and severe pain, respectively.

Before and after surgery, the vertebral segment kyphosis Cobb angle was assessed by X-ray images, with the patient in a standing position. An extension cord was drawn along the upper end plate of the centrum prior to the symptomatic vertebrae, and another extension cord was drawn along the lower end plate of the centrum next to the symptomatic vertebrae. The angle between the two lines was defined as the Cobb angle.

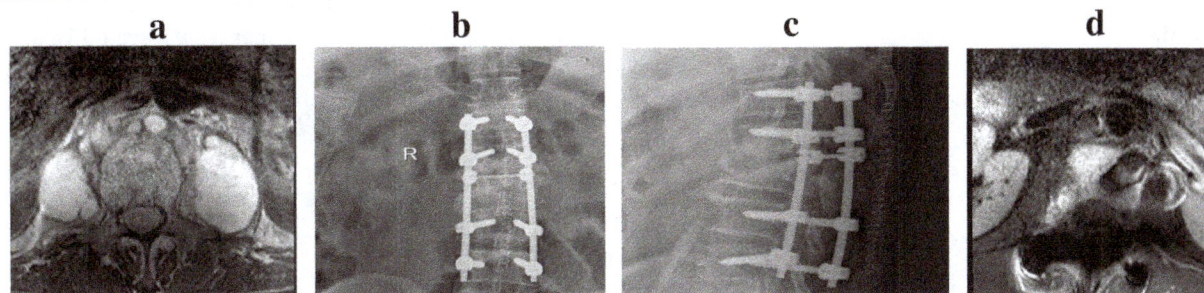

Fig. 2 A 39-year-old male patient with tuberculosis of the L1/2 lumbar vertebrae and PA underwent posterior pedicle screw fixation and anterior debridement, with bone graft fusion. **a.** Preoperative MRI showed lumbar tuberculosis, with abscess formation. **b, c.** The X-ray image 3 days after surgery showed good internal fixation and bone grafting. **d.** Postoperative MRI at the 3-month follow-up showed complete debridement and no obvious abscess

The Frankel grade was used to evaluate the status of spinal cord injury before surgery and at the final follow-up. Grade A denoted complete motor and sensory function disorder; grade B denoted complete function and incomplete sensory function; grade C denoted motor function disorder and incomplete sensory function; grade D denoted useful motor function, with or without auxiliary tools; and grade E denoted no motor or sensory function disorder, with a pathological reflex.

The lumbar vertebral function of the patients was estimated using the Japanese Orthopaedic Association (JOA) score.

Postoperative management
All patients were postoperatively treated with antituberculosis and liver protection drugs. A compound glycyrrhizin injection was used as the liver protection drug, which was administered via an intravenous injection (20 ml) once a day. Patients with severe anemia and hypoalbuminemia received an erythrocyte suspension and albumin. Pyrazinamide was discontinued 3 months after the operation. After bed rest and immobilization for 12 weeks, all the patients could gradually walk under a protective load.

Postoperative follow-up and complications evaluation
Sixty-eight patients had a mean follow-up time of 13 months (range 6~ 21 months). The condition of sinus tract formation in group A and group B was analyzed. Six months after surgery, the status of the sequestrum and abscess were assessed through CT examination. Other complications such as mixed infection, recurrence of tuberculosis, pedicle screw loosing, and screw pulling out were evaluated.

Statistical analysis
Statistical analyses of all data were performed using SPSS, version 16.0 (IBM, Chicago, IL, USA). The measurement data were expressed as the mean ± standard deviation (SD) and compared using Student's t test. A chi-square test was performed to compare the enumeration data. A value of $P < 0.05$ was taken as statistically significant.

Results
Of 72 cases, four patients with mental illness in group B were excluded due to noncompliance. The other 68

patients had a mean follow-up time of 13 months (range 6–21 months). The average blood loss ($P = 0.005$), duration of the surgery ($P = 0.003$), anterior incision length ($P = 0.00$), and postoperative anal exhaust time ($P = 0.017$) in group A were remarkably lower than those in group B (Table 2). In addition, sinus tract formation was noted in one case in the group and in five cases in group B (Table 2, $P = 0.002$).

The ESR and CRP of patients in group A were clearly increased 1 week postsurgery but dramatically decreased 1 month and 6 months postsurgery (Table 3, all $P < 0.05$). Variations in the ESR and CRP trends at different follow-up times in group B were in accordance with those observed in group A (Table 3, all $P < 0.05$). As shown in Table 3, the ESR and CRP levels in group A were remarkably lower than those in group B after 3 weeks of antituberculosis therapy and 1 month after surgery. However, there was no statistically significant between-group difference in these parameters 1 month and 6 months postsurgery (Table 3, all $P < 0.05$).

The results of the VAS indicated that the pain index of the patients in group A and group B was largely improved 1 month following surgery as compared with the preoperative data (Table 4, $P < 0.05$). However, there was no statistically significant between-group difference in the VAS 1 month postsurgery (Table 4, $P = 0.087$). As compared with the measurements before surgery, the Cobb angle of the patients in the two groups was clearly reduced 1 month after surgery ($P < 0.05$), with no significant between-group difference (Table 4, $P = 0.63$).

At the final follow-up, the status of spinal cord injury in the patients was evaluated by the Frankel grade. As compared with the preoperative Frankel grades, the spinal cord injury grades of the patients in group A and group B were notably improved at the final follow-up ($P < 0.01$), with no significant between-group difference ($P > 0.05$, Table 5). These findings revealed that the spinal cord injury of all the patients was migrated at the final follow-up.

The JOA scores, which indicated the lumbar vertebral function of the patients, are displayed in Table 6. In group A, the JOA scores were markedly elevated 1 month postsurgery and at the final follow-up as compared with the presurgery scores ($P < 0.05$). Likewise, the JOA scores

Table 2 Comparison of anterior blood loss, duration of surgery, anterior incision length, postoperative anal exhaust time, and sinus tract formation in the two groups ($\bar{x}\pm s$)

Groups	Cases (n)	Intraoperative blood loss (ml)	Duration of surgery (minutes)	Incision length (cm)	Anal exhaust time (hours)	Sinus tract formation (n)
A	36	156.3 ± 24.7	67.6 ± 13.2	11.7 + 2.6	22.3 ± 5.12	1
B	32	206.5 ± 39.2	105.7 ± 16.3	20.3 + 2.9	30.3 ± 5.69	5
Statistic		$t = 8.875$	$t = 3.280$	$t = 9.058$	$t = 5.013$	$\chi^2 = 7.696$
P value		0.005	0.003	0	0.017	0.002

Table 3 Comparison of the ESR and CRP level in different follow-up times postsurgery in the two groups ($\bar{x}\pm s$)

	Group A	Group B	t value	P value
Cases (n)	36	32		
ESR (mm/h)				
3 weeks after anti-TB treatment	37.1 ± 3.2	43.5 ± 5.0	3.012	0.005
1 week after surgery	78.7 ± 0.6	79.3 ± 0.5	3.180	0.003
1 month after surgery	29.1 ± 0.4	28.5 ± 0.7	1.210	0.235
6 months after surgery	9.9 ± 0.7	10.3 ± 0.6	1.794	0.090
CRP (mg/L)				
3 weeks after anti-TB treatment	70.8 ± 0.6	74.2 ± 0.7	3.107	0.004
1 week after surgery	84.3 ± 8.0	93.8 ± 9.1	3.214	0.003
1 month after surgery	15.6 ± 0.8	16.1 ± 0.6	1.816	0.079
6 months after surgery	3.1 ± 0.5	2.8 ± 0.6	1.571	0.126

ESR erythrocyte sedimentation rate, *CRP* C-reactive protein, *anti-TB* antituberculous

Table 5 Frankel grading in the two groups with lumbar spinal tuberculosis before and after surgery (cases)

	Before surgery		The final follow-up									
			Group A (grades)					Group B (grades)				
Grades	Group A	Group B	A	B	C	D	E	A	B	C	D	E
Grade A	0	0										
Grade B	0	0										
Grade C	6	4			2		4			2		2
Grade D	4	4					4					4
Grade E	26	24					26					24
Summation	36	32			2		34			2		30

of the patients in group B were much higher 1 month postsurgery and at the final follow-up as compared with the scores prior to surgery ($P < 0.05$). When compared with group B, the JOA scores were significantly higher in group A 1 month postsurgery ($P = 0.036$), whereas there was no statistically significant difference in the scores of the two groups at the final follow-up ($P = 0.782$, Table 6). All the patients had recovered lumbar vertebral function 1 month after surgery.

Postoperative MRI performed at the 3-month follow-up indicated complete debridement and no obvious abscess near symptomatic vertebrae. The CT examination 6 months post-surgery revealed no sequestra and abscess formation in any of the patients, with excellent bone fusion. Up until the final follow-up, there were no cases with mixed infection, recurrence of tuberculosis, pedicle screw loosening, or screw pull out. Typical cases are shown in Figs. 1 and 2.

Discussion

Clinically, patients with lumbar spinal tuberculosis combined with PA often require surgical treatment to remove the tuberculous lesion, relieve spinal cord compression, enhance the stability of bone grafting and the reconstructed spine, and promote functional recovery [12, 13]. Recently, accumulating evidence has strongly

implied that surgical treatment performed during the exudative phase of lumbar spine tuberculosis significantly increased the incidence of abscess recurrence, unhealed lesions, and sinus tract formation [14]. Hence, preoperative antituberculosis therapy has become a necessity for patients with lumbar spinal tuberculosis with PA [15]. In the present study, all the patients were treated with antituberculosis drugs for 3 weeks prior to surgery. As shown by the findings, after antituberculosis therapy for 3 weeks, the ESRs and CRP levels were higher in group A as compared with those in group B, implying that the efficacy of preoperative antitubercular treatment may be influenced by preoperative PCD.

In most cases, antituberculosis drugs administered prior to surgery fail to induce a therapeutic concentration likely to benefit surgical outcomes [16]. In recent years, emerging evidence has suggested that a satisfactory clinical outcome can be obtained by percutaneous abscess drainage puncture guided by ultrasound [17, 18]. The latter is attributed to abscess drainage eliminating inflammatory cytokines, thereby preventing tuberculosis from eroding the tissues around the abscess and improving the outcomes of preoperative antitubercular treatment [19, 20]. Relative to group B, the patients in group A had shorter operative time, less bleeding, and shorter incision length during anterior spine surgery. The aforementioned may be due to preoperative PCD triggering an outflow of large amounts of pus; therefore, the scope of the operation, the difficulty of the surgery, and the surgical trauma were reduced. In addition, the postoperative anal exhaust

Table 4 Comparison of the VAS and Cobb angle before and after surgery in the two groups ($\bar{x}\pm s$)

Groups	Cases (n)	VAS scoring		Cobb angle (°)	
		Before surgery	1 month after surgery	Before surgery	1 month after surgery
A	36	8.4 ± 0.8	3.2 ± 0.7	18.5 ± 5.5	11.3 ± 4.7
B	32	8.3 ± 0.7	3.5 ± 0.2	17.9 ± 6.1	10.9 ± 5.1
Statistic		0.016	1.725	1.062	0.283
P value		0.984	0.087	0.300	0.630

VAS visual analog scale

Table 6 Comparison of JOA scores in different periods in the two groups ($\overline{x}\pm$s)

Groups	Cases (n)	JOA scoring		
		Before surgery	1 month after surgery	The final follow-up
A	36	6.37 ± 0.51	19.03 ± 3.57	26.71 ± 3.91
B	32	6.41 ± 0.61	16.82 ± 2.75	27.23 ± 5.23
Statistic		0.06	0.128	0.279
P value		0.952	0.036	0.782

JOA Japanese Orthopaedic Association (JOA)

time and sinus tract formation rate of patients in group A were lower than those in group B. These findings indicate that the reduction in operative trauma in anterior spinal surgery might lead to reduced postoperative complications and improved clinical efficacy. Furthermore, PCD can be completed with the assistance of only a general sonographer. Thus, the procedure can be performed without the need for highly skilled hospital staff, suggesting that the use of PCD could be extended in the clinical setting.

Sometimes, percutaneous PCD fails to thoroughly drain an abscess due to the existence of s thick fester, calcified and caseous tissue in lesions, and a free sequestrum in a partial abscess, which are leading causes of the recurrence of PA. In such cases, anterior focal debridement should be redone. In the present study, we used drainage tubes with a diameter ≥ 3 cm for PCD because undersized drainage tubes are easily blocked by caseous necrotic tissues and surrounding soft tissues, both of which hamper abscess drainage [21]. During surgery, strict implementation of aseptic operative conditions can avoid cross-infection, as well as blood vessel and organ injury, thereby preventing the spread of tuberculosis.

The current study had some limitations. First, the sample size was relatively small. Second, we did not consider the effects of irrigation and local administration of antitubercular agents on the clinical outcome. Lastly, follow-up time was relatively short. Long-term multicenter studies with large sample sizes are needed to objectively and accurately evaluate the outcomes of preoperative PCD.

Conclusion

We conclude that preoperative PCD is a safe and feasible option for the treatment of lumbar spinal tuberculosis with PA and that PCD could enhance the effect of antituberculosis treatment administered prior to surgery, reduce surgical trauma, and reduce postoperative complications. This study provides support for the use of preoperative PCD in treating lumbar spinal tuberculosis with PA to enhance clinical outcomes.

Abbreviations
CRP: C-reactive protein; ESR: Erythrocyte sedimentation rate; PA: Psoas abscess; PCD: Preoperative percutaneous catheter drainage

Acknowledgements
Not applicable.

Funding
None.

Authors' contributions
SS put forward the concept of the study, designed the study, prepared the manuscript, and contributed to the statistical analysis. JF contributed to the data acquisition. GH contributed to the quality control of data and algorithms. SH analyzed the data and interpretation. ZL edited the manuscript. All authors read and approved the final manuscript.

Competing interests
The authors declare that they have no competing interests.

References
1. Zhang X, Zhang Z, Zhang Y, Wang J, Lu M, Hu W, et al. Minimally invasive retroperitoneoscopic surgery for psoas abscess with thoracolumbar tuberculosis. Surg Endosc. 2015;29(8):2451–5.
2. Khorgade RR, Bhise PR, Deshmukh MM. Psoas abscess due to mycobacterium tuberculosis: a case report. Int J Res Med Sci. 2017;5(7): 3251–3253.
3. Jain AK. Magnetic resonance evaluation of tubercular lesion in spine. Int Orthop. 2012;36(2):261–9.
4. Liu P, Zhu Q, Jiang J. Distribution of three antituberculous drugs and their metabolites in different parts of pathological vertebrae with spinal tuberculosis. Spine. 2011;36(20):E1290.
5. Ding WY, Yan-Lei HE, Bao-Jun LI. Brachy segament posterior fixation combined with anterior debridement used in the treatment of lumbar tuberculosis. J Cervicodynia Lumbodynia. 2010;31(2):38–42.
6. Huo H, Xing W, Yang X. Surgical management of thoracic and lumbar tuberculosis. Chin J Spine Spinal Cord. 2011;21(10):819–24.
7. Li J, Li XL, Zhou XG, Zhou J, Dong J. Surgical treatment for spinal tuberculosis with bilateral paraspinal abscess or bilateral psoas abscess: one-stage surgery. J Spinal Disord Tech. 2014;27(8):309–14.
8. Matsumoto T, Yamagami T, Morishita H, Iida S, Asai S, Masui K, et al. CT-guided percutaneous drainage within intervertebral space for pyogenic spondylodiscitis with psoas abscess. Acta Radiol. 2012;53(1):76.
9. Dinç H, Ahmetoğlu A, Baykal S, Sari A, Sayil O, Gümele HR. Image-guided percutaneous drainage of tuberculous iliopsoas and spondylodiskitic abscesses: midterm results. Radiology. 2002;225(2):353.
10. Dave BR, Babu KR, Dipak S, Devanand D, Nitu B, Ajay K. Outcome of percutaneous continuous drainage of psoas abscess: a clinically guided technique. Indian J Orthopaedics. 2014;48(1):67–73.
11. Ye F, Zhou Q, Feng D. Comparison of the anteroposterior and posterior approaches for percutaneous catheter drainage of tuberculous psoas abscess. Med Sci Monit. 2017;23:5374.
12. Ma YZ, Cui X, Li HW, Chen X, Cai XJ, Bai YB. Outcomes of anterior and posterior instrumentation under different surgical procedures for treating thoracic and lumbar spinal tuberculosis in adults. Int Orthop. 2012;36(2): 299–305.
13. Jain AK, Jain S. Instrumented stabilization in spinal tuberculosis. Int Orthop. 2012;36(2):285–92.
14. Gui QH, Bo LI, Yu YU, Yi-Ming QU, Min-Peng LU. Anterior approach operation for thoracic and lumbar spinal tuberculosis: the cause of recurrence and revision. J Clin Orthopaedics. 2016;19(2):11–14.

15. Qin SB. Thinking about the diagnosis and treatment of tuberculosis and the choice of operation time for spinal tuberculosis. Zhongguo gu shang = China journal of orthopaedics and traumatology. 2013;26(26):533–5.
16. Oguz E, Sehirlioglu A, Altinmakas M, Ozturk C, Komurcu M, Solakoglu C, et al. A new classification and guide for surgical treatment of spinal tuberculosis. Int Orthop. 2008;32(1):127.
17. Huang F, Zhang M, Liu Y, Spine DO. One-stage anterolateral debridement, bone graft and internal fixation combined with local closed irrigation drainage for lumbar spinal tuberculosis with abscess. Chin J Spine Spinal Cord. 2014;24(5):422–6.
18. Chen X, Ma Y. Percutaneous catheter drainage combined with antituberculosis chemotherapy in the management of tuberculous iliopsoas abscesses. Chin J Minim Invasive Surg. 2003;3(4):359–361.
19. Jin ZM, Wang P, Tang ZY. Ultrasound-guided percutaneous catheter drainage in the treatment of abdominal abscess. Med Innov China. 2013; 10(9):119–122.
20. Huang XR. Percutaneous catheter drainage combined with local chemotherapy in the treatment of spinal tuberculous abscesses. Contemp Med. 2010;16(17):79–83.
21. Wang Q, Hu M, Ma YZ, Luo XB. Case-control studies of two kinds of method for the treatment of lumbar tuberculosis with psoas abscess. Zhongguo gu shang = China journal of orthopaedics and traumatology. 2016;29(1):33.

26

Posterior hemivertebra resection with unilateral instrumented fusion in children less than 10 years old: preliminary results at minimum 5-year follow-up

Xuhong Xue and Sheng Zhao[*]

Abstract

Background: The main treatment for congenital hemivertebra is posterior hemivertebrectomy with bilateral transpedicular fixation. To date, studies describing posterior unilateral fusion are few, especially in younger children. The modified method by posterior hemivertebrectomy combined with unilateral transpedicular instrumentation and fusion was described. The purpose was to present the clinical and radiological outcome of children less than 10 years treated for congenital scoliosis with posterior hemivertebrectomy and unilateral instrumented fusion.

Methods: A study of 43 consecutive patients through Jan. 2006 to Mar. 2013 for hemivertebrae in children less than 10 years was performed. Patients undergoing hemivertebrectomy and posterior convex short-segment fusion, which had been followed up for at least 60 months, were included. Coronal main curve, kyphosis, T1-S1 height, fused vertebra height, and concave height were measured at preoperation, immediate postoperation, and final follow-up. The outcome and efficacy of the correction provided and growth of the non-fused concave side of the spine was investigated.

Results: The average follow-up period was 73.88 ± 16.77 months. The mean Cobb angle of the coronal curve was improved from 46.1 to 8.1° (correction rate 82.4%). At final follow-up, there was 7.8% loss of correction. The average concave height, fusion segment height, and T1-S1 height were 60.1 ± 19.7 mm, 56.9 ± 22.9 mm, and 326.6 ± 64.5 mm in immediate postoperation, which improved to 73.1 ± 23.7 mm, 71.2 ± 22.0 mm, and 388.7 ± 78.9 mm at the last follow-up. These parameters were significantly different between the immediate postoperation and at final follow-up. The rate of reoperation was 9.3% (4/43), mainly in PJK and curve progression after surgery.

Conclusions: Despite with some complications, posterior hemivertebrectomy and unilateral instrumented fusion are commendable procedures. We concluded that it is a simple, secure, reliable, less-invasive, and well-tolerated technique that can successfully resolve this kind of congenital scoliosis in children.

Keywords: Hemivertebrae, Unilateral fusion, Hemivertebrectomy, Congenital scoliosis

* Correspondence: zhaosheng0807@163.com
Department of Orthopedics, The Second Hospital of Shanxi Medical University, Taiyuan, No. 382 Wuyi Road, Taiyuan 030001, Shanxi, People's Republic of China

Background

Congenital scoliosis encompasses a continuous bending of spinal deformities, which result from the localized imbalance in the longitudinal growth of the spine caused by asymmetrical development of one or more vertebras [1]. It may be classified into failures of formation, failures of segmentation, or mixed deformities [2]. The most common anomaly caused by failure of formation is the hemivertebra. Based on pathological features, hemivertebra has been described to three types including (1) the fully segmented, (2) the semi-segmented, and (3) the incarcerated types [3]. Incarcerated hemivertebra and a balanced trunk usually have a benign result, while non-incarcerated hemivertebra has a normal-growth plate leading to progression of a wedge-shaped deformity. Scoliosis caused by non-incarcerated hemivertebra is more rigid than other types, which is difficult to correct by conservative treatment such as back brace and cast, which often requires surgery for correction [4, 5].

Posterior or anterior convex growth arrest (CGA) has been used to the treatment of early-onset congenital scoliosis [6]. Although successful results have been reported with the technique, the failure rates ranging from 8 to 21% have also been reported [7]. Several drawbacks of the classic CGA have also been described. On the one hand, the need for an additional anterior procedure has been one of the most worrisome drawbacks of the procedure. On the other hand, some problems such as being unable to obtain acute correction and unpredictability of gradual correction after surgery have been reasons of failure in CGA [8].

To negate the previously mentioned drawbacks, the technique has been modified. We applied pedicle screws through the posterior approach on the convex short-segment instrumentation aiming to control convex growth. Meanwhile, hemivertebra resection via the posterior approach was adopted aiming to achieve acute correction. Personalized hemivertebra excision was introduced to balance the growth potential in both sides of the spine. It can achieve convex growth arrest and preserve concave growth potential at the same time. The outcome and efficacy of this technique has been investigated in the present study.

Methods

With the approval of the institution's Institutional Review Board, 43 consecutive patients with hemivertebrae younger than 10 years of age were treated using hemivertebrectomy and posterior convex short-segment fusion through Jan. 2006 to Mar. 2013 at a single spine center. They had been followed up for at least 60 months. There were 23 boys and 20 girls. There were 22 fully segmented and 21 semi-segmented hemivertebra. The hemivertebra was located within the thoracic spine (T1–

T11) in 27 cases, within the thoracolumbar region (T12–L1) in seven cases, and within the lumbar spine (L2–L5) in 11 cases. Three patients had contralateral bar formation and synostosis of the ribs. Most of abnormal vertebra was located at the right side, only three cases within the left side. We used a 4.5-mm rod with polyaxial pediatric posterior instrumentation screws of 4.0-mm diameter in six patients whose ages were below 3 years, and we used a 5.5-mm rod with a 4.75- or 5.0-mm-diameter pediatric posterior instrumentation screws in the remaining 37 patients (Bonovo Orthopedics, Inc).

Preoperative evaluation included a thorough neuromuscular examination, routine radiographs, 3-dimensional computed tomography scan, and magnetic resonance imaging due to increased incidence of intraspinal abnormalities associated with congenital scoliosis. Cardiovascular and urogenital examinations were performed to detect congenital heart diseases and abnormalities of the renal system. None of the patients had undergone a prior operation. None had a neurologic deficit or cord anomaly. Surgery was indicated by proved or expected deterioration of the deformity.

Preoperation, immediate postoperation, and final follow-up standing posteroanterior and lateral radiograms were evaluated. Coronal main curve was recorded for the instrumented segment. Global thoracic kyphosis was measured between T2 and T12 on a sagittal plane. These values were compared preoperatively, postoperatively, and at last follow-up. The height between T1 and S1 was determined by the vertical distance from the midpoint of the superior endplate of T1 to the midpoint of the superior endplate of S1 (Fig. 1a). The height of fusion segment was determined by the vertical distance from the midpoint of the superior endplate of the upper instrumented vertebra (UIV) to the midpoint of the superior endplate of the lowest instrumented vertebra (LIV) (Fig. 1b). The height between the concave side pedicles of the upper- and lower-end vertebra of the main curve was also determined and recorded as the concave height (Fig. 1b). These measurements of the height on the radiograph are done digitally in early postoperative and at final follow-up X-rays. Operative reports were reviewed to determine the presence of any intraoperative complication. Medical records were reviewed to identify any complication in the perioperative and follow-up periods. Measurements were taken from standing long-cassette anterior-posterior and lateral radiographs.

Surgical technique

The patients were positioned prone on the operating table. A standard midline skin incision was used, and subperiosteal dissection was performed on the convex side only to expose the hemivertebra and the vertebrae

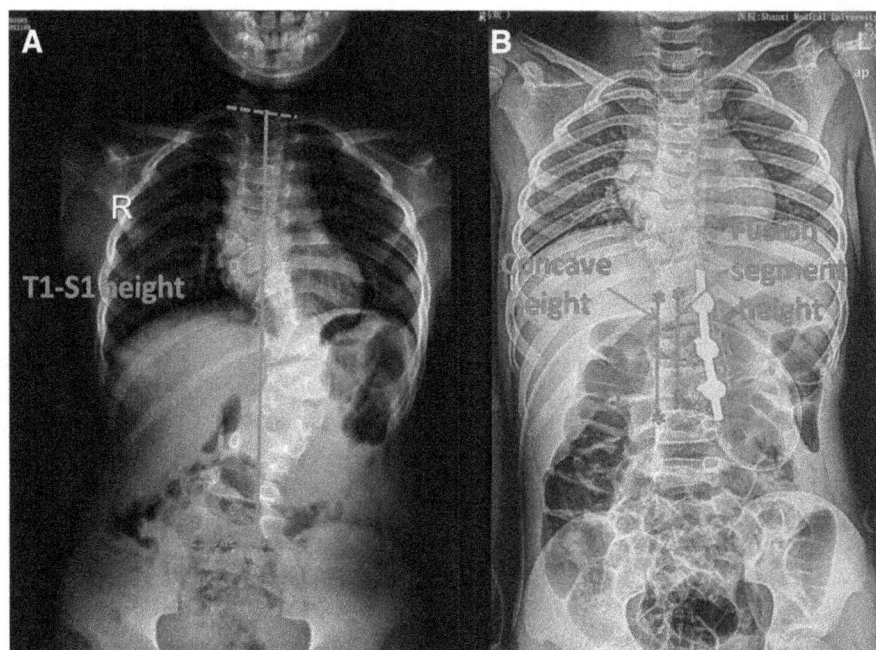

Fig. 1 T1-S1 height: the vertical distance from the midpoint of the superior endplate of T1 to the midpoint of the superior endplate of S1 (**a**); fusion segment height: vertical distance from the midpoint of the superior endplate of upper UIV to the midpoint of the superior endplate of LIV; concave height: the height between the concave side pedicles of the upper and lower end vertebra of the main curve (**b**)

just above and below, including the lamina, transverse processes, and facet joints. Fluoroscopy was used for the determination of instrumentation levels. Unilateral pedicle screws were inserted into the vertebra above and the vertebra below using the funnel technique described by Viau et al. [9]. Briefly speaking, the posterior cortex of the lamina overlying the top of the pedicle is removed by a rongeur to make a 6–8-mm-diameter opening in the cortex. The cancellous isthmus of the pedicle is directly visualized by removing the cancellous bone from the upper part of the pedicle with a small curette. After further removal of the cancellous bone, enlargement of the pedicle funnel leads the curette into the upper part of the pedicle isthmus. The cortical margins of the upper part of the pedicle then act as a funnel to permit safe insertion of the pedicle probe through the pedicle isthmus. Firstly, careful probing of the pedicle is then performed with the 2-mm probe, and then, if the pedicle inner diameter allows it, with the larger pedicle probe. At last, a ball-tip probe is used to inspect the depth of the opening as well as all four walls of the pedicle for a perforation (Fig. 2a).

The posterior parts of the pedicle were removed; inferior half of the lamina above was excised including the inferior articular process, and then, the superior articular process of the hemivertebra was excised (Fig. 2b). This was followed by excision of the inferior articular process of the hemivertebra and the superior articular process of the vertebra below. If in the thoracic spine, the rib head

was also removed. The spinal cord and the nerve roots were identified and protected, as well as the pleura. Epidural veins were cauterized by bipolar cautery to allow clear visualization. The remnants of the vertebral body of the hemivertebra and the adjacent disks were removed. The vertebral end plates of the convex side were debrided down to the bone, and the contralateral end plate was retained (Fig. 2c). The concave side was not exposed as continued spinal growth on this side will improve the correction in 40 patients. Subsequently, a pre-contoured rod was connected to the screws on the convex side. Gradual compression was applied until the gap was closed. Bones retrieved during osteotomy were used as graft material for fusion of the posterior elements. In cases with contralateral bar formation and multiple rib anomalies, unilateral exposure is not sufficient and bilateral exposure is necessary to cut off the bar or synostosed rib heads. Three cases involved a double hemivertebra or concave bar and multiple rib anomalies, which required extension of the fusion to more segments (Fig. 3). In one patient aged 2.8 years, no appropriately sized pedicle screw was available; therefore, 3.0-mm, cortical screws combined with wires were used as an alternative (Fig. 4). For lumbar or lumbosacral hemiveterbra, unilateral short-segment instrumentation combined with hemivertebra resection was also very applicable.

After surgery, all patients were fitted with a rigid brace to protect the instrumentation for at least 6 months.

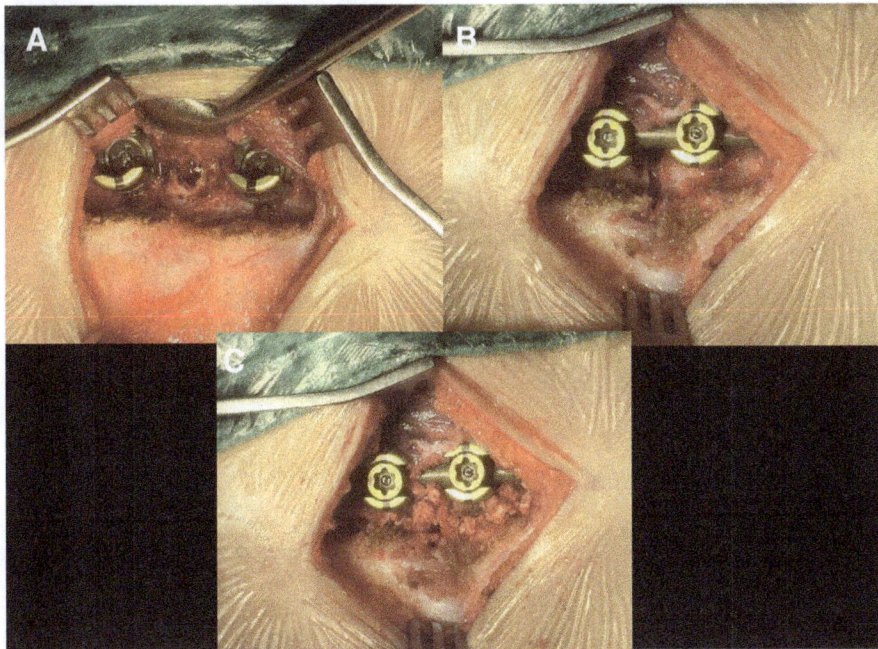

Fig. 2 Interoperation image: convex side only to expose the hemivertebra, and unilateral pedicle screws were inserted into the vertebra using the funnel technique (**a**). Hemivertebra resection: the vertebral end plates of the convex side were excised (**b**). Gradual compression until the gap was closed. Bone graft for fusion of the posterior elements (**c**)

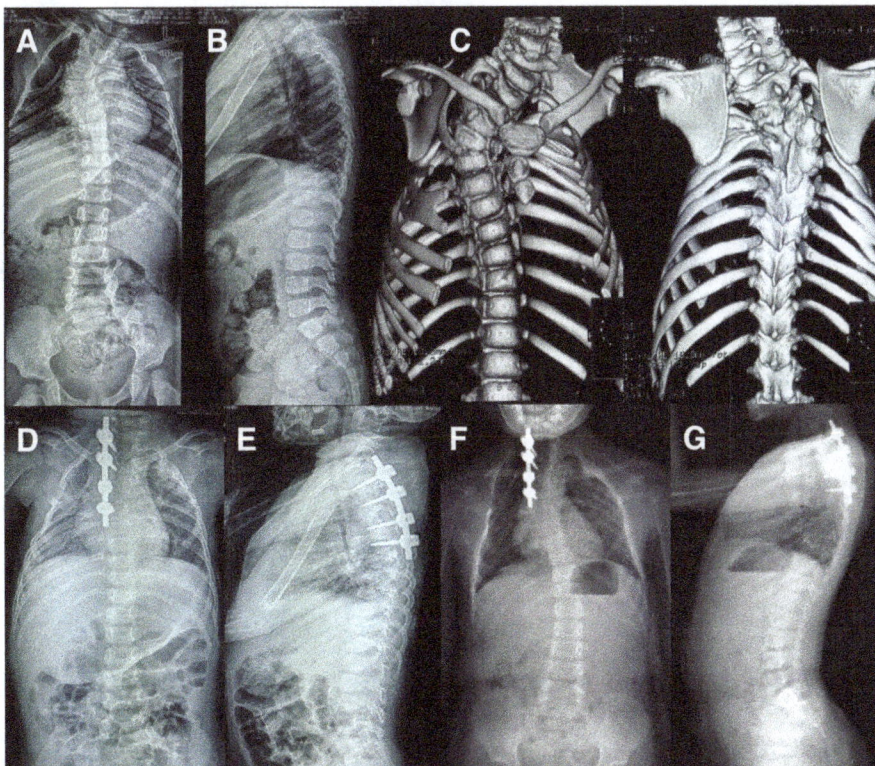

Fig. 3 A 2 years and 4 months old girl with congenital scoliosis. Radiographs and 3D-computed tomography images obtained preoperatively (**a**, **b**, **c**), postoperatively (**d**, **e**), and at the latest follow-up visit, 60 months later (**f**, **g**)

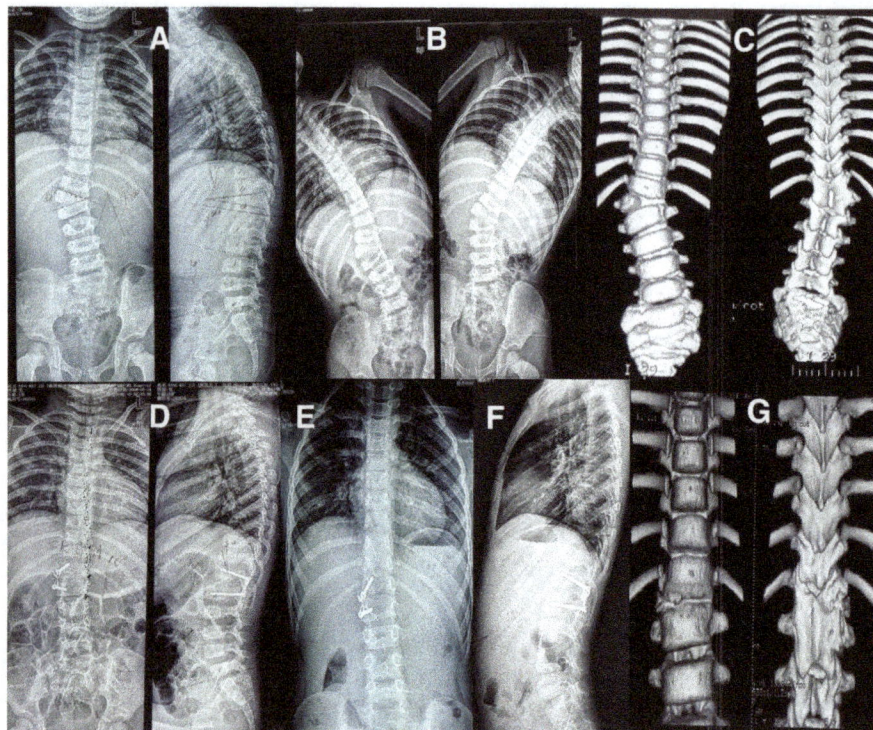

Fig. 4 A 2 years 9 months old girl with T12 hemivertebra. Radiograph images and 3D-computed tomography images obtained preoperatively (**a–c**), postoperatively (**d**), and at the latest follow-up visit, 69 months later (**e**, **f**, **g**)

Statistics

Paired *t* test was used to analyze the difference of coronal curve angle, thoracic kyphosis, segmental kyphosis, T1-S1 height, fusion segment height, and concave height at preoperation, postoperation, and final follow-up. SPSS version 17.0 (SPSS Inc., Chicago, IL) was used in all statistical analyses. The differences with a *P* value less than 0.05 were considered as statistically significant.

Results

Of the 43 patients, 10 had rib anomalies, 3 had concave unsegmented bar, 1 had congenital cardiac anomalies,

and 6 had intraspinal anomalies. No intraoperative complications were noticed. There were no neurologic complications. No implant failure was found at the final radiographic evaluations. Four patients experienced reoperation, and the overall rate of reoperation was 9.3%; demographic data are summarized in Table 1. The reasons of reoperation included two proximal junctional kyphosis (Fig. 5) and two curve progressions in the distal junction. In total, the average follow-up period was 73.88 ± 16.77 months (range, 60 to 112 months). Average age of the patients at surgery was 6 years and 7 months (range, 2 to 10 years).

Table 1 Patients' demographic data in revision surgery

Patients	Sex	Age	Abnormality	Association anomalies	Revision reason	Initial surgery	Duration time (months)	Revision surgery	Final F/U (months)
1	M	8	HV:T5; Unsegment T3–7	Sprengel deformity	PJK	T5 HV resection with T4–7 convex fusion	11	T2 PSO with T1–3 convex fusion	112
2	M	2	HV:T12	–	PJK due to T11 pedicle fracture	T12 HV resection with T10-L2 convex fusion	12	T11 Y-shape osteotomy with T9-L2 convex fusion	45
3	F	7	HV:T6; Unsegment T5–9	Fused rib in concave (9–10)	Curve progression in distal junction	T6 HV resection with T5–7 convex fusion	27	T7 PSO with T5–10 convex fusion	80
4	M	5	HV:T6; BF:T10; Unsegment L2–3	–	Curve progression	T6 HV resection with T3–9 convex fusion	78	Bilateral fusion from T3 to L3	90

F female, *M* male, *HV* hemivertebra, *BF* butterfly vertebra

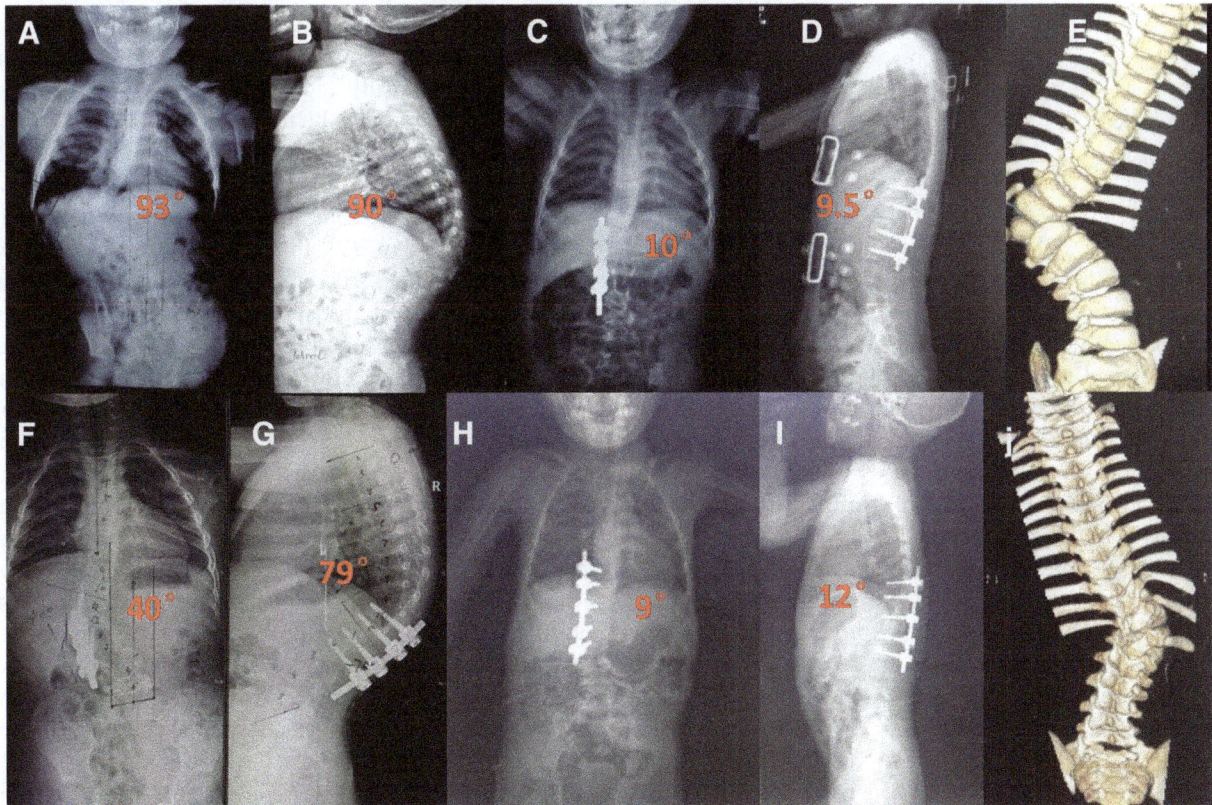

Fig. 5 A 2.5-year-old boy with T12 hemivertebra. Radiograph images and 3D-computed tomography images obtained preoperatively (**a**, **b**, **e**, **j**), postoperatively (**c**, **d**), and at the latest follow-up visit, 12 months later (**f**, **g**) and revision surgery (**h**, **i**)

There were no major vascular or neurological complications.

When all the patients were evaluated together, the average coronal curve magnitude was 46.1 ± 19.6° (range, 21 to 93°) preoperatively, 8.1 ± 9.6° (range, 0 to 37°) immediate postoperatively, and 11.7 ± 12.2° (3 to 49°) at last follow-up. The difference between the preoperative and early postoperative main curve Cobb angle measurements was significant (P = 0.000). At the latest follow-up, there was 7.8% (3.6°) loss of correction. The global thoracic kyphosis was 35.5 ± 21.7° (range, 18 to 72°) preoperatively, 34.9 ± 7.7° (15 to 41.5°) immediate postoperatively, and 37.6 ± 7.5° (19 to 44°) at last follow-up. The segmental kyphosis was 23.3 ± 27.2° (3 to 90°) preoperatively, 10.1 ± 3.1° (9 to 15°) immediate postoperatively, and 7.4 ± 7.2° (1 to 22°) at the last follow-up assessment resulting in a mean improvement of 13.2° postoperatively, and this improvement continued at the latest follow-up with a mean increase of 2.7°(Table 2).

The average concave height was 60.1 ± 19.7 mm in the immediate postoperative period and 73.1 ± 23.7 mm at last follow-up. There was a significant difference between immediate postoperative and at last follow-up measurements (P = 0.003). The average fusion segment height was 56.9 ± 22.9 mm in the immediate postoperative period and 71.2 ± 22.0 mm at last follow-up (P = 0.002). The average T1-S1 height was 326.6 ± 64.5 mm in the immediate postoperative period and 388.7 ± 78.9 mm at last follow-up (P = 0.001) (Table 3). The average fusion segment was 2.9 ± 1.8 levels (2–6 levels).

Discussion

The natural history of congenital scoliosis is still unknown. There is no treatment algorithm because of the variability of surgical solutions. The coronal and sagittal deformities, as well as the patient age and type and location of the anomaly, should be taken into consideration. As the most frequent cause of congenital scoliosis, most untreated fully segmented and semi-segmented non-

Table 2 Summary of radiographic parameters preoperatively and postoperatively

	Preoperation	Postoperation	P value
Coronal curve cobb(°)	46.1 ± 19.6	8.1 ± 9.6	0.000
Thoracic kyphosis(°)	35.5 ± 21.7	34.9 ± 7.7	0.951
Segmental kyphosis(°)	23.3 ± 27.2	10.1 ± 3.1	0.007
T1-S1 height(mm)	322.9 ± 63.4	356.9 ± 60.3	0.088

Table 3 Summary of radiographic parameters postoperatively and at the last follow-up

	Postoperation	Last follow-up	P value
Coronal curve cobb(°)	8.1 ± 9.6	11.7 ± 12.2	0.031
Thoracic kyphosis(°)	36.7 ± 8.3	37.6 ± 7.5	0.523
Segmental kyphosis(°)	10.1 ± 3.1	7.4 ± 7.2	0.346
T1-S1 height (mm)	326.6 ± 64.5	388.7 ± 78.9	0.001
Concave height (mm)	60.1 ± 19.7	73.1 ± 23.7	0.003
Fusion segment height (mm)	56.9 ± 22.9	71.2 ± 22.0	0.002

incarcerated hemivertebra will progress and create a wedge-shaped deformity during the spinal growth period [10]. In this situation, the conditions of most patients cannot be controlled with nonsurgical treatments like wearing orthosis. Thereby, most spine surgeon had reached a consensus on surgical treatment for congenital scoliosis due to hemivertebra.

At present, the recommended surgical options mainly include in situ fusion, convex growth arrest, and hemivertebra excision via a combined anterior and posterior approach in one or two stages [2, 11–13]. Currently, the one-stage posterior hemivertebra resection combined with bilateral transpedicular screw instrumentation has become the commonly adopted procedure for the correction of congenital scoliosis. The use of pedicle screws is a powerful method which allows excellent deformity correction in the coronal and sagittal planes, and is safe, even in very young children [10]. The pedicle screw instrumentation can effectively transmit the correction torque to the anterior and middle columns of the spine, increasing the compressive resistance of the anterior and middle columns [14]. Thereby, it helps retard the growth of vertebrae and prevents the crankshaft phenomenon.

Despite the major improvements in the treatment of congenital scoliosis due to hemivertebra, described, simple, and less-invasive methods were more acceptable and popular. The posterior unilateral transpedicular screw fixation could be an advisable alternative to further minimize the trauma in children and decrease the growth arrest of the concave side. Moreover, short-segment fusion can be performed to preserve more growing segments and motor units. Most of the concave pedicle was anomaly and tiny in malformed vertebra; thus, pedicle screw placement is very difficult, having to extend the instrument segment if bilateral transpedicular screw fixation was selected.

In the present study, the mean correction rates of the segmental curve and segmental kyphosis were 82.4% and 56.2%, respectively. Deformities were satisfactorily corrected, and there were no significant losses during the follow-up, suggesting that unilateral transpedicular fixation can provide sufficient force for correction in children. These correction rates are in accordance with previous reports of posterior bilateral fixation describing

similar case series [13, 15]. For these patients with scoliosis progression in follow-up, including two curve progression in the proximal junction and two cases in the distal junction, insufficient fusion levels and complex congenital scoliosis may be the main cause.

Unilateral short-segment fixation requires pedicle screw strength. Pedicle fracture, which requires revision surgery, is the most common complication reported in previous studies [16, 17]. In our series, only one patient experienced pedicle fracture that was revised. The patient with severe kyphoscoliosis due to T12 hemivertebrea shows proximal junction kyphosis in 7 months after initial hemivertebrectomy and unilateral fusion. The rigid curve, poor flexibility for kyphoscoliosis, and poor adherence for brace may be the cause. Many studies have confirmed that pedicle fractures are related to the surgical technique rather than to the weakness of the pedicle [15]. Therefore, we adopted the funnel technique in all cases to guarantee accuracy of the pedicle screw placement. Most important of all, the use of a brace post operation is very necessary, not only to protect the instrumentation, but also to maintain further correction. We recommend the minimum 6-month duration of brace use, even after the bone fusion is complete.

The safety of the pedicle screws in the pediatric spine and their effect on vertebral growth have been the topic of controversy in the literature, as some experimental studies have shown growth retardation secondary to pedicle screw instrumentation in immature animals [18, 19]. However, prior clinical studies have shown no growth-retardation effect of the pedicle screws in the pediatric spine [20]. A recent study by Xue et al. has also observed no negative effects of the pedicle screw instrumentation on vertebral bodies' growth. No spinal stenosis existed in an average of 7 years after instrumentation on CT axial images. In their study, 35 patients less than 7 years were consisted undergoing pedicle screw instrumentation [21].

The limitation of this study was that it is a retrospectively reviewed study with a small number of patients included; more patients are needed in the future. The other drawback was that all patients have been followed-up for at least 60 months, which are very young and far from mature bone; thus, continuous follow-up is needed in the future. In addition, this study does not contain results about life quality in the follow-up. Further trials about life quality, especially spinal mobilization and mental health status, are needed to be evaluated in the future.

Conclusions

Despite having some complications, posterior hemivertebrectomy and unilateral instrumented fusion are commendable procedures for early correction in young children. The safety and efficacy of the correction were proved by radiographic measurements. The growth of the non-fused concave side of the spine was observed. We concluded that it is a simple, secure, reliable, less-invasive, and well-tolerated technique that can successfully resolve this kind of congenital scoliosis in children.

Abbreviations
CGA: Convex growth arrest; LIV: Lowest instrumented vertebra; PJK: Proximal junction kyphosis; MRI: Magnetic resonance imaging; SPSS: Statistic Package for Social Science; CT: Computed tomography; UIV: Upper instrumented vertebra

Acknowledgements
Many thanks are given to our center colleagues and the devotion of the patients.

Funding
This work is supported by the National Natural Science Foundation of China (no. 81702212).

Authors' contributions
XXH and ZS conceived and designed the study. XXH measured and recorded the data. XXH and ZS wrote the paper. ZS reviewed and edited the manuscript. Both authors read and approved the final manuscript.

Competing interests
The authors declare that they have no competing interests.

References
1. McMaster MJ, Ohtsuka K. The natural history of congenital scoliosis. A study of two hundred and fifty-one patients. J Bone Joint Surg Am. 1982;64:1128–47.
2. Winter RB, Moe JH, Eilers VE. Congenital scoliosis. A study of 234 patients treated and untreated. Part I: natural history. J Bone Joint Surg Am. 1968;50:1–15.
3. Kose KC, Inanmaz ME, Altinel L, Bal E, Caliskan I, Isik C, et al. Convex short segment instrumentation and hemi-chevron osteotomies for Putti type 1 thoracic hemivertebrae: a simple treatment option for patients under 5 years old. J Spinal Disord Tech. 2013;26(6):E240–7.
4. Ruf M, Harms J. Posterior hemivertebra resection with transpedicular instrumentation: early correction in children aged 1-6 years. Spine. 2003;28:2132–8.
5. Chu G, Huang J, Zeng K, Guo Q, Zhang H. A modified surgical procedure for congenital kyphoscoliosis: selective partial hemivertebrectomy via posterior-only approach. Childs Nerv Syst. 2015;31(6):923–9.
6. Andrew T, Piggot H. Growth arrest for progressive scoliosis: combined anterior and posterior fusion of the convexity. J Bone Joint Surg Br. 1985;67:193–7.
7. Uzumcugil A, Cil A, Yazici M, Acaroglu E, Alanay A, Aksoy C, et al. Convex growth arrest in the treatment of congenital spinal deformities: revisited. J Pediatr Otrhop. 2004;24:658–66.
8. Demirkiran G, Yilmaz G, Kaymaz B, Akel I, Ayvaz M, Acaroglu E, et al. Safety and efficacy of instrumented convex growth arrest in treatment of congenital scoliosis. J Pediatr Orthop. 2014;34(3):275–81.
9. Viau M, Tarbox BB, Wonglertsiri S, Karaikovic EE, Yingsakmongkol W, Gaines RW. Thoracic pedicle screw instrumentation using the "Funnel Technique": part 2. Clinical experience. J Spinal Disord Tech. 2002;15(6):450–3.
10. Ruf M, Harms J. Hemivertebra resection by a posterior approach: innovative operative technique and first results. Spine. 2002;27:1116–23.
11. Callahan BC, Georgopoulos G, Eilert RE. Hemivertebral excision for congenital scoliosis. J Pediatr Orthop. 1997;17:96–9.
12. Holte DC, Winter RB, Lonstein JE, Denis F. Excision of hemivertebrae and wedge resection in the treatment of congenital scoliosis. J Bone Joint Surg Am. 1995;77:159–71.
13. Chang DG, Kim JH, Ha KY, Lee JS, Jang JS, Suk SI. Posterior hemivertebra resection and short segment fusion with pedicle screw fixation for congenital scoliosis in children younger than 10 years: greater than 7-year follow-up. Spine. 2015;40(8):E484–91.
14. Burton DC, Asher MA, Lai SM. Scoliosis correction maintenance in skeletally immature patients with idiopathic scoliosis. Is anterior fusion really necessary? Spine. 2000;25(1):61–8.
15. Zhang J, Shengru W, Qiu G, Yu B, Yipeng W, Luk KD. The efficacy and complications of posterior hemivertebra resection. Eur Spine J. 2011; 20:1692–702.
16. Hicks JM, Singla A, Shen FH, Arlet V. Complications of pedicle screw fixation in scoliosis surgery: a systematic review. Spine. 2010;35(11):E465–70.
17. Di Silvestre M, Parisini P, Lolli F, Bakaloudis G. Complications of thoracic pedicle screws in scoliosis treatment. Spine. 2007;32(15):1655–61.
18. Cil A, Yazici M, Daglioglu K, Aydingoz U, Alanay A, Acaroglu RE, et al. The effect of pedicle screw placement with or without application of compression across the neurocentral cartilage on the morphology of the spinal canal and pedicle in immature pigs. Spine. 2005;30(11):1287–93.
19. Fekete TF, Kleinstück FS, Mannion AF, Kendik ZS, Jeszenszky DJ. Prospective study of the effect of pedicle screw placement on development of the immature vertebra in an in vivo porcine model. Eur Spine J. 2011;20(11):1892–8.
20. Olgun ZD, Demirkiran G, Ayvaz M, Karadeniz E, Yazici M. The effect of pedicle screw insertion at a young age on pedicle and canal development. Spine. 2012;37:1778–84.
21. Xue X, Shen J, Zhang J, Li S, Wang Y, Qiu G. X-ray assessment of the effect of pedicle screw on vertebra and spinal canal growth in children before the age of 7 years. Eur Spine J. 2014;23(3):520–9.

27

Combined detection of COMP and CS846 biomarkers in experimental rat osteoarthritis: a potential approach for assessment and diagnosis of osteoarthritis

Tianwen Ma, Zhiheng Zhang, Xiaopeng Song, Hui Bai, Yue Li, Xinran Li, Jinghua Zhao, Yuanqiang Ma and Li Gao[*]

Abstract

Background: To comprehensively evaluate the diagnostic value of serum cartilage oligomeric matrix protein (COMP) and chondroitin sulfate 846 epitope (CS846) biomarkers in osteoarthritis (OA), longitudinal and combined measurement of serum COMP and CS846 were performed at different stages in the pathological process of OA in a rat model of anterior cruciate ligament transection (ACLT).

Methods: Sixty male Sprague-Dawley rats were randomly divided into two groups, including a model group ($n = 30$) and a control group ($n = 30$). Rat models were established by ACLT surgery, and sham operations were performed on rats in the control group. Prior to surgery and at 2, 4, 6, 8, and 10 weeks after ACLT surgery, serum levels of COMP and CS846 biomarkers were determined using an enzyme-linked immunosorbent assay approach. Five rats per group were euthanized at 2, 4, 6, 8, and 10 weeks after surgery, after which tibial plateau specimens were collected. Macroscopic observation and histological examination were employed for rat tibial plateau. Histological changes in articular cartilage were evaluated according to Osteoarthritis Research Society International (OARSI) scoring criteria. The area under the curve (AUC) of COMP, CS846, and combined biomarkers was compared using receiver operating characteristic (ROC) curve.

Results: Within 10 weeks after surgery, serum levels of COMP and CS846 in the model group were significantly higher when compared to those in the control group. Moreover, a significant correlation was observed between changes in COMP and CS846 levels. At each time point, macroscopic observations and OARSI scores were significantly increased in the development of OA. The AUC of combined biomarkers was higher compared to that of COMP and CS846 alone. Finally, a positive relationship was found between levels of COMP and CS846 and the OARSI score.

Conclusions: In this study, we found that combined detection of serum CS846 and COMP levels can be used for diagnosis and monitoring of OA progression.

Keywords: Osteoarthritis, COMP, CS846, Serum, Biomarkers

* Correspondence: gaoli43450@163.com
Heilongjiang Key Laboratory for Laboratory Animals and Comparative Medicine, College of Veterinary Medicine, Northeast Agricultural University, Harbin 150030, China

Background

Osteoarthritis (OA) is a progressive degenerative joint condition that is estimated to affect over 250 million individuals worldwide [1]. Currently, there is no effective cure to treat OA [2]. Presently, the diagnosis of OA is based on clinical symptoms and traditional radiology. Magnetic resonance imaging (MRI) not only assesses changes in cartilage during OA development, but also assesses joint tissue damage. However, due to financial constraints and the lack of an internationally validated assessment scale, the use of MRI in the routine diagnosis of OA is limited [3], and X-rays remain the routine diagnostic method. Although the accuracy and sensitivity of these approaches are relatively high, these methods fail to distinctively identify the developmental stages of OA. Similarly, most of the current OA treatments are largely palliative until the articular cartilage has been severely damaged; during the development of OA, the joints become completely dysfunctional and prosthetic replacement becomes necessary [4]. Therefore, an effective method for early diagnosis of OA is imperative, and early changes in OA may be reversed by effective therapeutic drugs.

OA is often not detected until the middle or end stage [5–7]. In recent years, OA biomarkers have received increased attention as an objective indicator for early diagnosis of OA and for assessment of the disease process [8]. OA biomarkers can be detected at an early stage of OA, prior to the presence of radiographic signs. Cartilage oligomeric matrix protein (COMP) is a non-collagenous component of cartilage, which accounts for roughly 1% of the wet weight of articular tissue [9]. COMP promotes the combination of type II collagen fibers and stable fiber networks. Chondroitin sulfate (CS) is a glycosaminoglycan (GAG) that is covalently attached to specific proteins to form proteoglycans, which are abundant components of the extracellular matrix (ECM) [10]. CS 846 epitope (CS846) is a CS synthetic marker and inseparable from the degree of joint injury in patients with OA. CS846 is a by-product of proteoglycan metabolism and has been detected in serum and synovial fluid (SF) [11]. Therefore, CS846 and COMP as sensitive and specific biomarkers reflecting degradation of cartilage and synovial tissues have increasingly been used as helpful promising tools in early OA diagnosis before irreversible damage has occurred.

However, in many studies of early OA diagnosis, only one biomarker in the pathological process of OA was measured at a single time point [12, 13]. In verifying our hypothesis that COMP and CS846 can be used as a joint biomarker for knee OA, a longitudinal study of the combined measurement of serum levels of COMP and CS846 was performed using an anterior cruciate ligament transection (ACLT) rat models in which the relationship between COMP and CS846 levels and the degradation of articular cartilage were evaluated. The area under the curve (AUC) of COMP, CS846, and combined biomarkers in the evaluation and diagnosis of osteoarthritis was analyzed by ROC curve analysis. When promising, combined biomarkers that were identified for clinical use may have a beneficial effect on both patient health and the medical economy.

Methods

Animals

A total of 60 male Sprague-Dawley rats (11–12 weeks old, 300–350 g) were purchased from the Animal Experimental Center of the Second Affiliated Hospital of the Harbin Medical University (Harbin, China) and housed in a controlled environment (light/dark, 12/12 h; temperature 23 ± 1 °C). Rats had access to water and food ad libitum. Ethical treatment of animals in this study was approved by the Animal Welfare Committee protocol (#NEAU-2017-02-0252-11) at Northeast Agricultural University (Harbin, China). All efforts were made to minimize animal suffering and to reduce the number of animals used.

Surgically induced osteoarthritis in rats

Prior to use, animals were acclimated for 1 week. Then, rats were randomly assigned to the model group ($n = 30$) or control group ($n = 30$). Rats in the model group were anesthetized by inhalation of 2% isoflurane (catalog no. C008170801, Yipin Pharm-hebei, China) in oxygen/nitrous oxide, and the right knee was shaved and scrubbed to prepare for surgery. Rats underwent ACLT via an incision on the medial aspect of the right knee joint capsule, anterior to the medial collateral ligament. The anterior cruciate ligament (ACL) was transected using a microsurgical knife using a surgical microscope (Corder Optics ad electronics Co., Ltd., Chengdu, China). After irrigation with saline to remove tissue debris, the patella was relocated. Next, a positive anterior drawer test was performed to ensure complete transection of the ligament. The wound was closed with braided, absorbable polyglycolide absorbable suture 6/0 (Jinhuan Medical Products Co., Ltd., Shanghai, China). During surgery, close attention was paid not to damage the articular cartilage. No surgery was performed on the left hind knee. After surgery, rats were allowed to walk freely. Rats were administered intramuscular injections of penicillin (400,000 units) once daily for three consecutive days. Rats in the control group were sham-operated using the same approach but without any ligament transection or meniscectomy.

Sample collection and storage

In this study, right knee joints and serum were harvested at 0, 2, 4, 6, 8, and 10 weeks after surgery ($n = 5$ rats per group). Animals were euthanized using an overdose of diethyl ether, and right knee joints were collected. Blood samples were obtained from the orbital vein, and serum was collected in Eppendorf tubes without additives. Next, blood was centrifuged at 1000×g for 20 min at room temperature. Supernatant was collected and stored at − 80 °C until future analysis.

Macroscopic observation

For macroscopic observation, rat tibial plateaus were collected. Cartilage degradation on the surface of tibial plateau was evaluated using a dissecting microscope, and the degree of degradation was graded on a scale of 0–4 as follows: 0 = surface smooth with normal color; 1 = surface rough with minimal fibrillation or a slight yellowish color; 2 = cartilage erosion extending into superficial or middle layers; 3 = cartilage ulceration extending into deeper layers; and 4 = cartilage depletion with subchondral bone exposed [14]. Macroscopic observations were conducted by an observer who was blinded to the groups.

Safranin O staining, OARSI score, and histopathological evaluation

Safranin O is a basic stain that binds proteoglycans present in cartilage with a high affinity [15]. In brief, knee joints from rats were fixed for 72 h in 10% buffered formalin and decalcified for 3 weeks in 10% EDTA solution at 4 °C. Then, joints were embedded in paraffin blocks and cut into 5-μm-thick sections. Subsequently, knee joints were stained with Safranin O to evaluate cartilage destruction, which was graded using the Osteoarthritis Research Society International (OARSI) scoring system for medial tibial plateaus [16]. OARSI scores were graded on a scale of 0–6. All sections were stained in a single batch, and two experienced observers, who were blinded to the study, performed the scoring.

COMP and CS846 biomarker analysis

Serum levels of COMP and CS846 of the rats in each group were determined using a sandwich enzyme-linked immunosorbent assay (ELISA) (catalog nos. EHJ-96099r and EHJ-96089r, Huijia Biological Technology Co., Ltd., Amoy, China). ELISA was performed according to the manufacturer's instructions. A linear regression curve was drawn using the standards provided with the kit and was used to calculate the COMP and CS846 concentrations in each sample. All analyses were performed by the Heilongjiang Key Laboratory for Laboratory Animals and Comparative Medicine in Harbin.

Statistics

SPSS software (version 19.0 for Windows, SPSS, Chicago, IL, USA) was used for all statistical analyses. Values are expressed as the mean ± SD. One-way analysis of variance (ANOVA) analysis was used for statistical comparisons between multiple groups. Correlations were analyzed using Spearman's rank correlation analyses. AUC of the receiver operating characteristic (ROC) curve was used to assess the predictive value of COMP, CS846, and the combination thereof for OA. Multivariate regression analysis was employed to establish the diagnostic mathematical model. Based on this model, the prediction value was calculated, followed by ROC curve analysis. $P < 0.05$ was considered statistically significant.

Results

Macroscopic observation

In the model group, all knees demonstrated cartilage degenerative changes of varied degrees (Fig. 1). Cartilage on the tibial plateau in the control group appeared macroscopically normal with a smooth surface, and no cartilage defects or osteophytes were observed (Fig. 1a). With the development of OA, the degree of articular surface ulceration in rats was increased and was gradually accompanied with a loss of luster. Two weeks after induction of OA, the joint surface had a slightly rough appearance (Fig. 1b). In addition, 4 weeks after induction of OA (Fig. 1c), the cartilage surface of ACLT rats was rough and uneven, the joint surface was dull, and local ulcers were formed. At 6 weeks after induction of OA, the middle layer of articular cartilage was eroded (Fig. 1d). Moreover, the articular cartilage surface was dark red in color and was severely damaged at 8 and 10 weeks after OA induction (Fig. 1e, f). In addition, the ulcerated area was increased, and the lower part of the cartilage was exposed. Accordingly, macroscopic observation (Fig. 2) showed that OA-related cartilage degradation increased with time after ACLT surgery. At each time point, the macroscopic observation scores in the model group were significantly higher when compared to those in the control group ($P < 0.05$).

Histological analysis

Figure 3 presents representative images of safranin O-stained rat joint tissues at 2, 4, 6, 8, and 10 weeks after ACLT surgery. In the control group, the articular surface was smooth, safranin O was evenly distributed, and chondrocytes were arranged in a regular manner (Fig. 3a). The different stages of OA in the model group showed different degrees of articular cartilage pathology. Two weeks after induction of OA, the surface of articular cartilage was partially rough, the matrix was intact, and chondrocytes in the superficial zone were arranged unevenly (Fig. 3b). At 4 weeks after surgery, the surface of articular cartilage was rough, staining intensity of the matrix was reduced, chondrocytes in the middle area were disordered, and chondrocytes were enlarged in size (Fig. 3c). In addition, at 6 weeks after surgery, surface

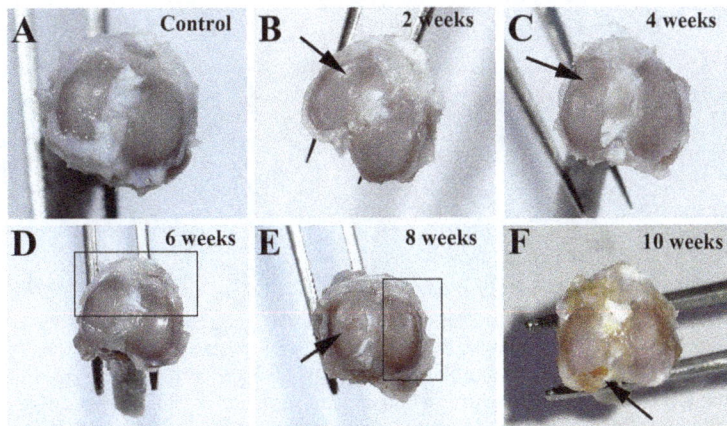

Fig. 1 Macroscopic observation of tibial plateau. **a** Tibial plateau of rats in the control group showed a smooth cartilage surface, and no cartilage defects or osteophytes. **b** After 2 weeks of surgery, the joint surface was slightly rough (arrow). **c** The joint surface was partially recessed at 4 weeks of after surgery (arrow). **d** The joint surface was rough and matte at 6 weeks of after surgery (rectangle frame). **e** The articular cartilage was severely damaged at 8 weeks after surgery (rectangle frame). **f** The joint surface showed a large area of ulcers, and subchondral bone was exposed at 10 weeks after surgery (arrow)

irregularity, a decrease in safranin O staining, and disordered chondrocytes were observed (Fig. 3d). Knee joints from rats in the model group at 8 weeks after OA induction showed chondrocyte death, loss of the intercellular matrix, and thinning or destruction of the cartilage layer (Fig. 3e). Additionally, the matrix showed a loss of staining, and an unequivocal dissipation of chondrocytes was observed at the lesion area at 10 weeks after surgery (Fig. 3f). The OARSI scores of rats in the model group increased with the progression of OA. The OARSI score for cartilage degeneration showed a significant higher score in rats in the model group when compared to rats in the control groups ($P < 0.05$) (Fig. 4).

COMP and CS846 levels

The concentration of COMP and CS846 in knee joints of rats of the control and model groups at various time points are summarized in Fig. 5a, b. The levels of COMP and CS846 continuously increased over 10 weeks after ACLT surgery (COMP standard linear regression curve $r^2 = 0.99106$; CS846 standard linear regression curve $r^2 = 0.99350$). Compared with the control joint, COMP and CS846 levels significantly increased from the second to the tenth week after OA induction ($P < 0.05$). In addition, a positive correlation was observed between serum COMP levels and serum CS846 levels ($r = 0.879$, $P < 0.001$) (Fig. 6).

Correlation between COMP and CS846 concentration and the OARSI score

A positive correlation was observed between changes in rat serum COMP levels and corresponding articular cartilage OARSI scores ($r = 0.915$, $P < 0.001$) (Fig. 7). In addition, a positive correlation was observed between changes in rat serum CS846 levels and corresponding articular cartilage OARSI scores ($r = 0.912$, $P < 0.001$) (Fig. 8).

ROC curve analysis of single and combined biomarkers

The ROC curve diagram showed that the area of COMP, CS846 and the combination thereof were > 0.5 (above the reference line), respectively, indicating that both single detection and combined detection were important for the diagnosis of OA (Fig. 9). Among them, the AUC of serum COMP, CS846, and combined biomarkers was 0.851, 0.868, and 0.926, respectively. Among all, the combined biomarkers yielded an ROC value, which was significantly higher when compared to that of single

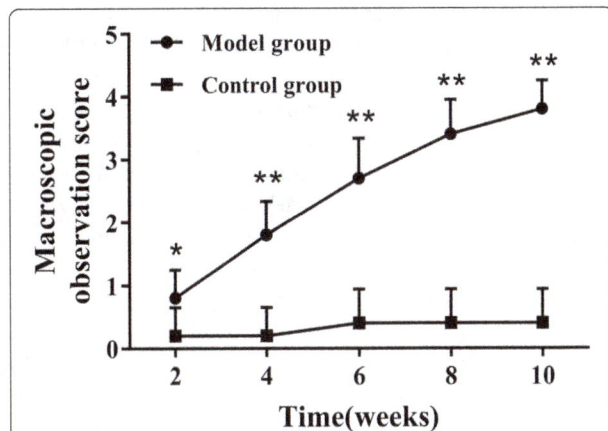

Fig. 2 Macroscopic observation score of tibial plateau of rats in the model and control groups at various time points. Data are shown as the mean ± standard error of the mean. *$P < 0.05$ or **$P < 0.01$ compared with the control group

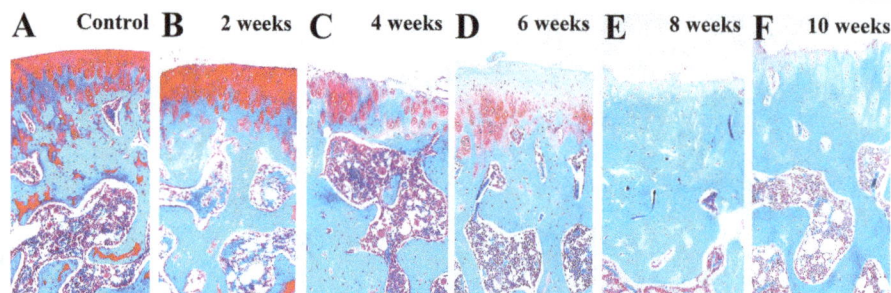

Fig. 3 Representative safranin O-stained sections of articular cartilage. **a** In the control group, the cartilage surface was smooth and safranin O staining was uniform. **b** At 2 weeks after surgery, chondrocytes arranged at the surface area were uneven and the matrix was intact. **c** At 4 weeks after surgery, the intensity of proteoglycan staining decreased, whereas that of chondrocytes increased. **d** Irregular cartilage surface and chondrocyte disturbance were observed at 6 weeks after surgery. **e** Chondrocyte death and proteoglycan loss were observed at 8 weeks after surgery. **f** The extracellular matrix showed a loss in staining intensity; unequivocal dissipation of chondrocytes were observed at the lesion area at 10 weeks after surgery. Magnification × 10

biomarkers ($P < 0.05$) and would be ideal for the diagnosis of OA.

Discussion

In this study, we combined the expression of serum levels of COMP and CS846 in OA rats to provide a reference for early diagnostic criteria of OA. A sensitive and stable biochemical indicator was established. In the past few years, the importance of serum biomarkers in OA, synovitis, joint effusion, and the progression of cartilage damage has become increasingly appreciated and has been proven helpful for monitoring disease progression and clinical therapy [1, 17]. However, studies focusing on the magnitude and timing of the effects of OA on serum marker levels are limited. To our knowledge, this is the first study in which the value of combined detection of serum levels of CS846 and COMP was evaluated

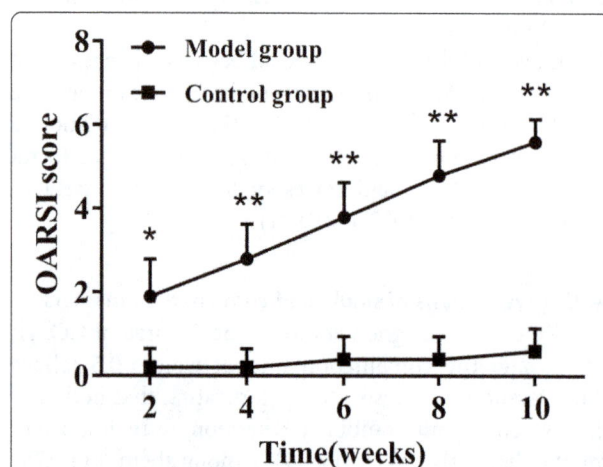

Fig. 4 OARSI score of articular cartilage of rats in model and control groups at various time points. Data are shown as the mean ± standard error of the mean. *$P < 0.05$ or **$P < 0.01$ compared with rats in the control group

in early OA diagnosis. In addition, the ACLT model, in which permanent instability in the articular cartilage knee joint occurs, is a frequently used and well-accepted OA model [15, 18]. Thus, the rat OA model used in this study is an excellent translational model for estimating intra-articular inflammation with outcomes that are relevant to human OA [19].

Articular cartilage is composed of hyaline cartilage, which is composed of an abundant ECM and chondrocytes embedded therein, and with mechanical properties [2]. Degradation of the network of collagen and proteoglycans in OA cartilage leads to a loss in tensile strength and shear properties of cartilage [20]. COMP is a tissue-specific protein that binds to the type II collagen network. When articular cartilage is destroyed, COMP is released into the SF and subsequently absorbed in the serum [21]. COMP has shown promising effects as a prognosticator of rapid joint destruction in humans with levels in both serum and SF being increased in patients with OA when compared to those without joint disease [22]. Interestingly, Geng et al. reported that COMP deficiency enhanced the early onset and development of chronic arthritis but does not affect collagen II autoimmunity [23]. In addition, in a study performed by Fernandes et al., it was suggested that COMP could be used as a diagnostic marker for early OA as shown by elevated serum COMP levels in patients with knee pain symptoms without any radiological abnormalities, thereby indicating early cartilage damage in patients when compared to healthy controls [24]. Moreover, in a study by Huebner et al., SF levels of keratin sulfate (KS) and COMP increased, which was coincident with histological OA, and correlated positively with the severity of histological damage in guinea pig [25]. In our study, we showed that at 2 weeks after ACLT surgery, rats in the model group had significantly higher serum levels of COMP when compared to rats in the control group that

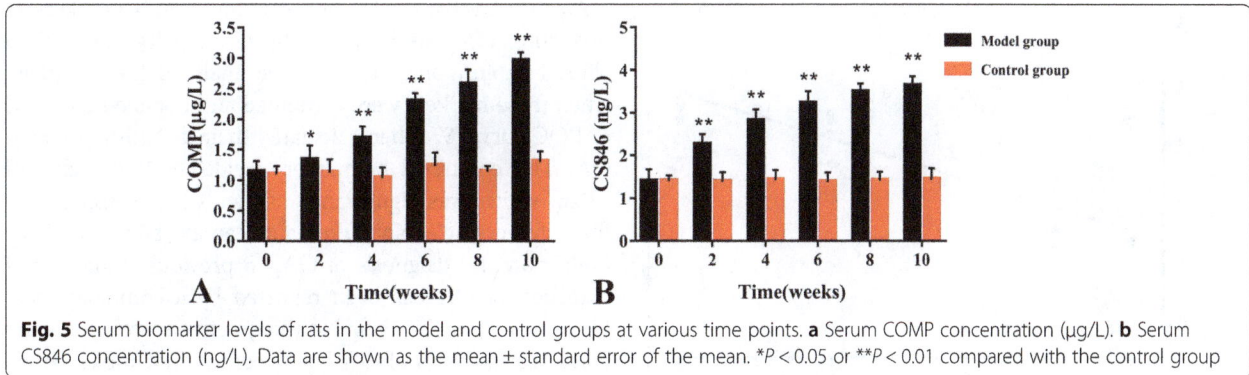

Fig. 5 Serum biomarker levels of rats in the model and control groups at various time points. **a** Serum COMP concentration (μg/L). **b** Serum CS846 concentration (ng/L). Data are shown as the mean ± standard error of the mean. *$P < 0.05$ or **$P < 0.01$ compared with the control group

at 4 weeks after surgery, they started to rapidly increase. In addition, at other time points, serum COMP levels of rats in the OA group were also higher when compared to those in the control group. In a previous study, similar results were obtained in rabbits with ACLT-induced OA [26]. These results indicated that serum COMP levels in rats in the model group increased early in OA development and gradually increased within 10 weeks after ACLT surgery. The increased release of COMP into serum during early OA is likely due to series of catabolic events that occur in articular cartilage, resulting in a high turnover rate by chondrocytes to repair the cartilage matrix. This process first led to dismantling of the cartilage matrix and subsequently a net loss of tissue. This inference is supported by our histological results, which indicated minor damage in the articular cartilage in rats in the model group at week 2 after surgery. Similar results were obtained by Bin et al. [27]. Also, the increase in SF COMP levels correlated with the length of time post injury, suggesting that COMP may be a suitable marker for longitudinal studies to evaluate its role in joint healing [28]. Georgiev et al. observed higher serum COMP levels in knee OA patients when compared to controls, and COMP correlated positively with

Whole-Organ MRI Score, suggesting that COMP may reflect structural damage of the knee joint [29].

CS846 is a synthetic CS marker and inseparable from the degree of joint injury in patients with OA [10]. CS846 levels were found to be significantly increased in serum and SF of experimental equine OA models when compared to healthy controls, and levels further increased in response to exercise [30]. Levels of CS and CS846 were significantly increased in patients with juvenile idiopathic arthritis [31]. Previous studies have indicated that CS846 was almost absent from mature adult cartilage; however, CS846 is present at increased levels following OA [32, 33] and joint injury [34]. In a previous study, Svoboda et al. reported that changes in serum levels of CS846 from baseline to follow-up were significantly different between ACL-injured patients and uninjured controls [35]. In our study, we found that at all time points after surgery, serum levels of CS846 in rats in the model group were higher when compared to those in the control group. In addition, we found that CS846 serum levels increased significantly at 2 weeks after ACLT surgery. This may explain the degradation of proteoglycans observed in the early onset of OA. These

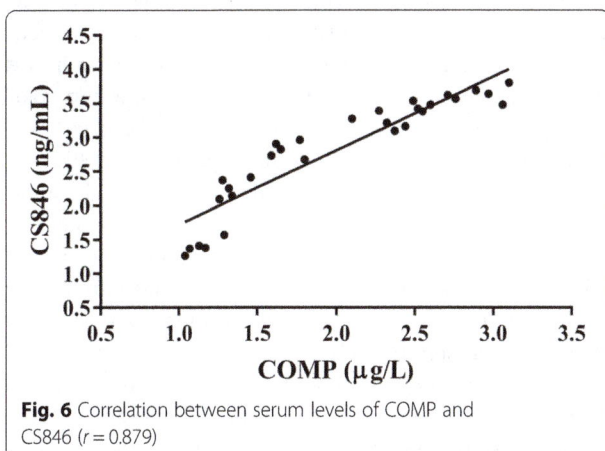

Fig. 6 Correlation between serum levels of COMP and CS846 ($r = 0.879$)

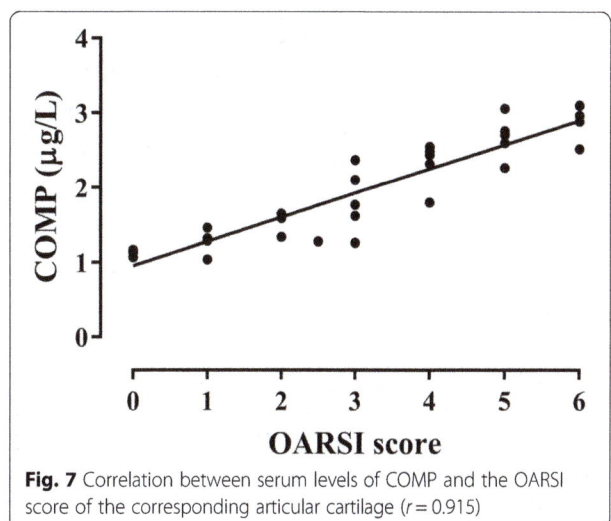

Fig. 7 Correlation between serum levels of COMP and the OARSI score of the corresponding articular cartilage ($r = 0.915$)

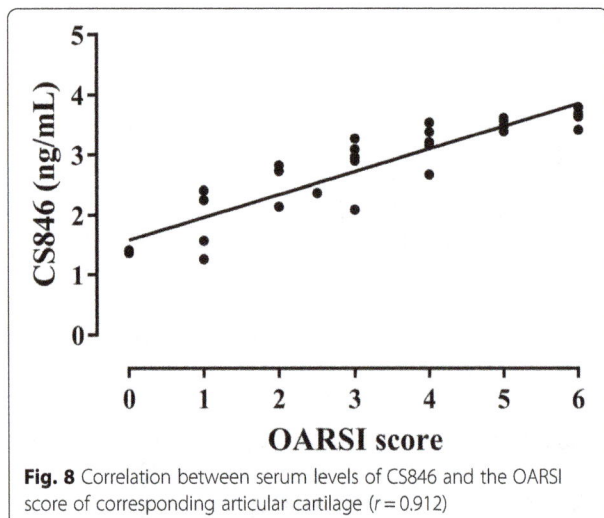

Fig. 8 Correlation between serum levels of CS846 and the OARSI score of corresponding articular cartilage ($r = 0.912$)

findings were supported by our macroscopic observation and histological results, indicating that there was minor damage of articular cartilage in the model group at 2 weeks after surgery. Nevertheless, in the present study, post injury changes in CS846 between ACL-injured cases and uninjured controls were comparable with those observed between OA patients and healthy controls as reported by Svoboda et al. [35]. In previous studies, it has been suggested that the combination of urinary CTX-II, serum COMP, and serum CS846 levels is indicative of the amount of joint damage in patients with hemophilic arthropathy [36]. Based on the data obtained from prior studies and ours, we hypothesized that CS846 can be used as an OA biomarker to assess the extent of articular cartilage damage. In addition, we found that serum levels of CS846 and COMP increased with the development of OA, and the peak value was not detected at 10 weeks after ACLT surgery.

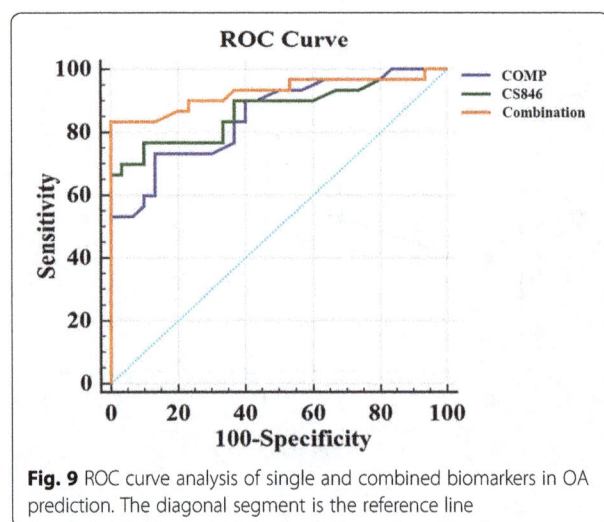

Fig. 9 ROC curve analysis of single and combined biomarkers in OA prediction. The diagonal segment is the reference line

As the sensitivity of a single serum OA biomarkers in predicting OA was low, thereby limiting its potential in clinical application. Therefore, we analyzed the sensitivity when these markers were combined and obtained the AUC of ROC curve. We then calculated their diagnostic value in OA. The combined biomarkers yielded a ROC value of 0.926, which was significantly higher when compared to that of the single biomarker and can be better used for evaluation and diagnosis of OA. In previous studies, early detection of OA has been reported by a combination of biomarkers [26, 27, 37]. Nowadays, the search for early diagnostic markers of OA has become a hot topic. To investigate the correlation between levels of COMP and CS846 and the severity of articular cartilage degeneration, histological changes in articular cartilage at various time points were evaluated based on the OARSI scoring system. In this study, the OARSI scores of rats in the model group were significantly higher regarding both OARSI scores and macroscopic observation scores when compared to the control group. There was a highly positive correlation between COMP and CS846 levels and the OARSI scores ($r = 0.915$, $r = 0.912$, $P < 0.001$). We found that the higher the levels of COMP and CS846 in the serum of ACLT rats, the more severe the degree of articular cartilage lesions. The correlation of COMP was higher compared to that of CS846. Histological examination showed that within 10 weeks after the induction of OA, the surface roughness of articular cartilage gradually increased and the chondrocytes first became hypertrophied and then decreased. In addition, chondrocyte disorganization gradually increased, the intensity of safranin O staining decreased, and the matrix gradually degraded. At 10 weeks after surgery, the stroma showed almost no staining, and clear dissociation of chondrocytes was observed in the lesion area. Histology showed that at 2 weeks after ACLT surgery, the joint surface was rough and after 4 weeks, the degree of joint unevenness was aggravated. Similarly, macroscopic observations also demonstrated that the articular surface was rough at 2 weeks after surgery, and depression appeared on the articular surface at 4 weeks after ACLT surgery, followed by gradual increase of joint surface ulceration and destruction. In the ACLT model used in this study, articular cartilage degeneration was a slow and gradual process, which was in accordance with the true histological processes of OA. These findings indicated that the OA model established in this study was successful. Moreover, we found a positive correlation between changes in levels of COMP and CS846 in rat serum over the course of 10 weeks. As a biomarker, the serum concentration of COMP can reflect the degree of denaturation of type II collagen, whereas serum levels of CS846 can reflect the degree of proteoglycan degradation [35]. Together, these results showed that the degradation of both collagen and proteoglycans resulted in loss of the ECM, thereby causing progressive degeneration of articular cartilage. Synovial hyperplasia, fibrosis, secretion of inflammatory mediators, and cartilage degrading enzymes can lead to acceleration of OA, which intensifies the degradation of proteoglycans and the presence of aggrecan fragments bearing the CS846 epitope. The destruction of cartilage further degrades the collagen network and exacerbates the release of COMP into the SF, which is absorbed by the blood. ECM degradation of chondrocytes is a result of the combined action of type II collagen and proteoglycans [38]. The combined detection of COMP and CS846 fully reflects the degeneration of cartilage. This also indicated that the two indicators of early lesions in response to OA can be used as joint biomarkers for the diagnosis of OA. These results supported the idea that a combination of biomarkers may relate significantly better to the severity of joint damage than individual biomarkers do.

A single test for CS846 or COMP only partially reflected ECM degradation. Combined detection of serum CS846 and COMP concentrations predicted overall degradation of type II collagen and proteoglycans, thereby assessing the degree of OA and early diagnosis of OA. Although the results are promising, our study also has some limitations. Both macroscopic observational histological tests at 10 weeks after OA induction in rats in the model group showed that the degree of OA was significant and that the longitudinal study of 10 weeks was not sufficient. Accordingly, the peak value of CS846 and COMP levels in serum could not be determined at the end of this study. We only performed histological analysis of the tibial plateau, not including the femoral condyle. However, the results were reliable because OA caused articular cartilage degradation in the tibial plateau within 10 weeks after ACLT surgery.

Conclusions

This study provides valuable information on the relationship between serum levels of COMP and CS846, and the degree of OA. Within 10 weeks after ACLT, levels of COMP and CS846 increased significantly, and a positive correlation was observed between the two biomarkers. Serum levels of COMP and CS846 positively correlated with the OARSI score during the OA progression. The combined biomarkers yielded a ROC value, which was significantly higher when compared to that of the single biomarker and would be better if used for the diagnosis of OA. In conclusion, combined detection of serum levels of COMP and CS846 has potential in assessing the degree of OA and OA diagnosis.

Abbreviations

ACL: Anterior cruciate ligament; ACLT: Anterior cruciate ligament transection; COMP: Cartilage oligomeric matrix protein; CS: Chondroitin sulfate; CS846: Chondroitin sulfate 846 epitope; ECM: Extracellular matrix; GAG: Glycosaminoglycan; KS: Keratin sulfate; OA: Osteoarthritis; SF: Synovial fluid

Acknowledgements
Not applicable

Funding
This work was financially supported by the National Key Research and Development Program of China (2017YFD050220).

Authors' contributions
All authors were involved in the conception and design of the study, or in acquisition analysis and interpretation of data, and in revising it critically for important intellectual content. The experiments were designed by TM and LG. The experiments were performed by TM, ZZ, XS, HB, YL, XL, JZ, and YM. TM, ZZ, XS, HB, and LG collected and analyzed data. TM, ZZ, and LG interpreted the data. TM wrote and edited the manuscript. All authors critically reviewed the content and approved final version for publication.

Competing interests
The authors declare that they have no competing interests.

References
1. Hunter DJ, Nevitt M, Losina E, Kraus V. Biomarkers for osteoarthritis: current position and steps towards further validation. Best Pract Res Clin Rheumatol. 2014;28:61–71.
2. Dubey NK, Mishra VK, Dubey R, Syed-Abdul S, Wang JR, Wang PD, et al. Combating osteoarthritis through stem cell therapies by rejuvenating cartilage: a review. Stem Cells Int. 2018;2018:5421019.
3. Pelletier JP, Cooper C, Peterfy C, Reginster JY, Brandi ML, Bruyere O, et al. What is the predictive value of MRI for the occurrence of knee replacement surgery in knee osteoarthritis? Ann Rheum Dis. 2013;72:1594–604.
4. Arabelovic S, Mcalindon TE. Considerations in the treatment of early osteoarthritis. Curr Rheumatol Rep. 2005;7:29–35.
5. Bijlsma JW, Berenbaum F, Lafeber FP. Osteoarthritis: an update with relevance for clinical practice. Lancet. 2011;377:2115–26.
6. Carlson AK, Rawle RA, Adams E, Greenwood MC, Bothner B, June RK. Application of global metabolomic profiling of synovial fluid for osteoarthritis biomarkers. Biochem Biophys Res Commun. 2018;499:182–8.
7. Kang SJ, Kim JW, Kim KY, Ku SK, Lee YJ. Protective effects of calcium gluconate on osteoarthritis induced by anterior cruciate ligament transection and partial medial meniscectomy in Sprague-Dawley rats. J Orthop Surg Res. 2014;9:14.
8. Tanishi N, Yamagiwa H, Hayami T, Mera H, Koga Y, Omori G, et al. Usefulness of urinary CTX-II and NTX-I in evaluating radiological knee osteoarthritis: the Matsudai knee osteoarthritis survey. J Orthop Sci. 2014;19: 429–36.
9. Lai Y, Yu XP, Zhang Y, Tian Q, Song H, Mucignat MT, et al. Enhanced COMP catabolism detected in serum of patients with arthritis and animal disease models through a novel capture ELISA. Osteoarthr Cartil. 2012;20:854–62.
10. Garvican ER, Vaughan-Thomas A, Clegg PD, Innes JF. Biomarkers of cartilage turnover. Part 2: non-collagenous markers. Vet J. 2010;185:43–9.
11. Bakker MF, Verstappen SM, Welsing PM, Jacobs JW, Jahangier ZN, van der Veen MJ, et al. The relation between cartilage biomarkers (C2C, C1,2C, CS846 and CPII) and the long-term outcome of rheumatoid arthritis patients within the CAMERA trial. Arthritis Res Ther. 2011;13:1–8.
12. Sugiyama S, Itokazu M, Suzuki Y, Shimizu K. Procollagen II C propeptide level in the synovial fluid as a predictor of radiographic progression in early knee osteoarthritis. Ann Rheum Dis. 2003;62:27–32.
13. Coyle CH, Henry SE, Haleem AM, O'Malley MJ, Chu CR. Serum CTXii correlates with articular cartilage degeneration after anterior cruciate ligament transection or arthrotomy followed by standardized exercise. Sports Health. 2012;4:510–7.
14. Pelletier JP, Jovanovic D, Fernandes JC, Manning P, Connor JR, Currie MG, et al. Reduced progression of experimental osteoarthritis in vivo by selective inhibition of inducible nitric oxide synthase. Arthritis Rheum. 1998;41:1275–86.

15. Kim JE, Song DH, Kim SH, Jung Y, Kim SJ. Development and characterization of various osteoarthritis models for tissue engineering. PLoS One. 2018;13: e0194288.

16. Pritzker KP, Gay S, Jimenez SA, Ostergaard K, Pelletier JP, Revell PA, et al. Osteoarthritis cartilage histopathology: grading and staging. Osteoarthr Cartil. 2006;14:13–29.

17. Wu J, Wang K, Xu J, Ruan G, Zhu Q, Cai J, et al. Associations between serum ghrelin and knee symptoms, joint structures and cartilage or bone biomarkers in patients with knee osteoarthritis. Osteoarthr Cartil. 2017;25:1428–35.

18. Kuyinu EL, Narayanan G, Nair LS, Laurencin CT. Animal models of osteoarthritis: classification, update, and measurement of outcomes. J Orthop Surg Res. 2016;11:1–27.

19. Hayami T, Pickarski M, Zhuo Y, Wesolowski GA, Rodan GA, Duong LT. Characterization of articular cartilage and subchondral bone changes in the rat anterior cruciate ligament transection and meniscectomized models of osteoarthritis. Bone. 2006;38:234–43.

20. Setton LA, Elliott DM, Mow VC. Altered mechanics of cartilage with osteoarthritis: human osteoarthritis and an experimental model of joint degeneration. Osteoarthr Cartil. 1999;7:2–14.

21. Vilim V, Olejarova M, Machacek S, Gatterova J, Kraus VB, Pavelka K. Serum levels of cartilage oligomeric matrix protein (COMP) correlate with radiographic progression of knee osteoarthritis. Osteoarthr Cartil. 2002;10: 707–13.

22. Lohmander LS, Saxne T, Heinegard DK. Release of cartilage oligomeric matrix protein (COMP) into joint fluid after knee injury and in osteoarthritis. Ann Rheum Dis. 1994;53:8–13.

23. Geng H, Carlsen S, Nandakumar KS, Holmdahl R, Aspberg A, Oldberg A, et al. Cartilage oligomeric matrix protein deficiency promotes early onset and the chronic development of collagen-induced arthritis. Arthritis Res Ther. 2008;10:R134.

24. Fernandes FA, Pucinelli ML, da Silva NP, Feldman D. Serum cartilage oligomeric matrix protein (COMP) levels in knee osteoarthritis in a Brazilian population: clinical and radiological correlation. Scand J Rheumatol. 2007;36:211–5.

25. Huebner JL, Kraus VB. Assessment of the utility of biomarkers of osteoarthritis in the guinea pig. Osteoarthr Cartil. 2006;14:923–30.

26. Zuo H, Jiang L, Qu N, Wang J, Cui X, Yao W. The biomarkers changes in serum and the correlation with quantitative MRI markers by histopathologic evaluation of the cartilage in surgically-induced osteoarthritis rabbit model. PLoS One. 2015;10:e0124717.

27. Bai B, Li Y. Combined detection of serum CTX-II and COMP concentrations in osteoarthritis model rabbits: an effective technique for early diagnosis and estimation of disease severity. J Orthop Surg Res. 2016;11:149.

28. Skioldebrand E, Heinegard D, Eloarnta ML, Nilsson G, Dudhia J, Sandgren B, et al. Enhanced concentration of COMP (cartilage oligomeric matrix protein) in osteochondral fractures from racing thoroughbreds. J Orthop Res. 2005;23:156–63.

29. Georgiev T, Ivanova M, Kopchev A, Velikova T, Miloshov A, Kurteva E, et al. Cartilage oligomeric protein, matrix metalloproteinase-3, and Coll2-1 as serum biomarkers in knee osteoarthritis: a cross-sectional study. Rheumatol Int. 2018;38:1–10.

30. Frisbie DD, Al-Sobayil F, Billinghurst RC, Kawcak CE, McIlwraith CW. Changes in synovial fluid and serum biomarkers with exercise and early osteoarthritis in horses. Osteoarthr Cartil. 2008;16:1196–204.

31. Winsz-Szczotka K, Kuźnik-Trocha K, Komosińska-Vassev K, Jura-Półtorak A, Olczyk K. Laboratory indicators of aggrecan turnover in juvenile idiopathic arthritis. Dis Markers. 2016;2016:1–7.

32. Rizkalla G, Reiner A, Bogoch E, Poole AR. Studies of the articular cartilage proteoglycan aggrecan in health and osteoarthritis. Evidence for molecular heterogeneity and extensive molecular changes in disease. J Clin Invest. 1992;90:2268–77.

33. Glant TT, Mikecz K, Roughley PJ, Buzas E, Poole AR. Age-related changes in protein-related epitopes of human articular-cartilage proteoglycans. Biochem J. 1986;236:71–5.

34. Lohmander LS, Ionescu M, Jugessur H, Poole AR. Changes in joint cartilage aggrecan after knee injury and in osteoarthritis. Arthritis Rheum. 1999;42:534–44.

35. Svoboda SJ, Harvey TM, Owens BD, Brechue WF, Tarwater PM, Cameron KL. Changes in serum biomarkers of cartilage turnover after anterior cruciate ligament injury. Am J Sports Med. 2013;41:2108–16.

36. Jansen NW, Roosendaal G, Lundin B, Heijnen L, Mauser-Bunschoten E, Bijlsma JW, et al. The combination of the biomarkers urinary C-terminal telopeptide of type II collagen, serum cartilage oligomeric matrix protein, and serum chondroitin sulfate 846 reflects cartilage damage in hemophilic arthropathy. Arthritis Rheum. 2009;60:290–8.

37. Saberi Hosnijeh F, Siebuhr AS, Uitterlinden AG, Oei EH, Hofman A, Karsdal MA, et al. Association between biomarkers of tissue inflammation and progression of osteoarthritis: evidence from the Rotterdam study cohort. Arthritis Res Ther. 2016;18:81.

38. Sun Z, Yin Z, Liu C, Liang H, Jiang M, Tian J. IL-1β promotes ADAMTS enzyme-mediated aggrecan degradation through NF-κB in human intervertebral disc. J Orthop Surg Res. 2015;10:1–9.

28

Risk assessment and management of preoperative venous thromboembolism following femoral neck fracture

Ze-Nan Xia, Ke Xiao, Wei Zhu, Bin Feng, Bao-Zhong Zhang, Jin Lin, Wen-Wei Qian, Jin Jin, Na Gao, Gui-Xing Qiu and Xi-Sheng Weng[*] ⬦

Abstract

Background: Limited studies are available to investigate the prevalence of preoperative venous thromboembolism (VTE) in elderly patients with femoral neck fractures. Our primary aim was to determine the incidences of VTE and its risk or protective factors in such patient population. The secondary objective was to evaluate the need of therapeutic anticoagulation for isolated calf muscular venous thrombosis (ICMVT) prior to femoral neck fracture surgery.

Methods: This is a retrospective case-control study, including 301 femoral neck fracture patients who were admitted to our institution between January 2014 and March 2017. Bilateral Doppler ultrasonography was performed in each of the patients as a preoperative VTE screening. The event rate of VTE was calculated, and significant risk or protective factors were determined by using a multivariate logistic regression model. Patients with ICMVT were divided into anticoagulation and no anticoagulation groups to assess the efficacy and safety of preoperative therapeutic anticoagulation. Intraoperative blood loss, drainage volume, blood transfusion, perioperative hemoglobin change, and rate of thrombosis extension were compared between the two groups.

Results: The overall preoperative incidence of VTE in patients with femoral neck fracture was 18.9% (57/301), in which deep vein thrombosis (DVT) was 18.9% and pulmonary embolism (PE) was 1%. Among the DVT cases, 77.2% (44/57) were ICMVTs. Multiple fractures (odds ratio [OR] = 9.418; 95% confidence interval [CI] = 2.537 to 34.96), coexisting movement disorder (OR = 3.862; 95% CI = 1.658 to 8.993), bed rest for more than 7 days (OR = 2.082; 95% CI = 1.011 to 4.284) as well as elevated levels of D-dimer (OR = 1.019; 95% CI = 1.002 to 1.037) and fibrinogen (OR = 1.345; 95% CI = 1.008 to 1.796) led to an increase in the risk of VTE, while the recent use of antiplatelet drug (OR = 0.424; 95% CI = 0.181 to 0.995) and prophylactic anticoagulation (OR = 0.503; 95% CI = 0.263 to 0.959) decreased the risk of VTE. For the 39 patients with ICMVT undergoing femoral neck fracture surgery, there were no significant differences in the rate of thrombosis extension between anticoagulation and no anticoagulation groups, but significantly decreased postoperative hemoglobin was observed in the anticoagulation group.

Conclusion: Our findings showed a high prevalence of preoperative VTE in elderly patients with femoral neck fracture, with risk factors identified. We found that the most detected VTE were ICMVTs. Our study suggested that a direct surgery without preoperative use of therapeutic anticoagulation for ICMVT would not reduce the risk of thrombus extension, and the therapeutic use of anticoagulation may worsen postoperative anemia.

* Correspondence: xshweng@medmail.com.cn
Department of Orthopaedics, Peking Union Medical College Hospital, Chinese Academy of Medical Sciences, Shuaifuyuan 1#, Wangfujing, Dongcheng District, Beijing 100730, People's Republic of China

Introduction

Hip fractures have posed a significant health care problem worldwide as the elderly population is increasing. It was estimated that the number of hip fractures is approximately 1.7 million each year, and the number is expected to surpass 6 million by the year 2050 [1, 2]. Patients with hip fractures are at high risk of venous thromboembolism (VTE), including deep vein thrombosis (DVT) and pulmonary embolism (PE), which is a major cause of morbidity and mortality [3, 4]. A number of literature have focused on the risk factors and incidence of VTE developed after hip fracture surgery. The reported event rate of DVT and PE varied from 1.18 to 6% and 0.25 to 4.6%, respectively, when prophylaxis was used [5–8]. However, there was limited information on the prevalence of preoperative VTE in hip fracture patients waiting for surgery. Previous studies reported a great variation in the preoperative incidence of VTE after hip fracture ranging from 6 to 62%. These studies had several limitations including the highly selected population, small sample size, lack of thrombosis status in unaffected limbs, failure to detect calf muscular venous thrombosis by venography, and the lack of details of specific risk factors for assessment [9–15]. Identification of risk factors for VTE following hip fracture would provide important information on the prevention of thrombosis events and preoperative optimization, leading to a decreased rate of death and complications during the perioperative period. Several studies have reported that delayed admission or surgical intervention, elevated levels of D-dimer, female patients, pulmonary disease, and previous VTE were associated with an increased risk of VTE prior to hip fracture surgery [9, 11–14]. In the elderly population, femoral neck fractures occur frequently. Patients often have multiple comorbidity and concomitant medication, and we hypothesize that additional risk factors would contribute to the relatively high preoperative incidence of VTE, despite thromboprophylaxis is received.

Isolated calf muscular venous thrombosis (ICMVT) is confined to the gastrocnemius and soleal veins and accounts for 5.6 to 31.3% of DVT in lower extremities [16]. The latest American College of Chest Physicians (ACCP) guidelines recommend serial imaging of the deep veins for 2 weeks over anticoagulation in patients with isolated distal DVT without severe symptoms or risk factors for thrombosis extension and consider ICMVT is associated with a lower risk of extension than that of calf axial vein thrombosis [17]. However, the treatment protocols concerning ICMVT remain unclear, particularly in patients with hip fractures awaiting surgical treatment [18]. Preoperative therapeutic anticoagulation could effectively prevent thrombosis extension but, on the other hand, may increase the risk of perioperative bleeding and bed rest-related complications such as pneumonia, urinary infection, and decubitus ulcer. While immediate surgery without anticoagulation for ICMVT is beneficial to the earlier recovery of walking ability, the major concern remains on the possibility of proximal extension. It is important to take into consideration both the effectiveness and safety of the regimen when deciding whether therapeutic anticoagulation for ICMVT is necessary for patients awaiting elective hip fracture surgery. To date, there are no studies evaluating the outcomes of low molecular weight heparin (LMWH) treatment for ICMVT in the elderly patient population with femoral neck fracture. The purpose of the present study was to investigate the preoperative prevalence of VTE in patients with femoral neck fractures and identify associated risk or protective factors in these patients. Furthermore, this study compared the outcomes of two regimens for ICMVT and evaluated the necessity of therapeutic anticoagulation in patients waiting for femoral neck fracture surgery.

Materials and methods

Study population

This study was approved by the Ethics Committee of Peking Union Medical College Hospital (PUMCH), and written informed consent was obtained from all the participants prior to enrollment into the study. We conducted a retrospective review of all patients with femoral neck fracture, identified by hip joint X-ray in our institution between January 2014 and March 2017. Thirty-eight patients were excluded from the study due to the absence of evaluation information for the status of the deep venous system in lower extremities, which led to a total of 301 patients included in this study. Bilateral Doppler ultrasonography was routinely performed in each of the included patients after admission, if a DVT was identified, therapeutic anticoagulation was administrated according to the ACCP guidelines (2016, 10th edition). The insertion of an inferior vena cava filter (IVCF) before surgery was indicated when patients were at high risk of developing a life-threatening PE. Computed tomography pulmonary angiogram (CTPA) was applied to confirm a diagnosis of PE if patients presented with suggestive symptoms such as dyspnea, unexplained tachycardia, chest pain, decreased pulse oximetry, or abnormal arterial blood gas.

Outcome measures

To determine the risk factors for the occurrence of preoperative VTE following femoral neck fracture, associated clinical-pathological characteristics were collected, including age, gender, BMI, classification of fracture, duration of bed rest, comorbidities, smoking, long-term use of steroid or immunosuppressant, recent use of antiplatelet drug (within one week before injury), prophylactic anticoagulation prior to VTE diagnosis, and preoperative level of D-dimer, fibrinogen, and inflammation markers. Investigative comorbidities included hypertension, diabetes, malignancy, ischemic heart disease, atrial fibrillation, cerebrovascular disorder, chronic kidney disease, chronic pulmonary disease, autoimmune disease, movement disorder, Alzheimer's disease, and multiple fractures. Movement disorder was defined as a status of impaired or diminished movement in lower extremities caused by various diseases involving nervous, muscular, or skeletal system, such as hemiparalysis after stroke, myasthenia gravis, Parkinson's disease, and advanced osteoarthritis.

Patients with ICMVT undergoing fracture surgery were divided into anticoagulation and no anticoagulation groups. In the anticoagulation group, patients received therapeutic anticoagulation after detection of ICMVT from at least 12 h before surgery. In the no anticoagulation group, patients were arranged for surgery directly without anticoagulation after ICMVT diagnosis. Postoperative anticoagulation was initiated 12 h after surgery in both groups. LMWH was used as antithrombotics in each study patient at a two thirds to full dose of 100 U/kg twice daily during admission and turned to rivaroxaban after discharge for at least 3 months. Repeated Doppler ultrasonography was employed for suspected DVT if a patient developed sudden onset of lower limb swelling, pain, warmth, or erythema during 2 weeks of follow-up from the date of surgery. Baseline characteristics, efficacy, and safety of LMWH therapy were compared between the two groups. Intraoperative blood loss, drainage volume, blood transfusion, and perioperative hemoglobin change were measured to assess the safety of anticoagulation, while the rate of thrombosis extension was served as the parameter to judge whether anticoagulation was effective.

Statistical analysis

The SPSS 19.0 software (Chicago, IL, USA) was used for statistical analysis. Categorical variables were presented as proportions and continuous variables were presented as the mean ± standard error. Chi-square test and Fisher's exact test were used for comparisons between categorical variables, and Wilcoxon two-sample test and Student's t test were used for continuous variables. Univariate analysis was performed on numerous possible risk factors associated with preoperative VTE following femoral neck fracture. Factors with significant difference (combined movement disorder, multiple fractures, fibrinogen, bed rest time, and antiplatelet therapy) were included in the multivariate logistic regression model to generate adjusted odds ratios (OR) with 95% confidence intervals (CI) for further analysis. Besides, D-dimer and prophylactic anticoagulation employed as important potential risk factors were also forced into the model.

However, factors with data missing were excluded as erythrocyte sedimentation rate (ESR). Receiver operating characteristic (ROC) curve and area under the curve (AUC) analysis was used to evaluate the predictive value of risk factors. For all tests, $P < 0.05$ was considered statistically significant.

Results

Three hundred and thirty-nine patients with femoral neck fracture were admitted to our institution between January 2014 to March 2017. After excluding 38 patients in whom Doppler ultrasonography of deep vein in lower extremities was not performed, a total of 301 patients were included in this study. Of these patients, 57 (18.9%) were identified having DVTs by Doppler ultrasonography screening before surgery, and all of them were asymptomatic. Most of the DVTs ($n = 44$, 77.2%) were ICMVTs, 5 (7%) involved true distal deep veins (peroneal, tibial), and 8 (14%) involved proximal deep vein (external iliac, common femoral, superficial femoral); 35 DVTs (61.4%) were detected on the ipsilateral side of the fracture, 15 were detected on the contralateral side, and 7 occurred on both sides. PEs were diagnosed in 3 patients with proximal DVT using CTPA. After detection of VTE, 40 patients received therapeutic anticoagulation with LMWH, and 17 underwent fracture surgery without preoperative therapeutic anticoagulation. Surgeries for fracture under general anesthesia were performed in 50 patients, including hemi-arthroplasty in 40, total hip arthroplasty (THA) in 8, and closed reduction and internal fixation with cannulated screw in 2. Temporary or permanent IVCFs were implanted in 3 patients prior to surgery.

Associations of clinical-pathological parameters with preoperative VTE were listed in Table 1. In the univariate analysis, significantly elevated levels of fibrinogen and ESR were observed in patients with VTE. Although the level of D-dimer was higher in VTE group, there was no statistical difference. Duration of bed rest for more than 7 days was more commonly observed in patients with preoperative VTE, and the difference became more significant with the increase of time in bed (> 14 days). For patients with comorbidities and concomitant medication, movement disorder and multiple fractures were more frequently found in patients with VTE; in contrast, the recent use of antiplatelet drug was relatively less frequent. The proportion of prophylactic anticoagulation use tended to be higher in patients without VTE, but the difference was not significant. Notably, more patients received delayed chemoprophylaxis at more than 24 h after fracture in VTE group, and the difference became more significant when there was a delay on commencement of chemoprophylaxis for more than 48 h from the time of fracture (Fig. 1).

Seven selected variables were determined to be an independent risk or protective factors associated with

Table 1 Associations of clinical-pathological characteristics and preoperative VTE

Variable	No VTE (n = 244)	VTE (n = 57)	P value
Age (year)	76.30 ± 11.10	77.11 ± 9.38	0.764
Male gender	80 (32.79)	15 (26.32)	0.344
BMI (kg/m^2)	22.91 ± 3.69	22.91 ± 4.09	0.684
Garden typing			0.071
Type III and IV	216 (88.52)	55 (96.49)	
Type I and II	28 (11.48)	2 (3.51)	
Rockwood typing			0.280
Subcapital	186 (77.82)	47 (87.04)	
Transcervical	40 (16.74)	6 (11.11)	
Basicervical	13 (5.44)	1 (1.85)	
Bed rest time > 3 days	120 (49.38)	34 (59.65)	0.163
Bed rest time > 7 days	54 (22.22)	20 (35.00)	0.043
Bed rest time > 14 days	30 (12.35)	15 (26.32)	0.008
Smoking	20 (8.20)	7 (12.28)	0.331
Comorbidity			
Hypertension	144 (59.02)	27 (47.37)	0.110
Diabetes	71 (29.10)	10 (17.54)	0.077
Malignancy	30 (12.30)	7 (12.28)	0.998
Ischemic heart disease	57 (23.36)	8 (14.04)	0.123
Atrial fibrillation	19 (7.79)	5 (8.77)	1.000
Cerebrovascular disorder	44 (18.03)	6 (10.53)	0.170
Chronic kidney disease	12 (4.92)	3 (5.26)	1.000
Chronic pulmonary disease	10 (4.10)	3 (5.26)	0.978
Autoimmune disease	11 (4.51)	3 (5.26)	1.000
Movement disorder	18 (7.38)	14 (24.56)	< 0.001
Alzheimer's disease	7 (2.87)	4 (7.02)	0.267
Multiple fractures	6 (2.46)	7 (12.28)	0.003
Concomitant medication			
Steroid or immunosuppressant	14 (5.74)	2 (3.51)	0.728
Antiplatelet drug	66 (27.05)	8 (14.04)	0.040
Prophylactic anticoagulation	137 (56.85)	25 (43.86)	0.077
D-dimer (μg/mL)	10.11 ± 17.27	11.35 ± 22.88	0.067
Fbg (g/L)	3.92 ± 1.11	4.2 ± 1.28	0.035
ESR (mm/h)	37.35 ± 26.85	45.33 ± 25.97	0.035
hsCRP (mg/L)	42.84 ± 36.21	54.63 ± 48.69	0.142

Fbg fibrinogen, *ESR* erythrocyte sedimentation rate, *hsCRP* high-sensitive C-reactive protein

preoperative VTE following femoral neck fracture in the multivariate logistic regression analysis (Table 2). Elevated levels of D-dimer and fibrinogen were significantly associated with an increased risk of VTE. Bed rest for more than 7 days led to a twofold increase in the risk of VTE, and patients with comorbidity of movement disorder or multiple fractures were at four- to ninefold

higher risk for VTE. Conversely, the recent use of antiplatelet drug and prophylactic anticoagulation were found to be protective factors which significantly decreased the risk of VTE after femoral neck fracture.

ROC curve analysis was used to evaluate the potency of the identified seven risk or protective factors in predicting the occurrence of VTE following femoral neck fracture (Fig. 2). The AUC of D-dimer was 0.578 (95% IC 0.506–0.650), fibrinogen was 0.590 (95% IC 0.505–0.676), multiple fractures was 0.552 (95% IC 0.507–0.597), movement disorder was 0.578 (95% IC 0.519–0.636), antiplatelet drug use was 0.563 (95% IC 0.508–0.617), prophylactic anticoagulation was 0.566 (95% IC 0.493–0.639), and bed rest time for over 7 days was 0.563 (95% IC 0.495–0.631). Furthermore, the AUC of the established model containing all the seven factors was 0.731 (95% IC 0.657–0.806), indicating a moderate predictive value for the onset of preoperative VTE after femoral neck fracture.

Among the subpopulation of 44 patients with ICMVT, surgeries for femoral neck fracture were performed in 39 of them. Of these, 24 patients received preoperative therapeutic anticoagulation with LMWH after detection of ICMVT, and 15 underwent surgeries directly without preoperative anticoagulation. No significant differences were found in the baseline characteristics between the anticoagulation group and no anticoagulation group (Table 3). During the period of the 2-week follow-up, three ICMVTs extended into axial DVTs in the anticoagulation group; however, the difference in the rate of thrombosis extension was not statistically significant between the two groups. With respect to hemorrhage related safety assessment, intraoperative blood loss, postoperative drainage volume, and blood transfusion rate in the anticoagulation group were equivalent with those in the no anticoagulation group, but significantly decreased hemoglobin was observed after surgery in the presence of preoperative therapeutic anticoagulation. This result indicated that therapeutic anticoagulation for ICMVT prior to femoral neck fracture surgery seemed to not provide a significant reduction in the rate of thrombus extension, but in turn had a significant influence on postoperative hemoglobin.

Discussion

In this retrospective case-control study, we have made some major findings. Firstly, we observed the incidence of VTE following femoral neck fracture was 18.9%, independent of surgical treatment. Secondly, we identified fibrinogen, combined movement disorder, multiple fractures as new risk factors, and oral antiplatelet therapy and prophylactic anticoagulation as protective factors for the development of VTE after fractures. Finally, it is the first time that we evaluated the necessity of therapeutic anticoagulation for ICMVT in patients awaiting for femoral neck fracture surgery in terms of effectiveness and safety and revealed preoperative

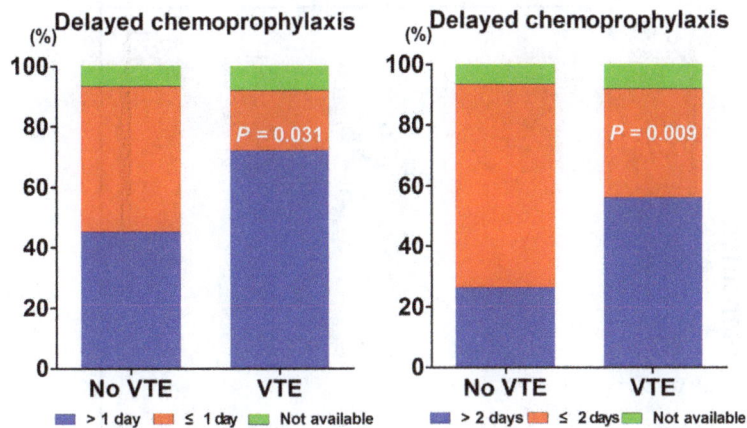

Fig. 1 Comparison of percentage of delayed chemoprophylaxis > 1 day and 2 days between patients with and without VTE (*n* = 162). Delayed chemoprophylaxis was defined as prophylactic anticoagulation initiated at more than 24 h after femoral neck fracture

anticoagulation might not significantly prevent postoperative thrombus progression, but increased the risk of hemorrhage to some extent.

Patients with hip fractures have a high risk for VTE events because of endothelial injury of adjacent blood vessels, hypercoagulability following coagulation cascade, and venous stasis resulting from immobilization [19]. To date, the understanding of the preoperative VTE rate occurred after hip fracture is limited. There are only several small studies investigated that, and the findings were not consistent [9–15]. The studies employed venography for diagnosis, and the overall rate of preoperative VTE was 9.8–11.1%, or it could be as high as 29.6% when the enrolled population was limited to patients identified as subcapital femoral neck fracture without chemical thromboprophylaxis with LMWH [9, 13, 14]. Other studies showed an 11.9–16.3% overall incidence of VTE event, when Doppler ultrasonography was used [12, 15]. With the developments in venous duplex technology, the ability to detect ICMVT has improved significantly. Doppler

ultrasonography has been demonstrated to be more sensitive and specific in detection of both proximal and distal DVT compared to venography, and given this, the event rate obtained by venography in earlier studies might be underestimated [20]. In addition, the highly selected population was likely to magnify or minify the real rate of thrombosis. Precluding these limitations, this study revealed the overall preoperative incidence of VTE after femoral neck fracture was 18.9% based on a larger sample size. In this respect, our result was considered to be more reliable.

Regarding the distribution of thrombosis, most were confined to calf intermuscular veins, but the proportion of 77.2% observed in this study was much higher than previous data. The variation could be mainly attributed to the different study population. We focused on the patients after femoral neck fracture who received ultrasonography screening, while population enrolled in earlier studies were patients presenting with symptoms and signs suspicious for DVT which undoubtedly led to a lower proportion of ICMVT [16]. Considering the high incidence of VTE and overwhelming percentage of asymptomatic ICMVT after femoral neck fracture, we proposed that routine screening for DVT in lower extremities with Doppler ultrasonography prior to fracture surgery be required. Notably, DVTs in our study were discovered mostly on the ipsilateral side of the fracture, and a similar finding has shown a significant tendency for DVTs to occur on the same side as the hip fracture, suggesting local vessel injury and immobility of affected limb may be more important than general hypercoagulability in causing DVT after hip fracture [21].

Although previous studies indicated the viability of incidence rate of VTE, there seemed to be a correlation between the period of delay in treatment and the incidence of perioperative thrombosis. It was observed that the rate of VTE event increased from 6 to 14.5% if patients were

Table 2 Multivariate logistic regression analysis for VTE

Variable	OR	95% CI		P value
		Lower limit	Upper limit	
D-dimer	1.019	1.002	1.037	0.0323
Fbg	1.345	1.008	1.796	0.0442
Multiple fractures (yes vs no)	9.418	2.537	34.960	0.0008
Movement disorder (yes vs no)	3.862	1.658	8.993	0.0017
Use of antiplatelet drug (yes vs no)	0.424	0.181	0.995	0.0487
Prophylactic anticoagulation (yes vs no)	0.503	0.263	0.959	0.0370
Bed rest time > 7 days (yes vs no)	2.082	1.011	4.284	0.0465

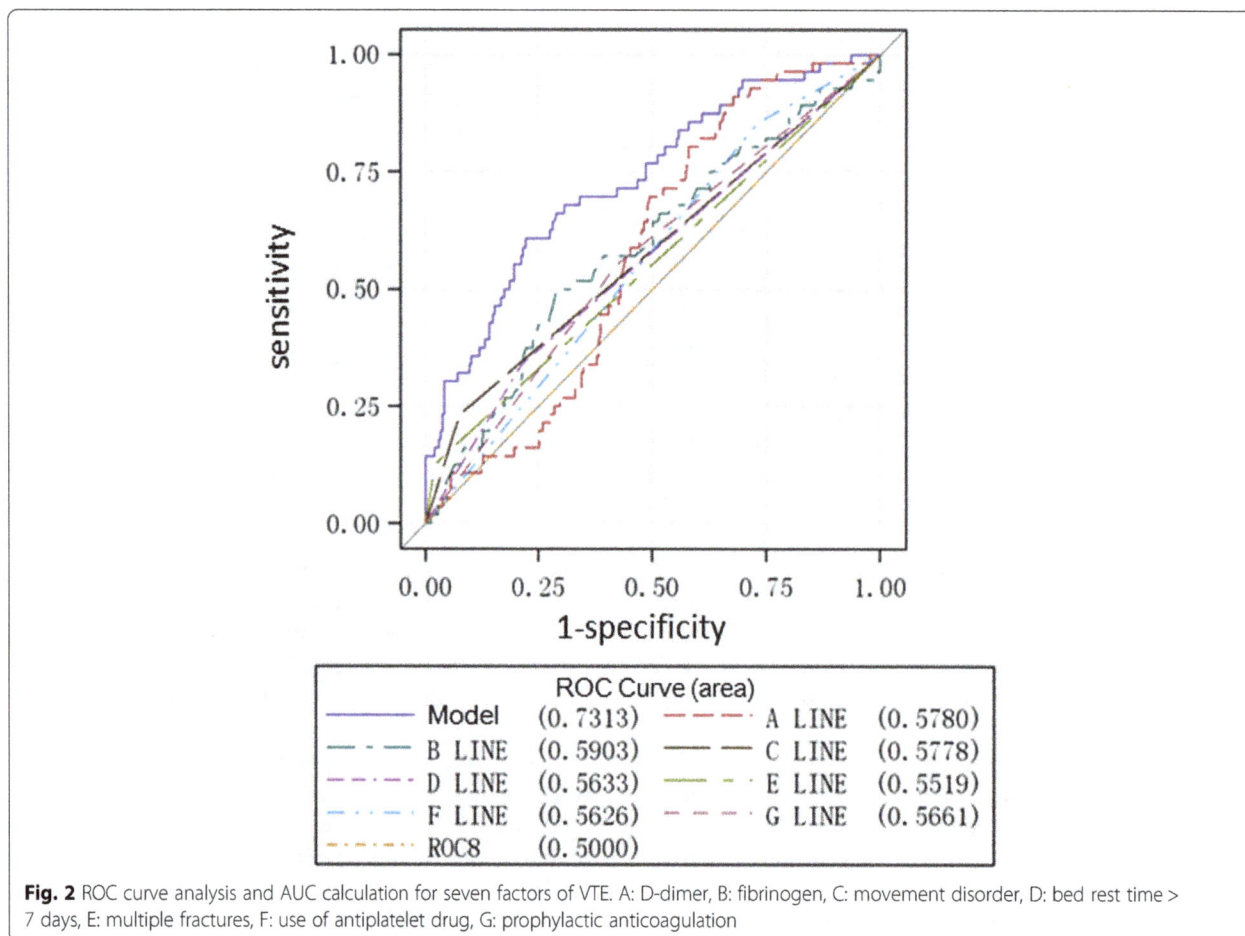

Fig. 2 ROC curve analysis and AUC calculation for seven factors of VTE. A: D-dimer, B: fibrinogen, C: movement disorder, D: bed rest time > 7 days, E: multiple fractures, F: use of antiplatelet drug, G: prophylactic anticoagulation

admitted or received surgery within 48 h to 17–62% when there was a delay for more than 48 h [9–12]. Delayed admission to hospital or surgical intervention was considered to increase the risk of preoperative VTE after hip fracture [9, 12]. Delay may result from preoperative

Table 3 Baseline characteristics of patients with ICMVT in anticoagulation and no anticoagulation groups

Variable	Anticoagulation (n = 24)	No anticoagulation (n = 15)	P value
Age (year)	76.17 ± 8.99	79.33 ± 10.66	0.188
Male gender	5 (20.83)	4 (26.67)	0.711
Garden typing			0.266
Type IV	20 (83.33)	10 (66.67)	
Type III	4 (16.67)	5 (33.33)	
Pre. HGB (g/L)	120.50 ± 16.82	119.80 ± 18.59	0.904
Prophylactic anticoagulation	9 (37.50)	8 (53.33)	0.508
Surgery			0.121
Hemiarthroplasty	17 (70.83)	14 (93.33)	
Others	7 (29.17)	1 (6.67)	

Pre. preoperative

medical evaluation and optimization as well as prolonged bed rest at home. Venous hypostasis associated with bed rest or prolonged immobilization was an important risk factor for the development of thrombosis in patients with leg injury, particularly hip fractures [13, 22], but no studies revealed the relation between the period of bed rest and risk of VTE events. We found bed rest for more than 7 days, as an independent risk, led to a twofold increase in the risk of preoperative VTE. Combined with previous findings, we believed that surgery should be performed as soon as possible, no longer than 7 days after femoral neck fracture if necessary medical optimization is required.

The present study has investigated a number of baseline characteristics and its relation to preoperative VET. We identified the elevated levels of D-dimer as one of the independent risk factors for VTE. This was consistent with another research in which the sensitivity and specificity of D-dimer in diagnosing preoperative DVT were 71.4 and 78.6% when the cutoff value was set at 2.79 mg/L [13]. D-dimer represented an applicable modality with a high sensitivity and poor specificity to detect acute DVT in nontraumatic settings. Since tissue injury caused by trauma also led to elevated levels of

D-dimer, the diagnostic reliability was not validated in patients after trauma [23]. In recent years, Yang et al. have reported a cutoff value of 3 mg/L for D-dimer to predict DVT event with a sensitivity of 88.37% and a specificity of 96.96% in patients after surgery for lower limb fractures [24], and Bakhshi et al. have found that D-dimer levels more than 1000 ng/mL were 100% sensitive and 71% specific for detecting DVT in the same population [25]. All these findings suggested a yet unexplored value for D-dimer to predict VTE in patients after trauma such as femoral neck fractures.

In addition to D-dimer, high level of fibrinogen was also recognized as one of the well-established risk factors for VTE [26, 27], and it was supported by our findings in patients with femoral neck fractures for the first time. It is possible that the elevated fibrinogen increases fibrin network density, blood viscosity, and the resistance of clots to fibrinolysis, thereby leading to a hypercoagulable state [27–29]. We hypothesized that hyperfibrinogenemia is not merely a biomarker of thrombotic risk, but also contributes to the etiology of VTE following femoral neck fracture [30].

To the best of our knowledge, the relationship between ESR and VTE has never been established in patients with hip fractures. In this study, a significantly elevated level of ESR was observed in patients with VTE. This could be regarded as a potential risk factor and warrants further investigation. Fibrinogen is referred as an acute phase reactant (APR) that accompanies inflammation and tissue injury, ESR is an indirect measure of the acute phase response and levels of APR, particularly with fibrinogen, and they both reflect the presence and intensity of an inflammatory process. The increase of both ESR and fibrinogen observed in the present study implicated that the enhanced acute phase response accompanied with acute inflammatory states may play a role in the occurrence of VTE after femoral neck fracture.

Different from the previous studies, we found the development of VTE after hip fracture was not influenced by patient's gender, type of fractures, or pulmonary disease [14], but it was significantly correlated with the coexisting movement disorder or multiple fractures. Patients with movement disorder or multiple fractures were at four- to ninefold higher risk for VTE, and it means they may need a more aggressive initial treatment and close surveillance.

LMWH or aspirin was recommended to use in patients undergoing hip fracture surgery according to the latest ACCP guidelines [18]. Sufficient evidences confirmed that chemical thromboprophylaxis resulted in a lower risk of VTE after hip fracture surgery [18, 31]. Consistently, we determined the recent use of antiplatelet drug and prophylactic anticoagulation to be protective factors which significantly reduced the risk of preoperative VTE after

femoral neck fracture. For the timing of commencement of VTE prophylaxis, the guidelines recommended the initiation of LMWH therapy either from at least 12 h before surgery, or at least 12 h after surgery, but no precise protocol was given [18]. On the ground of proofs that hypercoagulable state occurred in the early phase of injury and the risk of VTE increased with the delayed period of surgical intervention, it is reasonable to initiate the thromboprophylaxis as early as possible [12, 32]. Delayed initiation of prophylaxis has been well demonstrated to contribute to the development of symptomatic VTE and fatal PE in patients with traumatic brain injury [33, 34]. A similar phenomenon was noted in this study that delayed chemoprophylaxis at more than 24 h from the time of injury was positively correlated with the occurrence of VTE, and more significant correlation was present when the delayed time was over 48 h. Thus, we suggested the use of LMWH or antiplatelet drug for VTE prophylaxis, when hip fracture surgery was delayed. The initial prophylactic anticoagulation with LMWH within 24 h appeared beneficial, while further studies are needed to determine the optimal timing of prophylactic anticoagulation commencement.

ICMVT was considered to have a lower risk of extension than thrombosis that involved the axial veins, as suggested by the ACCP guidelines [17]. However, the treatment options for ICMVT remains controversial in regard to the use of controversies monitoring with duplex examinations versus therapeutic anticoagulation. Despite the multiple trials that showed the potential benefit of anticoagulation use in the treatment of ICMVT [16, 35], a latest meta-analysis demonstrated insignificant outcomes of anticoagulation use in decreasing the rate of thrombosis progression, as well as increasing the rate of complete recanalization when compared with the no anticoagulation [36] (Table 4). The present study provided novel findings on the assessment of efficacy and safety of therapeutic anticoagulation for ICMVT in patients after femoral neck fracture. We found preoperative therapeutic anticoagulation for ICMVT may

Table 4 Comparison of outcomes between anticoagulation and no anticoagulation groups in patients with ICMVT

Variable	Anticoagulation (n = 24)	No anticoagulation (n = 15)	P value
Intra. blood loss (mL)	277.08 ± 173.19	230.00 ± 154.46	0.287
Total drainage volume	204.00 ± 114.01	226.25 ± 156.75	0.911
Intra./post. blood transfusion	9 (37.50)	4 (26.67)	0.728
Post. lowest HGB	88.88 ± 13.91	98.87 ± 13.84	0.035
Peri. HGB change	31.63 ± 14.75	20.93 ± 16.92	0.044
Post. VTE extension	3 (12.50)	0 (0.00)	0.271
Post. infection	6 (25.00)	2 (13.33)	0.450

Intra. intraoperative, *Post.* postoperative, *Pre.* preoperative

not effectively decrease the risk of thrombus progression, but may worsen postoperative anemia. As such, direct surgery for femoral neck fracture regardless of the status of ICMVT seems appropriate. We speculated that these patients could not benefit from the preoperative therapeutic anticoagulation, possibly due to the prolonged duration of bed rest, delayed recovery of walking ability, and extended inpatient time accompanied by treatment of ICMVT.

This study had several limitations. Firstly, it was a retrospective study that relied on data from the electronic medical record system. Inferior accuracy and integrity of collected clinical information was inherent to retrospective nature compared with the prospective study. Because some data were missing such as BMI, ESR, high sensitive C-reactive protein (hsCRP), we chose to use available case analysis and to disregard some data. History of previous VTE, traction therapy, and plaster immobilization were not analyzed as associated variables due to information default. The incomplete information may affect our result to some extents. Secondly, because the data were from a single institution, selection biases was inevitable; however, the interpretation of the results would not be complicated by the heterogeneity of practices that are commonly found in a multicenter study. Thirdly, the target sample size of ICMVT was small. Lastly, we followed up thrombus progression for only 2 weeks after surgery and then performed ultrasonography only in patients with suspicious symptoms. Any long-term and asymptomatic thrombus progression events might be missed. A further study with a larger population on the evaluation of therapeutic anticoagulation for ICMVT before hip fracture surgery is greatly needed.

Conclusion

In conclusion, we showed that the overall preoperative incidence of VTE following femoral neck fracture was high, and most of which were ICMVTs. The elevated levels of D-dimer and fibrinogen, coexisting movement disorder, and multiple fractures, as well as bed rest for more than 7 days, were identified as risk factors of VTE, while the recent use of antiplatelet drug and prophylactic anticoagulation were considered as protective factors. When ICMVT is observed after femoral neck fracture, direct surgery without therapeutic anticoagulation seems appropriate. The absence of preoperative use of therapeutic anticoagulation would not reduce the risk of thrombus extension, but it may provide less effect on postoperative anemia. This study proposed intervention strategies to lower the VTE risk and, of importance, opens a new prospect to the time of prophylactic anticoagulation commencement and management option of ICMVT.

Abbreviations
ACCP: American College of Chest Physicians; AUC: Area under the curve; CI: Confidence intervals; CTPA: Computed tomography pulmonary angiogram; DVT: Deep vein thrombosis; ESR: Erythrocyte sedimentation rate; hsCRP: High sensitive C-reactive protein; ICMVT: Isolated calf muscular venous thrombosis; IVCF: Inferior vena cava filter; LMWH: Low molecular weight heparin; OR: Odds ratios; PE: Pulmonary embolism; ROC: Receiver-operating characteristic; THA: Total hip arthroplasty; VTE: Venous thromboembolism

Acknowledgements
National High-tech R&D Program (863 Program) with grant no. 2015AA020316 and no. 2015AA033601 from the People's Republic of China. L. S. Thanks for the financial support from China.

Funding
No funding was received for this study.

Authors' contributions
ZNX, KX, and XSW contributed to the conception and design of the study. WZ, BZZ, and BF contributed to the acquisition of data. JL, WWQ, and JJ contributed to the analysis of data. NG, GXQ, and ZNX wrote the manuscript. All authors reviewed and approved the final version of the manuscript.

Competing interests
The authors declare that they have no competing interests.

References
1. Miyamoto RG, Kaplan KM, Levine BR, Egol KA, Zuckerman JD. Surgical management of hip fractures: an evidence-based review of the literature. I: femoral neck fractures. J Am Acad Orthop Surg. 2008;16(10):596–607 PubMed PMID: 18832603.
2. Kannus P, Parkkari J, Sievanen H, Heinonen A, Vuori I, Jarvinen M. Epidemiology of hip fractures. Bone. 1996;18(1 Suppl):57S–63S PubMed PMID: 8717549.
3. Geerts WH, Code KI, Jay RM, Chen E, Szalai JP. A prospective study of venous thromboembolism after major trauma. N Engl J Med. 1994;331(24): 1601–6. https://doi.org/10.1056/NEJM199412153312401 PubMed PMID: 7969340.
4. Anderson FA Jr, Spencer FA. Risk factors for venous thromboembolism. Circulation. 2003;107(23 Suppl 1):I9–16. https://doi.org/10.1161/01.CIR. 0000078469.07362.E6 PubMed PMID: 12814980.
5. Prevention of pulmonary embolism and deep vein thrombosis with low dose aspirin: Pulmonary Embolism Prevention (PEP) trial. Lancet. 2000; 355(9212):1295–302 PubMed PMID: 10776741.
6. Eriksson BI, Lassen MR, Investigators PEiH-FSP. Duration of prophylaxis against venous thromboembolism with fondaparinux after hip fracture surgery: a multicenter, randomized, placebo-controlled, double-blind study. Arch Intern Med. 2003;163(11):1337–42. https://doi.org/10.1001/archinte.163. 11.1337 PubMed PMID: 12796070.
7. Rosencher N, Vielpeau C, Emmerich J, Fagnani F, Samama CM, Group E. Venous thromboembolism and mortality after hip fracture surgery: the ESCORTE study. J Thromb Haemost. 2005;3(9):2006–14. https://doi.org/10. 1111/J.1538-7836.2005.01545.x PubMed PMID: 16102107.
8. Westrich GH, Rana AJ, Terry MA, Taveras NA, Kapoor K, Helfet DL. Thromboembolic disease prophylaxis in patients with hip fracture: a multimodal approach. J Orthop Trauma. 2005;19(4):234–40 PubMed PMID: 15795571.
9. Hefley FG Jr, Nelson CL, Puskarich-May CL. Effect of delayed admission to the hospital on the preoperative prevalence of deep-vein thrombosis

associated with fractures about the hip. J Bone Joint Surg Am. 1996;78(4): 581–3 PubMed PMID: 8609137.

10. Roberts TS, Nelson CL, Barnes CL, Ferris EJ, Holder JC, Boone DW. The preoperative prevalence and postoperative incidence of thromboembolism in patients with hip fractures treated with dextran prophylaxis. Clin Orthop Relat Res. 1990;255:198–203. PubMed PMID: 1693325.

11. Zahn HR, Skinner JA, Porteous MJ. The preoperative prevalence of deep vein thrombosis in patients with femoral neck fractures and delayed operation. Injury. 1999;30(9):605–7 PubMed PMID: 10707228.

12. Smith EB, Parvizi J, Purtill JJ. Delayed surgery for patients with femur and hip fractures-risk of deep venous thrombosis. J Trauma. 2011;70(6):E113–6. https://doi.org/10.1097/TA.0b013e31821b8768 PubMed PMID: 21817966.

13. Song K, Yao Y, Rong Z, Shen Y, Zheng M, Jiang Q. The preoperative incidence of deep vein thrombosis (DVT) and its correlation with postoperative DVT in patients undergoing elective surgery for femoral neck fractures. Arch Orthop Trauma Surg. 2016;136(10):1459–64. https://doi.org/10.1007/s00402-016-2535-4 PubMed PMID: 27535672.

14. Shin WC, Woo SH, Lee SJ, Lee JS, Kim C, Suh KT. Preoperative prevalence of and risk factors for venous thromboembolism in patients with a hip fracture: an indirect multidetector CT venography study. J Bone Joint Surg Am. 2016;98(24): 2089–95. https://doi.org/10.2106/JBJS.15.01329 PubMed PMID: 28002372.

15. Luksameearunothai K, Sa-Ngasoongsong P, Kulachote N, Thamyongkit S, Fuangfa P, Chanplakorn P, et al. Usefulness of clinical predictors for preoperative screening of deep vein thrombosis in hip fractures. BMC Musculoskelet Disord. 2017;18(1):208. https://doi.org/10.1186/s12891-017-1582-5 PubMed PMID: 28532441; PubMed Central PMCID: PMCPMC5440897.

16. Henry JC, Satiani B. Calf muscle venous thrombosis: a review of the clinical implications and therapy. Vasc Endovasc Surg. 2014;48(5–6):396–401. https://doi.org/10.1177/1538574414541704 PubMed PMID: 25027613.

17. Kearon C, Akl EA, Ornelas J, Blaivas A, Jimenez D, Bounameaux H, et al. Antithrombotic therapy for VTE disease: CHEST Guideline and Expert Panel Report. Chest. 2016;149(2):315–52. https://doi.org/10.1016/j.chest.2015.11.026 PubMed PMID: 26867832.

18. Falck-Ytter Y, Francis CW, Johanson NA, Curley C, Dahl OE, Schulman S, et al. Prevention of VTE in orthopedic surgery patients: Antithrombotic Therapy and Prevention of Thrombosis, 9th ed: American College of Chest Physicians Evidence-Based Clinical Practice Guidelines. Chest 2012;141(2 Suppl):e278S-e325S. doi: https://doi.org/10.1378/chest.11-2404. PubMed PMID: 22315265; PubMed Central PMCID: PMC3278063.

19. Bagot CN, Arya R. Virchow and his triad: a question of attribution. Br J Haematol. 2008;143(2):180–90. https://doi.org/10.1111/j.1365-2141.2008.07323.x PubMed PMID: 18783400.

20. Miller N, Satin R, Tousignant L, Sheiner NM. A prospective study comparing duplex scan and venography for diagnosis of lower-extremity deep vein thrombosis. Cardiovasc Surg. 1996;4(4):505–8 PubMed PMID: 8866090.

21. Protty MB, Aithal S, Hickey B, Pettit R, Johansen A. Mechanical prophylaxis after hip fracture: what is the risk of deep vein thrombosis? A retrospective observational study. BMJ Open. 2015;5(2):e006956. https://doi.org/10.1136/bmjopen-2014-006956 PubMed PMID: 25678543; PubMed Central PMCID: PMC4330328.

22. Lassen MR, Borris LC, Nakov RL. Use of the low-molecular-weight heparin reviparin to prevent deep-vein thrombosis after leg injury requiring immobilization. N Engl J Med. 2002;347(10):726–30. https://doi.org/10.1056/NEJMoa011327 PubMed PMID: 12213943.

23. Johna S, Cemaj S, O'Callaghan T, Catalano R. Effect of tissue injury on D-dimer levels: a prospective study in trauma patients. Med Sci Monit. 2002; 8(1):CR5–8 PubMed PMID: 11796959.

24. Yang Y, Zan P, Gong J, Cai M. D-dimer as a screening marker for venous thromboembolism after surgery among patients younger than 50 with lower limb fractures. Clin Appl Thromb Hemost. 2017;23(1):78–83. https://doi.org/10.1177/1076029615588784 PubMed PMID: 26045546.

25. Bakhshi H, Alavi-Moghaddam M, Wu KC, Imami M, Banasiri M. D-dimer as an applicable test for detection of posttraumatic deep vein thrombosis in lower limb fracture. Am J Orthop. 2012;41(6):E78–80 PubMed PMID: 22837995.

26. van Hylckama Vlieg A, Rosendaal FR. High levels of fibrinogen are associated with the risk of deep venous thrombosis mainly in the elderly. J Thromb Haemost. 2003;1(12):2677–8 PubMed PMID: 14675106.

27. Machlus KR, Cardenas JC, Church FC, Wolberg AS. Causal relationship between hyperfibrinogenemia, thrombosis, and resistance to thrombolysis in mice. Blood. 2011;117(18):4953–63. https://doi.org/10.1182/blood-2010-11-316885 PubMed PMID: 21355090; PubMed Central PMCID: PMC3100702.

28. Undas A, Zawilska K, Ciesla-Dul M, Lehmann-Kopydlowska A, Skubiszak A, Ciepluch K, et al. Altered fibrin clot structure/function in patients with idiopathic venous thromboembolism and in their relatives. Blood. 2009; 114(19):4272–8. https://doi.org/10.1182/blood-2009-05-222380 PubMed PMID: 19690336.

29. Lisman T, de Groot PG, Meijers JC, Rosendaal FR. Reduced plasma fibrinolytic potential is a risk factor for venous thrombosis. Blood. 2005; 105(3):1102–5. https://doi.org/10.1182/blood-2004-08-3253 PubMed PMID: 15466929.

30. Aleman MM, Walton BL, Byrnes JR, Wolberg AS. Fibrinogen and red blood cells in venous thrombosis. Thromb Res. 2014;133 Suppl 1:S38–40. https://doi.org/10.1016/j.thromres.2014.03.017 PubMed PMID: 24759140; PubMed Central PMCID: PMC4003903.

31. Marsland D, Mears SC, Kates SL. Venous thromboembolic prophylaxis for hip fractures. Osteoporos Int. 2010;21(Suppl 4):S593–604. https://doi.org/10.1007/s00198-010-1403-2 PubMed PMID: 21057999.

32. Shaz BH, Winkler AM, James AB, Hillyer CD, MacLeod JB. Pathophysiology of early trauma-induced coagulopathy: emerging evidence for hemodilution and coagulation factor depletion. J Trauma. 2011;70(6):1401–7. https://doi.org/10.1097/TA.0b013e31821266e0 PubMed PMID: 21460741; PubMed Central PMCID: PMC3131448.

33. Yablon SA, Rock WA Jr, Nick TG, Sherer M, McGrath CM, Goodson KH. Deep vein thrombosis: prevalence and risk factors in rehabilitation admissions with brain injury. Neurology. 2004;63(3):485–91. PubMed PMID: 15304579.

34. Reiff DA, Haricharan RN, Bullington NM, Griffin RL, McGwin G Jr, Rue LW 3rd. Traumatic brain injury is associated with the development of deep vein thrombosis independent of pharmacological prophylaxis. J Trauma. 2009; 66(5):1436–40. https://doi.org/10.1097/TA.0b013e31817fdf1c. PubMed PMID: 19430251.

35. Elfandi A, Anghel S, Sales C. Current management of isolated soleal and gastrocnemius vein thrombosis. J Vasc Surg Venous Lymphat Disord. 2015; 3(3):341–4. https://doi.org/10.1016/j.jvsv.2015.02.002. PubMed PMID: 26992317.

36. Huang XC, Hu XH, Wang XR, Zhou CX, Wang GY. Efficacy and safety of therapeutic anticoagulation for the treatment of isolated calf muscle vein thrombosis - a systematic review and meta-analysis. Vasa. 2016;45(6):478–85. https://doi.org/10.1024/0301-1526/a000569. PubMed PMID: 27598049.

29

High failure rate of proximal femoral locking plates in fixation of trochanteric fractures

Shuangjian He[1,2], Bin Yan[1], Jian Zhu[1], Xiaoyi Huang[1] and Jianning Zhao[2,3*]

Abstract

Background: The aim of this study was to report our previous results of treatments for trochanteric fractures with proximal femoral locking plates (PFLP) and to analyze the underlying mechanisms and possible risk factors associated with the high failure rate of this technique.

Methods: From January 2010 to October 2014, 273 consecutive patients with trochanteric femoral fractures were identified, and 95 patients (with 97 fractures) ultimately met the inclusion criteria. Clinical records regarding demographic features and intraoperative data including total incision length, operation time, blood loss, and failures detected in radiographs were documented and assessed. The collected data were analyzed with SPSS 19.0 software.

Results: The stable group (AO/OTA 31 A1 and A2.1) had less blood loss than the unstable group (AO/OTA 31 A2.2, A2.3, and A3). The ultimate failure rate was 36% in 97 fractures. The obvious complications in this study included nonunion in 7 (7.2%) fractures, implant breakage in 4 (4.1%) fractures, varus deformity in 34 (35%) fractures, and loosening of the proximal femoral screw in 21 (21.6%) fractures. Six patients received reoperations. The total failure rate in the stable group was 17% and was 50% in the unstable group. In patients greater than 60 years old in the unstable group, the failure rate was 60.5%.

Conclusions: High failure rates of PFLP were observed in patients with trochanteric fracture, especially in patients who were greater than 60 years old with unstable fracture types. PFLP was not an appropriate treatment for trochanteric fractures.

Keywords: Trochanteric fractures, Hip fracture, Locking plate, Mechanical failure, Complications

Background

With the increase in the aging population, trochanteric fractures including pertrochanteric, intertrochanteric, and subtrochanteric fractures also have a rising trend, and most of these fractures need surgical treatment [1–4]. For stable fracture types, either extramedullary or intramedullary implants such as the dynamic hip screw (DHS), the dynamic condylar screw (DCS), and proximal femoral nail anti-rotation (PFNA) are considered to be successful devices [1, 5]. According to published studies,

however, the most effective implant for the treatment of unstable trochanteric fractures is still being debated [6–11]. In most previous studies, intramedullary devices were recommended for patients with unstable fractures patterns and reportedly achieved better clinical results with lower complications than extramedullary implants. However, some authors suggested that the use of intramedullary devices had no significant advantage over extramedullary devices, especially in cases with highly comminuted fractures at the site of nail insertion and the lateral femoral wall both of which are considered major risks related to higher failure rates [12, 13].

As an extramedullary device, the proximal femoral locking plates (PFLP) has the advantage of angular stable fixation, and it can preserve more bone stock. The PFLP

* Correspondence: zhaojianning.0207@163.com
[2]Department of Orthopaedics, Jinling Clinical Medical College, Nanjing Medical University, Nanjing, Jiangsu, China
[3]Department of Orthopaedics, Jinling Hospital, Nanjing Medical University, No. 305, Zhongshan East Road, Nanjing 210002, Jiangsu, China
Full list of author information is available at the end of the article

Table 1 Perioperative variables plate

	Included (n = 95 patients/97 fractures)		
	n (%)	Mean (±SD)	Range
Number of patients	95		
Number of fractures	97		
Age (years)*		66.8 ± 14.7	32–92
< 60*	21 (22)		
60 or older*	74 (78)		
Gender*			
Male*	58 (61)		
Female*	37 (39)		
Mechanism of injury			
Ground level fall*	64 (67)		
Fall from a height*	22 (23)		
Traffic accident*	9 (10)		
AO fracture types†			
A1.1†	4 (4)		
A1.2†	15 (15)		
A1.3†	4 (4)		
A2.1†	18 (19)		
A2.2†	17 (18)		
A2.3†	7 (7)		
A3.1†	2 (2)		
A3.2†	3 (3)		
A3.3†	27 (29)		
Laterality†			
Left†	46 (47)		
Right†	51 (53)		
Time from fracture to surgery (days)		4.3 ± 2.1	1–11
Total incision length (cm)		16.6 ± 3.1	12–30
Operative time (min)		131.5 ± 38.9	60–230
Blood loss (ml)		477.7 ± 202.5	200–1500
Total failure of fractures†	35 (36)		
Breakage of implant†	4 (4)		
Loosening of proximal screw†	21 (22)		
Varus deformity†	34 (35)		
Nonunion†	7 (7)		
Reoperation†	6 (6)		

Quantitative data were presented as mean (SD)
*For included patients, values based on number of patients (n = 61 no failure, n = 34 failure)
†Values based on number of fractures (n = 62 no failure, n = 35 failure)

Table 2 Perioperative data in relation to fracture type

	Stable A1.1-A2.1	Unstable A2.2-A3.3	Total	p value
Number of fractures	41 (42%)	56 (58%)	97	
Mean operative time (min)	117 (39)	129 (35)	125 (37)	0.172*
Mean intraoperative blood loss (ml)	403 (101)	508 (218)	466 (187)	0.014*
Mean operative incision length (cm)	16 (2.1)	17 (3.4)	16.6 (3)	0.108*

Quantitative data were presented as mean (SD)
*Analyzed using a one-way ANOVA

attention to the higher than expected failure rates of PFLPs [11, 16, 17]. Unfortunately, few clinical data of case series are available to evaluate the use of PFLPs. The purpose of this study was to retrospectively report our previous results for trochanteric fractures treated with PFLPs and to analyze the underlying mechanisms as well as possible risk factors associated with the high failure rate of this technique.

Methods

Ethics statement

All clinical records and radiological data for this retrospective cohort study were approved by the ethics committee. Informed consent was obtained from all the patients.

Patient population and data collection

From January 2010 to October 2014, 273 consecutive patients with trochanteric femoral fractures who received a PFLP (5.0/6.0 Shanghai PuWei Medical Device Factory Co.) in our institutional orthopedic trauma center were identified. The inclusion criteria were the presence of pertrochanteric, intertrochanteric, or subtrochanteric fractures. Patients with pathological fractures (other than osteoporosis), previous fractures, open fractures, combined fractures

Table 3 Postoperative mechanical failure in relation to fracture type

	Included (n = 95 patients/97 fractures)			p value
	Stable* n (%)	Unstable* n (%)	Total* n (%)	
Number of fractures	41 (42)	56 (58)	97 (100)	
Nonunion	0 (0)	7 (12.5)	7 (7.2)	0.02†
Breakage of implant	0 (0)	4 (7.1)	4 (4.1)	0.135†
Varus deformity	6 (14.6)	28 (50)	34 (35)	0.001†
Loosening of proximal screw	4 (9.7)	17 (30.3)	21 (21.6)	0.023†
Total failure rate	7 (17)	28 (50)	35 (36)	

*Values based on number of fractures (n = 62 no failure, n = 35 failure)
†Analyzed using an x^2 test (continuity correction)

is considered an alternative fixation method for most complex proximal femoral fractures and even led to excellent results for management of unstable fractures [9, 10, 14, 15]. However, some studies have drawn

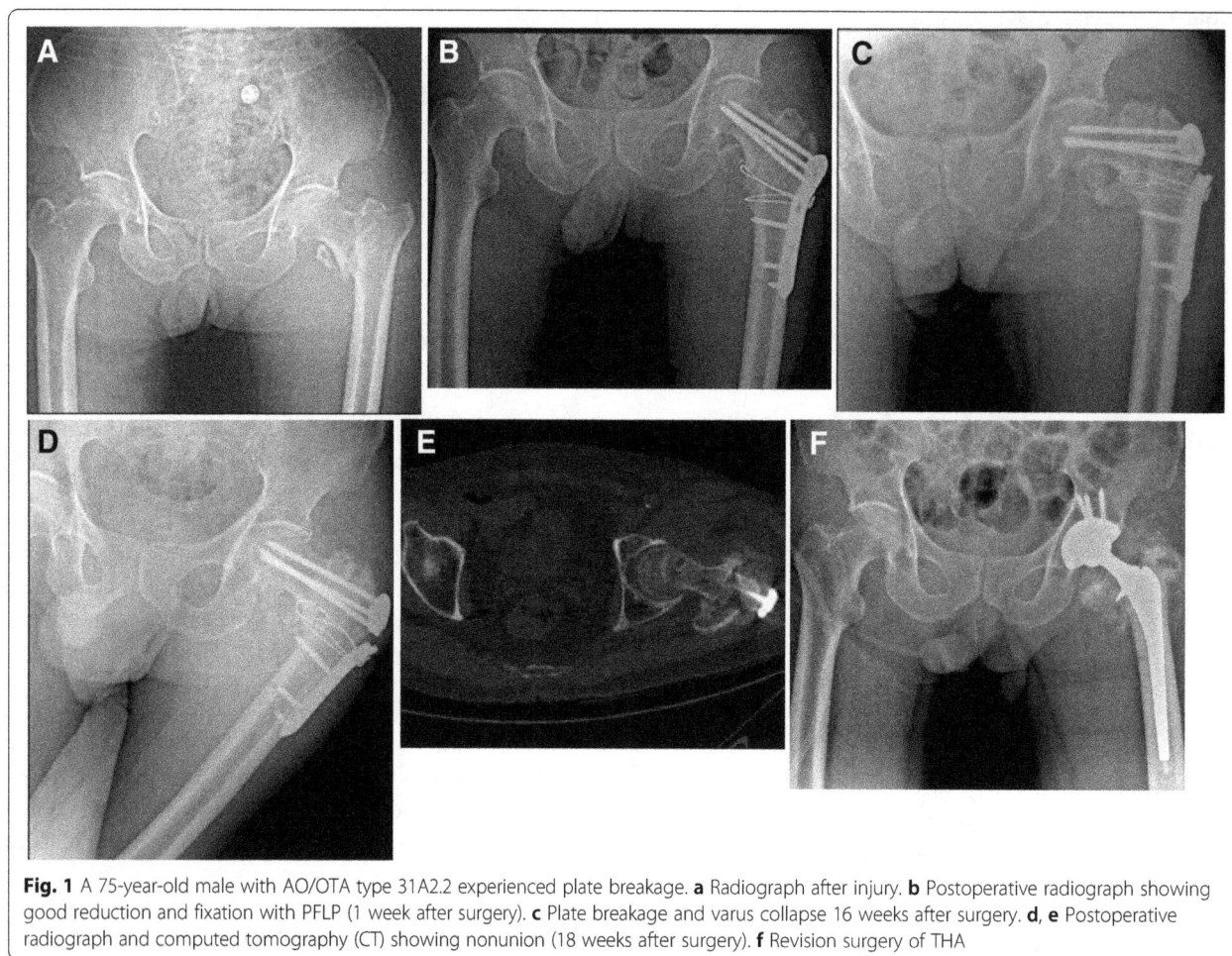

Fig. 1 A 75-year-old male with AO/OTA type 31A2.2 experienced plate breakage. **a** Radiograph after injury. **b** Postoperative radiograph showing good reduction and fixation with PFLP (1 week after surgery). **c** Plate breakage and varus collapse 16 weeks after surgery. **d, e** Postoperative radiograph and computed tomography (CT) showing nonunion (18 weeks after surgery). **f** Revision surgery of THA

on the ipsilateral side; patients with less than 12 months of follow-up; and patients with consecutive postoperative radiograph were excluded from this study.

All operations were performed by experienced surgeons who received training for using PFLPs. This plate has three proximal holes angled at 115° for 6.0 mm locking screw fixation into the femoral neck and head, and the remaining distal holes were inserted with either 4.5 mm nonlocking cortex screws or 5.0 mm locking screws to obtain femoral shaft fixation. Generally, a lateral subvastus approach to the proximal femur for open reduction and internal fixation was used for all cases. After the operation, partial and progressive weight bearing was encouraged based on how the callus formed on the radiograph.

Clinical data collected included patient age, gender, laterality, mechanism of injury, fracture pattern, time from fracture to surgery, total incision length, operation time, blood loss, revision procedure, and other data. Fractures were classified according to the AO/OTA (Orthopaedic Trauma Association) classification system. The stable fracture was defined as type of AO/OTA 31

A1 and A2.1, and the unstable fracture was defined as type of AO/OTA 31 A2.2, A2.3 and A3. The first postoperative radiograph and each follow-up anteroposterior and lateral radiographs were reviewed to assess fracture type, reduction status, screw position, neck-shaft angle, callus formation, and device failure.

Mechanical failure was defined as breakage of the implant, loosening of the proximal screw, varus deformity of the fracture, secondary loss of reduction, and shortening of the femoral neck. Additionally, nonunion and reoperations were quantified. Bone union was defined as the disappearance of the fracture line or radiological evidence of callus formation with no tenderness.

Statistical methods

All data were analyzed using SPSS 19.0 software. Chi-squared tests (continuity correction or linear-by-linear association) were used for comparison of categorical variables. Continuous variables were compared using an independent t test and one-way ANOVA. The difference between the groups was considered to be statistically significant when $p < 0.05$ in a two-sided test.

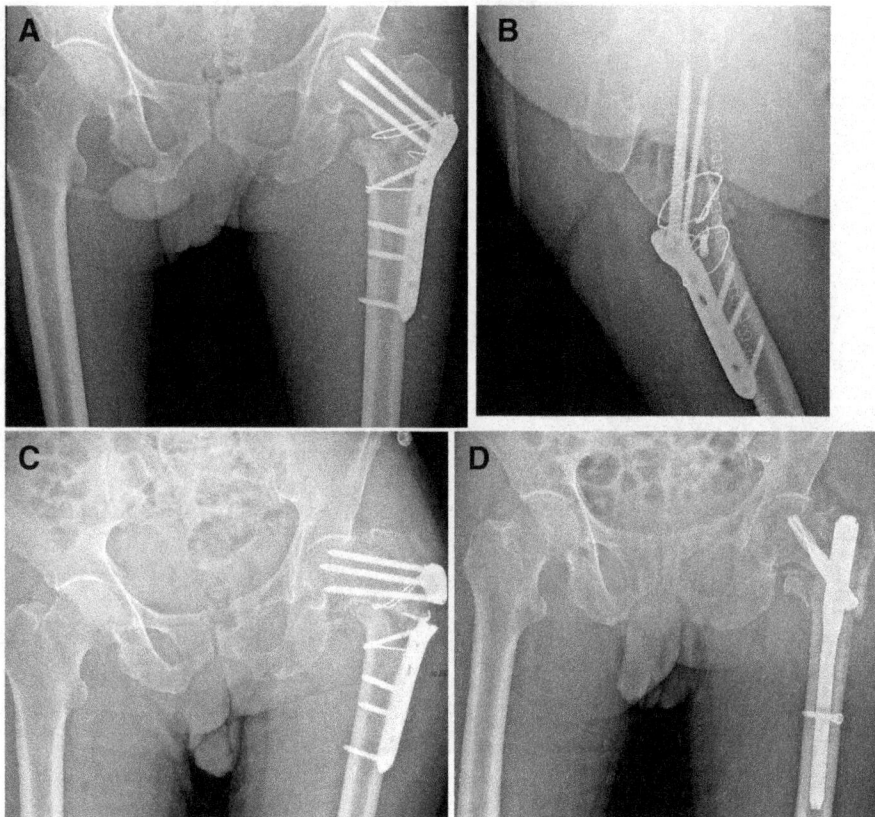

Fig. 2 A 78-year-old male with AO/OTA type 31A3.3 experienced plate breakage. **a, b** Postoperative anterio-posterior and lateral radiographs. **c** Plate breakage and varus collapse 10 weeks after surgery. **d** Postoperative radiograph of revision surgery of PFNA

Results

A total of 95 patients (58 males, 37 females; mean age 66.8 years, range 32–92 years) met the inclusion criteria and ultimately served as the reviewed study group. The causes of injury included a ground-level slip in 64 patients (67%), fall from a height in 22 patients (23%), and traffic accident in 9 patients (10%). Of these 95 patients, 2 patients had bilateral side trochanteric fractures, which resulted in 97 fractures that were classified as AO types (31 A1.1 = 4, A1.2 = 15, A1.3 = 4, A2.1 = 18, A2.2 = 17, A2.3 = 7, A3.1 = 2, A3.2 = 3, A3.3 = 27) (Table 1). Of the 97 fractures, 51 (53%) fractures involved the right side, and 46 (47%) fractures involved the left side. The mean time from fracture to surgery was 4.3 days (range 1–11). The mean total incision length was 16.6 cm (range 12–30). The mean operation time (from the beginning of the skin incision to the closure of wound) was 131.5 min (range 60–230), and the mean blood loss was 477.7 ml (range 200–1500) (Table 1).

Of the 95 patients (97 fractures) in this study, 21 (22%) patients were younger than 60 years old, and 74 (78%) patients were 60 years old or older. The stable group had less blood loss compared to the unstable group (403 ± 101 vs. 508 ± 218 ml; $p = 0.014$), while the

mean incision length and the operation time between two groups had no statistically significant difference ($p > 0.05$). The variables of the two groups are shown in Table 2.

Among 95 patients (97 fractures), 34 patients (35 fractures) suffered operation failure, which ultimately presented a high failure rate of 36%. The complications in this study included nonunion in 7 (7.2%) fractures, implant breakage in 4 (4.1%) fractures, varus deformity in 34 (35%) fractures, and loosening of proximal femoral screw in 21 (21.6%) fractures (Table 3; Figs. 1, 2, 3, 4, and 5).

In the 97 fractures included in this study, 41 (42%) were stable type fractures and 56 (58%) were unstable type fractures. The failure rates in relation to fractures types among groups of A1, A2, and A3 fractures were 13%, 38%, and 50%, respectively. The failure rates for nonunion implant breakage, varus deformity, and screw loosening in the stable group were 0%, 0%, 14.6%, and 9.7%, respectively, and the failure rates for patients in the unstable groups were 12.5%, 7.1%, 50%, and 30.3%, respectively. The total failure rate in the stable group was 17% compared to 50% in the unstable group (Table 3).

The total failure rates and the rates of nonunion, implant breakage, varus deformity, and screw loosening in

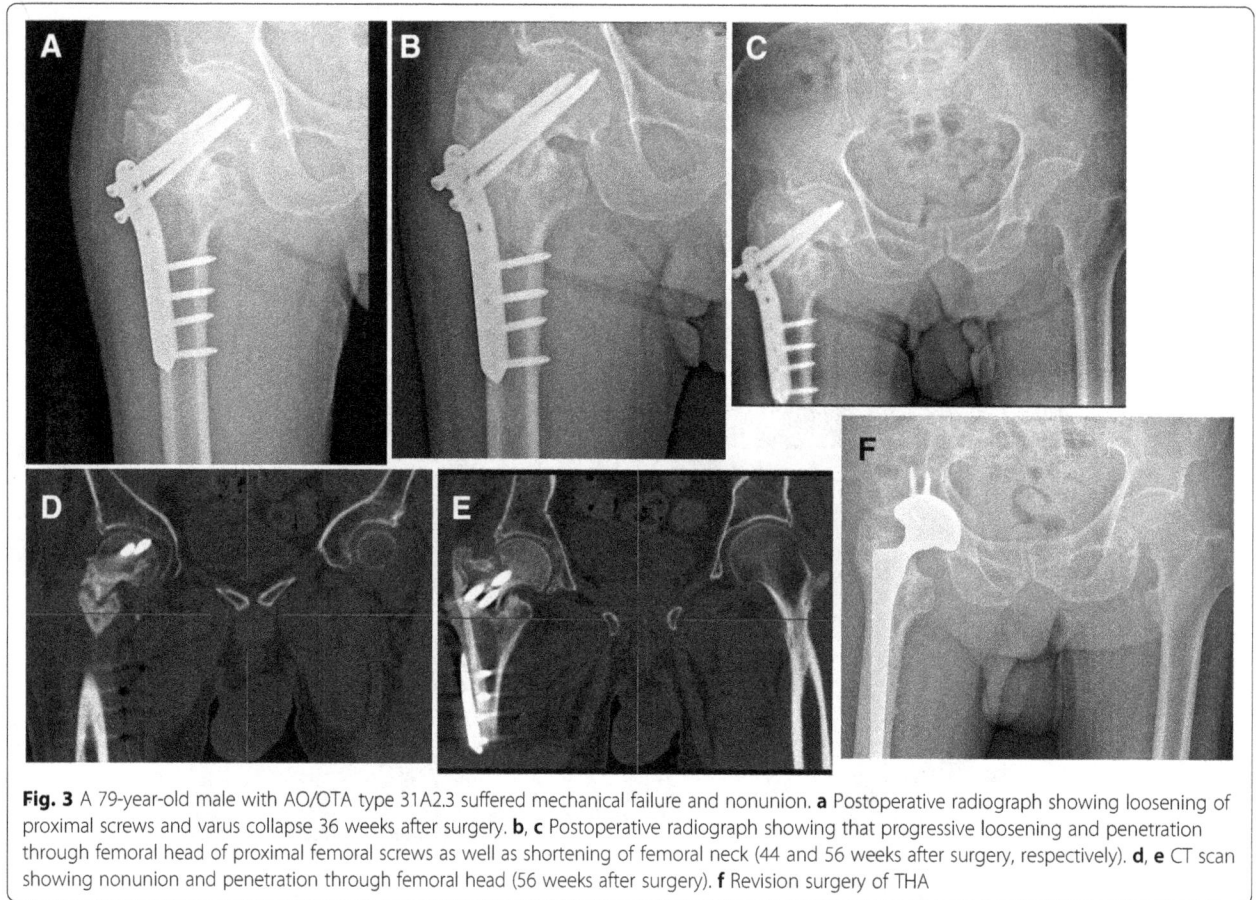

Fig. 3 A 79-year-old male with AO/OTA type 31A2.3 suffered mechanical failure and nonunion. **a** Postoperative radiograph showing loosening of proximal screws and varus collapse 36 weeks after surgery. **b**, **c** Postoperative radiograph showing that progressive loosening and penetration through femoral head of proximal femoral screws as well as shortening of femoral neck (44 and 56 weeks after surgery, respectively). **d**, **e** CT scan showing nonunion and penetration through femoral head (56 weeks after surgery). **f** Revision surgery of THA

patients older than 60 years old were significantly higher compared to patients less than 60 years old (44.5% vs. 9.5%; 9.5% vs. 0%; 5.4% vs. 0%; 43% vs. 9.5% and 27% vs. 0.5%, respectively). The variables for the two groups are shown in Table 4. Furthermore, the failure rate of PFLP in patients older than 60 years old with unstable fracture types was 60.5% (Table 5).

Six patients received revision operations, including reoperation with total hip arthroplasty (THA) in three patients, fixation of the PFNA in two patients, and a Gamma-nail procedure in one patient (Table 6).

Discussion

As an alternative implant for extramedullary devices, PFLP has become increasingly popular due to its advantage in proximal multiple angle-stable screws, which can enhance proximal femoral fixation and preserve more bone stock by leaving a smaller "footprint" after placement than other extramedullary plates with large proximal screws [18]. Furthermore, previous studies have shown that PFLP presented with equivalent biomechanical properties as other angularly stable implants or intramedullary nails [19–21]. Owing to biomechanical peculiarities, PFLP fixation has been recommended for fixation of complex proximal femoral fractures,

such as osteoporotic, comminuted, or unstable fractures as well as for revision fixation [22]. A series of studies have reported that the fixation with PFLP in cases of unstable trochanteric fractures can achieve satisfying radiological and clinical results with a higher union rate and fewer complications [9, 23]. Naiyer et al. demonstrated that for 25 patients with unstable intertrochanteric fractures treated with a proximal femoral locking compression plate, the failure rate was 16%, which was lower than the failure rate of 51% in the DHS group of 35 patients with the same type of fracture. However, recent studies have paid attention to the higher failure rate of PFLPs, especially in cases with unstable trochanteric fractures. Philipp et al. reported that in patients with unstable 31 A3 trochanteric fractures treated with a PFLP, incidences of reoperation (25%), mechanical failure (38%), and nonunion (19%) were observed whereas these percentages were 5%, 5%, and 5% in patients treated with cephalomedullary nailing (CMN) [12]. Similarly, Streubel et al. reported a total failure rate of 33% at the 12-month follow-up point in the presence of varus collapse with proximal screw loosening, screw "cutout," screw breakage, and plate fracture. Additionally, Wirtz et al. demonstrated the early results of PFLPs in the management of 19 patients with stable and unstable trochanteric fractures,

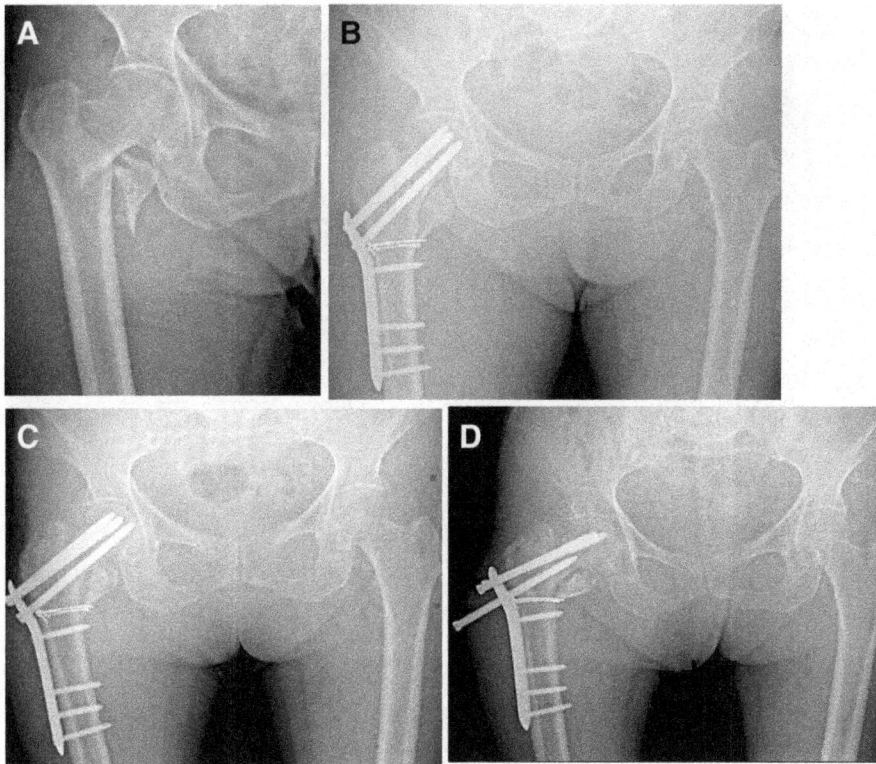

Fig. 4 A 81-year-old female with AO/OTA type 31A2.1 experienced loosening of proximal screws. **a** Radiograph after injury. **b** Postoperative radiograph showing good reduction and fixation (1 week after surgery). **c** Ten weeks postoperative radiograph showing loosening of proximal femoral screws, loss of reduction and varus collapse. **d** Progressive loss of reduction, screws loosening and varus collapse (24 weeks after surgery)

and 8 (42%) revision surgeries were required, including reosteosynthesis and THA because of secondary loss of reduction or implant removal [17].

In the present study, the cumulative failure rates of mechanical failure and nonunion in a consecutive cohort of patients with trochanteric fractures (AO/OTA type 31A1-A3) treated with PFLP, were reported. Furthermore, difference in intraoperative data, postoperative complications, and reoperations in relation to the patient's age and fracture types were analyzed to investigate the possible risk factors and underlying mechanisms associated with high failure rates when using this technique.

The overall failure rate was proximally 36% in 95 patients with 97 fractures after 12 months of follow-up. There was no difference in the number of complications according to gender and injury mechanism. The most frequent failure was varus deformity with a 35% failure rate, followed by loosening of the proximal screw with a failure rate of 22%. Based on prior studies and our present results, several factors seem to have played an important role in relation to high failure rates. First, the age of the patients may influence surgical outcomes. In the present study, the failure rate in patients 60 years old or older was 44.5%, which was significantly higher

than the 9.5% of patients who were younger than 60 years old. Among these observed failures, varus deformity (43%) and loosening of proximal screw (27%) in the elderly group were more likely to occur, which was probably due to the weakness of holding power resulting from poor bone quality especially in elderly patients with osteoporosis. Second, the type of fracture also make a great contribution to the failure. In our study, the failure rates among the groups with A1, A2, and A3 fractures were 13%, 38%, and 50%, respectively. The failure rate in the unstable group reached up to 50%, which was markedly higher than the 17% failure rate in the stable group. Additionally, in patients older than 60 years old with unstable fractures, the failure rate was as high as 60.5%, which was sufficient to suggest that the older patients who suffered unstable trochanteric fractures seemed to be the most important factor leading to a high failure rate. Third, the surgical technique, such as appropriate reduction and accurate placement of proximal screws as well as using a minimally invasive technique is also beneficial for reducing the incidence of failure. Ihab et al. compared the intraoperative differences and clinical outcomes between direct (open) reduction and indirect (biological) reduction groups with trochanteric fractures, and patients in the open group had a greater blood loss,

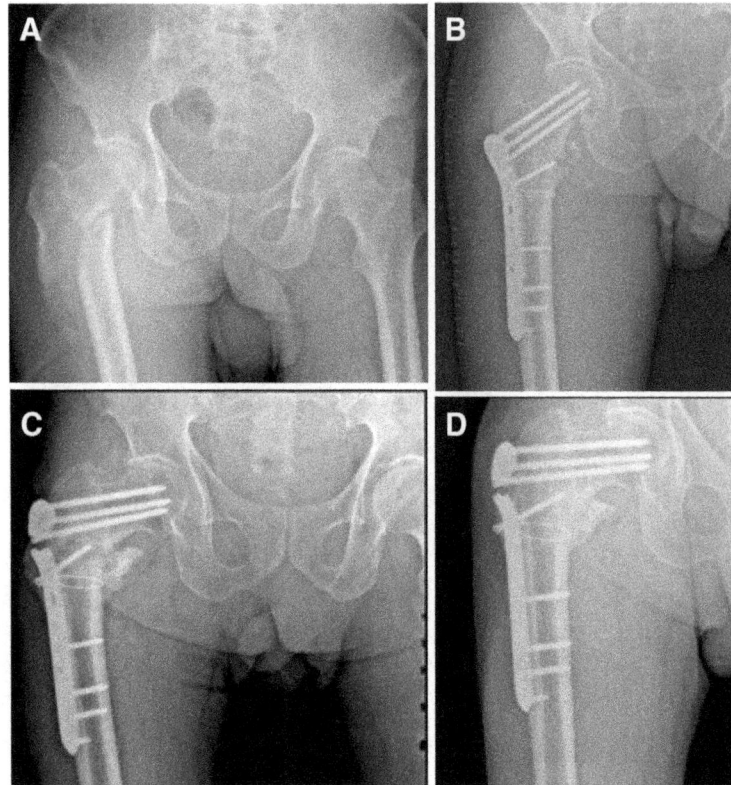

Fig. 5 A 71-year-old male with AO/OTA type 31A3.3 experienced plate breakage. **a** Radiograph after injury. **b** Postoperative radiograph showing good reduction and fixation with PFLP (1 week after surgery). **c** Plate breakage and varus collapse 36 weeks after surgery. **d** Seventy-two weeks postoperative radiograph showing malunion and varus deformity

longer operation time, and incision lengths. However, there was no difference in the healing rate or functional outcomes. In addition, closed reduction of unstable comminuted trochanteric fractures made it difficult to maintain sufficient reduction of the postero-medial region, which was one of the keys to avoiding mechanical failure. Although increasing clinical and biomechanical research has addressed the importance of the posteromedial buttress of the proximal femur, the results of other studies suggested that there was no robust evidence to confirm that the lower failure rate was associated with sufficient anatomical reduction of the medial buttress [10, 12, 17, 19, 24]. Similar results were observed in our studies in which most failure cases achieved good reduction of the medial buttress. However, in the present study, the mean intraoperative blood loss was statistically significantly lower in the stable group ($p = 0.014$). Furthermore, factors such as accurate placement of proximal screws and their appropriate position in the femoral head might also

Table 4 Mechanical failure rate in relation to age of patients

	Age less than 60	60 or older	Total
Number of patients	21 (22%)	74 (78%)	95 (100%)
Number of patients with failure (%)	2 (9.5)	33 (44.5)	35
Nonunion (%)†	0 (0)	7 (9.5)	7
Breakage of implant (%)†	0 (0)	4 (5.4)	4
Varus deformity (%)†	2 (9.5)	32 (43)	34
Loosening of proximal screw (%)†	1 (0.5)	20 (27)	21

†Values based on number of patients with fractures (n = 21 less than 60 years, n = 74 more than 60 years)

Table 5 Failure rates and reoperation in patients older than 60 years with unstable fracture types

Variables	Value (n)	Percentage (%)
Patients older than 60 years with unstable fractures	43	100%
Number of patients with failure	26	60.5%
Nonunion†	6	13.9%
Breakage of implant†	4	9.3%
Varus deformity (%)†	26	60.5%
Loosening of proximal screw †	16	37.3%
Number of reoperation	6	13.9%

Table 6 Data of reoperation cases

Case	Gender	Age (years)	Fracture type	Failure mode	Revision
1	M	61	A2.2	Severe varus collapse	THA
2	M	79	A2.3	Varus collapse, screw loosening, nonunion	THA
3	M	75	A2.2	Nonunion, breakage of implant	THA
4	M	78	A3.3	Nonunion, breakage of implant	PFNA
5	M	75	A3.3	Varus collapse, screw loosening, nonunion	PFNA
6	F	69	A3.3	Severe varus collapse, screw loosening;	Gamma-nail

contribute to enhancing the construct strength [12]. Previous biomechanical studies have shown that a screw deviation of 2° or more from the nominal locking axis angulations with the plate would significantly reduce the stiffness and fixation stability of the screw-plate constructs, resulting in early screw loosening, progressive varus of the fracture, and even implant breakage. Therefore, accurate placement of the proximal femoral locking screws was crucial for maintaining the stable and stiff biomechanical peculiarity of this device. Finally, the design features of PFLP affect the clinical effectiveness. It was generally acknowledged that the integrity of the lateral trochanteric wall was an important factor for maintaining the stability of the proximal femoral fractures and could greatly decrease the rate of malunion or nonunion. The locking screws of the PFLP could hold all the major proximal femoral fragments due to the angular and stable design. Therefore, several studies had suggested that it was useful to apply PFLP for treating trochanteric fractures of AO/OTA type 31A3, which was usually represented by comminuted fractures of the lateral wall that might lead to surgical failure due to secondary fracture or displacement of the proximal lateral fragments when using intramedullary nails or DHS. However, other studies had claimed that the weakness of high concentrations of stress at the junction of the PFLP and the proximal locking screws, as well as the small number and size of the proximal screws, was insufficient to resist cyclic axial or torsion loading and provide stable fixation to the proximal fragment, which likely resulted in hardware failure [24]. In order to reduce the risk of mechanical failure, avoiding early weight-bearing after treatment with PFLP was recommended by many researchers. In addition, increasing the size of the screws and providing a poly-axial position for the proximal locking screws might provide more stability for the proximal fragment [17].

There are several limitations to this study, including the lack of a control group treated with other methods such as PFNA, DHS, or percutaneous compression plate

(PCCP) fixation. Another drawback is the relatively small number of cases. Our group of patients ($n = 95$) may be small to achieve sufficient statistical relevance. To the best of our knowledge, however, to date, it seems to be one of the largest groups with clinical data on the results of fixation with a PFLP. In addition, this study did not include long-term follow-up of functional outcomes. Further studies should focus on the investigation of functional results from the PFLP and compare them to PFNA.

Conclusions

Our study revealed that PFLP resulted in high failure rate of trochanteric fractures, especially in patients older than 60 years old with unstable fracture types. PFLP was not an appropriate treatment for trochanteric fractures. However, we can still use it in stable trochanteric fractures with only two fragments. Advanced age and an unstable fracture type were major risk factors for the unsatisfactory outcomes of PFLP fixation.

Abbreviations
CMN: Cephalomedullary nailing; DCS: Dynamic condylar screw; DHS: Dynamic hip screw; PCCP: Percutaneous compression plate; PFLP: Proximal femoral locking plates; PFNA: Proximal femoral nail anti-rotation

Funding
This work was supported by the Clinical Science and Technology Project Foundation of Jiangsu Province (BL2012002), the Scientific Research Project of Nanjing Province (201402007), and the Natural Science Foundation of Jiangsu Province (BK20161385).

Authors' contributions
JZ designed the study. SH designed the study and wrote the manuscript. JZ was responsible for the data collection and analysis. XH and BY were responsible for follow-up. All authors read and approved the final manuscript.

Competing interests
The authors declare that they have no competing interests.

Author details
[1]Department of Orthopaedics, Taixing People's Hospital, Taixing, Jiangsu, People's Republic of China. [2]Department of Orthopaedics, Jinling Clinical Medical College, Nanjing Medical University, Nanjing, Jiangsu, China. [3]Department of Orthopaedics, Jinling Hospital, Nanjing Medical University, No. 305, Zhongshan East Road, Nanjing 210002, Jiangsu, China.

References

1. Shen J, Luo F, Sun D, Huang Q, Xu J, Dong S, Xie Z. Mid-term results after treatment of intertrochanteric femoral fractures with percutaneous compression plate (PCCP). Injury. 2015;46:347–57.
2. Miyamoto RG, Kaplan KM, Levine BR, Egol KA, Zuckerman JD. Surgical management of hip fractures: an evidence-based review of the literature. I: femoral neck fractures. J Am Acad Orthop Surg. 2008;16:596–607.
3. Kaplan K, Miyamoto R, Levine BR, Egol KA, Zuckerman JD. Surgical management of hip fractures: an evidence-based review of the literature. II: intertrochanteric fractures. J Am Acad Orthop Surg. 2008;16:665–73.
4. Shoda E. Hip fracture - epidemiology, management and liaison service. Surgical treatment of femoral proximal fracture. Clin Calcium. 2015;25:565–75.
5. Hou Z, Shi J, Ye H, Pan Z. Treatment of unstable intertrochanteric fractures with percutaneous non-contact bridging plates. Int J Surg. 2014;12:538–43.
6. Haidukewych GJ. Intertrochanteric fractures: ten tips to improve results. J Bone Joint Surg (Am Vol). 2009;91:712–9.
7. Anglen JO, Weinstein JN. Nail or plate fixation of intertrochanteric hip fractures: changing pattern of practice. A review of the American Board of Orthopaedic Surgery Database. J Bone Joint Surg (Am Vol). 2008;90:700–7.
8. Calderón A, Ramos T, Vilchez F, Mendoza-Lemus O, Peña V, Cárdenas-Estrada E, Acosta-Olivo C. Proximal femoral intramedullary nail versus DHS plate for the treatment of intertrochanteric fractures. A prospective analysis. Acta Ortop Mex. 2013;27:236–9.
9. Dhamangaonkar AC, Joshi D, Goregaonkar AB, Tawari AA. Proximal femoral locking plate versus dynamic hip screw for unstable intertrochanteric femoral fractures. J Orthop Surg (Hong Kong). 2013;21:317–22.
10. Asif N, Ahmad S, Qureshi OA, Jilani LZ, Hamesh T, Jameel T. Unstable intertrochanteric fracture fixation - is proximal femoral locked compression plate better than dynamic hip screw. J Clin Diagn Res. 2016;10:RC9–RC13.
11. Collinge CA, Hymes R, Archdeacon M, Streubel P, Obremskey W, Weber T, Watson JT, Lowenberg D, Members of the Proximal Femur Working Group of the Southeast Trauma Consortium. Unstable proximal femur fractures treated with proximal femoral locking plates: a retrospective, multicenter study of 111 cases. J Orthop Trauma. 2016;30:489–95.
12. Streubel PN, Moustoukas MJ, Obremskey WT. Mechanical failure after locking plate fixation of unstable intertrochanteric femur fractures. J Orthop Trauma. 2013;27:22–8.
13. Schneiderab K, Ohc J-K, Zderica I, Stoffelde K, Richardsa RG, Wolff S, Gueorguieva B, Norkg SE. What is the underlying mechanism for the failure mode observed in the proximal femoral locking compression plate? A biomechanical study. Injury. 2015;46:1483–90.
14. Hu S, Zhang S, Yu G. Treatment of femoral subtrochanteric fractures with proximal lateral femur locking plates. Acta Ortopédica Brasileira. 2012;20:329–33.
15. Kumar N, Kataria H, Yadav C, Gadagoli BS, Raj R. Evaluation of proximal femoral locking plate in unstable extracapsular proximal femoral fractures: surgical technique & mid term follow up results. J Clin Orthop Trauma. 2014;5:137–45.
16. Floyd MW, France JC, Hubbard DF. Early experience with the proximal femoral locking plate. Orthopedics. 2013;36:1488–94.
17. Wirtz C, Abbassi F, Evangelopoulos DS, Kohl S, Siebenrock KA, Krüger A. High failure rate of trochanteric fracture osteosynthesis with proximal femoral locking compression plate. Injury-Int J Care Injured. 2013;44:751–6.
18. Streubel P, Moustoukas M, Obremskey W. Locked plating versus cephalomedullary nailing of unstable intertrochanteric femur fractures. Eur J Orthop Surg Traumatol. 2016;26:385–90.
19. Floyd JC, O'Toole RV, Stall A, Forward DP, Nabili M, Shillingburg D, Hsieh A, Nascone JW. Biomechanical comparison of proximal locking plates and blade plates for the treatment of comminuted subtrochanteric femoral fractures. J Orthop Trauma. 2009;23:628–33.
20. Lee PY, Lin KJ, Wei HW, Hu JJ, Chen WC, Tsai CL, Lin KP. Biomechanical effect of different femoral neck blade position on the fixation of intertrochanteric fracture: a finite element analysis. Biomed Tech (Berl). 2016;61:331–6.
21. Jiang W, Liu Y, Yang L, Xu W, Liu S, Zhang D, Chen X, Wang H. Biomechanical comparative study on proximal femoral locking plate and Gamma3 for treatment of stable intertrochanteric fracture. Zhongguo xiu fu chong jian wai ke za zhi = Zhongguo xiufu chongjian waike zazhi = Chinese journal of reparative and reconstructive surgery. 2014;28:1096–9.
22. Pountos I, Giannoudis PV. The management of intertrochanteric hip fractures. Orthop Trauma. 2016;30:103–8.
23. Sasnur PA: Surgical outcome of proximal femoral fractures using proximal femoral - locking compression plate. 2015.
24. Wieser K, Babst R. Fixation failure of the LCP proximal femoral plate 4.5/5.0 in patients with missing posteromedial support in unstable per-, inter-, and subtrochanteric fractures of the proximal femur. Arch Orthop Trauma Surg. 2010;130:1281–7.

30

Is minimally invasive superior than open transforaminal lumbar interbody fusion for single-level degenerative lumbar diseases: a meta-analysis

Aimin Li*, Xiang Li and Yang Zhong

Abstract

Background: In recent years, the minimally invasive transforaminal lumbar interbody fusion (MI-TLIF) is increasingly used to manage the lumbar degenerative disease. However, whether MI-TLIF was superior than open transforaminal lumbar interbody fusion (O-TLIF) was controversial. The aim of this meta-analysis was to compare the clinical outcomes between the MI-TLIF and O-TLIF in single-level degenerative lumbar diseases.

Methods: Two reviewers independently searched EMBASE, PubMed, Web of Science, and Google database from inception to February 2018 for studies comparing the MI-TLIF and O-TLIF approach for single-level lumbar degenerative disease. The data were extracted and analyzed for primary outcomes such as total blood loss, visual analog score (VAS), and other secondary outcomes (length of hospital stay, operation time, fluroscopic time, and Oswestry Disability Index (ODI)). Meta-analysis was performed by Stata 12.0.

Results: Seven RCTs were finally included in this meta-analysis. Compared with O-TLIF, MI-TLIF was associated with significantly less blood loss (weighted mean difference (WMD) = − 291.46; 95% confidence interval (CI) − 366.66 to − 216.47; $P = 0.000$,). There was no significant difference between the length of hospital stay, postoperative VAS, and ODI. Compared with O-TLIF, MI-TLIF was associated with an increase of the fluroscopic time ($P < 0.05$).

Conclusion: The MI-TLIF showed significantly less blood loss compared with O-TLIF and more fluroscopic time. There was no significant difference between the length of hospital stay, postoperative VAS, and ODI. More high-quality studies and subsequent meta-analyses are needed in the future.

Keywords: Single-level, Degenerative lumbar disease, Transforaminal lumbar interbody fusion, Minimally invasive

Background

Minimally invasive transforaminal lumbar interbody fusion (MI-TLIF) was first introduced by Harms and Rolinger in the year of 1982 [1]. MI-TLIF has been used increasingly in lumbar degenerative diseases for decades based on the shorter length of hospital stay and blood loss than open TLIF (O-TLIF) [2–4]. O-TLIF requires wide dissection of the sacral spinalis, which causes severe soft tissue injuries and more perioperative blood loss [5].

O-TLIF was also associated with residual back pain for some patients after surgery [6, 7]. As a new technique, MI-TLIF exposes spinal joints and transverse processes directly through the space between sacrospinous muscles. Several studies show that MI-TLIF could reduce the injury of the iatrogenic soft tissue caused by muscle stripping and traction in surgery [8]. However, the MI-TLIF has some drawbacks. During the minimally invasive procedure, only one side of the articular process was removed. For patients with severe spinal stenosis, the central tube decompression could not be performed.

All of what mentioned above limited the application of this technique in such patients. The potential benefits of MI-TLIF versus O-TLIF for single-level lumbar degenerative diseases remain controversial.

* Correspondence: chengzou07@sina.com
Department of Orthopedics, The 5th Central Hospital of Tianjin, Tianjin 30000, People's Republic of China

The aim of the current meta-analysis was to assess the efficacy and safety of O-TLIF and MI-TLIF for single-level degenerative lumbar diseases in terms of total blood loss, the length of hospital stay, operation time, postoperative visual analog scale (VAS), and Oswestry Disability Index (ODI).

Methods

This study was undertaken in accordance with the Preferred Reporting Items for Systematic Reviews and Meta-Analyses (PRISMA) statement [9]. Ethical approval and written informed consent from patients were not necessary because our study was based on summaries and analyses of results of existing studies.

Search strategy

Two reviewers (Aimin Li and Yang Zhong) independently searched the EMBASE, PubMed, Web of Science, and Google database from inception to February 2018. Search core terms included "transforaminal lumbar interbody fusion," "TLIF," "minimally invasive spine surgery," "MIS," "minimally invasive," and "clinical outcome." We searched with the restricted language of English and only included articles published in the English language. Two reviewers (Aimin Li and Xiang Li) also manually searched the references of each retrieved papers for additional studies.

Study selection

A study was considered qualified for inclusion if studies were randomized controlled trials (RCTs) or no-RCT study, comparing MI-TLIF with O-TLIF for single-level degenerative lumbar diseases. And all studies reported data for at least one of the following index: total blood loss, length of hospital stay, operation time, fluroscopic time, postoperative VAS, and ODI.

Following studies were excluded from the meta-analysis: conference abstracts; unpublished studies; case report; studies not suitable with the inclusive criteria; duplicated reports; multi-level lumbar degenerative disease samples; samples of fracture, infection, tumor, or postoperative recurrence; and samples of severe osteoporosis and other metabolic diseases.

Study selection

All potentially relevant studies were imported into Endnote Software (Version X7, Thompson Reuters, CA, USA) and duplicated studies were excluded. Then, the two researchers who had searched the databases excluded studies based on titles and abstracts. The two researchers read the full text of the remaining studies and excluded those that were not suitable with the inclusive criteria. Disagreements were solved by checking the articles and contacting related authors if required.

Data extraction

The following data were extracted by two researchers independently from the final eligible studies. Extracted information includes first author, publication year, country, study design, and numbers of cases and controls. Data were collected on the following primary outcomes: estimated blood loss and visual analog score. Data were also collected on the following secondary outcomes: operative time, length of hospital stay, or ODI.

Quality assessment

The quality of each included study was assessed on the basis of the Cochrane Handbook for Systematic Reviews of Interventions, version 5.1.0 (http://handbook.cochrane.org/) [10]. It included the following sections: random sequence generation, allocation concealment, blinding of participant and personnel, blinding of outcome assessment, incomplete outcome data, selective reporting, and other bias. Each domain was measured as low bias, unclear bias, or high bias. Diversities between assessments by the two reviewers were resolved by discussion.

Statistical analysis

The extracted outcomes from data could not be compared directly because the included studies were comprehensive. Outcomes for which sufficient, equivalent data were meta-analyzed using Forest plots generated with Stata 12.0. We analyzed continuous data using weighted mean differences (WMD) and their 95% confidence interval (CI), such as estimated blood loss, operative time, length of hospital stay, VAS, and ODI. Analyses were undertaken if at least three studies comparing the same outcome for MI-TLIF and O-TLIF could be combined. Each meta-analysis was done using all available searches. Pooled results were assessed for heterogeneity using the I^2 tests. Heterogeneity was defined as good when I^2 was between 0 and 25%; low, between 25.1 and 50%; moderate, between 50.1 and 75%; or high, between 75.1 and 100%. Fixed-effects meta-analysis was performed when $P \geq 0.1$ and $I^2 \leq 50\%$; otherwise, random-effects meta-analysis was performed. Sensitivity analysis was done for all outcomes to analyze the reason for the formation of heterogeneity. All statistical analyses were undertaken using Stata 12.0. Additional "leave-one-out" sensitivity analyses will be performed to explore whether the results were dominated by a single study, which was investigated by omitting one study at each turn and examining the influence

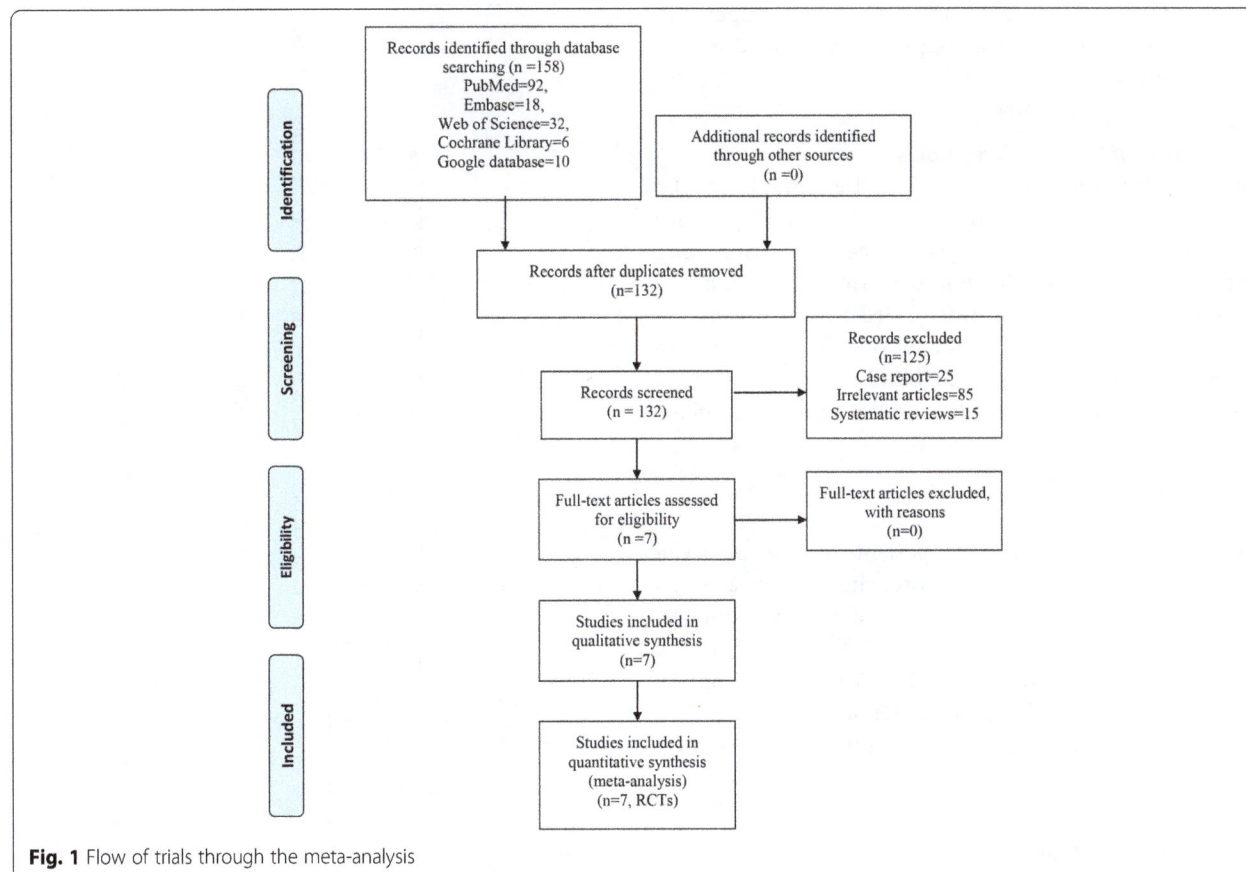

Fig. 1 Flow of trials through the meta-analysis

of each individual study on the final outcomes. Publication bias was performed by funnel plot and Begg's test. If the effect size was symmetrical and P value drawn from Begg's test was more than 0.05 indicated that there was no publication bias.

Results

Search results

After systematic search of the electronic databases, a total of 363 studies were identified, and no additional records were found during manual searches of review articles and relevant publications. After removing 244

duplicate studies using Endnote X7 (Version X7, Thompson Reuters, CA, USA), another 589 studies were excluded based on their titles and abstracts. The remaining 30 studies were read in full, and 20 were excluded because they failed to satisfy the selection criteria. In the end, 7 studies were included in this meta-analysis [11–17]. Flow of trials through the meta-analysis can be seen in Fig. 1.

General characteristics of the included studies

The general characteristics of the included studies are listed in Table 1. The publication year of the included

Table 1 The general characteristic of the included studies

Reference	Country	Mean age (years)	Sample size	Study type	Follow-up	O-TLIF	MI-TLIF
Singh et al. [11]	USA	51.67/49.85	33/33	RCTs	6 months	Midline incision	Unilateral approach
Kulkarni et al. [12]	India	51.55/50.40	36/25	RCTs	36.5 months	Posterior midline incision	Unilateral approach
Lee et al. [13]	Singapore	56.6/ 56.8	40/40	RCTs	24 months	NS	NS
Seng et al. [14]	Singapore	52.2/56.6	72/72	RCTs	60 months	Midline incision	Parasagittal incision
Serban et al. [15]	USA	51.3/ 50.1	24/23	RCTs	6 months	Midline skin	Parasagittal incision
Wang et al. [16]	China	56.4/ 54.2	42/39	RCTs	36.1 months	Midline open approach	NS
Wang et al. [17]	China	47.9/53.2	42/43	RCTs	26.3 months	Midline open approach	Unilateral approach

RCTs, randomized controlled trials, *MI-TLIF*, minimally invasive transforaminal lumbar interbody fusion, *O-TLIF*, open transforaminal lumbar interbody fusion, *NS* not stated

studies ranged from 2010 to 2017. The sample size ranged from 23 to 72. Follow-up duration ranged from 6 to 60 months.

Risk of bias of the included studies

Risk of bias summary and risk of bias graph can be seen in Figs. 2 and 3 respectively. Five studies performed proper random sequence generation, and the rest two studies did not perform proper random sequence generation and were listed as unclear risk of bias. Since these two operations could not be performed blinded, thus the blinding to the participants and personnel was all with unclear risk of bias.

	Random sequence generation (selection bias)	Allocation concealment (selection bias)	Blinding of participants and personnel (performance bias)	Blinding of outcome assessment (detection bias)	Incomplete outcome data (attrition bias)	Selective reporting (reporting bias)	Other bias
Kulkarni2016	+	?	?	?	+	+	+
Lee 2012	?	?	?	?	+	+	?
Seng 2013	+	?	?	?	+	+	–
Serban 2017	+	?	?	?	+	+	–
Singh 2014	?	?	?	?	+	+	+
Wang 2010	+	?	?	?	+	+	+
Wang 2014	+	?	?	?	+	+	+

Fig. 2 The risk of bias summary, +, no bias; –, bias; ?, bias unknown

Results of meta-analysis

Total blood loss

Seven studies including 532 patients investigated the total blood loss of two approaches. Meta-analysis showed that MI-TLIF was associated with a reduction of the total blood loss than O-TLIF (WMD = – 291.46; 95% CI – 366.66 to – 216.47; $P = 0.000$; Fig. 4). This meta-analysis involved a random-effects model because of high heterogeneity among the studies ($I^2 = 88.8\%$).

Length of hospital stay

Six studies including 522 patients reported data on the length of hospital stay. This meta-analysis showed that there was no significant difference between the MI-TLIF and O-TLIF in terms of the length of hospital stay (WMD = – 1.63, 95% CI – 3.76 to 0.49; $P = 0.132$; Fig. 5). Meta-analysis involved a random-effects model because of high heterogeneity among the studies ($I^2 = 99.2\%$).

Operating time

Six studies including 532 reported data on operating time. Meta-analysis result showed that there was no significant differences for operating time in MI-TLIF group and O-TLIF group (WMD = – 12.89, 95% CI – 44.53 to 18.76; $P = 0.425$; Fig. 6). This meta-analysis involved a random-effects model because of high heterogeneity among the studies ($I^2 = 97.6\%$).

Postoperative VAS score

Five studies involving 457 patients investigated the outcome of postoperative VAS. This meta-analysis showed that there was no significant difference between the postoperative VAS after MI-TLIF and O-TLIF (WMD = – 0.19, 95% CI – 0.63 to 0.25; $P =$ 0.389; Fig. 7). This meta-analysis involved a random-effects model because of high heterogeneity among the studies ($I^2 = 88.8\%$).

Postoperative ODI

Five studies investigated the outcome of postoperative ODI. This meta-analysis showed that there was no significant difference between the ODI between MI-TLIF and O-TLIF groups (WMD = 0.20, 95% CI – 1.18 to 1.58; $P = 0.778$; Fig. 8). This meta-analysis involved a random-effects model because of no significant heterogeneity among the studies ($I^2 =$ 50.2%).

Fluroscopic time

Three studies investigated the outcome of fluroscopic time. This meta-analysis showed that MI-TLIF was associated with an increase of the fluroscopic time than O-TLIF (WMD = 35.79, 95% CI 23.31 to 48.27; $P = 0.000$; Fig. 9). This meta-analysis involved a

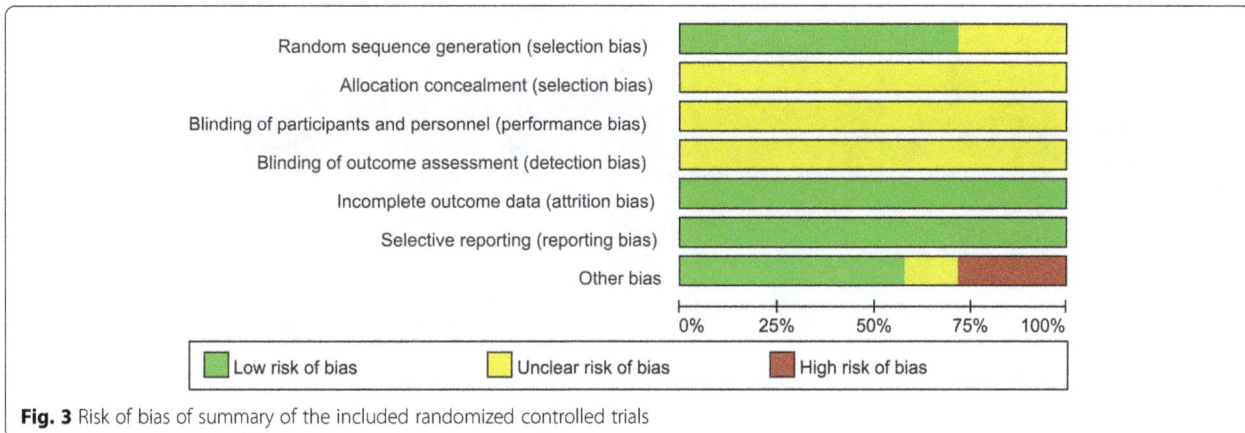

Fig. 3 Risk of bias of summary of the included randomized controlled trials

random-effects model because of no significant heterogeneity among the studies ($I^2 = 91.8\%$).

Sensitivity analysis and publication bias
Additional leave-one-out sensitivity analyses show that the overall effects were not altered and thus the results were relatively robust (Fig. 10). Publication bias was measured by funnel plot and the effects size was symmetrical; thus, there was no publication bias for total blood loss (Fig. 11). Then, Begg's test was performed and the *P* value was 0.985 indicating that there was no publication bias (Fig. 12).

Discussion
Main finding
Our meta-analysis comprehensively and systematically reviewed the current available literature and

found that (1) MI-TLIF have experienced less intra-operative blood loss than those in O-TLIF patients; (2) there was no significant difference between the length of hospital stay, operating time, postoperative ODI, and VAS; (3) and MI-TLIF was associated with an increase of the fluroscopic time than O-TLIF.

Comparison with other meta-analyses
Several meta-analyses on the topic have been published [18–20]. Although the main finding of our meta-analysis was consistent with previous meta-analyses, differences between ours and the previous ones should be noted. First, these previous meta-analyses included retrospective comparison studies and thus may cause large selection bias. In comparison, our current meta-analysis only included

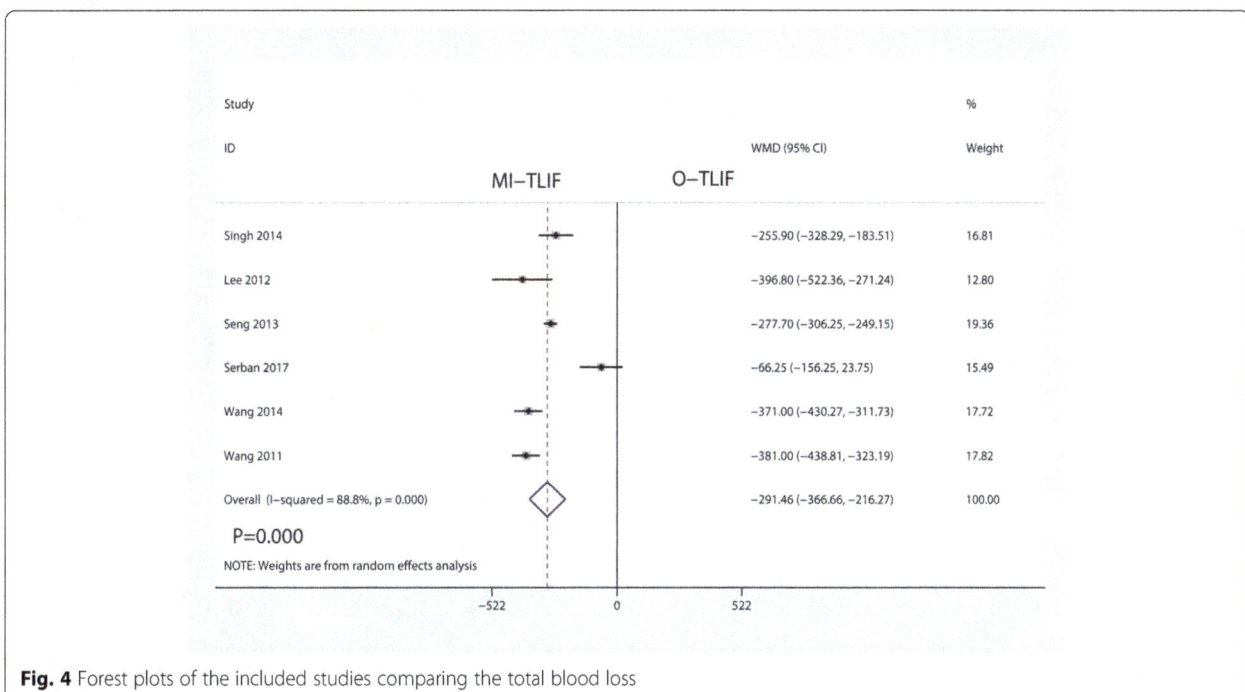

Fig. 4 Forest plots of the included studies comparing the total blood loss

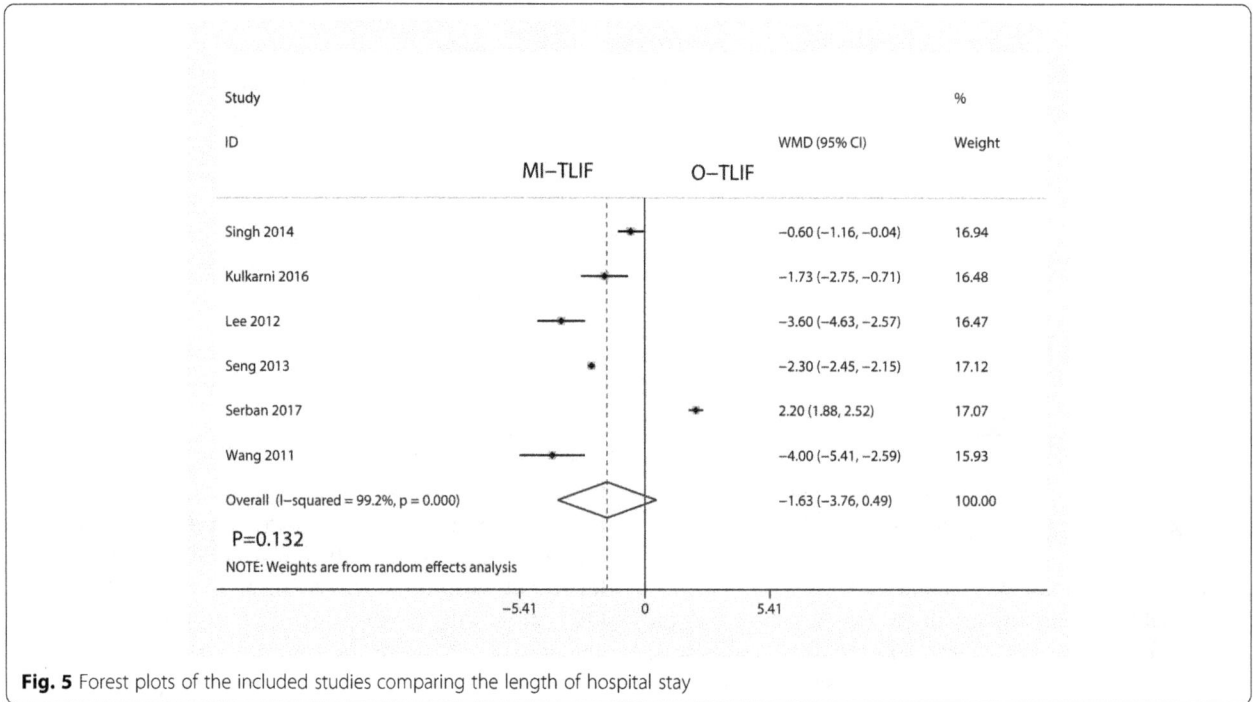

Fig. 5 Forest plots of the included studies comparing the length of hospital stay

prospective observe studies and thus could avoid this bias. Second, we also evaluated the effect of fluroscopic time between the two methods and provided a new insight into the advantage of these two methods.

This meta-analysis is the latest one to evaluate the efficacy and safety of MI-TLIF and O-TLIF for single-level degenerative lumbar diseases and to determine which surgical technique is superior. A few studies [12, 13] have described a superior or comparative outcome for patients undergoing MI-TLIF approach for single-level degenerative lumbar diseases. Singh et al. [11] showed MI-TLIF demonstrated reductions of operative time, length of stay,

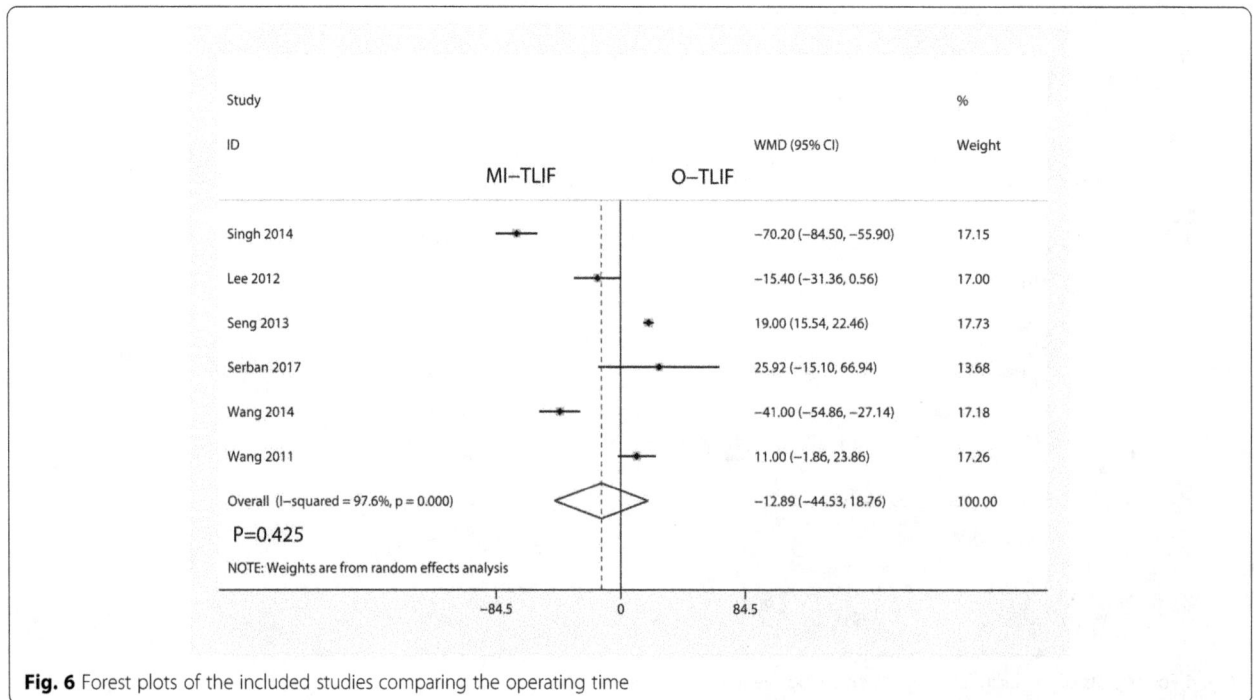

Fig. 6 Forest plots of the included studies comparing the operating time

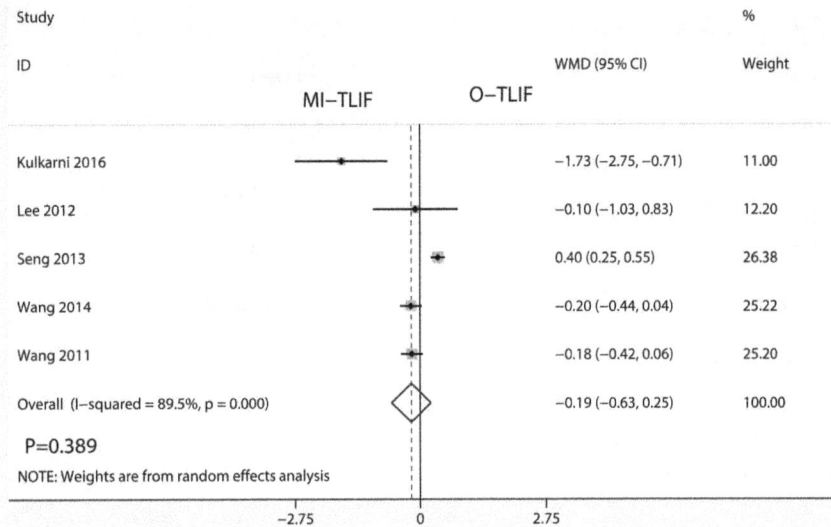

Fig. 7 Forest plots of the included studies comparing the postoperative VAS score

anesthesia time, VAS scores, and estimated blood loss compared with the open method. Lee et al. [5] verified the safety of MI-TLIF approach and similar operative duration, good clinical outcomes. Wang et al. [16] demonstrated that minimally invasive TLIF has similar surgical efficacy with the traditional open TLIF in treating one-level degenerative lumbar diseases. Serban et al. [15] justified the two techniques provided similar clinical and radiological outcomes. Seng et al. [14] showed MI-TLIF is comparable with open TLIF in terms of midterm clinical outcomes and fusion rates.

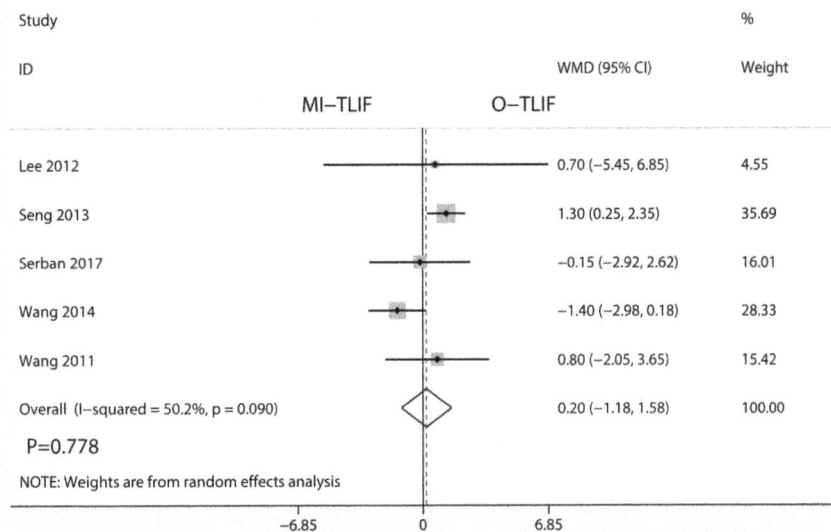

Fig. 8 Forest plots of the included studies comparing the postoperative ODI

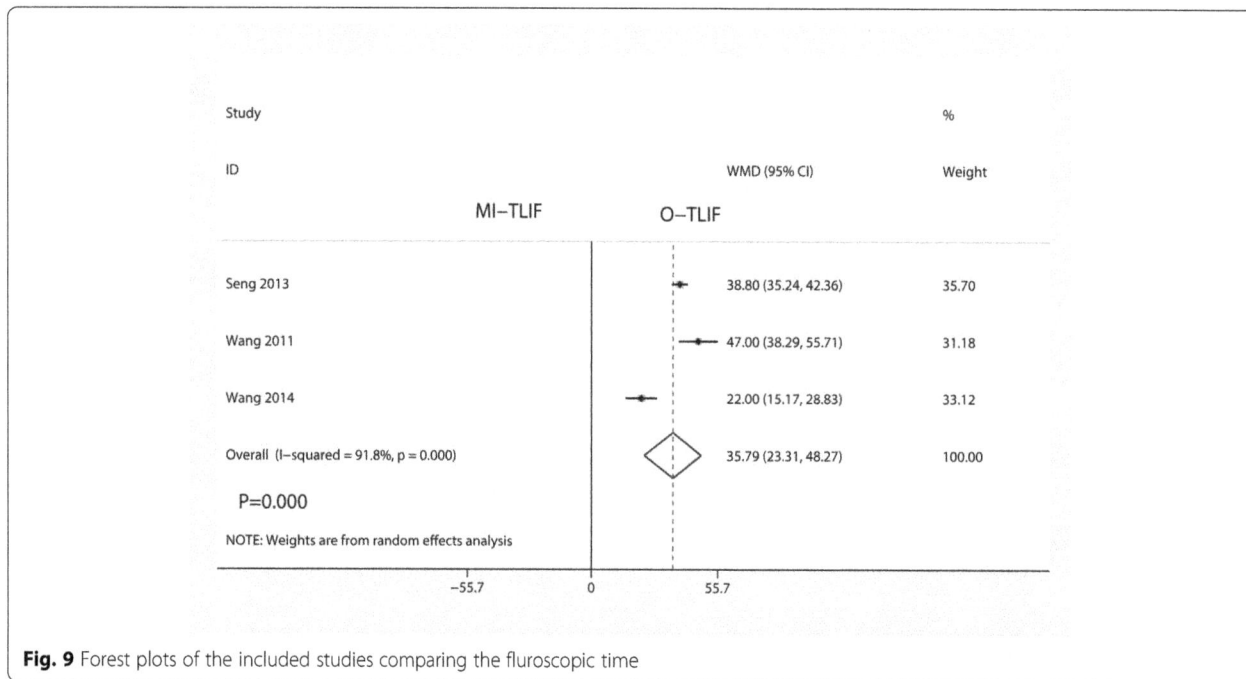

Fig. 9 Forest plots of the included studies comparing the fluroscopic time

Furthermore, a meta-analysis carried out in 2015 concluded that MI-TLIF is associated with decreased complication rates, and increased radiation exposure [21]. Current meta-analysis indicated that MI-TLIF was associated with an increase of the radiation exposure than O-TLIF. And the conclusion was consistent with previous meta-analysis. The two approaches for single-level degenerative lumbar diseases appear to be associated with similar results on operative time and postoperative ODI. Due to the limited number of studies available, we did not

investigate other clinical outcomes such as risk of complications and fusion rates.

Theoretically, many doctors prefer performing MI-TLIF because it may be associated with small incisions and more rapid recovery. However, the learning curve for MI-TLIF was always longer than O-TLIF. Park et al. [22] revealed that perioperative complications occurred more often in the early period of a surgeon's experience with MI-TLIF. Thus, MI-TLIF need for more learning time than O-TLIF. Nandyala et al. [23] identified that MI-TLIF is a

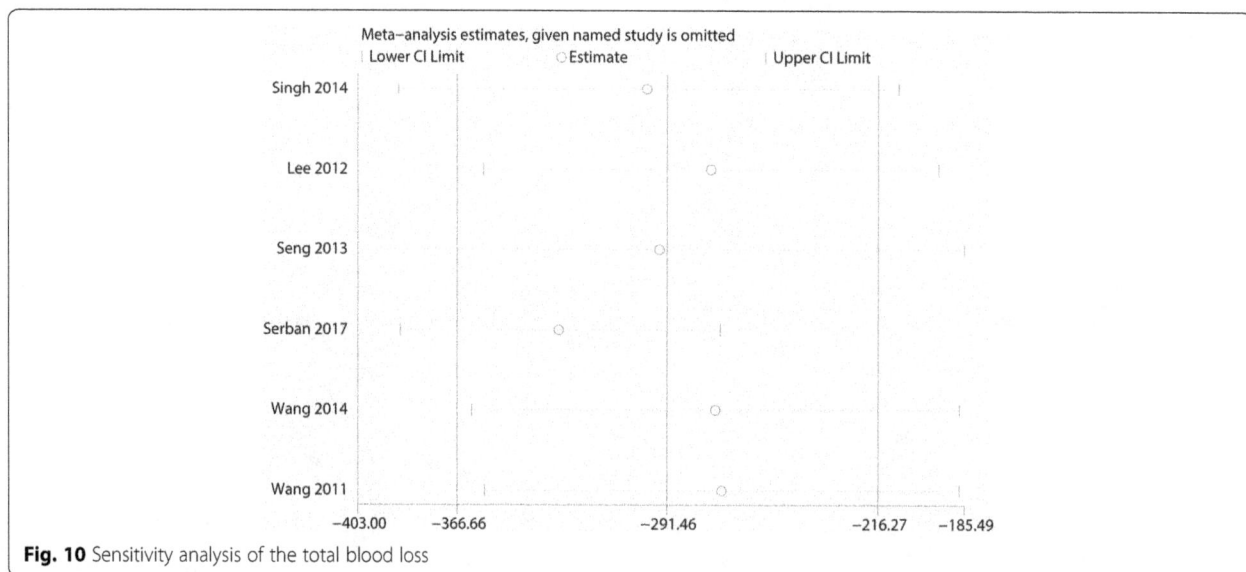

Fig. 10 Sensitivity analysis of the total blood loss

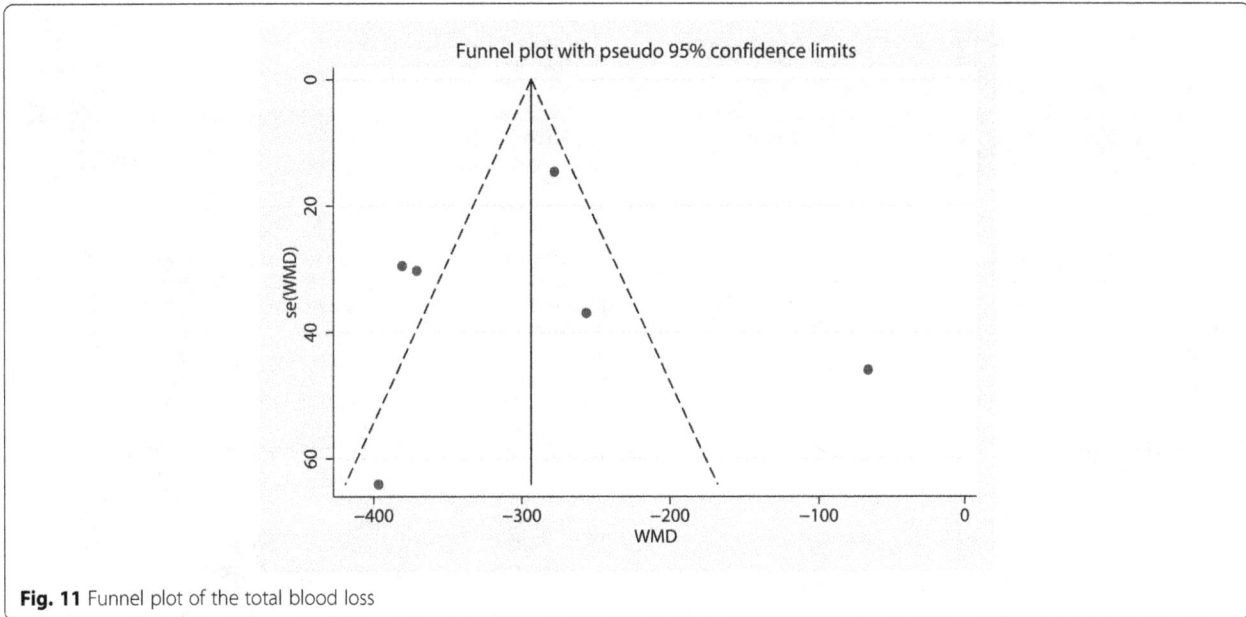

Fig. 11 Funnel plot of the total blood loss

technically difficult procedure to the practicing spine surgeon and further studies are warranted to delineate the methods to minimize the complications associated with the learning curve.

There were several limitation of current meta-analysis: (1) there was a large heterogeneity between the included outcomes, though we performed a sensitivity analysis; however, we could not found the heterogeneity. (2) There were some missed data and we could not obtained the original data and thus may cause the bias. (3) The number of enrolled patients was relatively small, which may limit the statistical effects of the data. (4) Follow-up in some studies were

relatively short and long-term effects of O-TLIF versus MI-TLIF need further study.

Conclusion

In conclusion, this meta-analysis suggests that MI-TLIF appeared to achieve less blood loss than O-TLIF. However, the two procedures, MI-TLIF and O-TLIF, were comparable in clinical efficacy and fusion rates. Due to the limited number of the included RCTs, more well-designed multicenter RCTs with larger sample sizes and long-term follow-up are still needed to compare the clinical efficacy and safety of MI-TLIF and O-TLIF.

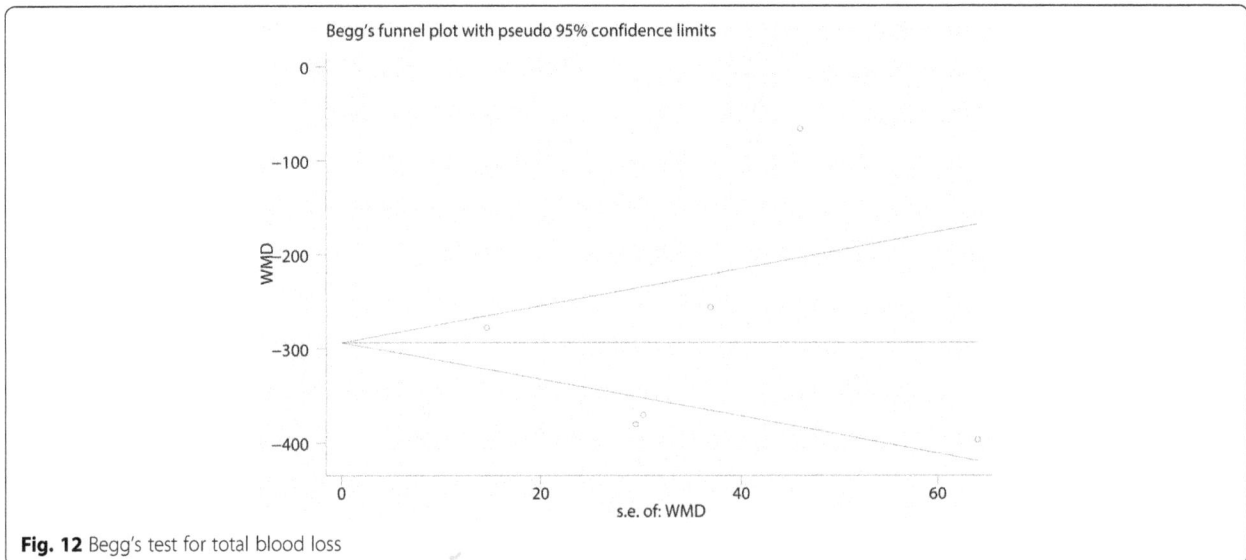

Fig. 12 Begg's test for total blood loss

Abbreviations

df: Degrees of freedom; fixed: Fixed-effects modeling; IV: Inverse variance; MI-TLIF: Minimally invasive transforaminal lumbar interbody fusion; ODI: Oswestry Disability Index; O-TLIF: Open transforaminal lumbar interbody fusion; random: Random-effects modeling; RCTs: Randomized controlled trials; SD: Standard deviation; TLIF: Transforaminal lumbar interbody fusion; VAS: Visual analog score

Authors' contributions

AML and XL conceived the study design. YZ performed the study, collected the data, and contributed to the study design. AML and XL prepared the manuscript. AML edited the manuscript. All authors read and approved the final manuscript.

Competing interests

The authors declare that they have no competing interests.

References

1. Harms J, Rolinger H. A one-stager procedure in operative treatment of spondylolistheses: dorsal traction-reposition and anterior fusion (author's transl). Z Orthop Ihre Grenzgeb. 1982;120(3):343–7.
2. Hackenberg L, et al. Transforaminal lumbar interbody fusion: a safe technique with satisfactory three to five year results. Eur Spine J. 2005;14(6):551–8.
3. Houten JK, et al. Clinical and radiographically/neuroimaging documented outcome in transforaminal lumbar interbody fusion. Neurosurg Focus. 2006; 20(3):E8.
4. Kobayashi K, et al. Reoperation within 2 years after lumbar interbody fusion: a multicenter study. In: Eur Spine J; 2018.
5. Lee MJ, Mok J, Patel P. Transforaminal lumbar interbody fusion: traditional open versus minimally invasive techniques. J Am Acad Orthop Surg. 2018; 26(4):124–31.
6. Kawaguchi Y, Matsui H, Tsuji H. Back muscle injury after posterior lumbar spine surgery. A histologic and enzymatic analysis. Spine (Phila Pa 1976). 1996;21(8):941–4.
7. Styf JR, Willen J. The effects of external compression by three different retractors on pressure in the erector spine muscles during and after posterior lumbar spine surgery in humans. Spine (Phila Pa 1976). 1998;23(3):354–8.
8. Schwender JD, et al. Minimally invasive transforaminal lumbar interbody fusion (TLIF): technical feasibility and initial results. J Spinal Disord Tech. 2005;18(Suppl):S1–6.
9. Liberati A, et al. The PRISMA statement for reporting systematic reviews and meta-analyses of studies that evaluate healthcare interventions: explanation and elaboration. Bmj. 2009;339:b2700.
10. GS HJ. Cochrane handbook for systematic reviews of interventions version 5.1.0. 2011. http://handbook.cochrane.org. [Epub ahead of print]
11. Singh K, et al. A perioperative cost analysis comparing single-level minimally invasive and open transforaminal lumbar interbody fusion. Spine J. 2014; 14(8):1694–701.
12. Kulkarni AG, et al. Minimal invasive transforaminal lumbar interbody fusion versus open transforaminal lumbar interbody fusion. Indian J Orthop. 2016; 50(5):464–72.
13. Lee KH, et al. Clinical and radiological outcomes of open versus minimally invasive transforaminal lumbar interbody fusion. Eur Spine J. 2012;21(11):2265–70.
14. Seng C, et al. Five-year outcomes of minimally invasive versus open transforaminal lumbar interbody fusion: a matched-pair comparison study. Spine (Phila Pa 1976). 2013;38(23):2049–55.
15. Serban D, Calina N, Tender G. Standard versus minimally invasive Transforaminal lumbar interbody fusion: a prospective randomized study. Biomed Res Int. 2017;2017:7236970.
16. Wang J, et al. Comparison of the clinical outcome in overweight or obese patients after minimally invasive versus open transforaminal lumbar interbody fusion. J Spinal Disord Tech. 2014;27(4):202–6.
17. Wang J, et al. Comparison of one-level minimally invasive and open transforaminal lumbar interbody fusion in degenerative and isthmic spondylolisthesis grades 1 and 2. Eur Spine J. 2010;19(10):1780–4.
18. Xie Q, et al. Minimally invasive versus open Transforaminal lumbar interbody fusion in obese patients: a meta-analysis. BMC Musculoskelet Disord. 2018; 19(1):15.
19. Imada AO, Huynh TR, Drazin D. Minimally invasive versus open laminectomy/discectomy, transforaminal lumbar, and posterior lumbar interbody fusions: a systematic review. Cureus. 2017;9(7):e1488.
20. Xie L, Wu WJ, Liang Y. Comparison between minimally invasive transforaminal lumbar interbody fusion and conventional open transforaminal lumbar interbody fusion: an updated meta-analysis. Chin Med J. 2016;129(16):1969–86.
21. Khan NR, et al. Surgical outcomes for minimally invasive vs open transforaminal lumbar interbody fusion: an updated systematic review and meta-analysis. Neurosurgery. 2015;77(6):847–74 discussion 874.
22. Park Y, et al. Perioperative surgical complications and learning curve associated with minimally invasive transforaminal lumbar interbody fusion: a single-institute experience. Clin Orthop Surg. 2015;7(1):91–6.
23. Nandyala SV, et al. Minimally invasive transforaminal lumbar interbody fusion: one surgeon's learning curve. Spine J. 2014;14(8):1460–5.

Permissions

All chapters in this book were first published in JOSR, by BioMed Central; hereby published with permission under the Creative Commons Attribution License or equivalent. Every chapter published in this book has been scrutinized by our experts. Their significance has been extensively debated. The topics covered herein carry significant findings which will fuel the growth of the discipline. They may even be implemented as practical applications or may be referred to as a beginning point for another development.

The contributors of this book come from diverse backgrounds, making this book a truly international effort. This book will bring forth new frontiers with its revolutionizing research information and detailed analysis of the nascent developments around the world.

We would like to thank all the contributing authors for lending their expertise to make the book truly unique. They have played a crucial role in the development of this book. Without their invaluable contributions this book wouldn't have been possible. They have made vital efforts to compile up to date information on the varied aspects of this subject to make this book a valuable addition to the collection of many professionals and students.

This book was conceptualized with the vision of imparting up-to-date information and advanced data in this field. To ensure the same, a matchless editorial board was set up. Every individual on the board went through rigorous rounds of assessment to prove their worth. After which they invested a large part of their time researching and compiling the most relevant data for our readers.

The editorial board has been involved in producing this book since its inception. They have spent rigorous hours researching and exploring the diverse topics which have resulted in the successful publishing of this book. They have passed on their knowledge of decades through this book. To expedite this challenging task, the publisher supported the team at every step. A small team of assistant editors was also appointed to further simplify the editing procedure and attain best results for the readers.

Apart from the editorial board, the designing team has also invested a significant amount of their time in understanding the subject and creating the most relevant covers. They scrutinized every image to scout for the most suitable representation of the subject and create an appropriate cover for the book.

The publishing team has been an ardent support to the editorial, designing and production team. Their endless efforts to recruit the best for this project, has resulted in the accomplishment of this book. They are a veteran in the field of academics and their pool of knowledge is as vast as their experience in printing. Their expertise and guidance has proved useful at every step. Their uncompromising quality standards have made this book an exceptional effort. Their encouragement from time to time has been an inspiration for everyone.

The publisher and the editorial board hope that this book will prove to be a valuable piece of knowledge for researchers, students, practitioners and scholars across the globe.

List of Contributors

Ya-Zhou Zhang, Xu-Yang Cao, Xi-Cheng Li, Jia Chen, Yue-Yuan Zhao, Zhi Tian and Wang Zheng
Department of Orthopedics, Heibei General Hospital, No. 348 Heping East Road, Shijiazhuang 050051, Hebei, China

Ying-Cheng Huang
Department of Orthopedics, Kaohsiung Veterans General Hospital, No. 386, Dazhong 1st Rd., Zuoying Dist., Kaohsiung City 81362, Taiwan, Republic of China
Department of Orthopedic Surgery, National Defense Medical Center, Taipei, Taiwan, Republic of China

Chien-Jen Hsu, Jenn-Huei Renn, Kai-Cheng Lin, Shan-Wei Yang, Yih-Wen Tarng and Wei-Ning Chang
Department of Orthopedics, Kaohsiung Veterans General Hospital, No. 386, Dazhong 1st Rd., Zuoying Dist., Kaohsiung City 81362, Taiwan, Republic of China

Chun-Yu Chen
Department of Orthopedics, Kaohsiung Veterans General Hospital, No. 386, Dazhong 1st Rd., Zuoying Dist., Kaohsiung City 81362, Taiwan, Republic of China
Department of Orthopedic Surgery, National Defense Medical Center, Taipei, Taiwan, Republic of China
Department of Occupational Therapy, Shu-Zen Junior College of Medicine and Management, Kaohsiung, Taiwan, Republic of China

Xiaoyue Zhu
Baoshan Center for Disease Control and Prevention, Shanghai, People's Republic of China

Lingli Sang and Dandong Wu
Department of Epidemiology, School of Public Health, Nantong University, Nantong, Jiangsu Province, People's Republic of China

Jiesheng Rong
Department of Orthopedics Surgery, The Second Affiliated Hospital of Harbin Medical University, Harbin, Heilongjiang Province, People's Republic of China

Liying Jiang
Shanghai Key Laboratory for Molecular Imaging, Shanghai University of Medicine and Health Sciences, Shanghai, People's Republic of China

Andres Keller, Guillermo Izquierdo, Jorge Cabrolier, Nathaly Caicedo and Emilio Wagner
Department of Orthopedics, Universidad del desarrollo - Clinica Alemana de Santiago, Vitacura 5951, 7650568 Santiago, Chile

Pablo Wagner
Department of Orthopedics, Universidad del desarrollo - Clinica Alemana de Santiago, Vitacura 5951, 7650568 Santiago, Chile
Universidad de los Andes - Hospital Militar de Santiago, Santiago, Chile

Nicola Maffulli
Centre for Sports and Exercise Medicine, Barts and The London School of Medicine and Dentistry, Mile End Hospital, London, UK

Wen-Chao Li, Rui-Jiang Xu, Gang Cai and Hui Chen
Department of Pediatric Surgery, Chinese People's Liberation Army General Hospital, Beijing 100853, China

Qing-Xu Meng
Department of Basic Surgery, Affiliated Hospital of Hebei University, Baoding 071002, China

Hong-Juan Li
Department of Orthopaedic, Yu Huang Ding Hospital of Yantai, Yantai 370600, China

Andrea L. Grant, Jodie L. Morris, Peter McEwen, Kaushik Hazratwala and Matthew Wilkinson
The Orthopaedic Research Institute of Queensland (ORIQL), 7 Turner St, Pimlico, Townsville, Queensland 4812, Australia
Heart, Trauma and Sepsis Research Laboratory, College of Medicine and Dentistry, James Cook University, 1 James Cook Drive, Townsville, Queensland 4811, Australia

Geoffrey P. Dobson and Hayley L. Letson
Heart, Trauma and Sepsis Research Laboratory, College of Medicine and Dentistry, James Cook University, 1 James Cook Drive, Townsville, Queensland 4811, Australia

Tao Wang and Xi-Jiang Zhao
Department of Orthopedic Surgery, Affiliated Hospital of Jiangnan University, 200 Huihe Rd, Wuxi 214062, Jiangsu, China

Jun-Ying Sun, Jun-Jun Zha and Chao Wang
Department of Orthopedic Surgery, The First Affiliated Hospital of Soochow University, 188 Shizi Street, Suzhou 215006, Jiangsu, China

Cheng-Ta Wu and Shih-Hsiang Yen
Department of Orthopaedic Surgery, Kaohsiung Chang Gung Memorial Hospital, 123, Ta Pei Road, Niao Sung District, Kaohsiung, Taiwan, Republic of China

Bradley Chen
Institute of Public Health, National Yangming University, Taipei, Taiwan, Republic of China

Jun-Wen Wang
Department of Orthopaedic Surgery, Kaohsiung Chang Gung Memorial Hospital, 123, Ta Pei Road, Niao Sung District, Kaohsiung, Taiwan, Republic of China College of Medicine, Chang Gung University, 123, Ta Pei Road, Niao Sung District, Kaohsiun0067, Taiwan, Republic of China

Chung-Cheng Huang
Department of Radiology, Kaohsiung Chang Gung Memorial Hospital, Kaohsiung, Taiwan, Republic of China

Kyung Cheon Kim, Kyu-Woong Yeon and Sun-Cheol Han
Shoulder Center, Department of Orthopedic Surgery, TanTan Hospital, Daejeon, South Korea

Hyun Dae Shin and Woo-Yong Lee
Department of Orthopedic Surgery, Regional Rheumatoid and Degenerative Arthritis Center, Chungnam National University Hospital, Chungnam National University School of Medicine, 266 Munwha-ro, Jung-gu, Daejeon 35015, South Korea

Keisuke Komiyama, Satoshi Hamai, Daisuke Hara, Kensei Yoshimoto, Kyohei Shiomoto and Yasuharu Nakashima
Department of Orthopedic Surgery, Graduate School of Medical Sciences, Kyushu University, 3-1-1 Maidashi, Higashi-ku, Fukuoka 812-8582, Japan

Satoru Ikebe
Department of Creative Engineering, National Institute of Technology, Kitakyushu College, 5-20-1 Shii, Kokuraminami-ku, Kitakyushu, Fukuoka 802-0985, Japan

Hidehiko Higaki, Hirotaka Gondo and Yifeng Wang
Department of Life Science, Faculty of Life Science, Kyushu Sangyo University, 2-3-1 Matsugadai, Higashi-ku, Fukuoka 813-0004, Japan

Liqing Yang, Yuefeng Sun and Ge Li
Department of orthopedics, Shengjing Hospital of China Medical University, Shenyang 110004, China

Jiajun Wu, Xiuhui Wang and Xiaoxiao Zhou
Department of Orthopedics, Zhoupu Hospital Affiliated to Shanghai University of Medicine and Health Sciences, No. 1500 Zhouyuan Road, Pudong New Area, Shanghai 201318, China

Changqing Zhang
Department of Orthopedics, Shanghai Sixth People's Hospital Affiliated to Shanghai Jiao Tong University, No. 600 Yishan Road, Xuhui District, Shanghai 201306, China

Yang Yang
Department of Orthopedics, Taizhou Hospital Affiliated to Wenzhou Medical University, Zhejiang, China

Rene Burchard
Department of Health, University of Witten/Herdecke, Witten, Germany
Department of Trauma and Orthopaedic Surgery, Kreisklinikum Siegen, Weidenauer Str. 76, 57076 Siegen, Germany
School of Science and Technology, University of Siegen, Siegen, Germany

Robin Massa
Department of Trauma and Orthopaedic Surgery, Kreisklinikum Siegen, Weidenauer Str. 76, 57076 Siegen, Germany

Christian Soost
Department of Statistics an Econometrics, University of Siegen, Kohlbettstr, 15, 57072 Siegen, Germany

Wolfgang Richter, Gerhard Dietrich, Arne Ohrndorf, Hans-Jürgen Christ and Claus-Peter Fritzen
Department of Mechanical Engineering, University of Siegen, Paul-Bonatz-Str. 9-11, 57076 Siegen, Germany

Jan Adriaan Graw
Department of Anesthesiology and Operative Intensive Care Medicine, Charité—Universitätsmedizin Berlin, Campus Virchow-Klinikum, Augustenburger Platz 1, 13353 Berlin, Germany
Berlin Institute of Health, Berlin, Germany

Jan Schmitt
Department of Orthopaedics and Trauma Surgery, Lahn-Dill-Kliniken Wetzlar, Forsthausstraße 1, 35578 Wetzlar, Germany

Ayman El-Menyar
Department of Surgery Clinical Research Unit, Westchester Medical Center Health Network, Valhalla, New York, USA
Trauma Surgery, Clinical Research, Hamad General Hospital, Doha, Qatar
Clinical Medicine, Weill Cornell Medical School, Doha, Qatar

Mohammed Muneer
Department of Surgery, Hamad General Hospital, Doha, Qatar

David Samson
Department of Surgery Clinical Research Unit, Westchester Medical Center Health Network, Valhalla, New York, USA

Hassan Al-Thani
Department of Surgery, Trauma and Vascular Surgery, Hamad General Hospital, Doha, Qatar

Ahmad Alobaidi
Department of Surgery, Orthopedic Surgery, Al Wakrah Hospital, Doha, Qatar

Paul Mussleman
Distributed eLibrary, Weill Cornell Medical School, Doha, Qatar

Rifat Latifi
Department of Surgery, Westchester Medical Center Health Network and New York Medical College, Valhalla, New York, USA

Zhiqiang Wang, Yi Yin, Qingshan Li, Guanjun Sun, Xu Peng, Hua Yin and Yongjie Ye
Department of Orthopaedics Surgery, Suining Central Hospital, Suining 629000, Sichuan, China

Hisaki Aiba, Hideyuki Goto, Satoshi Yamada, Hideki Okamoto, Masahiro Nozaki, Shinji Miwa, Makoto Kobayashi, Kojiro Endo, Shiro Saito and Takanobu Otsuka
Department of Orthopedic Surgery, Nagoya City University Graduate School of Medical Sciences, 1, Kawasumi, Mizuho-cho, Mizuho-ku, Nagoya 467-8601, Japan

Masaaki Kobayashi
Department of Orthopedic Surgery, Nagoya City University Graduate School of Medical Sciences, 1, Kawasumi, Mizuho-cho, Mizuho-ku, Nagoya 467-8601, Japan
Department of Orthopedic Surgery, Ogaki Municipal Hospital, 4-86 Minaminokawa-cho, Ogaki 503-8502, Japan

Yuko Waguri-Nagaya
Department of Joint Surgery for Rheumatic Diseases, Nagoya City University Graduate School of Medical Sciences, 1, Kawasumi, Mizuho-cho, Mizuho-ku, Nagoya 467-8601, Japan

Jun Mizutani and Hiroto Mitsui
Department of Rehabilitation Medicine, Nagoya City University Graduate School of Medical Sciences, 1, Kawasumi, Mizuho-cho, Mizuho-ku, Nagoya 467-8601, Japan

Taeko Goto
Department of Radiology, Nagoya City University Graduate School of Medical Sciences, 1, Kawasumi, Mizuho-cho, Mizuho-ku, Nagoya 467-8601, Japan

Chenhao Pan and Zubin Zhou
Department of Orthopaedic Surgery, Shanghai Jiao Tong University Affiliated Sixth People's Hospital, Shanghai 200233, China

Xiaowei Yu
Department of Orthopaedic Surgery, Shanghai Jiao Tong University Affiliated Sixth People's Hospital, Shanghai 200233, China
Department of Orthopaedic Surgery, Shanghai Sixth People's Hospital East Campus, Shanghai University of Medicine and Health Sciences, Shanghai 201306, China

Meinald T. Thielsch and Patrick Boertz
Department of Psychology, University of Münster, Fliednerstr. 21, 48149 Münster, Germany

Georg Gosheger
Universitätsklinikum Münster, Münster, Germany

Mark Wetterkamp and Tobias L. Schulte
St. Josef-Hospital, Ruhr University Bochum, Bochum, Germany

Xiaojie Li, Wenli Xue, Yong Cao, Yanming Long and Mengsheng Xie
Department of Prosthodontics, College and Hospital of Stomatology, Guangxi Medical University, 10th Shuangyong Road, Nanning 530021, China

Patrick Haubruck
HTRG—Heidelberg Trauma Research Group, Center for Orthopedics, Trauma Surgery and Spinal Cord Injury, Trauma and Reconstructive Surgery, Heidelberg University Hospital, Schlierbacher Landstrasse 200a, 69118 Heidelberg, Germany
Raymond Purves Bone and Joint Research Laboratories, Kolling Institute of Medical Research, Institute of Bone and Joint Research, University of Sydney, St Leonards, New South Wales 2065, Australia

Anja Solte, Raban Heller, Michael Tanner, Gerhard Schmidmaier and Christian Fischer
HTRG—Heidelberg Trauma Research Group, Center for Orthopedics, Trauma Surgery and Spinal Cord Injury, Trauma and Reconstructive Surgery, Heidelberg University Hospital, Schlierbacher Landstrasse 200a, 69118 Heidelberg, Germany

Volker Daniel
Department of Transplantation Immunology, Institute of Immunology, University of Heidelberg, Im Neuenheimer Feld 305, 69120 Heidelberg, Germany

Arash Moghaddam
HTRG—Heidelberg Trauma Research Group, Center for Orthopedics, Trauma Surgery and Spinal Cord Injury, Trauma and Reconstructive Surgery, Heidelberg University Hospital, Schlierbacher Landstrasse 200a, 69118 Heidelberg, Germany
ATORG—Aschaffenburg Trauma and Orthopedic Research Group, Center for Trauma Surgery, Orthopedics and Sports Medicine, Am Hasenkopf 1, 63739 Aschaffenburg, Germany

Shiqi Cao
Department of Rehabilitation, Minimally Invasive Spine Center, Navy General Hospital, No. 6, Fucheng Road, Haidian District, Beijing 100048, People's Republic of China
Joint Surgery and Sports Medicine Department, Changzheng Hospital, Navy Medical University, No. 415, Fengyang Road, Huangpu District, Shanghai 200003, People's Republic of China

Jia Cao and Qirong Qian
Joint Surgery and Sports Medicine Department, Changzheng Hospital, Navy Medical University, No. 415, Fengyang Road, Huangpu District, Shanghai 200003, People's Republic of China

Sirui Li
College of Basic Medicine, Army Medical University, Chongqing 400038, People's Republic of China

Wei Wang
Department of Orthopaedics, Chengdu Military General Hospital, No. 270, Tianhui Road, Jinniu District, Chengdu 610083, People's Republic of China

Yu Ding
Department of Rehabilitation, Minimally Invasive Spine Center, Navy General Hospital, No. 6, Fucheng Road, Haidian District, Beijing 100048, People's Republic of China

Jian-qiao Hong, Yang-xin Wang, Si-hao Li, Guang-yao Jiang, Bin Hu, Yu-te Yang, Jia-hong Meng and Shi-gui Yan
Department of Orthopaedic Surgery, The Second Affiliated Hospital, Zhejiang University School of Medicine, No.88 Jiefang Road, Hangzhou 310009, People's Republic of China

Shun-Wun Jhan, Wen-Yi Chou, Kuan-Ting Wu and Ya-Ju Yang
Department of Orthopedic Surgery, Kaohsiung Chang Gung Memorial Hospital and Chang Gung University College of Medicine, 123 Ta Pei Road, Niao Sung Dist, Kaohsiung, Taiwan

Ching-Jen Wang and Jih-Yang Ko
Department of Orthopedic Surgery, Kaohsiung Chang Gung Memorial Hospital and Chang Gung University College of Medicine, 123 Ta Pei Road, Niao Sung Dist, Kaohsiung, Taiwan
Center for Shockwave Medicine and Tissue Engineering, Department of Medical Research, Kaohsiung Chang Gung Memorial Hospital and Chang Gung University College of Medicine, Kaohsiung, Taiwan

Zhao Meng, Chen Wang and Yan Zou
Department of Orthopaedics, Children's Hospital of Hebei Province, No.133, Jianhua Street, Yuhua District, Shijiazhuang 050031, China

Li-Jun Tian
Department of Orthopaedics, the Third Hospital of Shijiazhuang, No. 15 South of Tiyu Street, Shijiazhuang 050011, Hebei, China

Xue-Jun Zhang and Dong Guo
Department of Orthopaedics, Beijing Children's Hospital, Capital Medical University, No. 56 Nan-li-shi Road, Beijing 100045, China

Zhen Lai, Shiyuan Shi, Jun Fei, Guihe Han and Shengping Hu
Department of Orthopedics, Hospital of Integrated Traditional Chinese and Western medicine in Zhejiang Province, 208 Huancheng E.Rd, Hangzhou 310003, Zhejiang Province, People's Republic of China

Xuhong Xue and Sheng Zhao
Department of Orthopedics, The Second Hospital of Shanxi Medical University, Taiyuan, No. 382 Wuyi Road, Taiyuan 030001, Shanxi, People's Republic of China

Tianwen Ma, Zhiheng Zhang, Xiaopeng Song, Hui Bai, Yue Li, Xinran Li, Jinghua Zhao, Yuanqiang Ma and Li Gao
Heilongjiang Key Laboratory for Laboratory Animals and Comparative Medicine, College of Veterinary Medicine, Northeast Agricultural University, Harbin 150030, China

Ze-Nan Xia, Ke Xiao, Wei Zhu, Bin Feng, Bao-Zhong Zhang, Jin Lin, Wen-Wei Qian, Jin Jin, Na Gao, Gui-Xing Qiu and Xi-Sheng Weng
Department of Orthopaedics, Peking Union Medical College Hospital, Chinese Academy of Medical Sciences, Shuaifuyuan 1, Wangfujing, Dongcheng District, Beijing 100730, People's Republic of China

Shuangjian He
Department of Orthopaedics, Taixing People's Hospital, Taixing, Jiangsu, People's Republic of China
Department of Orthopaedics, Jinling Clinical Medical College, Nanjing Medical University, Nanjing, Jiangsu, China

Bin Yan, Jian Zhu and Xiaoyi Huang
Department of Orthopaedics, Taixing People's Hospital, Taixing, Jiangsu, People's Republic of China

Jianning Zhao
Department of Orthopaedics, Jinling Clinical Medical College, Nanjing Medical University, Nanjing, Jiangsu, China
Department of Orthopaedics, Jinling Hospital, Nanjing Medical University, No. 305, Zhongshan East Road, Nanjing 210002, Jiangsu, China

Aimin Li, Xiang Li and Yang Zhong
Department of Orthopedics, The 5th Central Hospital of Tianjin, Tianjin 30000, People's Republic of China

Index